CURRENT ISSUES AND FUTURE DIRECTION IN KIDNEY TRANSPLANTATION

Edited by **Thomas Rath**

Current Issues and Future Direction in Kidney Transplantation
http://dx.doi.org/10.5772/45909
Edited by Thomas Rath

Contributors

Farzad Kakaei, Silvio Tucci Jr, Wai Hon Lim, Hung Do Nguyen, Rebecca Williams, Germaine Wong, Bhadran Bose, Jean-Paul Squifflet, Slawomir Dariusz Szajda, David William Mudge, Kimberley Oliver, Siddharth Sharma, Philippe Saas, Jamal Bamoulid, Cécile Courivaud, Béatrice Gaugler, Didier Ducloux, Stefan Reuter, Mihai Lucan, Phuong-Thu Pham, Rashad Hassan Rashad Hassan, Ahmed Akl, Shyam Dheda, Siew Chong, Katrien De Vusser, Rubina Naqvi, Marco Antonio Ayala-Garcia, Beatriz Gonzalez Yebra, Eduardo Guani Guerra, Éctor Jaime Ramírez Barba, Iris Lee, Mythili Ghanta, Jeanne Dreier, Raji Jacobs, Abdul Razack Amir, Salwa Sheikh, Rawan Amir, Thomas Rath, Maria Jose Herrero, Ana Luisa Robles Piedras, Minarda De La O Arciniega, Josefina Reynoso Vázquez

Published by InTech

Janeza Trdine 9, 51000 Rijeka, Croatia

Publishing Process Manager Danijela Duric
Technical Editor InTech DTP team
Cover InTech Design team

Additional hard copies can be obtained from orders@intechopen.com

Current Issues and Future Direction in Kidney Transplantation, Edited by Thomas Rath
p. cm.
ISBN 978-953-51-0985-3

For EU product safety concerns:
IN TECH d.o.o., Prolaz Marije Krucifikse Kozulić 3, 51000 Rijeka, Croatia,
info@intechopen.com or visit our website at intechopen.com.

Meet the editor

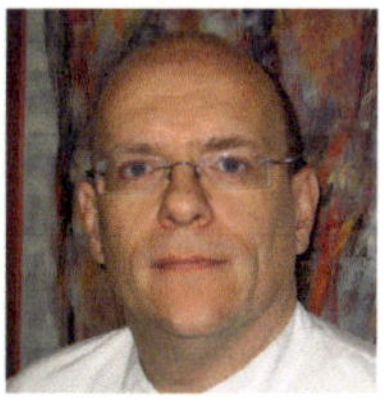

Dr. Thomas Rath completed his Internal Residency at Westpfalz-Klinikum in Kaiserslautern, Germany in 1998. Afterwards he gained the certified speciality of Nephrology which was followed by the additional certification for Infectiology. In 1998 he joined the Transplant Team in Kaiserslautern, where he became Senior Physician of the Department. Since 2006 he is Head of the Department of Nephrology and Transplantation in Kaiserslautern with more than 1000 renal transplants since its official approval. He is also responsible for the Outpatient Clinics for Infectious Diseases at the Westpfalz-Klinikum, Kaiserslautern. Dr. Rath is member of different international and national medical societies. He gives lectures at the Technical University of Kaiserslautern about "impaired function of human organs and artificial organ support".

Contents

Preface

Renal transplantation is the treatment of choice for patients with end-stage renal disease and until now half a million renal transplants are done by surgeons, nephrologists, immunologists, nurses and patients.

This open-access book covers diagnostic methods as well as clinical aspects and advances in transplantation immunology. The area covered spans from imaging methods, impact of donor factors, clinical comorbidities to recent developments in HLA-Matching and Antibody-Mediated rejection.

The authors are all experienced clinicians and scientists from different regions of the world. So, this book may help us all by giving useful information to improve care for our patients.

Dr. med. Thomas Rath
Department of Nephrology and Transplantation Medicine
Westpfalz-Klinikum, Kaiserslautern, Germany

Section 1

Diagnostic Methods in Renal Transplantation

Chapter 1

Medical Evaluation of the Adult Kidney Transplant Candidate

Phuong-Thu Pham, Son V. Pham,
Phuong-Anh Pham and Phuong-Chi Pham

Additional information is available at the end of the chapter

http://dx.doi.org/10.5772/54736

1. Introduction

1.1. Patient education

Prior to the formal evaluation process, all potential transplant candidates are encouraged to attend a "patient education" session. At the meeting, patients are informed about the medical and surgical risks and benefits of renal transplantation, the necessity for frequent outpatient visits in the early postoperative period, the potential adverse effects of immunosuppression, and the importance of compliance with immunosuppressive therapy. The potential advantages and disadvantages of deceased *versus* living donor renal transplantation are discussed with the patients, and when possible, with their family members, significant others, and/or friends. Other issues that are addressed include prolonged waiting time for a deceased donor transplant due to the critical shortage of donor organ and adverse effects of waiting time on patient and graft survival. In addition, patients are forewarned that various medical and psychosocial conditions may preclude a patient from being a transplant candidate. Absolute and relative contraindications to kidney transplantation are outlined in table (1).

1.2. General assessment

1.2.1. Medical / urological evaluation

The routine assessment of a renal transplant candidate includes a detailed history and a thorough physical exam. In particular, it is important to search for the etiology of the original kidney disease as it can predict the transplant course and outcome and the risk for disease recurrence. When available, the kidney biopsy report should be reviewed and the risk of

Absolute contraindications
Active malignancy
Active infection
Severe irreversible extrarenal disease
Life expectancy < 2 years
Liver cirrhosis[1] (unless combined liver and kidney transplant)
Primary oxalosis (unless combined liver and kidney transplant)
Limited, irremediable rehabilitative potential
Poorly controlled psychiatric illnesses
Active substance abuse
Relative contraindications
Active peptic ulcer disease[2]
Medical noncompliance
Active hepatitis B virus infection[3]
Morbid obesity
Special considerations
ABO incompatibility[4]
Positive T cell crossmatch[4]
Post-percutaneous coronary intervention (PCI) patients. Transplant surgery not recommended:
Within 4 weeks of coronary revascularization with balloon angioplasty
Within 3 months of bare metal stent placement
Within 12 months of drug eluting stent placement

[1]Kidney alone transplant may be safe in end-stage kidney disease patients with compemsated HCV cirrhosis and hepatic portal vein gradient < 10 mmHg (see text)
[2]Should be treated prior to transplantation
[3]Liver biopsy and pretransplant antiviral therapy recommended. Hepatology consult.
[4]Pretransplant desensitization protocols may allow successful transplantation across these barriers

Table 1. Contraindications for renal transplantation

recurrent disease should be discussed with the transplant candidate. Patients with end-stage kidney disease (ESKD) secondary to congenital or genitourinary abnormalities should undergo a voiding cystourethrogram and appropriate urological evaluation, preferably by the kidney transplant surgeon. Documentation of the patients' residual urine volume from the native kidneys is invaluable in the assessment of graft function in the posttransplant period. A history of familial or hereditary renal disease must be obtained if living related kidney donation is an option. The patients's surgical history should be elicited with special emphasis on previous abdominal operations. The surgical evaluation of the transplant candidate is discussed elsewhere.

A complete physical exam should include a careful assessment for the presence of carotid and peripheral vascular disease. Patients should preferably have a body mass index below 30-35 as obesity is associated with a higher incidence of postoperative complications. In addition to a thorough history and physical exam, patients should also undergo a number of routine laboratory testings and imaging studies as outlined in table 2.

http://dx.doi.org/10.5772/54736

Laboratory evaluation
Serologies: HIV, hepatitis B and C, CMV, EBV, HSV, RPR (FTA-ABS if positive)
Comprehensive metabolic panel, CBC with differential and platelet count, PT/INR, PTT
Urinalysis, urine culture
PSA in men > 50 years of age[1]
Immunofixation electrophoresis in candidates > 60 years of age
Other evaluation
ECG
Chest x-ray
Colonoscopy if > 50 years of age[2]
Abdominal ultrasound in diabetics to evaluate for gall stones
Native renal ultrasound to assess for acquired cystic disease or masses
Pap smear (for women)[2]
Mammogram for women > 40 years of age[2] or with family history of breast cancer
Cardiac evaluation (see text)
Urologic evaluation if history of bladder /voiding dysfunction, recurrent urinary tract infections (see text)
Immunologic studies
Blood group and HLA typing
HLA antibodies
Crossmatching

CMV: cytomegalovirus; *EBV*: Epstein-Barr virus; *HSV*: herpes simplex virus; *RPR*: rapid plasmin reagin; FTA-ABS: fluorescin treponemal antibodies; *PSA*: prostate specific antigen; ECG: electrocardiogram

1High-risk patients should be screened at an earlier age (African-Americans, those with two or more first-degree relatives with prostate cancer).

2Part of routine health maintenance, not required for listing unless deemed necessary by the clinician at the time of evaluation.

Table 2. Assessment of renal transplant candidate

1.2.2. Psychiatric evaluation

Coexisting psychiatric disorders have been suggested to be associated with poor transplant outcomes due in part to behavioral factors such as nonadherence to medical therapy as well as physiologic factors such as modification of immunologic and stress responses (Danovitch, 2010). Patients should be inquired about mood or anxiety disorders, alterations in perceptions, morbid destructive or violent thoughts directed to self or others, medical adherence, risk taking, substance abuse, and environmental and interpersonal stressors (Danovitch, 2010). Positive prognostic factors include strong family and social support, good insight, sound spirituality, and the ability to cope with various stressors. It should also be noted that neurocognitive symptoms may masquerade as depression hence assessment of organic brain dysfunction should not be overlooked. Oftentimes, the psychiatric evaluation for transplant candidacy can be complex and would require referral to subspecialty service for diagnosis and treatment. A comprehensive discussion of psychiatric issues is beyond the scope of this chapter.

The following section describes specific medical and urological issues that should be addressed during the transplant evaluation process.

2. Evaluation of risk factors by specific organ system disease

2.1. Recurrence of glomerular disease of the native kidneys

Recurrence of glomerular disease is the third most common cause of graft loss after chronic allograft injury and death with a functioning graft. Currently available data on the incidence of recurrent disease and resultant graft loss are heterogeneous due to different study design, follow-up durations, patient samples, and the variable use of surveillance biopsies among centers. The reported incidence of recurrent renal disease after renal transplantation and the risk of graft loss from disease recurrence are shown in table 3. The clinical course and impact on graft survival vary between different types of glomerulonephritis (Colgert et al., 2008; Kasiske et al., 2009). Nonetheless, with the exception of primary focal segmental glomerulosclerosis (FSGS), recurrent glomerular disease is usually a late complication after transplantation. FSGS secondary to reflux nephropathy or obesity does not recur after transplantation. In patients with hypertensive renal disease or other causes of chronic kidney disease, focal segmental sclerosis may be found on histologic evaluation and must be differentiated from the primary disorder. Suggested risk factors for recurrence of primary FSGS include history of recurrence in a previous transplant, younger age at diagnosis, rapid progression to end stage renal disease from the time of initial diagnosis (< 3 years), presence of mesangial proliferation in the native kidneys, older donor kidneys, Caucasian ethnicity, and the collapsing variant. Living donor kidneys (versus deceased donor) have not consistently been demonstrated to be associated with an increased risk of recurrence. Familial and sporadic forms of FSGS with podocin mutation, slow progression to end stage kidney disease (ESKD), and non-nephrotic range proteinuria in the native kidney disease are associated with low risk of recurrence (Ponticelli et al., 2010).

Despite the propensity for certain kidney disease to recur, the risk generally does not preclude transplantation and recurrence rarely results in early graft loss. However, systemic primary amyloidosis (AL amyloidosis) and light chain deposition disease are associated with high rates of disease recurrence and increased morbidity and mortality after transplantation and are considered contraindication to transplantation by most centers. In rare selected patients with sustained complete remission of the hematological disorder kidney transplantation can be performed at the discretion of the transplant nephrologist and hematologist/oncologist (Bridoux et al., 2011; Canaud et al., 2012).

2.2. Cardiovascular disease and peripheral vascular disease

Cardiovascular disease (CVD) is the leading cause of death after renal transplantation. Deaths with a functioning graft occurring within 30 days after transplantation are due to ischemic heart disease in nearly half of the cases. Cardiovascular screening is considered by most

http://dx.doi.org/10.5772/54736

	Recurrence rates (%)	Graft loss from disease recurrence (%)
FSGS	20-50	50
Ig A nephropathy	20-60	10-30
MPGN I	20-50	30-35
MPGN II	80-100	10-20
Membranous GN	3-30	30
HUS[2]	10-40	10-40
Anti-GBM disease	15-50	< 5
ANCA-associated Vasculitis	7-25	< 5
SLE	3-10	< 5

FSGS: focal segmental glomerulosclerosis; *MPGN*: membranoproliferative glomerulonephritis; *GN*: glomerulonephropathy; *HUS*: hemolytic uremic syndrome; *SLE*: systemic lupus erythematosus.

1Only selected renal disease are listed.

2Diarrhea (+) HUS usually does not recur; Diarrhea (-) or familial may recur in 21-28%; Factor H or I mutation may recur in 80% to 100%; Patients with mutation membrane cofactor protein does not have recurrence (reference Kasiske et al., 2009)

Table 3. Rates of recurrent renal disease after transplantation and risk of graft loss from disease recurrence[1]

transplant centers as an essential component of the transplant evaluation process. A detailed cardiovascular history not only predicts the operative risk but also helps in postoperative cardiac management to improve short- and long-term cardiac outcomes. Over the years there has been much controversy over the best strategy for pre-transplant assessment and management of coronary artery disease (CAD) to prevent adverse peri-operative cardiac events. Recently, the American Heart Association / American College of Cardiology (AHA/ACC) have developed the 2012 AHA/ACC guidelines for "Cardiac Disease Evaluation and Management Among Kidney and Liver Transplantation Candidates" based on a comprehensive review of the literature pertinent to perioperative cardiac evaluation of potential kidney or liver transplant recipients (Lentine et al., 2012). These guidelines are endorsed by the American Society of Transplant Surgeons, American Society of Transplantation, and the National Kidney Foundation (discussed below). The AHA/ACC classifications of evidence to perform a test or therapy is shown in table 4.

a. Determining whether the transplant candidate has an active cardiac condition

The primary goal of pre-operative evaluation is to determine whether potential transplant candidates have any active cardiac condition both during the initial evaluation and immediately before an anticipated transplantation procedure. "Active" cardiac conditions are defined as unstable coronary syndromes (eg, unstable angina, severe angina, or recent myocardial infarction (MI), decompensated heart failure, significant arrhythmias, and severe valvular disease). The presence of one or more of these conditions is associated with high rates of perioperative cardiovascular morbidity and mortality, hence delay or cancellation of the

Evidence Class: Magnitude of procedure/treatment effect	
	I Conditions for which there is evidence for and/or general agreement that the procedure/therapy is useful and effective
	II Conditions for which there is conflicting evidence and/or a divergence of opinion about the usefulness/efficacy of performing the procedure/therapy
	IIa Weight of evidence/opinion is in favor of usefulness/efficacy
	IIb Usefulness/efficacy is less well established by evidence/opinion
	III Conditions for which there is evidence and/or general agreement that the procedure/therapy is not useful/effective and in some cases may be harmful
Evidence Level: Estimate of certainty (precision) of procedure/treatment effect	
	A Consistent direction and magnitude of effect from multiple randomized controlled trials
	B Consistent retrospective cohort, exploratory cohort, ecological, outcome research, or case-control studies, or extrapolation from level A studies
	C Case-series studies or extrapolations from level B studies

Table 4. Evidence Grading

surgical procedure may be required. The 2012 AHA/ACC guidelines recommend that a thorough history and physical examination be performed in all patients preoperatively to identify any active cardiac conditions (Class I; Level of Evidence C). In prospective transplant candidates with chronic cardiac conditions, re-assessment of their cardiac status before surgery may be necessary. The former is defined as chronic limiting angina, an MI that is < 30 days old but without symptoms of unstable angina, prior history of coronary artery bypass graft (CABG) or percutaneous coronary intervention (PCI), decompensated heart failure, moderate valvular disease or prior valve surgey, or stable arrhythmias.

b. Noninvasive stress testing in kidney transplant candidates without active cardiac conditions

The AHA/ACC recommend noninvasive stress testing in kidney transplant candidates with no active cardiac conditions based on the presence of multiple CAD risk factors regardless of functional status. Eight relevant risk factors among transplant candidates –as defined in the Lisbon Conference report include: diabetes, prior cardiovascular disease, dialysis duration of greater than 12 months, left ventricular hypertrophy, age > 60 years, smoking, hypertension, and dyslipidemia (Abbud-Filho et al., 2007). Although the exact number of risk factors required to initiate noninvasive stress testing has not been well defined, the AHA/ACC Committee suggests that the presence of 3 or more risk factors should prompt further evaluation with noninvasive stress testing (Class IIb; Level of Evidence C) (Lentine et al., 2012)

Noninvasive stress testing for CAD may be performed with exercise or with a pharmacological agent, and gauged by electrocardiography (EKG) changes (exercise stress test), myocardial perfusion distribution (myocardial perfusion imaging), or left ventricular wall motion (stress echocardiogram). Myocardial perfusion studies (MPS) and dobutamine stress echocardiogram (DSE) are more commonly used due to the frequent abnormalities detected on baseline EKGs in patients with ESKD. In addition, dialysis patients may not be able to achieve an adequate level of exercise during an exercise stress test because of their sedentary lifestyles. However,

http://dx.doi.org/10.5772/54736

it should also be noted that in ESKD patients both myocardial perfusion study (MPS) and DSE have reduced sensitivity and specificity compared with that of the general population. In the general population, abnormalities on myocardial perfusion study has been suggested to correlate well with the presence of coronary artery disease (CAD) with mean weighted sensitivity of 88% and specificity of 74% (Klocke et al., 2003). In patients with stage 5 CKD (GFR < 15 ml/min or dialysis dependent) DSE and MPS have been reported to have sensitivities ranging from 44% to 89%, and 29% to 92%, respectively, and specificities ranging from 71% to 94% and 67% to 89%, respectively, for identifying ≥ 1 coronary stenosis > 70% (Lentine et al. 2009, Lentine et al, 2012). Furthermore, abnormal MPS and DSE test results have not been consistently shown to be associated with prognostic value for cardiac events and mortality in ESKD patients. In a meta-analysis of 12 studies involving either thallium-201 scintigraphy or DSE, Rabbat *et al*. demonstrated that ESKD patients with inducible ischemia had 6 times higher risk of MI and 4 times higher risk of cardiac death than patients without inducible ischemia (Rabbat et al., 2003). In contrast, in a small prospective study of 106 kidney transplant candidates clinically classified as moderate (age ≥50 years) or high (diabetes mellitus, extra-cardiac vascular disease, or known CAD) coronary risk who underwent MPS, DSE, and coronary angiography, De Lima *et al.* found that clinical risk stratification and coronary angiographic findings of CAD (defined as ≥70% stenosis in ≥1 epicardial arteries by visual estimation by 2 observers) predicted major adverse cardiac events (MACEs) [defined as sudden death, myocardial infarction, arrhythmia, heart failure, unstable angina, or revascularization] after a median follow-up of 46 months but results of MPS and DSE did not predict MACEs (De Lima et al., 2003).

Given the wide ranges of sensitivities and specificities of the MPS and DSE and the inconsistent associations of angiographically defined CAD with subsequent survival in ESKD patients, the AHA/ACC Writing Committee acknowledges that there are currently no definitive data to support or refute screening for myocardial ischemia among potential kidney transplant candidates without active cardiac conditions. However, it is recommended that until further data are available, it may be useful to use aggregate CAD risk factors to target screening of patients with the highest pretest probability of having significant CAD. Suggested algorithm for pretransplant cardiac evaluation based on the 2012 AHA/ACC guidelines is shown in figure 1.

In general, high cardiac risk candidates should undergo a formal evaluation by cardiology. If necessary, percutaneous coronary intervention or coronary bypass surgery and cardiac rehabilitation should be performed prior to transplantation. If coronary intervention is indicated, caution should be made especially if stenting is planned. The 2012 AHA/ACC guidelines do not recommend transplant surgery within 3 months of bare metal stent (BMS) and within 12 months of DES placement, particularly if the anticipated time of poststent dual antiplatelet therapy will be shortened (Class III; level of Evidence B). Transplant surgery is also not advisable in patients within 4 weeks of coronary revascularization with balloon angioplasty (Clas III; Level of Evidence B) (Lentine et al., 2012).

In patients with established CVD or in those at risk for CV events, aggressive risk factor modification and treatment *per* ACC/AHA guidelines (Pearson et al., 2002) are recommended. The cardioprotective effects of statins, aspirin, ACE inhibitors, and/or β blockers have been

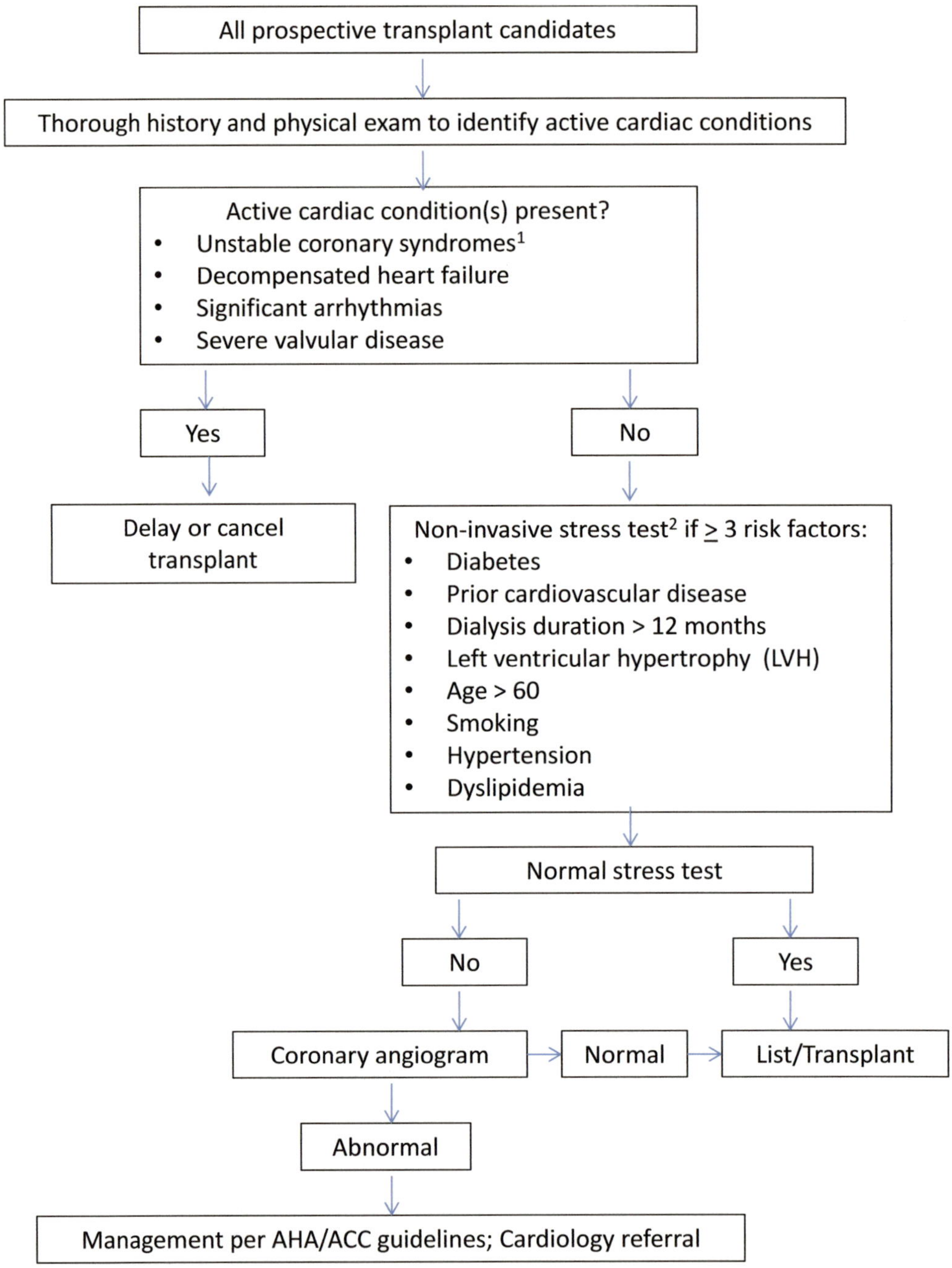

[1]Unstable coronary syndromes: unstable angina, severe angina, recent myocardial infarction
[2]Myocardial perfusion study or dobutamine stress echocardiogram (center specific).

Figure 1. Suggested algorithm for pretransplant cardiac evaluation

well-described. Omega-3 fatty acid consumption from fish or fish oil has also been suggested to confer a cardioprotective effect. If feasible, β1 cardioselective agents should be given several weeks prior to a planned living donor renal transplant. This allows time to maximize the efficacy of beta blockers and time to slowly titrate beta blockers, avoiding bradycardia and hypotension. Avoidance of these adverse effects may decrease the risk of stroke and all-cause mortality, leading to a positive net clinical benefit (Deveraeaux et al., 2008, Harte et al. 2008).

2.2.1. *Biomarkers for cardiac risk assessment*

In recent years, cardiac troponin T (cTnT) has been suggested to provide prognostic information in the cardiac evaluation of patients with ESKD. Independent investigators have demonstrated an association between increased levels of cardiac toponin T isoforms and all-cause and cardiac death risk in asymptomatic patients with ESKD (Lentine et al., 2009, Khan et al., 2005). In a study consisting of 644 wait-listed renal transplant candidates, Hickson *et al.* demonstrated that increasing cTnT levels were associated with progressively reduced survival independent of low serum albumin and history of stroke. The survival of patients with cTnT levels between 0.01 and 0.03 ng/mL did not differ from that of patients with levels < 0.01 ng/mL. In contrast, cTnT levels between 0.03 and 0.09 ng/mL were associated with significantly increased mortality (hazard ratio, HR=3.01, p=0.040). Notably, mortality was further increased in patients with cTnT levels >0.1 ng/mL (HR=4.085, p=0.009) whereas in patients with normal cTnT, excellent survival was achieved independent of other risk factors (Hickson et al., 2008). The 2012 AHA/ACA guidelines support the use of cTnT level at the time of evaluation for kidney transplantation as an additional prognostic marker (Class IIb; Level of Evidence B) (Lentine et al., 2012). However, the routine use of cTnT as adjunctive tools in cardiac risk assessment in renal transplant candidates remains to be studied.

2.3. Nonischemic cardiomyopathy

Patients with CKD frequently suffer from nonischemic cardiac abnormalities including left ventricular hypertrophy (LVH), left ventricular dilatation, left ventricular systolic and/or diastolic dysfunction. Renal transplantation has variably been shown to improve left ventricular dysfunction and ameliorate LVH (Zolty et al., 2008). Hence, the presence of such abnormalities does not necessarily preclude transplantation. Nonetheless, patients with an ejection fraction of 40% are considered moderate to high risk candidates and warrant a formal Cardiology consultation. An ejection fraction below 40% generally precludes transplantation. It is our practice to refer these patients to Cardiomyopathy Center for further diagnostic and therapeutic interventions. The presence of advanced irreversible cardiomyopathy is a contraindication to solitary kidney transplantation and patients should be referred for possible combined kidney-heart transplantation.

2.4. Peripheral vascular disease

Patients with a history of transient ischemic attacks or cerebrovascular accidents should undergo carotid Doppler studies. Duplex ultrasonography may be considered in asymptomatic patients with symptomatic peripheral arterial disease (PAD), CAD, or atherosclerotic aortic aneurysm (Class IIb). Patients without clinical evidence of atherosclerosis may also be screened if they have 2 or more risk factors including hypertension, hyperlipidemia, cigarette smoking, family history of atherosclerosis manifested before age 60 in a first-degree relative, or family history of ischemic stroke (Class IIb). It is also reasonable to screen asymptomatic patients with a carotid bruit (Class IIa). Lastly, asymptomatic patients with known or suspected carotid artery disease are recommended to undergo duplex ultrasonography studies (Class I) (Lentine et al., 2012). Evidence of significant stenosis requires vascular surgery consultation. If necessary, carotid endarterectomy should be performed prior to transplantation and patients should be symptom free for at least six months prior to transplantation. For those with milder carotid disease, neurology consultation and optimal medical management may be sufficient.

Peripheral vascular disease is present in a significant number of renal transplant recipients and is associated with increased morbidity and mortality. Vascular imaging with either a Doppler ultrasound, computed tomography (CT) scan or magnetic resonance angiography (MRA) of the pelvic vasculature is indicated in patients with a history of claudication and/or signs of diminished peripheral arterial pulses (particularly in diabetics) on physical exam. Our single-center experience reveals that in asymptomatic patients with diminished pedal pulses but good femoral pulses, screening has not resulted in intervention in any cases. Angiogram should be considered if noninvasive studies suggest the presence of large-vessel disease. Significant aortoiliac disease requires evaluation by the surgical transplant team and may preclude transplantation.

In transplant candidates with autosomal dominant polycystic kidney disease, screening for intracranial aneurysm with either CT scan or MRA is probably warranted in all patients with a history of headaches, stroke and/or family history of intracranial aneurysm or cerebrovascular accident.

2.5. Infections

All patients should be assessed for common latent or active infections and questioned for a history of infectious exposures. Active infections including diabetic foot ulcers and osteomyelitis must be fully treated prior to transplantation. A prior history of tuberculosis or untreated tuberculosis exposure requires appropriate posttransplant prophylactic therapy. Patients with an established history of systemic coccidioidomycosis or histoplasmosis or those from an endemic area should undergo appropriate antibody testing. In addition, these patients should be informed of possible disease reactivation with immunosuppressive therapy and indefinite posttransplant azole prophylactic therapy. A history of immunization should also be obtained to assure adequate immunizations for common infections prior to transplantation (e.g. hepatitis B, pneumovax, and other standard immunization appropriate for age). Immunization update is mandatory for those who have undergone surgical splenectomy. Up-to-date recommendations for routine adult immunizations are available through the Centers for Disease Control and Prevention website www.cdc.gov/vaccines/schedules/downloads/adult/adult-schedule.pdf. Ideally, all potential transplant candidates should complete all recommended immunizations at least 4 to 6 weeks before transplantation to achieve optimal immune response and to minimize the possibility of live vaccine-derived infection in the posttransplant period. Household members, close contacts, and health care workers should also be fully immunized.

Infection with influenza A (H1N1) virus has emerged as an important cause of morbidity and mortality in the general and dialysis population worldwide. More importantly, infected patients on chronic dialysis treatment were found to have a 10-fold higher mortality rate compared to the general population (Marcelli et al., 2009). Recipients of solid organ transplants have also been suggested to be at risk for more severe disease (Kumar et al., 2010). In a multicenter cohort study consisting of 237 adult and pediatric solid organ transplant recipients with microbiological-confirmed influenza A H1N1 infection, 71% required hospitalization. Among 230 patients for whom data on complications were available, 32% had pneumonia, 16% were admitted to the intensive care units, and ten (4%) died.(Kumar et al., 2010) Hence, unless contraindicated, influenza A (H1N1) vaccine should be considered in all prospective transplant candidates.

Hepatitis B antigenemia does not preclude transplant candidacy. However, patients should be referred for a liver biopsy to assess the severity of liver disease because liver enzymes may be spuriously normal despite necroinflammatory changes on biopsy (Fabrizi et al., 2010). Transplant candidacy should be based on both liver histology and serologic evidence of HBV replication (i.e. HBV DNA and HBeAg positivity). In transplant candidates with active HBV replication, antiviral therapy should be initiated pretransplantation. The presence of histologically mild liver disease does not preclude transplantation. However, patients should be forewarned that the introduction of immunosuppressive therapy in the posttransplant period can lead to progression of liver disease even in patients with histologically mild disease before transplantation. All patients with HBV should be placed on antiviral therapy after transplantation to prevent HBV reactivation and replication and progression of liver disease. Similar to HBV infection, liver biopsy is essential in the evaluation of transplant candidate with HCV because clinical and biochemical findings are unreliable indicators of the severity of liver disease in the dialysis population. The presence of minimal to mild chronic hepatitis (stages I and II) does not preclude transplantation. Pretransplantation antiviral treatment should be considered to prevent the progression of liver disease and protect the graft against HCV-related glomerulonephritis (Fabrizi et al., 2010). It should be noted that there is currently no effective treatment for chronic hepatitis C in renal transplant recipients. Although treatment with interferon-α may result in clearance of HCV RNA in 25-50% of cases, rapid relapse following drug withdrawal is nearly universal. More importantly, interferon-α treatment has been shown to precipitate acute allograft rejection and graft loss and is currently not routinely recommended for renal transplant recipients with HCV infection. The use of interferon-α should be individualized at the discretion of the transplant nephrologist and hepatologist. Studies evaluating interferon-free regimens are currently underway (Yee et al., 2012). Hepatitis C positive transplant candidates should be given the option of receiving a HCV-positive donor kidney which may reduce deceased donor kidney waiting time considerably.

Histological evidence of liver cirrhosis has been regarded as a contraindication to solitary kidney transplantation due to the risk of frank hepatic decompensation after transplantation as a consequence of immunosuppression. However, recent studies suggest that kidney alone transplant may be safe in end stage kidney disease (ESKD) patients with compensated hepatitis C (HCV) cirrhosis and hepatic portal venous gradient (HPVG) of less than 10 mmHg. In a single center study consisting of 37 kidney alone HCV positive transplant recipients (n=9 with cirrhosis and n= 28 with no cirrhosis), none developed decompensation of their liver disease at 3-year follow-up although one patient in the non-cirrhosis group developed metastatic hepatocellular carcinoma 16 months after transplantation. One- and three-year graft survival rates were 75% and 75% *vs.* 92.1% and 75.1% for the cirrhosis and non-cirrhosis groups, respectively (P=0.72). The corresponding one- and three-year patient survival rates were 88.9% and 88.9% *vs.* 96.3% and 77.9%, respectively (P=0.76). Only recipient age and decreasing albumin levels were significantly associated with worse graft and patient survival. The authors concluded that kidney alone transplant may be safe in ESKD patients with compensated HCV cirrhosis and HPVG of less than 10 mmHg. (Paramesh et al., 2012). While limited studies suggest that combined liver-kidney transplant may be unnecessary in ESKD patients with compensated HCV cirrhosis and HPVG of less than 10 mmHg, patients with decompensated liver cirrhosis should be referred for combined liver-kidney transplant.

Infections with the human immunodeficiency virus (HIV) was once considered a contraindication to transplantation due to early report of serious infectious complications and death following HIV infection transmitted from a transplanted organ or inadvertent transplantation of HIV-infected patients. However, with the advent of highly effective highly active antiretroviral agents (HAART) regimen, there have been changing views regarding transplantation in HIV positive patients. Currently, a number of transplant centers would consider transplantation in stable HIV patients, defined as those with an undetectable HIV viral load, CD4 lymphocyte count greater than 300/mm^3, and absence of opportunistic infections in the previous year. Specific recommendations may vary from center to center and a formal consultation with infectious disease is recommended.

2.6. Malignancy

Transplant recipients are at greater risk of developing both *de novo* and recurrent malignancy due to the use of immunosuppressants. As the incidence of malignancy increases with the intensity and duration of immunosuppression, a history of immunosuppressive therapy for the native kidneys represents an added risk for posttransplant malignancy. For patients who have had a history of malignancy, consultation with oncology is advisable. Table 5 provides the general guidelines for minimum tumor-free waiting periods for common malignancies. Among the pre-transplant treated cancers, the highest recurrence rates have been observed with multiple myeloma (67%), non-melanoma skin cancers (53%), bladder carcinomas (29%), sarcomas (29%), symptomatic renal cell carcinomas (27%), and breast carcinomas (23%) (Penn I, 1997). In an analysis of the Israel Penn International Transplant Tumor Registry involving 90 patients with a history of pretransplant prostate adenocarcinoma (77 renal, 10 heart, and 3 liver transplant recipients), prostate cancer recurrences were shown to be related to the stage of disease at initial diagnosis (Woodle et al., 2005). Tumor recurrence rates were 14%, 16%, and 33% for stage I, II, and III diseases, respectively. Hence, a longer waiting time may be necessary for more advanced disease. Most transplant centers adhere to standard cancer surveillance appropriate for age for all transplant candidates although the utility of such screening has been challenged by experts in the field (Danovitch GM, 2003).

Of note, studies in end-stage kidney disease (ESKD) patients treated by dialysis or transplantation, and in patients with HIV/AIDS suggest that cancers can be categorized into ESKD-related, immune deficiency-related, not related to immune deficiency or of uncertain status. ESKD-related cancers include kidney, urinary tract, thyroid and multiple myeloma (Steward et al., 2008). Hence screening for malignancy in adult kidney transplant candidates should focus on kidney and urinary tract particularly in dialysis-dependent ESKD patients. Serum immunofixation electrophoresis should be performed in all transplant candidates older than 60 years of age. Chronic hepatitis B and C infected individuals should be screened for liver cancer. Although thyroid carcinoma has been observed at increased frequency in dialysis patients compared with the general population, thyroid ultrasound is not part of routine pretransplant screening. It has been suggested that regular thyroid ultrasound is justified in dialysis patients although there have been no studies to confirm or refute this recommendation. Therefore, screening prospective renal transplant candidates for thyroid cancer should be done at the discretion of the clinicians. All suitable renal transplant candidate should have a baseline renal ultrasound to screen for renal neoplasm (discussed further under urologic evaluation).

Most tumors: wait time ≥2 years	
No waiting time if cure at the time of transplantation	
Incidental renal cell carcinoma	
In situ carcinoma of bladder	
In situ carcinoma of cervix	
Basal cell carcinoma	
Squamous cell carcinoma (skin) [2,3]	
Waiting time ≥2-5 years[2]	
Melanoma[2,,4]	5 yrs
Wilms tumor	2 yrs
Renal cell carcinoma	2 yrs if < 5cm
	5 yrs if > 5 cm
Breast carcinoma[5]	2-5 yrs
Lymphoma	2-5 yrs
Colorectal carcinoma	2-5 yrs
Invasive bladder	2 yrs
Uterine body	2 yrs
Invasive cervical carcinoma	2-5 yrs

[1]Certain cancers may recur despite a tumor-free waiting period.

[2]Oncology evaluation or consultation with the Israel Penn International Transplant Tumor Registry at www.ipittr.org may be invaluable

[3]Surveillance

[4]In situ melanoma may require a shorter waiting period of 2 years (dermatology consultation is probably warranted)

[5]Early in situ (eg ductal carcinoma in situ) may only require 2-year wait. Individuals with advanced breast cancer (stage III or IV) should be advised against transplantation

Table 5. Malignancy and renal transplantation[1,2]

2.7. Specific gastrointestinal evaluation

There has been no consensus on whether all asymptomatic renal transplant candidates should be screened for cholelithiasis. Screening is warranted, however, in diabetics and patients with a history of cholecystitis. Pretransplant cholecystectomy is recommended for these patients if there is evidence of cholelithiasis due to the increased risk of life-threatening cholecystitis after transplantation.

2.8. Hypercoagulable states

Thrombophilia generally does not preclude transplantation but does mandate the initiation of preventive strategies to reduce thrombotic complications and early graft loss. All transplant candidates should have routine coagulation studies performed. In high-risk candidates such as those with a previous history of thrombotic events including recurrent thrombosis of arteriovenous grafts and fistulas, positive family history of thrombosis, or history of recurrent miscarriage in female transplant candidates, a more extensive hypercoagulability profile should be performed. These may include screening for activated protein C resistance ratio or factor V Leiden mutation, factor II 20210 gene mutation, antiphospholipid antibody, lupus anticoagulation, protein C or protein S deficiency, antithrombin III deficiency, and homocysteine levels. It is our center practice to screen for lupus anticoagulant and antiphospholipid antibodies in all renal transplant candidates with systemic lupus erythematosous (Pham et al., 2010). It should be noted that although a prior history of thromboembolism does not preclude transplantation, a history of extensive venous thrombosis that involve the inferior vena cava, iliac vein or both may contraindicate transplantation and warrants evaluation by the surgical transplant team.

There has been no consensus on the optimal management of recipients with abnormal hypercoagulability profile. However, unless contraindicated, perioperative and/or postoperative prophylactic anticoagulation should be considered, particularly in patients with a prior history of recurrent thrombotic events. Transplant of pediatric *en bloc* kidneys into adult recipient with a history of thrombosis should probably be avoided. The duration of anticoagulation has not been well defined, but lifelong anticoagulation should be considered in high-risk candidates (Pham et al., 2010).

2.9. Urologic evaluation

All renal transplant candidates on dialysis should be imaged with a renal ultrasound, CT, or MRI to evaluate for acquired cystic kidney disease and associated renal cell carcinoma. Although there has been no consensus on the frequency of screening for renal neoplasms in wait-listed patients, the frequency of screening should follow the guidelines set forth for dialysis patients. If there is no evidence of acquired cystic kidney disease at initial screening, repeat ultrasound can be done annually or biannually (Eitner et al., 2010). Annual screening in patients who have been on dialysis for three to five years has been advocated (Chapman et al. 2011).. Urinalysis and urine cultures should be performed in all patients with significant residual urine volume. Transplant candidates with a history of recurrent urinary tract

http://dx.doi.org/10.5772/54736

infections, voiding symptoms, or end stage renal disease secondary to congenital or genitourinary abnormalities should undergo a voiding cystourethrogram (VCUG). Persistent hematuria or sterile pyuria may warrant endoscopic evaluation and/or retrograde pyelography. Urodynamic studies may be helpful in patients with a history of lower urinary tract dysfunction and/or urinary incontinence. Patients with bladder dysfunction secondary to neurogenic bladder or chronic infections can often be managed without urinary diversion. In continent patients with lower urinary tract dysfunction, intermittent self-catheterization is a safe and effective alternative to urinary diversion. However, a formal urologic evaluation and patient education during the initial transplant evaluation process is mandatory. Augmentation cystoplasty or urinary diversion procedures may be necessary in patients in whom simple reimplantation into a dysfunctional bladder is not an option. Male transplant candidates with sufficient urine volume and symptoms of outflow tract obstruction due to benign prostatic hypertrophy should undergo prostate resection before transplantation, whereas in anuric patients, the procedure should be postponed until after a successful renal transplant.

2.10. Specific urologic considerations: Pretransplant nephrectomy

For most patients with autosomal dominant polycystic kidney disease (ADPKD) pretransplant nephrectomy is not routinely recommended. However, unilateral or bilateral pretransplant nephrectomy(ies) may be necessary for those with massively enlarged kidneys, recurrent infection, bleeding, and/or intractable pain. Table 6 lists the special indications for pretransplant native nephrectomy. Generally, a minimum of six weeks after nephrectomy is recommended prior to transplantation. For transplant candidates who undergo preemptive transplantation from a living donor, simultaneous native nephrectomy and transplantation may be performed.

Absolute indications
Chronic renal parenchymal infection
Recurrent infected stones
Reflux or obstructive megaureter complicated by infection or stone formation
Polycystic kidney disease[1]
Heavy proteinuria
Relative indications
Intractable hypertension[2]
Acquired renal cystic disease[3]

[1]Indicated for massively enlarged kidneys, recurrently infected or bleeding, intractable pain

[2]Should be individualized

[3]When there is suspicion for adenocarcinoma

Table 6. Indications for pretransplant native nephrectomy

3. Evaluation of risk factors related to specific patients' characteristics

3.1. Advanced age

There is no arbitrary age limit for transplantation. The United Network for Organ Sharing/ Organ Procurement Transplantation (UNOS OPTN) database revealed that the number of kidney transplants performed in patients ≥ 65 has more than tripled over the last decade (ww.unos.org). Similar to the younger population, transplantation in the older age group of 60 to 74 years has been shown to improve survival compared to their wait-listed counterparts. Graft loss from rejection is lower in older compared to younger recipients presumably due to the decreased immune responsiveness in the aged population. It must be noted, however, that older transplant recipients are at increased risks for infectious complications, malignancy related to immunosuppression, and deaths in the early posttransplant period, most often as a consequence of cardiovascular disease.

Although advanced age *per se* has not been regarded as contraindication to transplantation, kidney transplantation among recipients over 80 years of age is uncommonly performed. Analysis of the UNOS/OPTN database revealed that of the transplants performed between 2000 and 2007 in recipients ≥ 60 years of age, only 0.6% were older than 80 years of age. For statistical analysis purposes, patients were divided into three age groups, 60-69, 70-79, and > 80 years with recipients aged 60-69 years used as reference. Median ages for recipients aged 60-69, 70-79, and > 80 years were 64, 72, and 81 years, respectively. Most of the differences were seen between recipients aged 60-69 and > 80 years. The rates of living donor transplants were lower in recipients > 80 years compared to 60-69 years (18% vs. 32%, respectively). The acute rejection rate at 1-year among recipients > 80 years was comparable to that of recipients 60-69 years of age. Three-year patient survival was significantly lower in recipients older than 80 years compared to recipients aged 60-69 years (64% vs. 84%, respectively) with an unadjusted relative risk of death of 2.35 (95% CI 1.83-3.03). However, graft survival was excellent and did not differ significantly between the two groups (88% vs. 90%) (Poommipanit et al., 2010). Hence, the assessment of transplant candidacy for patients over 80 years of age remains a challenge for transplant physicians. Screening for covert cardiovascular disease and occult malignancy, and careful assessment of infectious risk in older prospective transplant candidates are crucial and mandatory.

Currently, the waiting time for a deceased donor transplant in the United States is such that many wait-listed older transplant candidates die while awaiting transplantation from a standard deceased donor kidney. Furthermore, the duration of pretransplant dialysis has been shown to confer a significant and progressive increase in the risk of death-censored graft loss and the risk for patient death after transplantation. Compared with preemptive renal transplantation, waiting time of 0-6 months, 6-12 months, 12-24 months, and over 24 months conferred a 17%, 37%, 55%, and 68% increase risk for death-censored graft loss after transplantation, respectively (Meier-Kriesche et al., 2000). Similarly, mortality risk after transplantation was significantly increased with increasing waiting time on dialysis. It is our center practice to offer the expanded criteria donor (ECD) program to all candidates 50 years of age or older. Patients should be informed that candidates for ECD kidneys are simultaneously listed for a standard and ECD kidney. Although living donor kidneys offer older transplant candidates the best chance of meaningful improved survival and quality of life, older patients are often reluctant to accept living donor kidneys from their children or grandchildren. These issues must be discussed with patients and their families with particular care and compassion to optimize the chance of a satisfactory outcome. Nonetheless, it should be noted that extreme recipient-donor age pair (e.g recipient > 80 years and donor aged 20-30 years) may represent a great challenge for the clinicians as well as patients and their families.

3.2. Obesity

Obesity is considered a contraindication to transplantation by some centers as it is associated with increased risks of posttransplant complications including delayed graft function, surgical wound infection, and death, particularly from cardiovascular disease. Although there has been no consensus on an acceptable upper limit body mass index (BMI), weight reduction to a BMI of 30-35kg/m^2 or less prior to transplantation is recommended. Morbidly obese candidates may benefit from surgery referral for gastric bypass surgery or gastric banding procedure, or more recently, laparoscopic sleeve gastrectomy. However, it should be noted that there has been limited data on the safety and efficacy of bariatric surgery (BS) in renal transplant candidates. The USRDS registry data (1991-2004) demonstrated a median excess body weight loss of 31%-61% after bariatric surgery, with thirty-day mortality rate of 3.5% (72 were performed on pre-listed, 29 on waitlisted, and 87 on posttransplant patients). One graft was lost within 30 days after BS. (Modanlou et al. 2009). The authors concluded that although peri-operative mortality was not negligible, the rate may be lower with experienced surgeons and comparable to trials involving patients without kidney disease.

Data on patient and graft survival in obese *versus* non-obese transplant recipients are variable and contradictory. Determination of transplant candidacy in obese patients should, therefore, be assessed on an individual basis rather than reliance on an absolute BMI index. Obese candidates with comorbid conditions such as known coronary artery disease and advanced age are at particularly high risk and may fare better receiving dialysis.

3.3. Managing the wait-list candidates

Whereas the number of patients on the transplant waiting list has steadily increased, the number of deceased donor kidneys has remained far below the growing need, leading to longer waiting time and increased wait-list deaths. Hence, managing the wait-list has been one of the greatest problems facing transplant centers. Periodic reassessment of transplant candidates' medical and psychosocial issues entails ongoing communication between the dialysis units, patients, and transplant coordinators and transplant programs. In the event of a significant intercurrent illness that may necessitate delisting or placing candidates on hold, pertinent medical records should be obtained and reviewed by a transplant physician. If necessary, patients must be seen to reassess their candidacy. Most transplant programs attempt to see transplant candidates on an annual basis to update their overall heatlh and demographic issues although older candidates may require more frequent visits at the discretion of the transplant physician. During the follow-up visit, routine health maintenance status and cancer screening appropriate for age and gender such as prostate specific antigen, mammography, pap smear, and colonoscopy are also reviewed. Although recommendations for cardiac surveillance of waitlisted patients varies among transplant centers, most transplant programs advocate annual cardiac screening in diabetic transplant candidates. In addition to reassessing patients'medical status, the availability of living donors should be re-addressed. Currently, in an effort to maximize the utilization of living kidney donors, our program has implemented an algorithm to evaluate crossmatch positive and ABO-incompatible donor-recipient pairs. Patients are advised of living donor options including paired exchange transplantation, positive crossmatch and ABO incompatible transplantation through desensitization protocols, and living donor kidney exchange for both ABO-incompatible and crossmatch positive donor-recipient combinations. Discussion of this topic is beyond the scope of this chapter. For older transplant candidates, the advantages and disadvantages of expanded criteria donor kidney transplantation should be addressed. Finally, effective communication between patients'primary nephrologists and transplant centers is invaluable in permitting wait-listed transplant candidates to be at their optimal medical health when a deceased donor kidney becomes available.

Author details

Phuong-Thu Pham[1*], Son V. Pham[2], Phuong-Anh Pham[3] and Phuong-Chi Pham[4]

*Address all correspondence to: PPham@mednet.ucla.edu

1 Department of Medicine, Nephrology Division, Kidney and Pancreas Transplant Program, David Geffen School of Medicine at UCLA, Los Angeles, CA, USA

2 Audie L. Murphy VA Medical Center and University of Texas Health Science Center, San Antonio, TX, USA

3 Memphis VA Medical Center and University of Tennessee Health Science Center, Memphis, TN, USA

4 Department of Medicine, Nephrology Division, UCLA-Olive View Medical Center, David Geffen School of Medicine at UCLA, Sylmar, CA, USA

References

[1] Abbud-Filho M, Adams PL, Alberu J, et al. A report of the Lisbon Conference on the care of the kidney transplant recipients. Transplantation 83(suppl): S1-22, 2007

[2] Bridoux F, Ronco P, Gillmore J. Renal transplantation in light chain amyloidosis: coming out of the cupboard. Nephrol Dial Transplant 26: 1766-1768, 2011

[3] Canaud G, Audard V, Kofman T, et al. Recurrence from primary and secondary glomerulopathy after renal transplantation. Transplant Int 25: 812-824, 2012

[4] Chapman AB. Acquired cystic disease of the kidney in adults. Upto Date 2011 www.uptodate.com

[5] Colgert WA, Appel GB, Hariharan S. Recurrent glomerulonephritis after renal transplantation: An unsolved problem. Clin J Am Soc Nephrol 3(3): 800-807, 2008

[6] Danovitch GM. Guidelines on the firing-line. Am J Transplant 3: 514-515, 2003

[7] Danovitch I. Psychiatric aspects of kidney transplantation. In: Handbook of Kidney Transplantation, 5th ed, ed. Danovitch GM,Lippincott Williams and Wilkins, . Philadelphia, PA, pp 389-408, 2010

[8] De Lima JJ, Sabbaga E, Vieir ML, et al. Coronary angiography is the best predictor of events in renal transplant candidates compared with noninvasive testing. Hypertension 42:263-268, 2003

[9] Deveraeaux PJ, Yang H, Yusuf S, Guyatt G, Laslie K, Villar JC, Xavier D, Chrolavicius S, Greenspar L, Poque J, Pais P, Liu L, Xu S, Malaga G, Avezum A, Chan M, Jacka M, Choi P. Effects of extended release metoprolol succinate in patients undergoing non cardiac surgery (POISE Trial): A randomized controlled trial. Lancet 371: 1839-1847, 2008

[10] Eitner F. Acquired cystic kidney disease and malignant neoplasms. In: Floege J, Johnson RJ, Feehally J (eds). Comprehensive Clinical Nephrology, 4th edn. Elsevier Saunders: St. Louis, Missouri, 2010: 1010-1015

[11] Fabrizi F, Bunnapradist S, Martin P. Kidney transplantation and liver disease. In: Handbook of Kidney Transplantation, Danovitch GM (ed), 5th edition, pp 280-290, Lippincot Williams and Wilkins, Philadelphia, PA 2010

[12] Harte B, Amir K. Jaffer. Perioperative beta-blockers in noncardiac surgery: Evolution of the evidence. Cleveland Clinic Journal of Medicine 75: 513-519, 2008

[13] Hickson LJ, Cosio FG, El-Zoghby ZM, et al. Survival of patients on the kidney transplantwait list: Relationship to cardiac Troponin T. Am J transplant 8: 2352-2359,2008

[14] Kasiske BL, Zeier MG and KDGO Work Group. KDIGO Clinical Practice Guidelines for the care of kidney transplant recipients: Recurrent kidney disease. Am J Transplant 9 (suppl 3): S33-S37, 2009

[15] Khan NA,Hemmelgarn BR,Tonelli M,et al.Prognosticvalue of troponinT and I among asymptomaticpatients with end-stage renal disease: A meta-analysis. Circulation 112: 3088-3096, 2005

[16] Klocke FJ, Baird MG, Lorell BH, Bateman TM, Messer JV, Berman DS, O'Gara PT, Carabello BA, Russell RO Jr, Cerqueiria MD, St John Sutton MG, DeMaria AN, Udelson JE, Kennedy JW, Verani MS, Williams KA, Antman EM, Smith SC, Alpert JS, Gregoratos

G, Anderson JL, Hiratzka LF, Faxon DP, Hunt SA, Fuster V, Jacobs AK, Gibbons RJ, Russell RO ACC/AHA/ASNC guidelines for the clinical use of cardiac radionuclide imaging –Executive summary: A report of the American College of Cardiology/ American Heart Association Task Force on Practice Guidelines (ACC/AHA/ASNC Committee to Revise the 1995 Guidelines for the Clinical Use of Cardiac Radionuclide Imaging). J Am Coll Cardiol 42: 1318-1333, 2003

[17] Kumar D, Michaels MG, Morris MI, et al. Outcomes from panendemic influenza A H1N1 infection in recipients of solid-organ transplants: a multicentre cohort study. Lancet Inf Dis 10:521-526, 2010

[18] Lentine KL, Costa SP, Weir MR, et al. Cardiac disease evaluation and management among kidney and libver transplantation candidates. A scientific statement from the American Heart association and the American college of Cardiology foundation. Circulation126:00-00, 2012 http://circ.ahajournals.org

[19] Lentine KL, Hurst FP, Jindal RM, Villines TC, Kunz JS, Yuan CM, Hauptman PJ, Abbott KC. Cardiovascular risk assessment among potential kidney transplant candidates: Approaches and controversies 55 (1): 152-167, 2009

[20] Marcelli D, Marelli C, Richards N. InfluenzaA(H1N1)v pandemic in the dialysis population: first wave results from an international survey. Nephrol Dial Transplant 24: 3566-3572, 2009

[21] Meier-Kriesche HU, Port FK, Ojo AO, Rudich SM, Hanson JA, Cibrik DM, Leichtman AB, Kaplan B. Effect of waiting time on renal transplant outcome. Kidney Int 58(3): 1311-1317, 2000

[22] Modanlou KA, Muthyala U, Xiao H, Schnitzler MA, Salvalaggio PR, Brennan DC, Abbott KC, Graff RJ, Lentine KL. Bariatric surgery among kidney transplant candidates and recipients: Analysis of the United States Renal Data System and literature review. Transplantation 87: 1167-1173, 2009

[23] Paramesh AS, Davis JY, Mallikarjun C, et al. Kidney transplantation alone in ESRD patients with hepatitis C cirrhosis. Transplantation 94(3): 250-254, 2012

[24] Pearson TA, Blair SN, Daniels SR, Eckel RH, fair JM, Fortmann SP, Franklin BA, Goldstein LB, Greenland P, Grundy SM, Hong Y, Miller NH, Lauer RM, Ockene IS, Sacco RL, Sallis JF, Smith SC Jr, Stone NJ, Taubert KA. AHA guidelines for primary prevention of cardiovascular disease and stroke: 2002 update: Consensus Panel Guide to Comprehensive Risk Reduction for Adults Patients without Coronary or Other Atherosclerotic Vascular Disease. American Heart Association Science Advisory and Coordinating Committee. Circulation 106: 388-391, 2002

[25] Pham PT, Pham PA, Pham PC, et al. Evaluation of the adult kidney transplant candidates. Seminars in Dialysis 23(6): 595-605, 2010

[26] Ponticelli C. Recurrence of focal segmental glomerulosclerosis (FSGS) after renal transplantation. Nephrol Dial Transplant 25(1): 25-31, 2010

[27] Poommipanit N, Sampaio M, Reddy P, Miguel M, Ye X, Wilkinson AH, Pham PT, Gritsch AH, Danovitch GM, Bunnapradist S. Outcomes of octogenarian kidney transplant recipients in the United States. Abstract, American Transplant Congress 2010, San Diego, CA

[28] Rabbat CG, Treleaven DJ, Russell JD, et al. Prognostic value of myocardial perfusion studies in patients with end-stage renal disease assessed for kidney or kidney-pancreas transplantation: a meta-analysis. J Am Soc Nephrol 14:431-439, 2003

[29] Steward JH, Vajdic CM, van Leeween MT, et al. The pattern of excess cáncer in dialysis and transplantation. Nephrol Dial Transplant 24: 3225-3231, 2008

[30] Woodle ES, Gupta M, Buell JF, Neff GW, Gross TG, First MR, Hanaway MJ, Trofe J: Prostate cancer prior to solid organ transplantation: the Israel Penn International Transplant Tumor Registry experience. Transplant Proc 37(2): 958-959, 2005

[31] Yee HS, Chang MF, Pocha C, et al. Update on the management and treatment of hepatitis C virus infection: Recommendations from the department of Veterans Affairs hepatitis C resource center program and the National Hepatitis C Program Office. Am J Gastroenterol 107: 669-689, 2012

[32] Zolty R, Hynes PJ, Vittoris TJ. Severe left ventricular systolic dysfunction may reverse with renal transplantation: uremic cardiomyopathy and cardiorenal syndrome. Am J Transplant 8(11): 2219-2224, 2008

Chapter 2

Imaging in Kidney Transplantation

Valdair Francisco Muglia, Sara Reis Teixeira, Elen Almeida Romão, Marcelo Ferreira Cassini, Murilo Ferreira de Andrade, Mery Kato, Maria Estela Papini Nardin and Silvio Tucci Jr

Additional information is available at the end of the chapter

http://dx.doi.org/10.5772/55074

1. Introduction

At the end-stage of renal failure, the best option for treatment is kidney transplantation, before starting any form of dialysis. The scarcity of organs from cadaveric donors and the comorbidity of the receptors patients, delay this treatment from being routinely performed prior to dialysis. Living-donor kidney transplantation can meet this objective perfectly, since it does not depend on waiting lists imposed by cadaveric donation [1]. In recent years, the expansion of genetically unrelated living donation has facilitated living-donor kidney transplantation as spouses, distant relatives, and even good friends have increased the pool of potential living donors. The living-donor transplants offer better survival than those of cadaveric-donor transplants, despite of HLA compatibility [2, 3].

For cadaver's donors, cause of brain death, age, plasma levels of creatinine and hemodynamic stability are the main factors for evaluating a potential donor. In contradistinction, the imaging methods constitute the initial assessment of the living donor in the kidney transplantation, with special attention to the kidneys (size, structure, lithiasis, arterial blood flow) and pelvis anatomy. The abdominal Color Doppler ultrasound, computed tomography (CT), selective kidney arteriography and Magnetic Ressonance (MR) with three-dimensional reconstruction and excretory phase study provide an anatomical assessment of the arterial vascularization (identification of the main artery, accessory or aberrant arteries or early divisions) of the venous system (number, situation, size and anatomic abnormalities) and the kidney parenchyma with the variations of collecting duct system, helping to choose the most appropriate organ to be removed [4, 5].

In the postoperative phase, many kinds of images methods (ultrasound, scintigraphy, CT and MR) may help in early diagnosis of complications, as described below. In this chapter we review the usual image evaluation techniques in kidney transplantation.

2. Imaging methods

2.1. Ultrasonography

Ultrasonography (US) is the first choice for evaluating kidney allograft either in acute, immediate post-transplantation period or in the long-term follow-up [6, 7]. US is non-invasive, innocuous and due to its availability has a key hole when assessing complications of any nature in renal transplants. As the transplanted kidney usually lies in a superficial position in the iliac fossa, it is possible to use high-frequency transducers enabling images of high spatial resolution. In addition, the ability of Color Doppler (CD) and Power Doppler (PD) to investigate blood flow helps to make the diagnosis of the most common functional complications as rejection acute tubular necrosis [8, 9].

2.2. Magnetic resonance imaging

When additional imaging is required, generally because the sonographic findings were indeterminate, Magnetic Resonance Imaging (MRI) emerges as the problem-solving method in kidney transplantation [10, 11]. MRI has several advantages when compared to Computed Tomography (CT); it has no ionizing radiation and the main contraindication to this method is the use of cardiac pacemakers. MRI has the highest contrast resolution among all imaging methods and is able to produce angiographic images (MR angiography) without the use of contrast media. And, when necessary the contrast media for MRI, Gadolinium-based salts, are safer than iodinated contrast media used in CT [12, 13]. In addition, the MRI technique to study the collecting system based on T2-weighted images, MR urography, has been used as an alternative to intravenous urography (IVU) and CT [14].

After initial concerning about the possible relation between gadolinium salts and Systemic Nephrogenic Fibrosis [15, 16], there is a consensus that some Gadolinium-based contrast media (GBCM), more stable, may be used in patients with depressed renal function, as long as recommendations regarding type and doses of contrast media were respected [17, 18]. The only absolute contraindication that still persists for GBCM is patients in a regular scheme of peritoneal dialysis [18].

2.3. Computed Tomography

Computed Tomography (CT) is scarcely used to evaluate kidney transplants, because MRI covers all the possible indications for CT, without ionizing radiation and the use of nephrotoxic contrast media [19]. Although CT angiography has great spatial resolution, this technique should be avoided whenever possible, due to the potential nephrotoxicity of iodinated contrast. CT will play a major role for evaluation potential donors for living transplantation as will be described later on in this chapter [20].

2.4. Digital Subtraction Angiography

Digital Subtraction Angiography (DSA) was commonly used to investigate vascular complications, e.g. renal artery transplant stenosis, suspected by US and is still considered the gold standard for such diagnoses [7, 21]. However, nowadays, with the possibility of using non-invasive methods with high accuracy for diagnosing vascular complications, such as MR angiography, DSA is practically reserved for therapeutic purposes only. The ability to guide minimally invasive procedures, as angioplasty and stenting of vascular stenosis makes DSA the ideal method to assess post-transplant patients avoiding more aggressive surgical procedures [21].

3. Radionuclides imaging

Functional imaging methods based on nuclear medicine, such as the dynamic renal study which use glomerular filtration agents and tubular secretion agents, are useful and routinely used tools for evaluation of renal transplants. Glomerular agents (^{99m}Tc-DTPA) are considered to be ideal ones, since glomerular filtration is defined as the main reflex of renal function and their mechanism of extraction occur through the process of ultrafiltration driven by Starling forces in the glomeruli. The most important regulatory mechanisms in glomerular filtration are renal blood flow and the peripheral vascular resistance of afferent and efferent glomerular arterioles. The normal distribution of these renal agents is intravascular, and they are elimi-

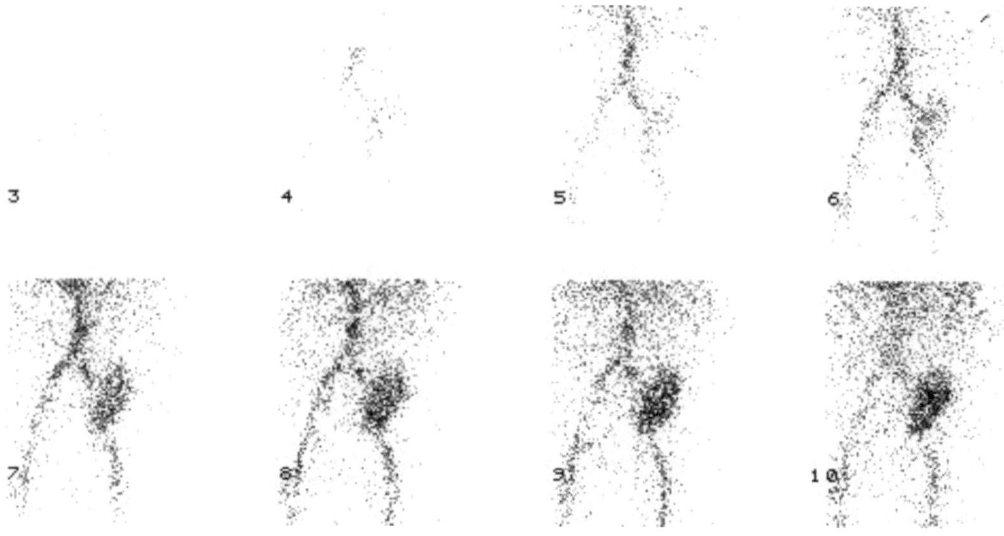

Figure 1. DTPA renal scintigraphy. Phase of preserved arterial blood flow.

nated by the renal parenchyma and excreted through the urinary pathways. The acquisition protocol involves the capture of sequential images within a short time interval immediately after the venous administration of the glomerular agent, providing information about renal perfusion (Figure 1), and of sequential images over a more prolonged period of time in order to obtain information about glomerular filtration and urine formation (Figure 2A). Semiquantitative analysis is performed based on the curves of the radioisotope renogram. These curves are obtained by drawing areas of interest in the kidneys and then tracing time count curves (Figure 2B).

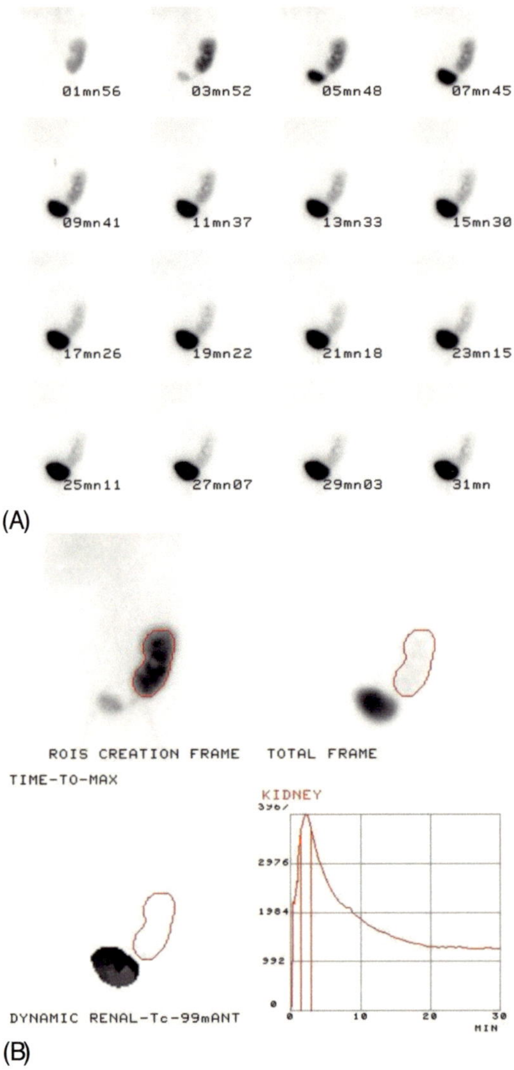

Figure 2. (A) and (B): ^{99mTc}-DTPA renal scintigraphy. Normal functional phase and renographic curve.

4. Post-transplant evaluation

4.1. Normal

Imaging methods are frequently used in patients with kidney transplantation, even when clinical parameters and laboratorial tests indicate a good evolution. As US is very sensitive, innocuous, and largely available, most of centers for renal transplantation include, at least, one US exam in the immediate prost-transplant period to detect possible subtle complications that otherwise could remain undetected until more severe symptoms [6, 22]. As mentioned early, US is performed with high frequency transducers, using scanners with Color and Power Doppler techniques.

The appearance of transplant kidney is quite similar to the native ones. But, in the immediate post-transplant period a mild dilatation of collecting system is expected due to hipotony (Figure 3).and edema in ureteral anastomosis [22]. A detailed examination is performed and, not rarely, incidental findings as kidney stones, cysts or small angiomiolipomas may be detected in first post-surgical examination. Besides, a careful search for perinephric collections is performed and CD and PD used for evaluation of vascular anastomosis. The renal transplant artery is usually anastomosed to the donor external iliac artery in an end-to-side way. Occasionally, the artery may be anastomosed in an end-to-end way to the internal iliac artery. The donor renal vein is anastomosed in an end-to-side way to the donor's external iliac vein [23].

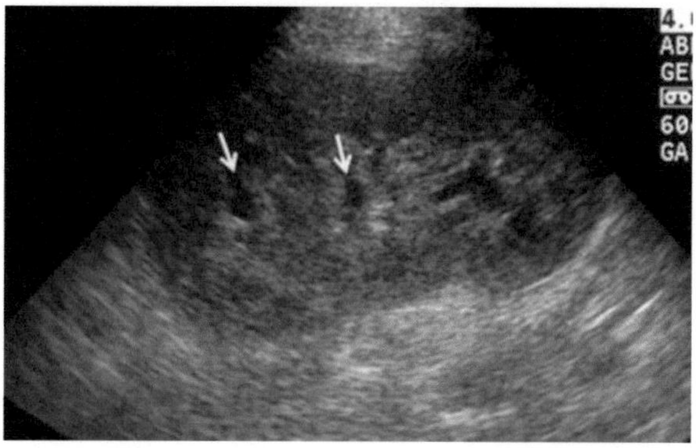

Figure 3. Normal sonographic appearance of a renal allograft in the immediate post-transplant period. Notice the mild dilatation of calyceal system (arrows).

5. Complications

Complications related to the graft following a renal transplant can be didactically divided into medical complications (MC), urological complications (UC) including fluid collections (FC), and vascular complications (VC). Neoplasms (NEO), and recurrent native renal disease are also complications that can occur but in minor incidence. The most common complications of renal transplantation are discussed bellow and listed in Table 1.

5.1. Medical complications

In the early post-transplant period, delayed graft function (DGF) occurs when the decline of the serum creatinine concentration is slower than wanted. The most common medical complications (MC) related to DGF are acute tubular necrosis (ATN), drug toxicity (mainly causes by calcineurin inhibitors - CNI), and rejection. In general, imaging tools in evaluating MC following renal transplantation are non-specific [24-26]. The major role of imaging in this setting is to exclude urologic, collections, and/or vascular complications. To date, quantitative criteria for the diagnosis of acute graft dysfunction with MR renography or nuclear medicine have not been adequately standardized. Promising techniques, especially using quantitative and functional MRI are objects of interest in this field [14, 27, 28].

5.1.1. Acute Tubular Necrosis (ATN)

ATN is the most common cause of DGF, defined as need for dialysis in the first week following transplantation. It is related to the cold ischemic time [29] and infrequently seen in patients whose transplants are from living donors [30, 31]. ATN occurs in the first days following transplantation, even in the first hours. Renal function usually recovers within 1-2 weeks, but can last abnormal up to 3 months [19, 31].

There is no imaging specific pattern for the diagnosis of ATN [10, 32]. Images can be completely normal depending on the severity of injury [33-35]. US can reveal swollen and globular kidneys, with increasing corticomedullary differentiation (CMD) [26]. The cortex is brightly echogenic, swollen, rendering medullary pyramids very prominent and compressing fat in the renal sinus. An elevated Resistance Index (RI > 0,80) measured in the intra-renal arteries is considered to be a non-specific marker of graft dysfunction, seen on both, ATN and rejection [8, 32, 36-40]. Serial measurements of RI and Pulsatile index (PI) combined with clinical and biochemical information is useful in monitoring the patient [31, 39]. At MRI, CMD tends to be preserved [41]. Dynamic functional MRI and perfusion show slightly delayed medullary enhancement, and markedly impaired contrast excretion [42, 43]. CT demonstrates decreased graft enhancement, eventually with no contrast media excretion [19].

With radionuclide imaging (iodine-131 orthoiodohippurate and Tc-99m MAG3), the most conspicuous findings are delayed transit with delayed time to maximal activity (T-max), delayed time from maximum to one-half maximal activity (T-1/2), and a high 20 to 3 minute ratio. On sequential images, marked parenchymal retention is seen [44, 45]. (Figure 4).

5.1.2. Rejection

Rejection can be classified according to the period of appearance as hyperacute (occurring within minutes), acute (occurring within days to weeks), late acute (occurring after 3 months), or chronic (occurring months to years after transplantation) [46]. When hyperacute rejection happens, graft dysfunction is usually irreversible. The humoral reaction of the patient leads

http://dx.doi.org/10.5772/55074

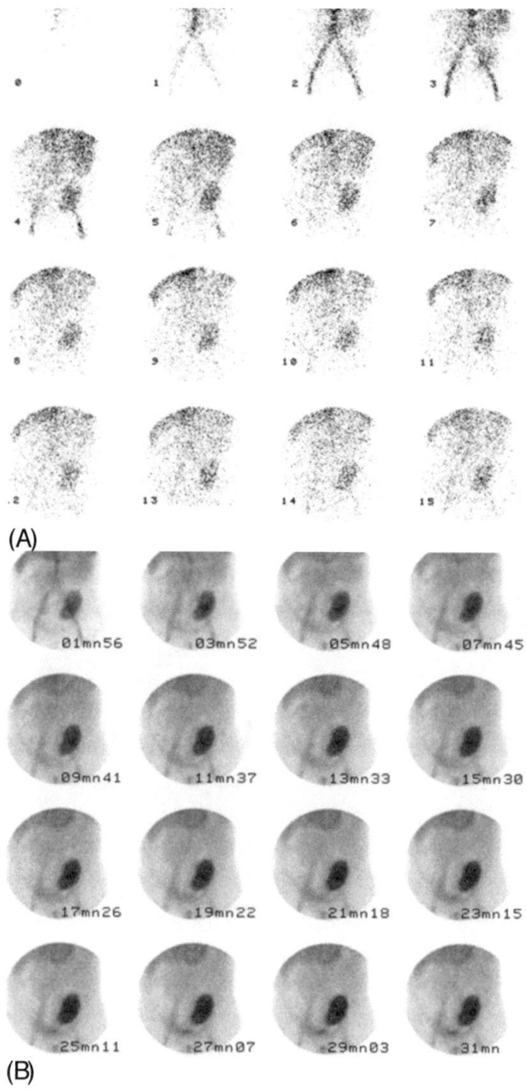

Figure 4. (A) and (B): 99mTc-DTPA renal scintigraphy. Postoperative period of 48 hours. Preserved arterial blood flow and glomerular function deficit, with minor urine formation during the study.

to a severe vascular lesion and to cortical necrosis. Imaging does not play any role. Absence of perfusion will be seen in Doppler, angiography or scintigrams [10]. Accelerated acute rejection occurs within the first week. The imaging features are the same as of acute rejection (AR). Cortical nephrocalcinosis may be seen in rejected transplants left in situ [10, 47].

Currently, the overall risk of acute rejection within 1 year after transplantation is less than 15% [46]. AR can be divided in acute-antibody mediated rejection and T-cell-mediated rejection. Acute-antibody mediated rejection is characterized by a rapid graft dysfunction due to inflammation. T-cell-mediated rejection can also present as an increasing creatinine level and diminished urinary output. Fever and graft tenderness now rarely occur. As mentioned before, imaging in AR is non-specific. Imaging findings superpose with other conditions such as ATN, drug nephrotoxicity, UC, and VC. The sonographic features are similar to those described for ATN [10, 33]. They include renal enlargement, heterogeneity of renal cortex, loss, increase or decrease of CMD, hypoechogenicity of renal pyramids, cortex and sinus, thickening of renal cortex and thickening of the walls of collecting system (figure 5). Although both ATN and AR cause PI and RI rise on Doppler US, the likelihood of AR is greater with high values [31]. An elevated RI (>0,9) is highly suggestive of AR, but is not specific [32, 36-38, 48, 49]. A PI of more than 1.5 is used in some centers for helping diagnosing rejection. Radionuclide studies show decreased renal perfusion and function [45, 50]. If the isotope study is normal in early post-operative phase and becomes abnormal subsequently, acute rejection can be diagnosed. MR findings are variable and include various degrees of swelling, globular morphology with indistinct margins of the graft, decrease or loss of the CMD are common findings [10, 14, 19, 28, 31]. Perfusion abnormalities are seen in contrast enhanced scans with marked decreased cortex and medulla enhancement, prolonged arterial phase, poor wash-out and patchy nephrogram [10, 14, 24, 28] (Figure 6).

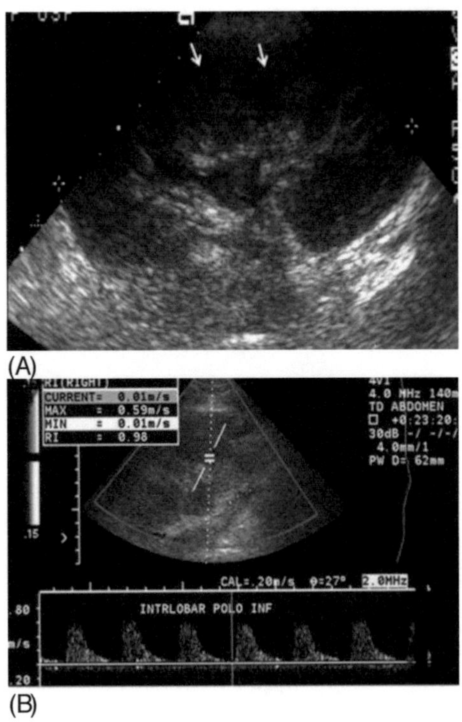

Figure 5. (A) Acute rejection, longitudinal scan. The cortex is swollen, extending into the renal sinus and compressing the fat. Medullary pyramids are prominent (arrows), indicative of an increase in cortical echogenicity. (B) Spectral Doppler shows a RI > 0,90 highly suggestive of AR.

Chronic rejection (CR) occurs after at least 3 months to years after transplantation. It happens due to an insufficient immunosuppression to control residual antigraft lymphocytes and antibodies. It presents as a progressive decline in renal function [46] and may be difficult to diagnose by a non-invasive techniques. RI measurements are not reliable for this diagnosis [24, 38, 40]. Initially, the graft is enlarged and shows increased cortical thickness, which later changes to a thin cortex and mild hydronephrosis on both US, CT, and MRI [19, 50] [28, 33]. A diminished uptake of radiopharmaceuticals and also a normal parenchymal transit with absent or minimal cortical retention is seen in scintigraphy studies. In advanced stages, parenchymal retention of radiotracers is present [45].

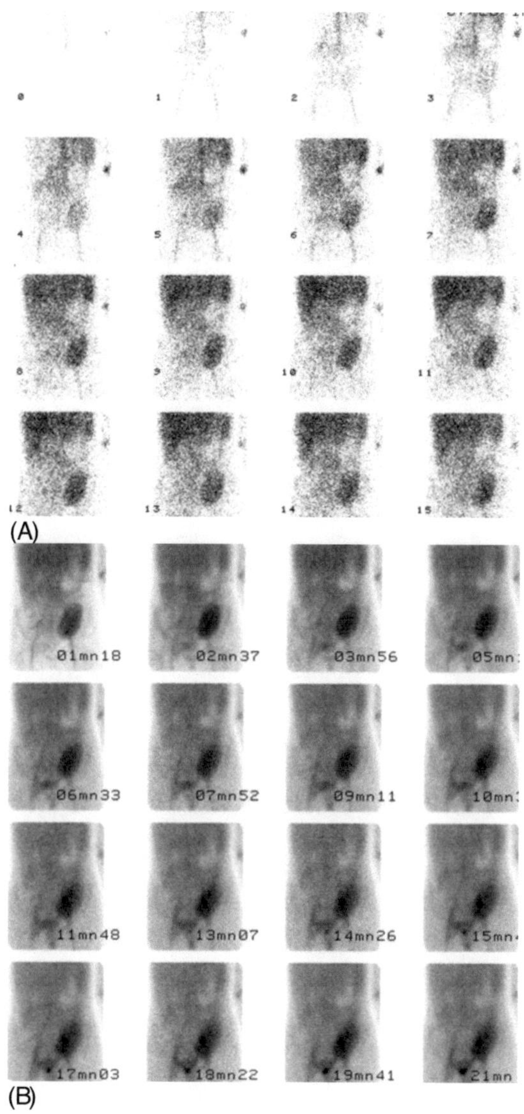

Figure 6. (A) and (B): 99mTc-DTPA renal scintigraphy. Two week follow up. Depressed arterial blood flow of a discrete degree and glomerular function deficit of moderate degree

5.1.3. Calcineurin Inhibitors (CNI) nephrotoxicity

CNI can cause renal vasoconstriction with ischemia. CNI toxicity is caused by afferent arteriolar vasoconstriction followed by a decrease in glomerular perfusion pressure and also by a tubulointerstitial injury independently from its vascular effects [51]. These physiological effects are similar between cyclosporine and tacrolimus. Monitoring the CNI serum levels is important to prevent the occurrence of nephrotoxicity and, on the other hand, to achieve the appropriate immunossupression. Moreover, nephrotoxicity of these drugs not related to their serum levels are described [52, 53].

When DGF occurs many experts prefer do not use CNI due to their possible detrimental effects in the ischemic damaged kidneys [54]. When creatinine level stabilizes without complete renal function recovery or when renal function deterioration occurs, a renal biopsy should be performed. Currently, no clinical findings are specific enough to differentiate allograft rejection from CNI nephrotoxicity. Imaging findings are also non-specific and superimposed with the other parenchymal complications. Cyclosporine toxicity may produce an enlarged kidney with increased cortical echogenicity and prominent medullary pyramids. On radionuclide images, acute cyclosporine toxicity resembles mild acute rejection, with depressed effective renal plasma flow and parenchymal retention [22, 45] Loss of the corticomedullary differentiation can be seen on MRI [55]. Findings should be correlated with cyclosporine levels. Sustained increasing in RI values (Figure 7), without a morphologic cause such as hydronephrosis, is indicative of graft dysfunction, but it´s non-specific and may be caused by acute or chronic rejection, ATN, or cyclosporine toxicity [56].

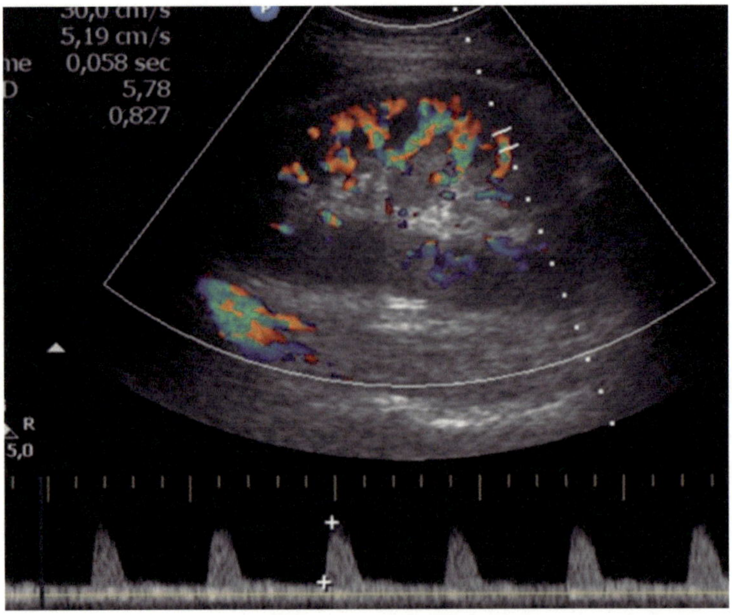

Figure 7. CNI toxicity. Spectral doppler evaluation with a mild elevatation of RI.

To date, no imaging or laboratory test has been found accurate enough to discriminate the parenchymal causes of graft dysfunction and renal biopsy remains as the gold standard [22, 49, 50, 57].

5.2. Urological complications

The clinical setting of most UCs is that of a decrease in graft function. Because many of the complications are treatable, it is extremely important to make an early diagnosis and separate from rejection or ATN. The first reports concerning renal transplantation showed a prevalence of UC varying from 10% to 25%, with a mortality rate ranging from 20% to 30%. Nowadays, due to advances in immunosuppressive therapy combined with careful surgical technique the incidence of UC decreased, ranging from 1% to 8% [58, 59]. The majority of the UC are seen during the first month to six months after transplant. Ureteric obstruction and urine leak are the most common [22, 60].

5.2.1. Obstructive uropathy

The major causes of ureteral obstruction are ureteral ischemia, edema at the uretero-vesical anastomotic site, infection, extrinsic compression of the ureter by fluid collections, and ureteral kinking. Other relatively rare causes are stones, papillary necrosis, clots, fungi, pelvic fibrosis, and herniation of the ureter [61]. Early-onset obstruction of the ureter is secondary to kinks, clots, edema, inflammation, or a tight submucosal tunnel. Percutaneous treatment is the best treatment option. Late-onset obstruction is caused by fibrosis, ischemia, or periureteral masses or may be secondary to rejection [19]. The transplanted ureter is relatively prone to ischemia due to limited blood supply [22, 24, 50, 58]. A large majority of the ureteral strictures occur in the distal third of the ureter, usually secondary to ischemia [22, 58].

Sonography shows dilated renal pelvis and calyces and is useful to determine the site of ureteral obstruction (Figure 8). This is a nonspecific finding because it is also seen in cases of diminished ureteral tonus resulted from denervation of the transplant [62], mild dilated collecting system in rejection, vesico-ureteral reflux, and secondary to overdistended bladder. In the later condition, it's important to repeat the US with an empty bladder.

When highly echogenic, weakly shadowing masses are present in the collecting system, fungus balls should be considered, whereas low-level echoes may suggest pyonephrosis or hemonephrosis [63]. Other abnormalities of the collecting system include calculi and urothelial tumors. In some cases of acute obstruction an increased RI and PI may be present, however, again they are nonspecific findings [37, 64].

At Nuclear Medicine, in patients with early partial obstruction, good perfusion and prompt uptake of the radiotracer may be seen; however, in patients with functionally significant hydronephrosis, radioactivity is retained in the collecting system. Delayed images are useful for differentiating an obstructed ureter from a dilated but unobstructed ureter, since a non-obstructed system shows clearance into the bladder. Diuretic renography and conventional

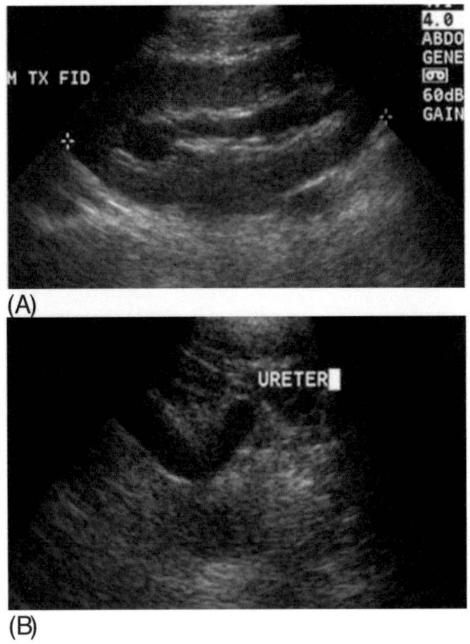

Figure 8. (A) and (B) - Mild hydronephrosis presumably, secondary to a tight submucosal tunnel.

clearance times can be used in the assessment of urinary tract patency [65]. The anterograde urography usually depicts the site of obstruction. The combination of normal results from the Whitaker test and anterograde pyelography virtually excludes the presence of obstruction [66]. If necessary, MDCT allows accurate imaging of the entire course of ureteral and periureteral diseases.

In pyelonephritis, diffuse thickening of the urothelium in the renal pelvis and proximal ureter may be seen, but it´s also seen in rejection. At MRI, an absent renal fat sinus and decrease in corticomedullary differentiation, along with striated nephrogram and multiple nonenhancing, round foci in the transplant renal parenchyma are the most frequent signs [43, 67].

Renal stones may either form in the transplant kidney or be incidentally carried from the donor kidney. Because the kidney and ureter are denervated, these patients do not present with a typical colic pain. The incidence and risk factors for calculus are the same as for a native kidney [10], in some reports ranging from 0,4% to 1,0% [68]. Lithiasis can lead to further complications such as obstruction or infection. Small stones are missed in plain films, since the transplant kidney overlies iliac bone. Unenhanced MDCT is the gold standard as can detect virtually 100% of stones.

Occasionally, gas may be seen in the collecting system, usually introduced from external sources, such as catheter or occasionally from needle biopsy or, very rarely, from emphysematous pyelonephritis. Evaluation of the collecting system and bladder may also show an abnormal position or condition of the stent.

5.2.2. *Perirenal collections*

In the early post transplant period, it is common to see fluid collections around the kidney in up to 50% cases. Common post-transplant fluid collections include urinome, hematoma, seroma, lymphocele, and abscess [33, 58, 62]. Rarely, they lead to a graft dysfunction or a collecting system obstruction.

US is very useful to assess the presence and size of perinephric fluid collections; however, it is not very specific for further differentiation among different types of content. The post-transplant time interval may suggest the nature of collections. Fluid collections seen in the immediate postoperative period are usually hematomas or seromas [50]. All fluid collection are identified with US and although solid echoes or septations may suggest specific diagnosis, correlation with clinical findings helps to restrict differential diagnosis, occasionally puncture with biochemical analysis of the fluid are required to final diagnosis

5.2.2.1. *Urinome / urinary leak*

Urinome occurs in up to 6% of transplant recipients [69] in the first weeks post-transplantation. It is believed to be caused by disruption of the vesicoureteric anastomosis or ischemic injury of the distal ureter [24]. It is normally preceded by increased abdominal pain, reduction in urine volumes and sometimes, urine leakage from the wound.

US is essential in the evaluation of perirenal collections, including urinomes. It is the modality of choice for diagnosis and guiding puncture. A cystogram may show leakage from the bladder and an isotope scan is often helpful. These collections are expected to show increased activity on radionuclide MAG-3 (Tc99 mercaptoacetyltriglycine) scans while other fluid collections usually result in photopenic defects [33] (Figure 9). The appearance on US is of a homogeneous anechoic collection, with thin walls, usually without echoes (Figure 10). CT and MRI show a clear fluid collection. Diagnostic aspiration may be required to confirm the nature of the collection. A communication between the fluid collection and urinary tract is required for final diagnosis.

5.2.2.2. *Hematoma*

Hematomas are seen mostly in the early post operative period. The overall incidence of significant postoperative hematomas from renal transplant varies from 4 to 8% [70, 71]. They have a complex appearance, poorly defined wall with internal echoes (Figure 11 A and B). Clots and debris appear as dense areas in unenhanced CT scans. Ultrasound and CT define the collection, but differentiation from abscess is difficult. Radionuclide scans demonstrate photopenic collection adjacent to the kidney, which do not fill up in delayed images. MRI signal depends on the stage of hematoma. Aspiration and imaging guided drainage are performed.

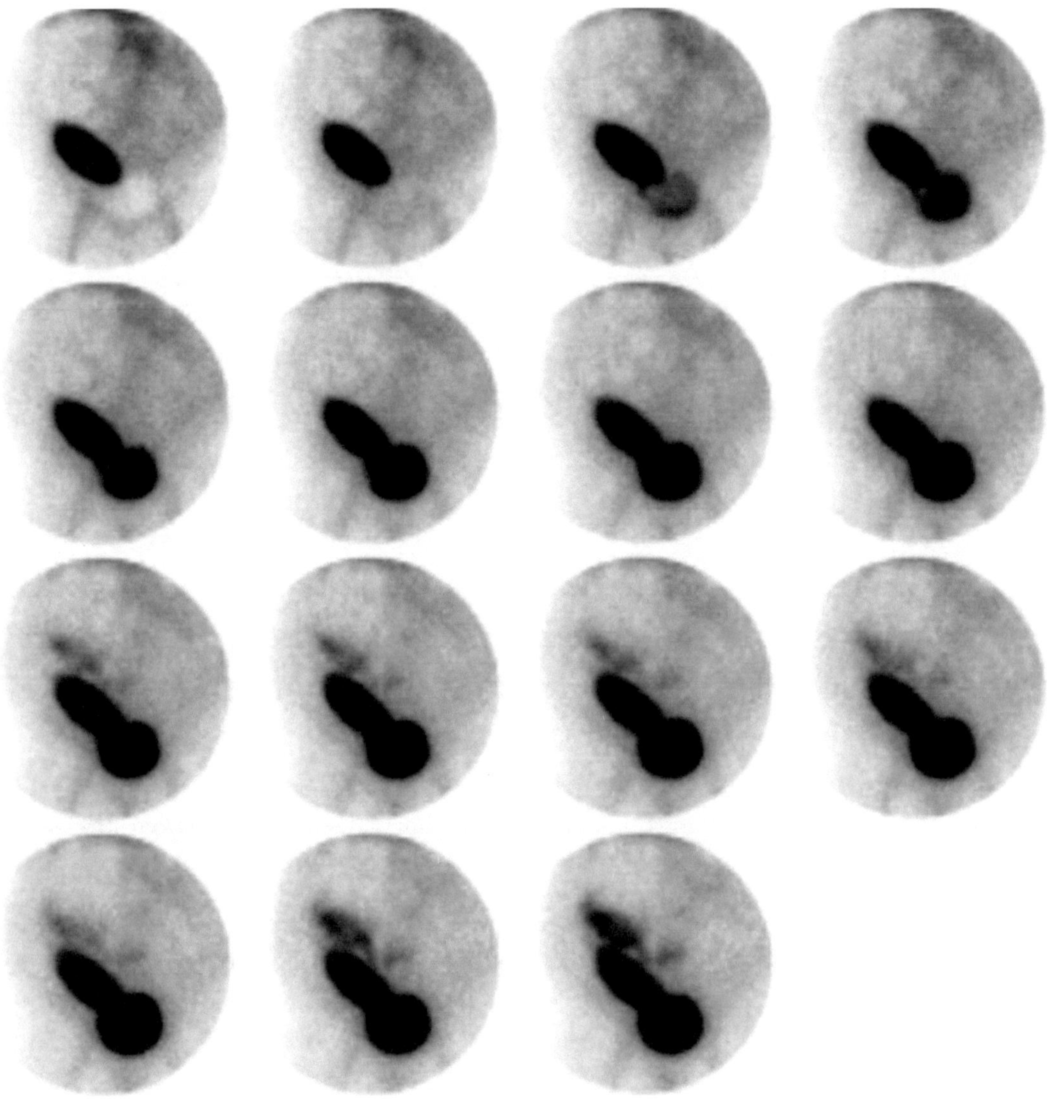

Figure 9. Anomalous accumulation of the glomerular agent (^{99mTc}-DTPA) above the renal pole compatible with a urinoma. ^{99mTc}-DTPA image showing accumulation of activity (arrow) outside the area of the kidney, ureter and bladder indicating urinary leakage.

5.2.2.3. Abscess

Abscess can be a complication of surgery, pyelonephritis or secondary to infections, urinomes, hematomas or lymphoceles. It can occur any time during the post transplant period. The appearance is the same as a hematoma, i.e. a complex collection. Parenchymal abscess manifests as a well defined hypoechoic mass on US, and nonenhancing, hypoattenuating collection on CT. On MR, it can show high signal intensity on DWI and peripheral enhancement after contrast media.

http://dx.doi.org/10.5772/55074

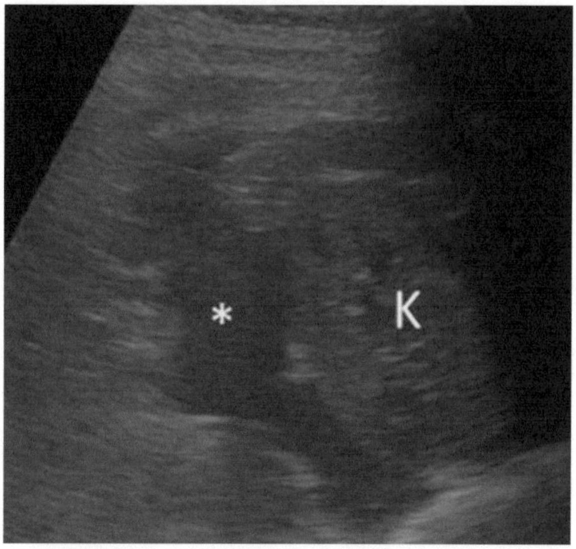

Figure 10. Urinoma. Gray-scale US shows a simple fluid collection around the kidney, anechoic (*). The biochemical analysis of the fluid after puncture revealed a high creatinine level.

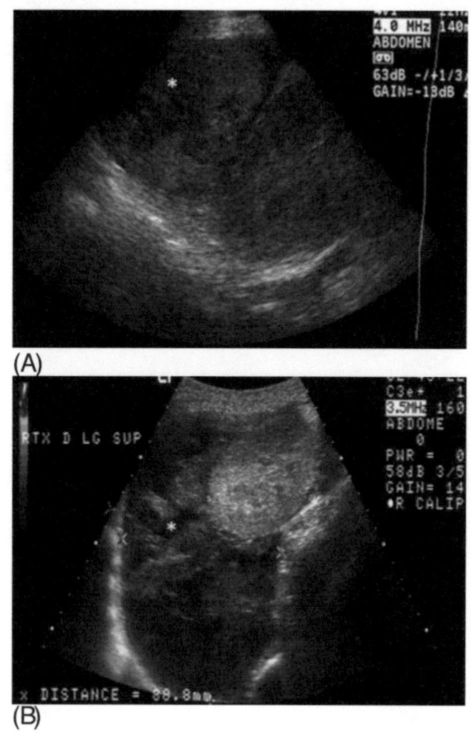

Figure 11. (A) Recent hematoma. Longitudinal US scan shows a complex, hyperechoic mass (*) around the graft. (B) Organizing hematoma. A complex collection (*) around the graft with hiper-and hypoechoic areas.

5.2.2.4. Lymphocele

Lymphoceles are lymph collection from the iliac lymphatic vessels of recipient or graft hilum that accumulates between the transplanted kidney and bladder. It results from surgical disruption of lymphatics and usually occur 4 to 8 weeks following transplantation [62, 70-72]. Usually these are small in size and asymptomatic; however, when large can cause hydronephrosis or lower extremity edema and may require drainage [33]. US shows an anechoic collection with fine septa within it, usually inferior to the region between the kidney and bladder (figure 12). Scintigraphy demonstrates a photopenic area which does not fill up with tracer on delayed images [73]. CT shows well defined round or oval collection of 0–20 HU. On MR images, an homogeneous and often minimal complex collection is depicted.

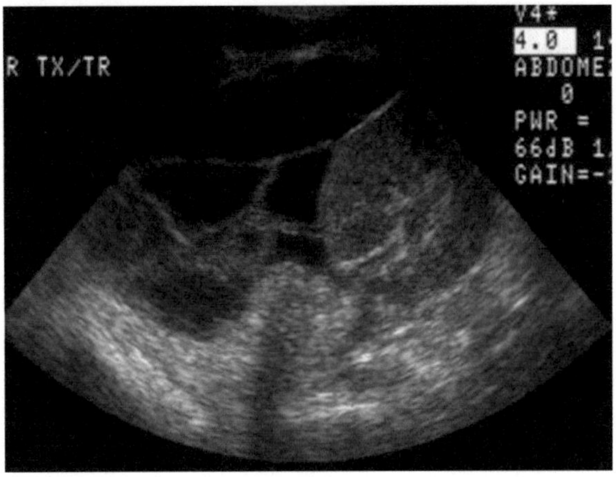

Figure 12. A minimal complex fluid collection around the graft extending to the pelvis, with fine septa, consistent with a lymphocele.

5.2.3. Vesicoureteral reflux

It seems to have a greater incidence in patients whom extravesical cystoureteral anastomosis was performed. However the clinical relevance is still not established, with a slightly increase in risk of infection. Cysto-uretrogram can easily make this diagnosis. Many technical modifications has been proposed to reduce the vesicoureteral reflux and urine leakage like modified Lich-Gregoir technic [74].

6. Other urological complications

- Ureteral necrosis: more common in the distal ureter and caused by a tight submucosal tunnel or vascular ischemia or rejection. It is a cause of urinary leak and is common in the first 6 months [75].

- Torsion: an extremely rare complication, more common in peritoneal location. It refers to rotation of the kidney transplant graft around its vascular pedicle resulting in vascular compromise and infarction [76]. On images the graft is with abnormal axis, enlarged, hypoechoic and with poor enhancement [77].
- Rupture: a rare complication of uncertain etiology. Biopsy, acute rejection, ATN, vascular occlusion, trauma, rejection, and renal cell cancer development are proposed etiologies [78-80]. Sonographic findings are extrarenal and subcapsular collections, laceration or hematomas within the perinephric space [79]. CT shows dense clot and perinephric collection. Radionuclide scans show photopenic defect. MR shows clots and an hemorrhagic perirenal collection.

6.1. Vascular complications

Vascular complications (VC) after renal transplantation are the most frequent type following urological complications, seen in less than 10% [81]. Early VC includes renal artery or vein thrombosis, lesions to the iliac vessels and cortical necrosis. Delayed complications mainly include renal artery stenosis, arteriovenous fistula and rarely pseudo-aneurysm. They have a high associated morbidity and mortality. Although DSA remains the gold standard for vascular complications, US with Doppler is the screening method for assessing blood supply of a kidney graft [49, 82]. MRI with angiography (MRA) has been used more often to confirm US diagnosis of vascular abnormalities in renal transplants [31]. With this combination, radionuclides are scarcely used to evaluate graft vascular complications.

6.1.1. Early vascular complications

Usually occurs in the first week post transplantation. Renal artery and vein thrombosis are generally related to the position of the graft, to a long vessel, to surgical techniques (anastomosis of the arteries), or to compression, e.g. hematoma compressing the renal vein. Renal vein thrombosis can also be secondary to extent of a thrombus in the iliac vein.

Arterial thrombosis is rare in the early transplant period. US and MRI show complete absence of flow in the main transplant renal artery and intrarenal arteries, no flow in the parenchyma with CD or PD (Figure. 13), and no parenchymal perfusion detectable at MRI. MRI can also demonstrate absence of renal artery enhancement. Occlusion of a lobar artery or a pedicle artery leads to a focal well-defined area of infarct, which consequences are dependent to the extension of this area [25]. In the ischemic area, the renal cortex has appearance of a wedge-based hypoechoic mass with echogenic walls, and no signal on CD [31]. MRI can better delimitate the zone of infarct. MRI and CT show a non-enhancing area with enhancing capsule. Scintigraphy may also be used to confirm arterial occlusion (Figure 14).

Renal vein thrombosis is a frequent cause of loss of the renal graft, occurring in 4-6% of the transplants in adults [83]. It´s a difficult diagnosis because it begins in the venules within the renal parenchyma, and initially, large veins remain normal [84]. Characteristic features of renal vein thrombosis include a dilated transplanted renal vein containing a thrombus with absent venous flow (Figure 15); lack of venous outflow that causes a very high resistance to arterial

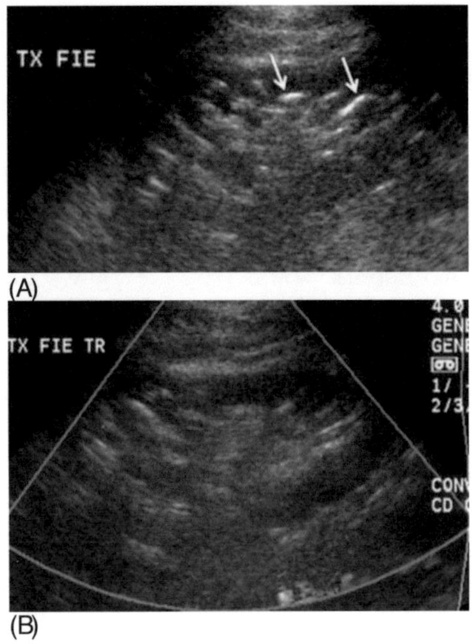

Figure 13. Acute renal artery thrombosis. (A) Gray-scale US shows gas within the collecting system (arrows). (B) Absence of signal at PD.

inflow; there may be no diastolic flow (RI = 1) or even diastolic flow reversal (Figure 16) [84]; absence of venous signals in the graft at CD or PD; decrease in the arterial sign at CD of the peripheric arteries [25]. These are non-specific findings, also present in ATN and rejection. Clinical and biochemical findings should take them apart. MRI can demonstrate the extent of the thrombus, but they must not delay the surgical approach.

6.1.2. Vascular thrombosis — Artery / vein

Lesions to the iliac or renal allograft vessels may occur during the transplantation and are associated with multiple arteries donors, anatomic variations, recipients ateromathosis, thrombophilia, obesity and other chronic diseases. They can lead to a non viable graft. Artery dissections, perforation, pseudoaneurysms, and thrombosis are the most common type of these complications [25]. Sonographic evaluation of such these lesions in the immediate post-transplant period may be limited and MRI/MRA might be necessary.

Cortical necrosis is extremely rare but severe. It can be secondary to a long cold ischemic time or rejection. Diagnosis is difficult because in the initial phase, arteries and veins remain patent. US can show a globular and heterogeneous graft with decrease in the CD sign of the cortical arteries. RI is elevated and progresses to absence of diastolic flow. Focal, patchy or diffuse zones of necrosis are better demonstrated by MRI. Biopsy is necessary to exclude rejection [25].

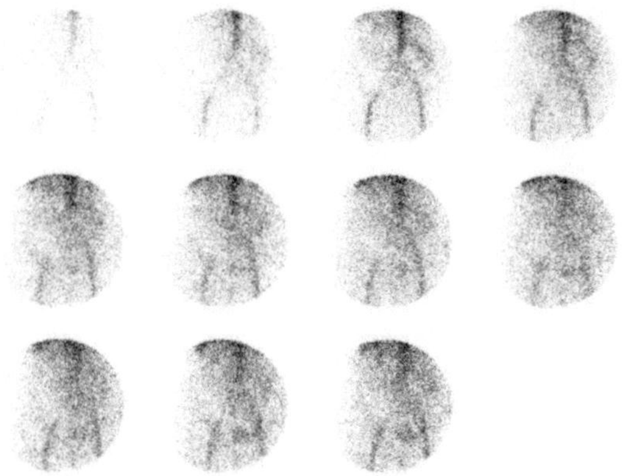
(A)

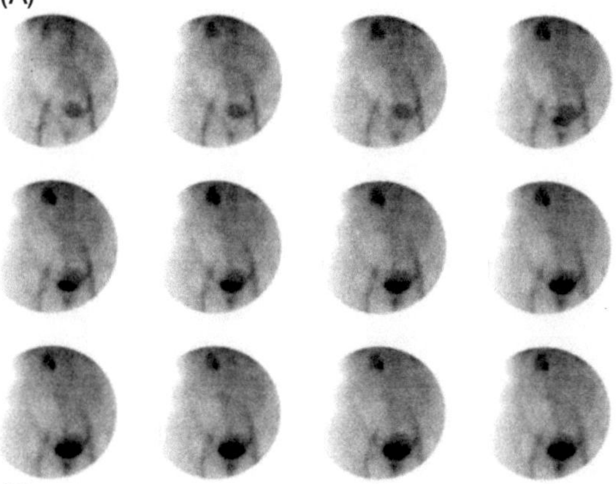
(B)

Figure 14. A and B: ^{99m}Tc-DTPA renal scintigraphy. Photopenic area in the left iliac fossa. Absence of arterial blood flow and of glomerular filtration in the transplanted kidney. Radionuclide angioscintipraphy performed with ^{99m}Tc-DTPA. The photon deficiency and no uptake of radioactivity at the site of the graft indicate non-viability.

6.2. Late vascular complications

Renal artery stenosis (RAS) is the most common VC. Stenosis can occur within a few months, most often caused by trauma to the donor's or recipient's vessel during clamping, or it may be delayed for few years, in which case atherosclerosis is usually the cause [84]. Kinking of the renal artery may cause a similar clinical condition, leading to an erroneous suspicion of RAS.

The patency of the renal artery should be performed in patients with severe hypertension refractory to medical therapy or with hypertension combined with either an audible bruit or unexplained graft dysfunction [50]. It usually occurs in the anastomosis or in the proximal donor artery, related to the surgery technique, media and intima injuries, and atherosclerosis, both from the donor or the recipient. They can occur in a short or long segment, multifocal or unifocal involvement. Flow disturbances resulting from a tight anastomosis are most readily detected in the site of the anastomosis.

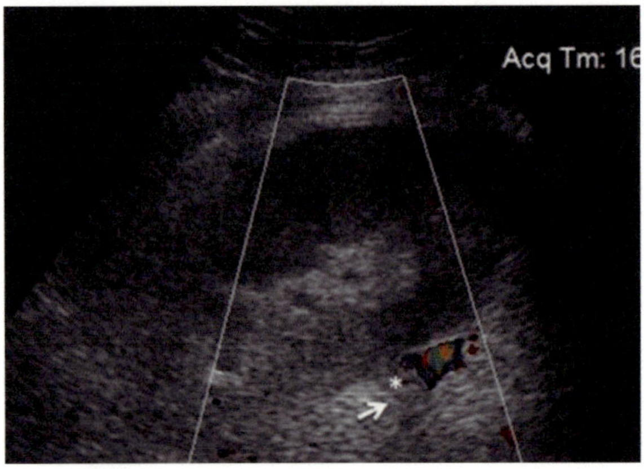

Figure 15. Renal vein thrombosis. The enlarged, occluded vein (arrow) is seen at the hilum, with a thrombus within (*).

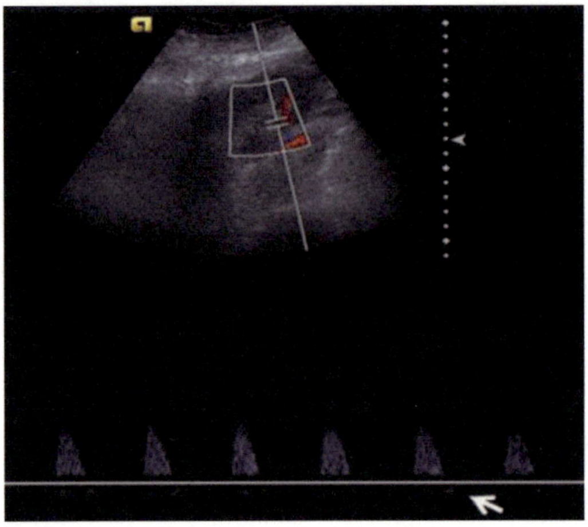

Figure 16. A reversal diastolic flow (arrow) and raising of the PSV in the interlobar artery as an indirect sign of renal vein thrombosis.

The Doppler criteria to diagnosis renal artery stenosis include: 1- high-velocity flow greater than 2 m/s measured in the renal artery (Figure 17A); 2- the ratio peak velocity in the transplant artery / peak velocity in the iliac artery close to the anastomosis higher than 2 (PVS RA/IA > 2); 3- velocity gradient between stenotic and pre-stenotic segments of more than 2:1; 4- marked distal turbulence [85, 86]. US with Doppler of the intra-renal arteries for detecting proximal artery stenosis shows a tardus parvus waveform; prolonged acceleration time, > 0.07 seconds (Figure 17B); diminished acceleration index (<3.0 m/s^2); decreased RI ($<0,56$); and loss of a normal early systolic compliance peak [85]. When US is inconclusive for RAS, MRA (preferable) and CT angiography may define the site and the degree of stenosis. The stenosis can also be confirmed by angiography, which also provides a good estimate of the vessel extent and helps in the planning of percutaneous transluminal angioplasty (Figure 18).

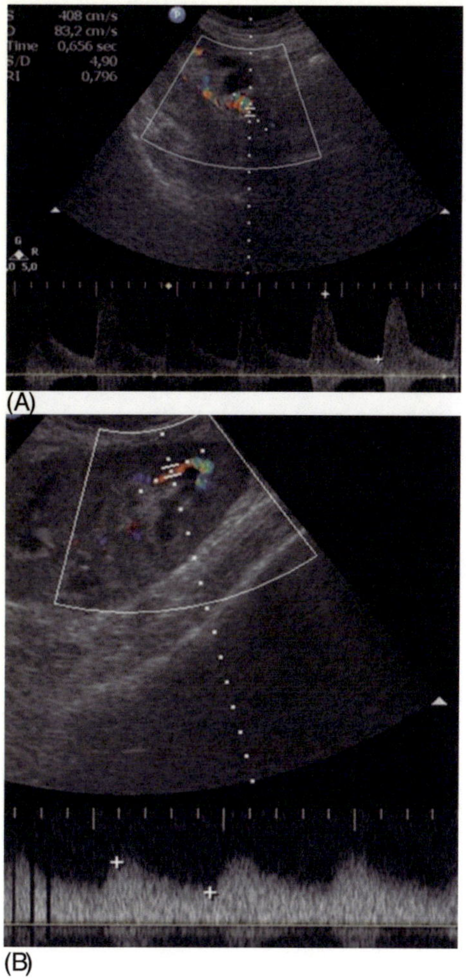

Figure 17. RAS. (A) Color-Doppler shows a focal stenosis near renal hilum with marked increase in PSV (4.0 m/s). (B) There is a tardus parvus waveform and a decreased RI at spectral Doppler.

Arteriovenous fistula (AVF) normally occurs secondary to transplant biopsy, with an incidence of 1-18% [84, 87]. Small lesions may resolve spontaneously; if not, they can be successfully treated with percutaneous embolization. They are usually asymptomatic, but can manifest with hypertension, hematuria, and graft dysfunction. Doppler US is the modality of choice for diagnosis. Focal high-velocity, low-impedance intrarenal arterial flow might suggest an arteriovenous fistula. An intense focus of high-velocity turbulent flow that is seen as a multicolored focus, persisting even with high pulse repetition frequency (or Doppler scale) at CDUS is also suspect. MRI and CT are used when US cannot define the vascular nature of the lesion. Visualization of a round abnormality in the renal parenchyma that enhances similar to the aorta at arterial-phase on MRI with an abnormal early venous drainage adjacent to the lesion is diagnostic for AVF [19]. DSA remains as the gold standard for such diagnosis and is also the method of choice for therapeutic (Figure 19).

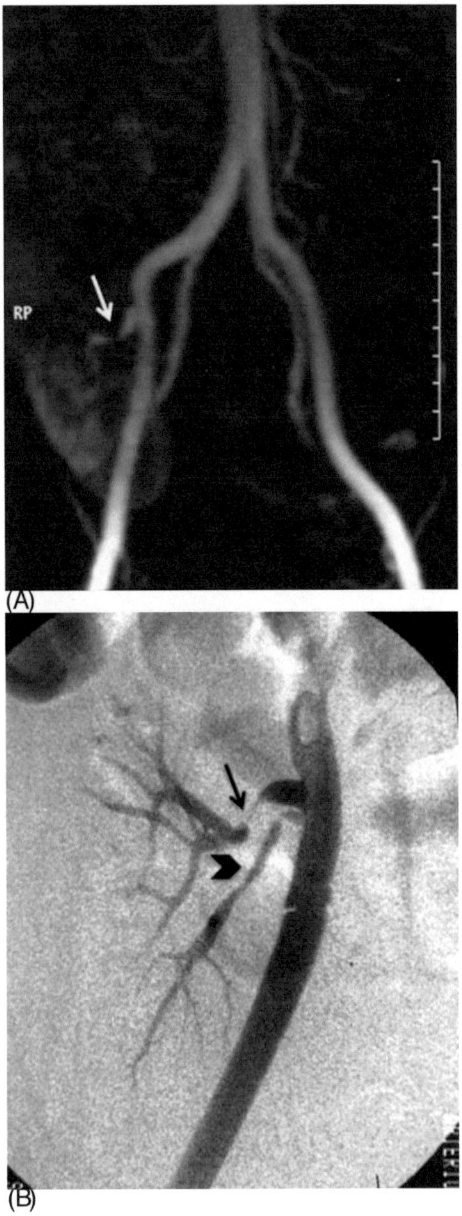

Figure 18. (A): MRA reconstructed with MIP nicely demonstrates the renal artery stenosis (arrow). (B): DSA of a different case showing multifocal stenosis in the renal artery (arrows) and a long segmental stenosis in the polar artery (arrowhead).

In general, pseudoaneurysms develop secondary to biopsy injury. Most of them resolve spontaneously within the first two months. However, if there were progressive enlargement, an unusual size (> 2 cm in diameter) or loss of renal function, intervention will be required [31]. US shows a simple or complex cyst. CD shows the to-and-fro yin and yang pattern seen in

http://dx.doi.org/10.5772/55074

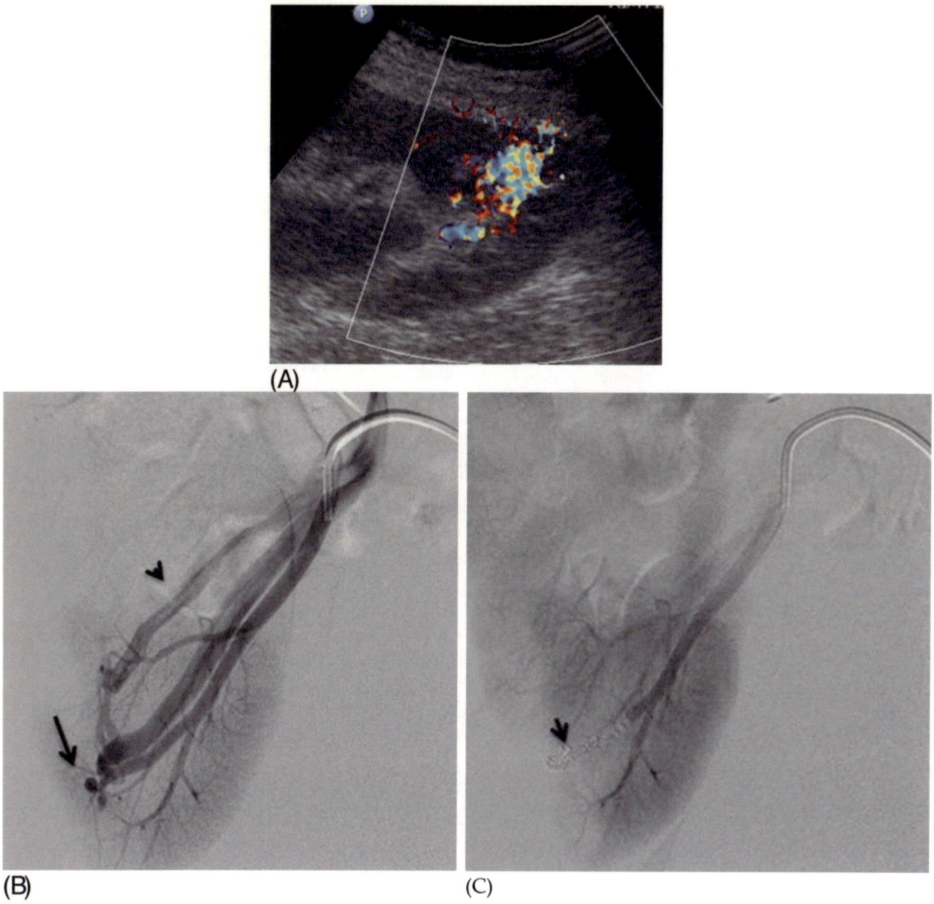

Figure 19. arteriovenous fistula. (A) US CD shows a vascular structure with troubling flow. (B) DSA pre- treatment showing a distal communication (arrow) between arterial and venous system with early drainage (arrowhead). (C) After coil placement (arrow) the AV fistula is no longer seen.

other sites of pseudoaneurysms. Extrarenal arterial pseudoaneurysm following renal transplantation is extremely rare.

Figure 20 shows an algorithm for initial evaluation of complications after kifney transplantation.

7. Other complications following renal transplantation

7.1. Malignancy after kidney transplantation

It is a known fact that patients submitted to renal replacement therapy, whether dialysis or transplantation, are at higher risk for cancer [88]. Among neoplasias, urologic tumors are about 4 to 5 times more frequent among renal transplant recipients and their characteristics differ

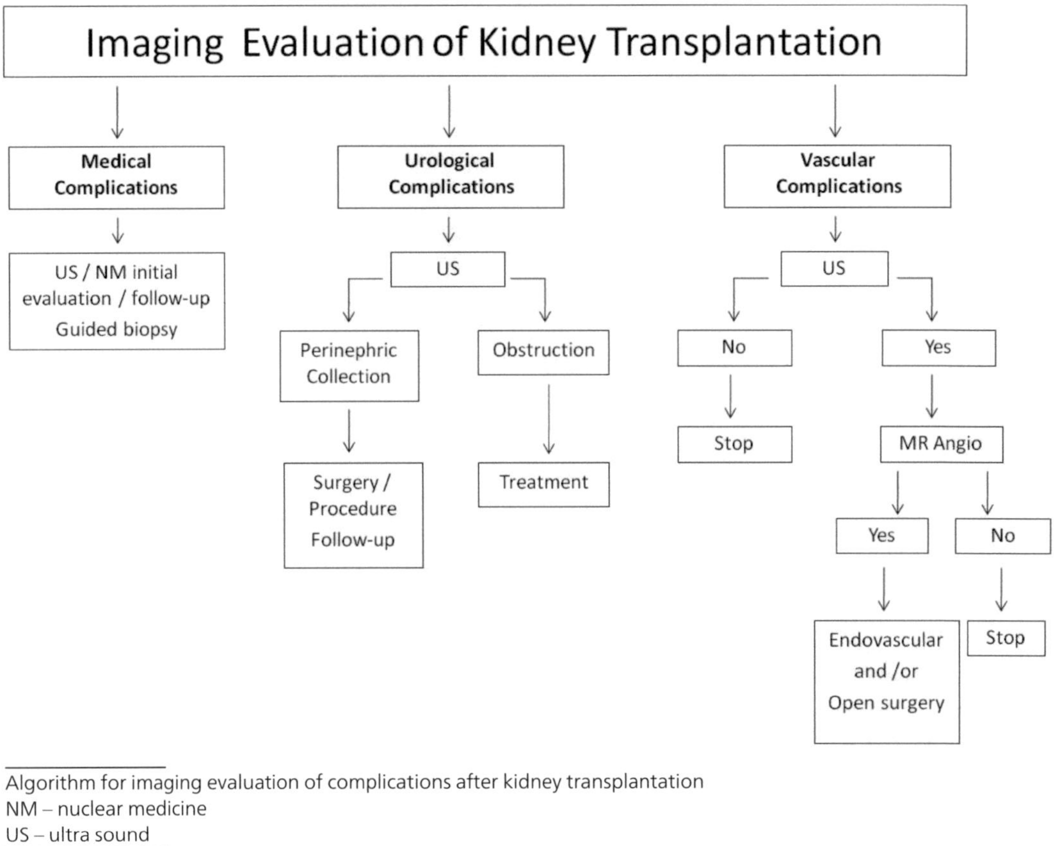

Figure 20. Algorithm for initial evaluation of kidney transplantation.

from those of tumors occurring in the general population. These neoplasias show three different presentations: de novo occurrence in the recipient, recurrence of a preexisting malignant neoplasia, or transfer of a malignant neoplasia together with the renal graft [89].

With increasing donor age, the use of marginal donors and the increased survival of renal grafts, malignant genitourinary neoplasms have become more common. Thus, post-renal transplant vigilance is important in order to obtain an early diagnosis and to institute appropriate treatment (Figure 21).

The imaging methods used for diagnostic confirmation are those cited earlier and their use varies according to the symptoms presented by the patient.

7.2. Disease recurrence

Disease recurrence in the graft has a greater prevalence in children than in adults, thereby increasing patient morbidity, graft loss and, sometimes, mortality rates. Indeed, the current overall graft loss is mainly due to primary glomerulonephritis (70–80%) and inherited metabolic diseases [7, 90-95]. It depends on the primary disease before transplantation. The

http://dx.doi.org/10.5772/55074

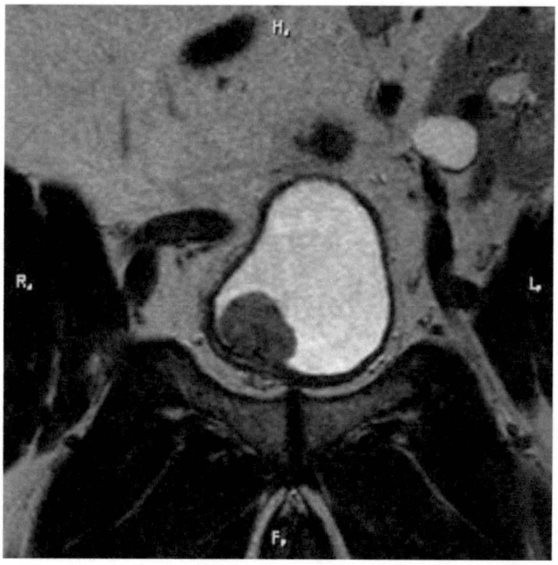

Figure 21. Vesical neoplasia in patient with renal allograft. A mass is seen in the bladder floor (arrow). Transplant kidney (TK) is in left inguinal fossa.

presentation of recurrence includes early massive proteinuria and sometimes graft failure and arterial hypertension [96]. Imaging has no specific pattern in these situations, and mainly plays a role in guiding biopsy.

7.3. End-stage disease

Nonfunctional renal grafts are often left in situ. As in chronic native renal parenchymal chronic disease the grafts are usually small, and can have fatty replacement, hydronephrosis, infarcts, hemorrhage, and calcifications [19].

7.4. Renal focal lesions

Focal lesions are seen as a less common complication after transplantation. Besides parenchymal abscess, and focal infarction, these may be secondary to recent surgery such as focal contusion or postbiopsy intrarenal hematoma. Focal lesions may be miscarried in surveillance [33].

8. Donors' evaluation

The number of people waiting for transplantation using cadaveric organs is usually very expressive, worldwide. Therefore kidney transplantation from living donors is becoming more and more frequent. Living donor kidney recipients have a significant increase in graft survival compared to deceased donor recipients. A living donor transplant has the advantage not to require a waiting list and can be performed in a preemptive manner (before the beginning of dialysis treatment). There is also evidence that patients who receive a preemptive transplant have a longer graft survival than patients who remain on dialysis before the transplant. In the past, only genetically related individuals were considered to be potential donors; however, the use of unrelated kidney donors is increasing and the recipients of these kidneys have a better graft survival than recipients of deceased kidney donors [97, 98].

The organ donor candidate must be an adult with the ability to decide, should have an affective relationship with the recipient and be free from coercion. He should be healthy from both a medical and psychic viewpoint and should be informed about the risks and benefits of donation [99].

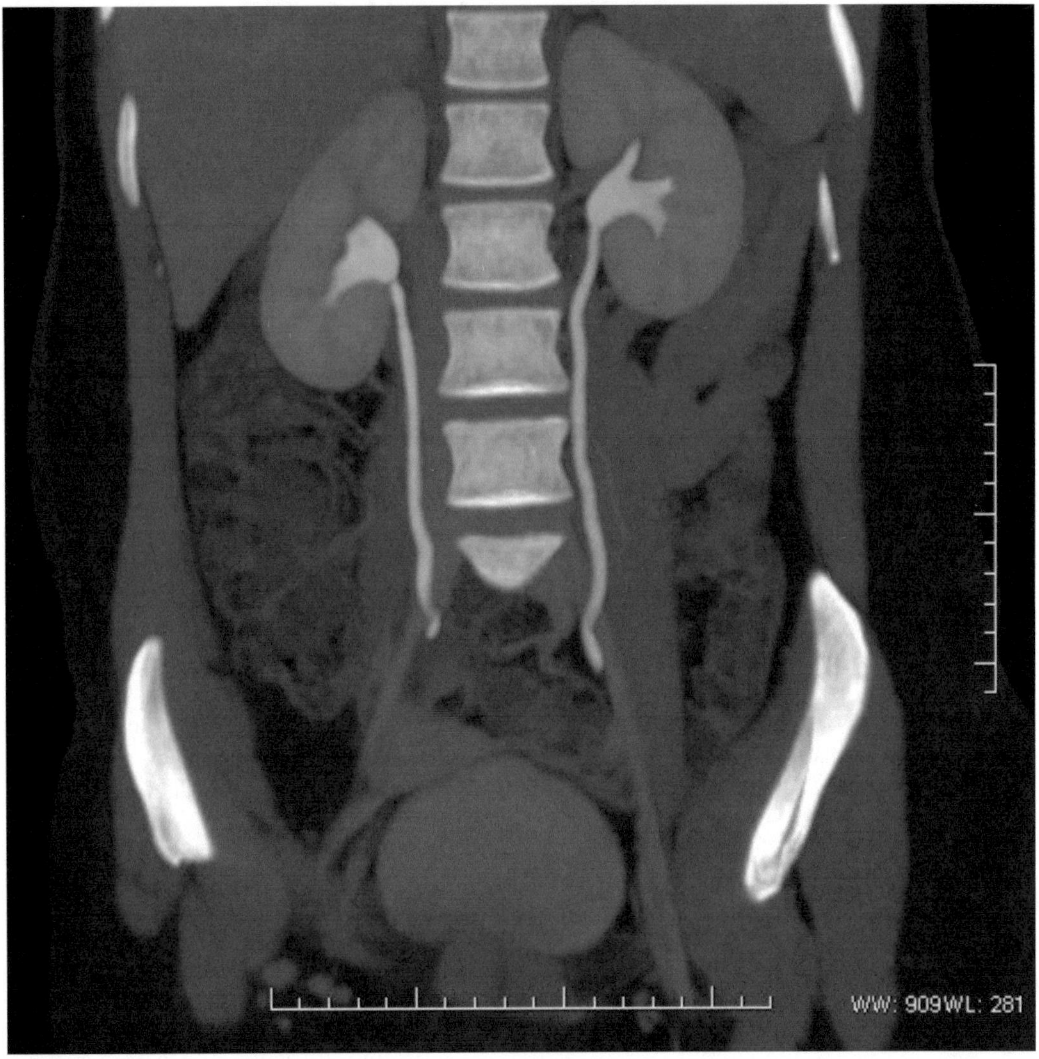

Figure 22. Split-bolus CT-Urography with MIP reconstruction allows evaluation of pelvicaliceal system and ureters fully distended, as well as renal parenchyma, in a potential kidney-donor.

http://dx.doi.org/10.5772/55074

The systematic evaluation of a living donor includes socioeconomic and psychological assessment, medical history and physical examination complemented with laboratory tests and imaging exams.

The evaluation of renal anatomy, mainly the vascular details of a living organ, is absolutely crucial, before removing it, surgically [18]. When living donors are considered, possible aortic and/or renal arterial, venous anatomical variants and/or congenital malformations are key factors to decide if a relative could be a potential donor, and moreover, which kidney will be removed, left or right. In addition, a detailed evaluation of collecting system and ureters may be obtained and may abbreviate decisions [82].

In the past, to obtain all the information required, urologist and nephrologists used to order at least 3 exams: 1- Intravenous urography (IVU) for evaluation of collecting system; 2- voiding cystourethrogram to detect a silent vesicoureteral reflux and its consequences to the kidneys and; 3- abdominal angiography to evaluate aorta and renal arteries. Nowadays, although there is a considerable variation of protocols for potential donors, all this information can be derived from only one technique, multidetector CT (MDCT). The fast scanners recently available allow timing-specific images, in other words it's possible to obtain early images, in the arterial phase, to depict arterial anatomy in detail and, later on, do another scanning during venous phase and later on, on excretory phase to depict pelvicaliceal system and ureters [15]. MDCT is reported to be as accurate as DSA for detecting supranummerary and polar arteries, as well as venous anatomical variations as circumaortic veins, double veins and so on. Some authors, in order to reduce ionizing radiation dose, suggest that the last (excretory) phase, could be replaced by a abdominal plain film, taking advantage of the contrast media in the collecting system and bladder, simulating an late film in IVU (Figure 22).

Voiding cystourethrogram (VCU) was commonly used for evaluating of living donors, however, several studies have shown that no clinically relevant information is provided for this examination in the great majority of cases. So, VCU is no longer used in most of individuals who are candidates for kidney donation [83].

Author details

Valdair Francisco Muglia[1], Sara Reis Teixeira[1], Elen Almeida Romão[2], Marcelo Ferreira Cassini[3], Murilo Ferreira de Andrade[3], Mery Kato[4], Maria Estela Papini Nardin[1] and Silvio Tucci Jr[3]

1 Department of Internal Medicine, Division of Radiology, University of Sao Paulo, Faculty of Medicine of Ribeirao Preto, Ribeirao Preto – SP, Brazil

2 Division of Nephrology, University of Sao Paulo, Faculty of Medicine of Ribeirao Preto, Ribeirao Preto – SP, Brazil

3 Division of Urology, University of Sao Paulo, Faculty of Medicine of Ribeirao Preto, Ribeirao Preto – SP, Brazil

4 Section of Nuclear Medicine, University of Sao Paulo, Faculty of Medicine of Ribeirao Preto, Ribeirao Preto – SP, Brazil

References

[1] Cecka, J. M. Kidney transplantation in the United States. Clin Transpl. (2008). , 2008, 1-18.

[2] Foss, A, Leivestad, T, Brekke, I. B, Fauchald, P, Bentdal, O, Lien, B, et al. Unrelated living donors in 141 kidney transplantations: a one-center study. Transplantation. (1998). Jul 15;, 66(1), 49-52.

[3] Collaborative Transplant Study (CTS)cited May (2010). Available from: www.ctstransplant.org/public/graphics/sample.shtml.

[4] Gluecker, T. M, Mayr, M, Schwarz, J, Bilecen, D, Voegele, T, Steiger, J, et al. Comparison of CT angiography with MR angiography in the preoperative assessment of living kidney donors. Transplantation. (2008). Nov 15;, 86(9), 1249-56.

[5] Turkvatan, A, Akinci, S, Yildiz, S, Olcer, T, & Cumhur, T. Multidetector computed tomography for preoperative evaluation of vascular anatomy in living renal donors. Surg Radiol Anat. (2009). Apr;, 31(4), 227-35.

[6] Friedewald, S. M, Molmenti, E. P, Friedewald, J. J, Dejong, M. R, & Hamper, U. M. Vascular and nonvascular complications of renal transplants: sonographic evaluation and correlation with other imaging modalities, surgery, and pathology. J Clin Ultrasound. [Review]. (2005). Mar-Apr;, 33(3), 127-39.

[7] Nankivell, B. J. Kuypers DRJ. Diagnosis and prevention of chronic kidney allograft loss. The Lancet. (2011). , 378(9800), 1428-37.

[8] Radermacher, J, Mengel, M, Ellis, S, Stuht, S, Hiss, M, Schwarz, A, et al. The renal arterial resistance index and renal allograft survival. N Engl J Med. [Research Support, Non-U.S. Gov't]. (2003). Jul 10;, 349(2), 115-24.

[9] Chow, L, Sommer, F. G, Huang, J, & Li, K. C. Power Doppler imaging and resistance index measurement in the evaluation of acute renal transplant rejection. J Clin Ultrasound. [Evaluation Studies]. (2001). Nov-Dec;, 29(9), 483-90.

[10] Rajiah, P, Lim, Y. Y, & Taylor, P. Renal transplant imaging and complications. Abdom Imaging. [Review]. (2006). Nov-Dec;, 31(6), 735-46.

[11] Sharfuddin, A. Imaging evaluation of kidney transplant recipients. Semin Nephrol. [Review]. (2011). May;, 31(3), 259-71.

[12] Haustein, J, Niendorf, H. P, Krestin, G, Louton, T, Schuhmann-giampieri, G, Clauss, W, et al. Renal tolerance of gadolinium-DTPA/dimeglumine in patients with chronic renal failure. Invest Radiol. [Clinical Trial]. (1992). Feb;, 27(2), 153-6.

[13] Liu, X, Berg, N, Sheehan, J, Bi, X, Weale, P, Jerecic, R, et al. Renal transplant: nonenhanced renal MR angiography with magnetization-prepared steady-state free precession. Radiology. (2009). May;, 251(2), 535-42.

[14] Kalb, B, Martin, D. R, Salman, K, Sharma, P, Votaw, J, & Larsen, C. Kidney transplantation: structural and functional evaluation using MR Nephro-Urography. J Magn Reson Imaging. [Review]. (2008). Oct;, 28(4), 805-22.

[15] Marckmann, P, Skov, L, Rossen, K, Dupont, A, Damholt, M. B, Heaf, J. G, et al. Nephrogenic systemic fibrosis: suspected causative role of gadodiamide used for contrast-enhanced magnetic resonance imaging. J Am Soc Nephrol. (2006). Sep;, 17(9), 2359-62.

[16] Grobner, T. Gadolinium--a specific trigger for the development of nephrogenic fibrosing dermopathy and nephrogenic systemic fibrosis? Nephrol Dial Transplant. (2006). Apr;, 21(4), 1104-8.

[17] Wang, Y, Alkasab, T. K, Narin, O, Nazarian, R. M, Kaewlai, R, Kay, J, et al. Incidence of nephrogenic systemic fibrosis after adoption of restrictive gadolinium-based contrast agent guidelines. Radiology. (2011). Jul;, 260(1), 105-11.

[18] Stacul, F, Van Der Molen, A. J, Reimer, P, Webb, J. A, Thomsen, H. S, Morcos, S. K, et al. Contrast induced nephropathy: updated ESUR Contrast Media Safety Committee guidelines. Eur Radiol. [Review]. (2011). Dec;, 21(12), 2527-41.

[19] Sebastia, C, Quiroga, S, Boye, R, Cantarell, C, Fernandez-planas, M, & Alvarez, A. Helical CT in renal transplantation: normal findings and early and late complications. Radiographics. [Review]. (2001). Sep-Oct;, 21(5), 1103-17.

[20] Chen, C. H, Shu, K. H, Cheng, C. H, Wu, M. J, Yu, T. M, Chuang, Y. W, et al. Imaging evaluation of kidney using multidetector computerized tomography in living-related renal transplantation. Transplant Proc. (2012). Jan;, 44(1), 7-10.

[21] Hagen, G, Wadstrom, J, Magnusson, M, & Magnusson, A. Outcome after percutaneous transluminal angioplasty of arterial stenosis in renal transplant patients. Acta Radiol. [Research Support, Non-U.S. Gov't]. (2009). Apr;, 50(3), 270-5.

[22] Irshad, A, Ackerman, S. J, Campbell, A. S, & Anis, M. An Overview of Renal Transplantation: Current Practice and Use of Ultrasound. Seminars in Ultrasound, CT, and MRI. (2009). , 30(4), 298-314.

[23] Kalble, T, Lucan, M, Nicita, G, & Sells, R. Burgos Revilla FJ, Wiesel M. EAU guidelines on renal transplantation. Eur Urol. [Consensus Development Conference Guideline Practice Guideline Review]. (2005). Feb;, 47(2), 156-66.

[24] Auriol, J. Urological and medical complications of renal transplant]. J Radiol. [Review]. (2011). Apr;, 92(4), 336-42.

[25] Ardelean, A, Mandry, D, & Claudon, M. Vascular complications following renal transplantation: diagnostic evaluation]. J Radiol. [Case Reports Review]. (2011). Apr;, 92(4), 343-57.

[26] Hricak, H, Terrier, F, & Demas, B. E. Renal allografts: evaluation by MR imaging. Radiology. (1986). May;, 159(2), 435-41.

[27] Yamamoto, A, Zhang, J. L, Rusinek, H, Chandarana, H, Vivier, P. H, Babb, J. S, et al. Quantitative evaluation of acute renal transplant dysfunction with low-dose three-dimensional MR renography. Radiology. [Clinical Trial In Vitro Research Support, Non-U.S. Gov't]. (2011). Sep;, 260(3), 781-9.

[28] Kalb, B, Votaw, J. R, Salman, K, Sharma, P, & Martin, D. R. Magnetic resonance nephrourography: current and developing techniques. Radiol Clin North Am. [Research Support, Non-U.S. Gov't Review]. (2008). Jan;v., 46(1), 11-24.

[29] Isoniemi, H. M, Krogerus, L, Von Willebrand, E, Taskinen, E, Ahonen, J, & Hayry, P. Histopathological findings in well-functioning, long-term renal allografts. Kidney Int. [Clinical Trial Randomized Controlled Trial Research Support, Non-U.S. Gov't]. (1992). Jan;, 41(1), 155-60.

[30] Shoskes, D. A, & Halloran, P. F. Delayed graft function in renal transplantation: etiology, management and long-term significance. J Urol. [Research Support, Non-U.S. Gov't Review]. (1996). Jun;, 155(6), 1831-40.

[31] Park, S. B, Kim, J. K, & Cho, K. S. Complications of renal transplantation: ultrasonographic evaluation. J Ultrasound Med. [Review]. (2007). May;, 26(5), 615-33.

[32] Neill, O, & Baumgarten, W C. DA. Ultrasonography in renal transplantation. Am J Kidney Dis. [Review]. (2002). Apr;, 39(4), 663-78.

[33] Irshad, A, Ackerman, S, Sosnouski, D, Anis, M, Chavin, K, & Baliga, P. A review of sonographic evaluation of renal transplant complications. Curr Probl Diagn Radiol. [Review]. (2008). Mar-Apr;, 37(2), 67-79.

[34] Swobodnik, W. L, Spohn, B. E, Wechsler, J. G, Schusdziarra, V, Blum, S, Franz, H. E, et al. Real-time ultrasound evaluation of renal transplant failure during the early post-operative period. Ultrasound Med Biol. [Comparative Study]. (1986). Feb;, 12(2), 97-105.

[35] Griffin, J. F, Short, C. D, Lawler, W, Mallick, N. P, & Johnson, R. W. Diagnosis of disease in renal allografts: correlation between ultrasound and histology. Clin Radiol. [Comparative Study]. (1986). Jan;, 37(1), 59-62.

[36] Grant, E. G, & Perrella, R. R. Wishing won't make it so: duplex Doppler sonography in the evaluation of renal transplant dysfunction. AJR Am J Roentgenol. [Comment]. (1990). Sep;, 155(3), 538-9.

[37] Perrella, R. R, Duerinckx, A. J, Tessler, F. N, Danovitch, G. M, Wilkinson, A, Gonzalez, S, et al. Evaluation of renal transplant dysfunction by duplex Doppler sonography: a prospective study and review of the literature. Am J Kidney Dis. [Review]. (1990). Jun;, 15(6), 544-50.

[38] Schwenger, V, Hinkel, U. P, Nahm, A. M, Morath, C, & Zeier, M. Color doppler ultrasonography in the diagnostic evaluation of renal allografts. Nephron Clin Pract. [Review]. (2006). c, 107-12.

[39] Zimmerman, P R. N, & Schiepers, C. Diagnostic imaging in kidney transplantation. In: GM D, editor. Handbook of kidney transplantation. 4th ed: Philadelphia: Lippincott Williams & Wilkins; (2005). , 347-368.

[40] Jimenez, C, Lopez, M. O, Gonzalez, E, & Selgas, R. Ultrasonography in kidney transplantation: values and new developments. Transplant Rev (Orlando). [Review]. (2009). Oct;, 23(4), 209-13.

[41] Neimatallah, M. A, Dong, Q, Schoenberg, S. O, Cho, K. J, & Prince, M. R. Magnetic resonance imaging in renal transplantation. J Magn Reson Imaging. [Research Support, Non-U.S. Gov't]. (1999). Sep;, 10(3), 357-68.

[42] Huang, A. J, Lee, V. S, & Rusinek, H. Functional renal MR imaging. Magn Reson Imaging Clin N Am. [Review]. (2004). Aug;vi., 12(3), 469-86.

[43] Fang, Y. C, & Siegelman, E. S. Complications of renal transplantation: MR findings. J Comput Assist Tomogr. [Review]. (2001). Nov-Dec;, 25(6), 836-42.

[44] Dubovsky, E. V, Russell, C. D, Bischof-delaloye, A, Bubeck, B, Chaiwatanarat, T, Hilson, A. J, et al. Report of the Radionuclides in Nephrourology Committee for evaluation of transplanted kidney (review of techniques). Semin Nucl Med. [Review]. (1999). Apr;, 29(2), 175-88.

[45] Dubovsky, E. V, Russell, C. D, & Erbas, B. Radionuclide evaluation of renal transplants. Semin Nucl Med. [Review]. (1995). Jan;, 25(1), 49-59.

[46] Nankivell, B. J, & Alexander, S. I. Rejection of the kidney allograft. N Engl J Med. Oct 7;, 363(15), 1451-62.

[47] Elsayes, K. M, Menias, C. O, Willatt, J, Azar, S, Harvin, H. J, & Platt, J. F. Imaging of renal transplant: utility and spectrum of diagnostic findings. Curr Probl Diagn Radiol. [Review]. (2011). May-Jun;, 40(3), 127-39.

[48] Dupont, P. J, Dooldeniya, M, Cook, T, & Warrens, A. N. Role of duplex Doppler sonography in diagnosis of acute allograft dysfunction-time to stop measuring the resistive index? Transpl Int. [Comparative Study]. (2003). Sep;, 16(9), 648-52.

[49] Baxter, G. M. Ultrasound of renal transplantation. Clin Radiol. [Review]. (2001). Oct;, 56(10), 802-18.

[50] Brown, E. D, Chen, M. Y, Wolfman, N. T, Ott, D. J, & Watson, N. E. Jr. Complications of renal transplantation: evaluation with US and radionuclide imaging. Radiographics. [Review]. (2000). May-Jun;, 20(3), 607-22.

[51] Benigni, A, Bruzzi, I, Mister, M, Azzollini, N, Gaspari, F, Perico, N, et al. Nature and mediators of renal lesions in kidney transplant patients given cyclosporine for more than one year. Kidney Int. (1999). Feb;, 55(2), 674-85.

[52] Scott, L. J, Mckeage, K, Keam, S. J, & Plosker, G. L. Tacrolimus: a further update of its use in the management of organ transplantation. Drugs. (2003). , 63(12), 1247-97.

[53] Seron, D, & Moreso, F. Preservation of renal function during maintenance therapy with cyclosporine. Transplant Proc. (2004). Mar;36(2 Suppl):257S-60S.

[54] Kanazi, G, Stowe, N, Steinmuller, D, Hwieh, H. H, & Novick, A. C. Effect of cyclosporine upon the function of ischemically damaged kidneys in the rat. Transplantation. (1986). Jun;, 41(6), 782-4.

[55] Ali, M. G, Coakley, F. V, Hricak, H, & Bretan, P. N. Complex posttransplantation abnormalities of renal allografts: evaluation with MR imaging. Radiology. (1999). Apr;, 211(1), 95-100.

[56] Browne, R. F, & Tuite, D. J. Imaging of the renal transplant: comparison of MRI with duplex sonography. Abdom Imaging. (2006). Jul-Aug;, 31(4), 461-82.

[57] Baxter, G. M. Imaging in renal transplantation. Ultrasound Q. [Review]. (2003). Sep;, 19(3), 123-38.

[58] Akbar, S. A, Jafri, S. Z, Amendola, M. A, Madrazo, B. L, Salem, R, & Bis, K. G. Complications of renal transplantation. Radiographics. [Review]. (2005). Sep-Oct;, 25(5), 1335-56.

[59] Kocak, T, Nane, I, Ander, H, Ziylan, O, Oktar, T, & Ozsoy, C. Urological and surgical complications in 362 consecutive living related donor kidney transplantations. Urol Int. (2004). , 72(3), 252-6.

[60] Azhar, R. A, Hassanain, M, Aljiffry, M, Aldousari, S, Cabrera, T, Andonian, S, et al. Successful salvage of kidney allografts threatened by ureteral stricture using pyelovesical bypass. Am J Transplant. Jun;, 10(6), 1414-9.

[61] Mukha, R. P, Devasia, A, & Thomas, E. M. Ureteral herniation with intermittent obstructive uropathy in a renal allograft recipient. Urol J. [Case Reports]. (2011). Spring; 8(2):98.

[62] Pozniak, M. A, & Dodd, G. D. rd, Kelcz F. Ultrasonographic evaluation of renal transplantation. Radiol Clin North Am. [Review]. (1992). Sep;, 30(5), 1053-66.

[63] Tublin, M. E, & Dodd, G. D. rd. Sonography of renal transplantation. Radiol Clin North Am. [Review]. (1995). May;, 33(3), 447-59.

[64] Tublin, M. E, Bude, R. O, & Platt, J. F. Review. The resistive index in renal Doppler sonography: where do we stand? AJR Am J Roentgenol. [Review]. (2003). Apr;, 180(4), 885-92.

[65] Tripathi, M, Chandrashekar, N, Phom, H, Gupta, D. K, Bajpai, M, Bal, C, et al. Evaluation of dilated upper renal tracts by technetium-99m ethylenedicysteine F+O diuresis renography in infants and children. Ann Nucl Med. [Clinical Trial Controlled Clinical Trial]. (2004). Dec;, 18(8), 681-7.

[66] Sperling, H, Becker, G, Heemann, U, Lummen, G, Philipp, T, & Rubben, H. The Whitaker test, a useful tool in renal grafts? Urology. (2000). Jul;, 56(1), 49-52.

[67] Winsett, M. Z, Amparo, E. G, Fawcett, H. D, Kumar, R, & Johnson, R. F. Jr., Bedi DG, et al. Renal transplant dysfunction: MR evaluation. AJR Am J Roentgenol. [Research Support, Non-U.S. Gov't]. (1988). Feb;, 150(2), 319-23.

[68] Stravodimos, K. G, Adamis, S, Tyritzis, S, Georgios, Z, & Constantinides, C. A. Renal transplant lithiasis: analysis of our series and review of the literature. J Endourol. [Review]. (2012). Jan;, 26(1), 38-44.

[69] Cranston, D. Urological complications after renal transplantation. J R Soc Med. (1996). Suppl 29:22.

[70] Silver, T. M, Campbell, D, Wicks, J. D, Lorber, M. I, Surace, P, & Turcotte, J. Peritransplant fluid collections. Ultrasound evaluation and clinical significance. Radiology. (1981). Jan;, 138(1), 145-51.

[71] Yap, R, Madrazo, B, Oh, H. K, & Dienst, S. G. Perirenal fluid collection after renal transplant. Am Surg. (1981). Jul;, 47(7), 287-90.

[72] Khauli, R. B, Stoff, J. S, Lovewell, T, Ghavamian, R, & Baker, S. Post-transplant lymphoceles: a critical look into the risk factors, pathophysiology and management. J Urol. (1993). Jul;, 150(1), 22-6.

[73] Kumar, R. Bharathi Dasan J, Choudhury S, Guleria S, Padhy AK, Malhotra A. Scintigraphic patterns of lymphocele in post-renal transplant. Nucl Med Commun. (2003). May;, 24(5), 531-5.

[74] Campos Freire J, de Goes GM, de Campos Freire JG. Extravesical ureteral implantation in kidney transplantation. Urology. (1974). Mar;, 3(3), 304-8.

[75] Browne, R. F, & Tuite, D. J. Imaging of the renal transplant: comparison of MRI with duplex sonography. Abdom Imaging. [Comparative Study Review]. (2006). Jul-Aug;, 31(4), 461-82.

[76] Lucewicz, A, Isaacs, A, Allen, R. D, Lam, V. W, Angelides, S, & Pleass, H. C. Torsion of intraperitoneal kidney transplant. ANZ J Surg. (2011). May 10.

[77] Wong-you-cheong, J. J, Grumbach, K, Krebs, T. L, Pace, M. E, Daly, B, Chow, C. C, et al. Torsion of intraperitoneal renal transplants: imaging appearances. AJR Am J Roentgenol. (1998). Nov;, 171(5), 1355-9.

[78] Millwala, F. N, Abraham, G, Shroff, S, Soundarajan, P, Rao, R, & Kuruvilla, S. Spontaneous renal allograft rupture in a cohort of renal transplant recipients: a tertiary care experience. Transplant Proc. [Case Reports]. (2000). Nov;, 32(7), 1912-3.

[79] Beek, F. J, Bax, N. M, Donckerwolcke, R, & Van Leeuwen, M. S. Sonographic findings in spontaneous renal transplant rupture. Pediatr Radiol. [Case Reports]. (1992). , 22(4), 313-4.

[80] Rahatzad, M, Henderson, S. C, & Boren, G. S. Ultrasound appearance of spontaneous rupture of renal transplant. J Urol. [Case Reports]. (1981). Oct;, 126(4), 535-6.

[81] Hohnke, C, Abendroth, D, Schleibner, S, & Land, W. Vascular complications in 1,200 kidney transplantations. Transplant Proc. [Review]. (1987). Oct;, 19(5), 3691-2.

[82] Lebkowska, U, Malyszko, J, Lebkowski, W, Brzosko, S, Kowalewski, R, Lebkowski, T, et al. The predictive value of arterial renal blood flow parameters in renal graft survival. Transplant Proc. (2007). Nov;, 39(9), 2727-9.

[83] Gao, J, Ng, A, Shih, G, Goldstein, M, Kapur, S, Wang, J, et al. Intrarenal color duplex ultrasonography: a window to vascular complications of renal transplants. J Ultrasound Med. (2007). Oct;, 26(10), 1403-18.

[84] Cosgrove, D. O, & Chan, K. E. Renal transplants: what ultrasound can and cannot do. Ultrasound Q. [Review]. (2008). Jun;quiz 141-2., 24(2), 77-87.

[85] Taylor, K. J, Morse, S. S, Rigsby, C. M, Bia, M, & Schiff, M. Vascular complications in renal allografts: detection with duplex Doppler US. Radiology. [Case Reports]. (1987). Jan;162(1 Pt 1):31-8.

[86] Snider, J. F, Hunter, D. W, Moradian, G. P, Castaneda-zuniga, W. R, & Letourneau, J. G. Transplant renal artery stenosis: evaluation with duplex sonography. Radiology. (1989). Sep;172(3 Pt 2):1027-30.

[87] Grenier, N, Claudon, M, Trillaud, H, Douws, C, & Levantal, O. Noninvasive radiology of vascular complications in renal transplantation. Eur Radiol. (1997). , 7(3), 385-91.

[88] Stewart, J. H, Vajdic, C. M, Van Leeuwen, M. T, Amin, J, Webster, A. C, Chapman, J. R, et al. The pattern of excess cancer in dialysis and transplantation. Nephrol Dial Transplant. (2009). Oct;, 24(10), 3225-31.

[89] Melchior, S, Franzaring, L, Shardan, A, Schwenke, C, Plumpe, A, Schnell, R, et al. Urological de novo malignancy after kidney transplantation: a case for the urologist. J Urol. Feb;, 185(2), 428-32.

[90] Cochat, P, Fargue, S, Mestrallet, G, Jungraithmayr, T, Koch-nogueira, P, Ranchin, B, et al. Disease recurrence in paediatric renal transplantation. Pediatr Nephrol. [Review]. (2009). Nov;, 24(11), 2097-108.

[91] Moroni, G, Tantardini, F, Gallelli, B, Quaglini, S, Banfi, G, Poli, F, et al. The long-term prognosis of renal transplantation in patients with lupus nephritis. Am J Kidney Dis. [Comparative Study Research Support, Non-U.S. Gov't]. (2005). May;, 45(5), 903-11.

[92] Ozdemir, B. H, Ozdemir, F. N, Demirhan, B, Turan, M, & Haberal, M. Renal transplantation in amyloidosis: effects of HLA matching and donor type on recurrence of primary disease. Transpl Int. (2004). Jun;, 17(5), 241-6.

[93] Seikaly, M. G. Recurrence of primary disease in children after renal transplantation: an evidence-based update. Pediatr Transplant. [Review]. (2004). Apr;, 8(2), 113-9.

[94] Ivanyi, B. A primer on recurrent and de novo glomerulonephritis in renal allografts. Nat Clin Pract Nephrol. [Review]. (2008). Aug;, 4(8), 446-57.

[95] Briganti, E. M, Russ, G. R, Mcneil, J. J, Atkins, R. C, & Chadban, S. J. Risk of renal allograft loss from recurrent glomerulonephritis. N Engl J Med. [Comparative Study]. (2002). Jul 11;, 347(2), 103-9.

[96] Newstead, C. G. Recurrent disease in renal transplants. Nephrol Dial Transplant. [Review]. (2003). Aug;18 Suppl 6:vi, 68-74.

[97] Spital, A. Increasing the pool of transplantable kidneys through unrelated living donors and living donor paired exchanges. Semin Dial. (2005). Nov-Dec;, 18(6), 469-73.

[98] Meier-kriesche, H. U, Port, F. K, Ojo, A. O, Rudich, S. M, Hanson, J. A, Cibrik, D. M, et al. Effect of waiting time on renal transplant outcome. Kidney Int. (2000). Sep;, 58(3), 1311-7.

[99] Israni, A. K, Halpern, S. D, Zink, S, Sidhwani, S. A, & Caplan, A. Incentive models to increase living kidney donation: encouraging without coercing. Am J Transplant. (2005). Jan;, 5(1), 15-20.

Chapter 3

Utility of Urinary Biomarkers in Kidney Transplant Function Assessment

Alina Kępka, Napoleon Waszkiewicz,
Sylwia Chojnowska, Beata Zalewska-Szajda,
Jerzy Robert Ładny, Anna Wasilewska,
Krzysztof Zwierz and Sławomir Dariusz Szajda

Additional information is available at the end of the chapter

http://dx.doi.org/10.5772/54746

1. Introduction

Kidney may undertake normal function immediately after transplantation or even several or over a dozen days delay. Absence of normal renal transplant function may lead to acute kidney injury (AKI), nephrotic syndrome (NS) and chronic kidney disease (CKD). **Acute kidney injury (AKI)** is characterized functionally by a rapid decline in the glomerular filtration rate (GFR), and biochemically by the resultant accumulation of nitrogenous wastes such as blood-urea nitrogen and creatinine (Devarajan, 2010). **Nephrotic syndrome (NS)** is a nonspecific disorder in which the kidneys damage is accompanied by a leak of large amounts of protein (proteinuria at least 3.5 grams per day per $1.73m^2$ body surface area) from the blood into the urine. Nephrotic syndrome is a disorder of the glomerular filtration barrier. The multiprotein complex between adjacent podocyte foot processes the slit diaphragm, is essential to the control of the actin cytoskeleton and cell morphology. Signaling from slit diaphragm proteins to the actin cytoskeleton is mediated via the Rho GTP-ases. These are thought to be involved in the control of podocyte motility, which has been postulated as a focus of proteinuric pathways (Hull & Goldsmith, 2008). It is common belief that nephrotic syndrome after transplantation results mainly from recurrence of renal disease in transplanted kidney and not defective graft function. **Chronic kidney disease (CKD)** – it is kidney damage for ≥3 months, defined by structural or functional abnormalities of the kidney, with or without decreased GFR, manifested by either pathological abnormalities or markers of kidney damage, including abnormalities of blood or urine or abnormalities in imaging tests (Ahmad et al., 2006).

2. Markers of nephrons damage

After kidney transplantation it is particularly important to monitor the biomarkers which allow to detect progress in disease process and determine which functional parts of kidney are going to be damaged, to enable application of a quick appropriate treatment (Lisowska-Myjak, 2010; Alachkar et al., 2010; Metzger et al., 2010). Administration of immunosuppressants for preventing renal graft rejection may lead to progressive damage to the renal tissue (interstitial fibrosis, tubular micro calcifications, atrophy of renal tubules) caused by high toxicity of suppressing drugs. Cyclosporine A(CsA), tacrolimus, mycophenolate mofetil, basiliximab, prednizon and sirolimus (rapamycin) are commonly used in immunosuppressive therapy following kidney transplantation. Cyclosporine A and tacrolimus generate immunosuppressive action by binding to cyclofiline and inhibiting the action of calcineurin 2, which stimulates proliferation and differentiation of lymphocytes T. Cyclosporine A inhibits synthesis of lymphokines by lymphocytes T. Lymphokines synthesized by lymphocytes T stimulate immunological system and have the ability to „kill" inflammatory and neoplastic cells. Mycophenolate mofetil selectively inhibits inosine monophosphate dehydrogenase, a basic enzyme in guanosine synthesis. Mycophenolate mofetil inhibits proliferation of lymphocytes T and B after stimulation with antigenes, cytokines and mitogens. Basiliximab similarly to Daclizumab, blocks receptors for IL-2.

Majority of renal pathological changes concern glomerules, proximal and distal tubules as well as vascular endothelium. At first renal proximal tubular cells (Fig.1.) demonstrating highest metabolic activity, possessing high amounts of mitochondries, lysosomes and peroxysomes are damaged. Remaining sections of nephron such as: Henle's loop, distal tubules and collecting tubules are usually damaged later. There are numerous biomarkers that identify injury the area of the renal nephron, such as the glomerulus, the proximal, and the distal tubule.

2.1. Biomarkers of renal glomeruli

The oldest biomarkers of renal glomeruli injure are serum urea and creatinine as well as clearance of endogenic creatinine, which similarly to inulin (gold standard in GFR determination) is excreted to urine and not absorbed in renal tubules. Clearance of endogenic creatinine is 10-20% higher than clearance of inuline, which is a result trace excretion of creatinine by renal tubules (Finney et al., 2000).

Cystatin C (CYC) is a cysteine protease inhibitor that is stably secreted from all nucleated cells, freely filtered through the glomerulus, and completely reabsorbed by the proximal tubules. During efficient function of proximal renal tubules there are traces of urinary CYC, independent of age and body mass. Given that cystatin C is not normally found in urine in significant amounts, the elevated level of urinary cystatin C may display dysfunction of tubular cells and tubulointerstitial disease. Concentration of CYC in normal urine accounts 0.03-0.3 mg/L (Filler et al., 2005). Increase in serum CYC is proportional to decrease in GFR (Campo et al., 2004). It was reported that serum CYC correlated better with GFR than creatinine (Filler et al., 2005; Schuck et al., 2004). After renal transplantation CYC concentration increased simultaneously to AKI development, because of decreased reabsorption from damaged tubules. Therefore

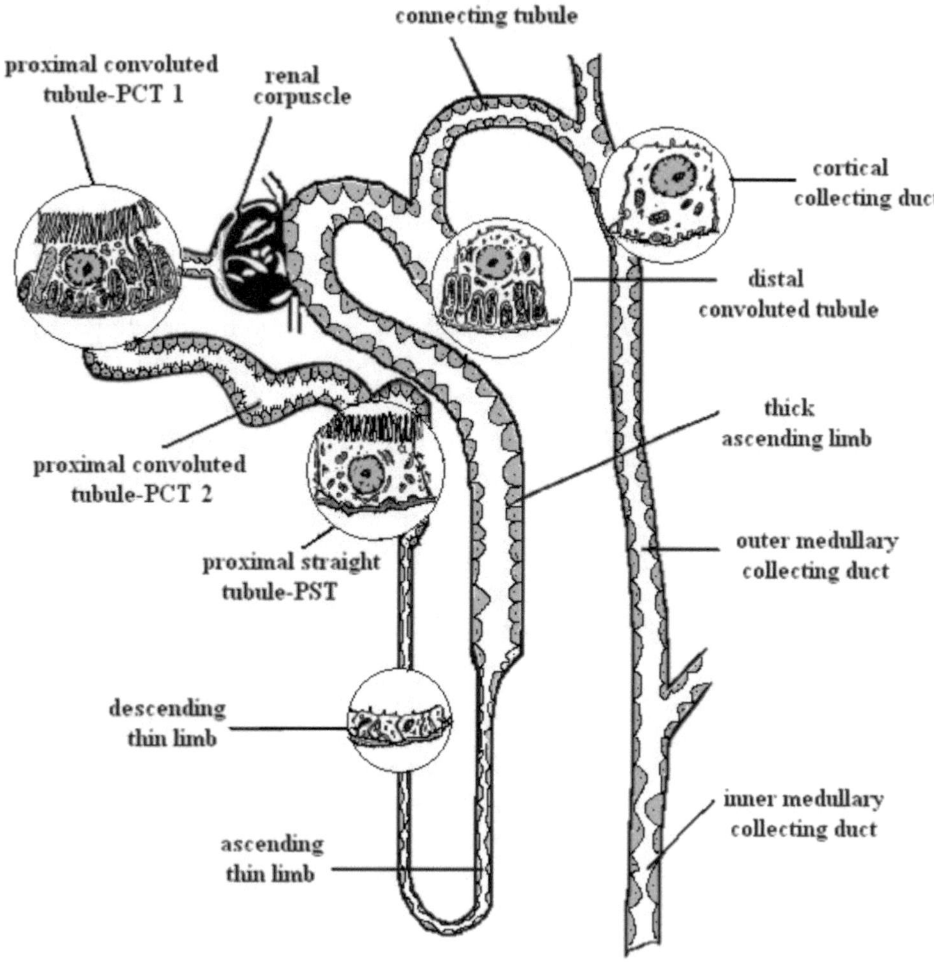

Figure 1. Nephron structure

urinary concentration of CYC may be treated as a good marker of the proximal tubules and effective biomarker of delayed renal graft function due to lack of diurnal changes, and high stability in routine conditions of urinary storage, urinary CYC may be determined in single urinary samples. Urinary CYC / creatinine ratio is a good indicator of renal tubules dysfunction as in disorders of renal tubules, urinary CYC concentration may increase even 200 fold (Uchida & Gotoh, 2002; Lisowska-Myjak, 2010). Two fully automated and quick immunological methods for CYC determination: turbidimetric PETIA (particle enhanced immunoturbidimetric assay) and nephelometric – PENIA (particle enhanced nephelometric immunoassay) were developed in 1994-1997. Presently measurements of urinary CYC are utilized mainly with a

PENIA method designed primary for CYC determination in serum (Herget-Rosenthal et al., 2004). PENIA method (particle enhanced nephelometric immunoassay)allows for a CYC detection at a concentration of 0.05-10.47 mg/L.

Proteinuria reflects increased filtration plasma proteins to tubular fluid and disturbed protein reabsorption by renal proximal tubular cells (Haraldsson & Sörensson, 2004; Halbesma et al., 2006; Giorgio et al., 2004). Proteinuria over 0.5g/24 hours is a marker the severity of the tubular damage, independent risk factor of progressive tubular-interstitial fibrosis and strong predictor of the end-stage renal insufficiency. Evident proteinuria is symptomatic for established renal damage significantly connected with decreased GFR (Abbate et al., 2006; Eddy, 2004; Tryggvason & Pettersson, 2003; Zoja et al., 2003; Ofstad & Iversen, 2005). Even minimal proteinuria lasting one year after renal transplantation is an indicator of a poor renal graft function and may be a risk factor for renal graft failure (Kang et al., 2009). Urinary protein is a non-invasive and easy to perform parameter. It was reported that proteinuria (<0.5 g/24 h) occurred in half of patients within 3 month after renal transplantation (Sancho Calabuig et al., 2009). Higher than standard doses of everolimus (EVL) resulted in an increase of proteinuria. Therefore the standard doses of EVL are recommended which seems to be suitable for protecting against an acute graft rejection with better prognosis of renal function in longer perspective (Loriga et al., 2010). As chronic allograft nephropathy (CAN) is the most frequent reason for late loss of graft, immunosuppression with mycophenolate mofetil significantly improves graft function and in such circumstances evaluation of proteinuria seems to have prognostic value (Grebe et al., 2004).

Albuminuria as a marker of glomerular filtration is more sensitive than proteinuria. Urinary albumin border value of 200 μg/min differentiates patients with albuminuria and proteinuria. Increase in urinary albumin excretion above 200 μg/min (macroalbuminuria) indicates damage to glomerular filtration membrane, a start of evident proteinuria, progression of kidney disease and cardiovascular changes (Ruggenenti & Remuzzi,2006). After exceeding maximal reabsorption capacity of proximal tubular cells, protein of primary urine appeared in final urine (Luke, 1999; Remuzzi et al., 2006; Zoja et al., 2003). Excessive accumulation, in proximal tubular cells, plasma proteins excreted to primary urine, induced increase in local expression of cytokines and chemokines, which presence in final urine is a specific indicator of development and extent of renal damage (Lisowska-Myjak, 2010; Alachkar et al., 2010). Renal tubular cells exposed to increased amounts of filtered plasma proteins resulting cell injury. Microalbuminuria predicts a loss of renal graft. Determination of urinary albumin and UACR-urine albumin-to-creatinine ratios (UACR) are particularly recommended indicators for detection of changes in transplanted kidney (Erman et al., 2011). Microalbuminuria is considered to be a better indicator of kidney transplant condition than proteinuria (Bandukwala et al., 2009). Albuminuria, the marker of renal glomeruli damage and chronic damage of transplanted kidney, which may also reflect interstitial inflammatory process, is considered a predictor of long-term allograft outcomes in a kidney graft recipient (Nauta et al., 2011).

http://dx.doi.org/10.5772/54746

2.2. Adhesion molecules connected podocytes with basement membrane

Integrin $\alpha 3$ and integrin $\beta 3$ are particularly recommended biomarkers for monitoring the function of transplanted kidney both at early and remote period after transplantation. The integrin family of cell adhesion proteins promotes the attachment and migration of cells on the surrounding extra cellular matrix (ECM). The signals initiated by integrin binding to ECM proteins are necessary to maintain cell survival, adhesion, migration and invasion. Integrins are transmembrane glycoproteins consisting of two units: α and β. Beta1 family of integrins represents the major class of cell substrate receptors with specificities primarily for collagens, laminins, and fibronectins (Srivastava et al., 2011).

Vascular cell adhesion molecule-1 (VCAM-1), sVCAM-1 (CD106) (soluble vascular cell adhesion molecule 1) and anti-intercellular adhesion molecule-1 (ICAM-1) The ICAM and VCAM – members of the immunoglobulin (Ig) superfamily, are the chief endothelial cell proteins that are recognized by the white cell integrins. Elevated urinary sVCAM-1, IL6, sIL6R and TNFR1 concentrations indicate an acute kidney transplant rejection in the first 2 weeks after transplantation (Reinhold et al., 2012). It was reported that increased urinary concentrations of sICAM-1, determined by ELISA, occured in patients with acute renal graft rejection (Teppo et al., 2001), and in people with proteinuria, high concentrations of sVCAM and sICAM were observed (van Ree et al., 2008). Recently a non-invasive monitoring of the acute renal graft rejection by determination of cell adhesion molecules has been recommended (Gwinner, 2007).

3. Biomarkers of proximal tubules

α_1-microglobulin (α_1M) is a 27 kDa glycoprotein related to retinol binding protein synthesized by liver cells, engaged in immunoregulation (binds lymphocytes T and B) and heme catabolism. Determination of α_1M (stable in acid urine) is a sensitive indicator of renal proximal tubules damage (Guder, 2008; Lisowska-Myjak, 2010; Câmara et al., 2009). (Teppo et al., 2004) reported that six month after transplantation, 32% of patients presented microalbuminuria. Evaluation of a damage to renal proximal tubules, on the basis of an increase in urinary α_1M concentration may be a consequence to a deterioration of glomerular filtration. Increase in α_1M /creatinine ratio is an early and sensitive indicator of a poor function of the transplanted kidney, and indicates a poor prognosis of long term survival of renal transplanted patients (Teppo et al., 2004).

Retinol binding protein (RBP), protein of the lipocalin family, synthesized mainly in a liver, supplies retinol to peripheral tissues. RBP removed from plasma by glomerular filtration is subsequently absorbed and catabolized in renal proximal tubules. Increased urinary RBP is caused by a disorder in glomerular filtration and reabsorption in renal proximal tubules (Guder, 2008; Kuźniar et al., 2006; Uchida & Gotoh, 2002; Câmara et al., 2009). It seems that urinary RBP is a better biomarker of proximal tubules damage than β_2M, as RBP has greater stability in acid urine than β_2M and renal insufficiency is only a clinical situation where an increase in urinary RBP concentration is observed.

Adenosine deaminase binding protein (ABP) is a glycoprotein (120-kDa) present in lungs, liver, placenta and brush border of renal proximal tubules. Increased expression in the urinary ABP is considered an early indicator of acute renal injury (AKI). Increase in urinary ABP was reported in patients with ischemia - without sepsis, after kidney transplantation, after toxic renal tubules damage, and in newborn with sepsis. Recently published opinion suggested that ABP to be the best marker of acute renal damage, better than β2-M or α1-M (Bagshaw, 2007). As ABP excretion was higher among kidney transplants recipients than in people with normal renal function, ABP is considered as a good indicator for detection of renal graft failure (Iglesias & Richard, 1994).

β_2-microglobulin (β_2M) is a membrane protein of major histocompatibility complex HLA. β_2M excretion is used for evaluation of nephrotoxic renal damage (aminoglycoside antibiotics, heavy metal salts) (Guder, 2008). It should be noted that determination β_2M for evaluation function of transplanted kidney may be ambiguous because of coexistence of many factors influencing its plasma and urinary concentration (e.g. toxic drugs action, ischemia reperfusion complications or renal graft rejection). Measurement of urinary β_2M may be helpful in evaluation of the condition of transplanted kidney, however the interpretation of result should be careful because of the plurality of factors influencing β_2M plasma concentration, renal filtration ability and tubular function (Kuźniar et al., 2006).

4. Markers of inflammatory reaction connected with acute renal failure

Neutrophil gelatinase-associated lipocalin (NGAL) is a glycoprotein expressed and secreted by immune cells, trachea, stomach, colon, and injured kidney epithelial cells as an monomer (22 kDa), dimer or trimer. NGAL may complex with collagenase type IV of human neutrophils named gelatinase B or metalloproteinase 9 (MMP-9) creating heterodimer (125 kDa) (Flower, 1996). NGAL binds and transports small lipophilic molecules e.g. free fatty acids, retinoids, arachidonic acid, and steroids (Mishra et al., 2003). NGAL is considered as provider iron to proximal renal tubules. Iron stimulates oxygenase synthesis which protects renal tubules cells. NGAL may be applied as a predictor of ischemic or toxic renal damage, before development of a full symptomatic renal insufficiency. Increase in urinary NGAL concentration is early, sensitive and non-invasive marker of renal damage correlating with intensity and time of ischemia and preceding increase in other markers such as hexosaminidase or β2-microglobulin. A strict correlation between NGAL concentration and degree of proteinuria was demonstrated (Flower, 1996). NGAL activated formation of nephrons in early step of renal development demonstrates a protective action in kidney (Mori & Nakao, 2007). Low molecular weight, resistant to degradation NGAL is easily excreted by cells of thick ascending arm of Henry loops and collective tubules into urine both free and in complex with MMP-9. Increase in urinary excretion of NGAL is observed several hours after stimuli of nephrotoxic factor. As concentration of urinary NGAL correlates with plasma NGAL concentration, NGAL may be an useful marker in diagnostics of renal diseases (Nickolas et al., 2008). There is an opinion that NGAL is the most promising biomarker for diagnosis of acute renal injury (AKI) in acute renal graft dysfunction (Halawa, 2011; Ting et al., 2012; Hollmen, 2011).

http://dx.doi.org/10.5772/54746

Kidney injury molecule-1 (KIM-1) is a transmembrane glycoprotein receptor (104 kDa) appearing as KIM-1a and KIM 1b. KIM-1 is produced in large quantities in renal proximal tubules after a toxic or ischemic damage. It is assumed that direct cause of KIM-1 induction is an increase of the protein concentration in glomerular ultrafiltration and presence of urinary protein casts favoring tubular obstruction, mechanical stress and an increase in glomerular pressure. An increase in urinary KIM-1 excretion is specific to the ischemic renal damage and is practically independent of chronic renal insufficiency or renal tract infection (Nickolas et al., 2008; Melnikov & Molitoris, 2008). It was reported that KIM-1 extracellular domain (fragment 90 kDa) reaches urine after cleavage by metalloproteinase (Han et al., 2002; Waanders et al., 2010). Urinary KIM-1 is particularly important in the diagnosis of the acute transplanted kidney insufficiency(AKI) (Halawa, 2011). As in renal graft recipients, contrary to urinary NGAL or IL-18, KIM determination gives better possibility for predicting a rate of the transplanted kidney deterioration (Szeto et al., 2010), KIM-1 was proposed as an independent predictor of the long term renal graft survival (Ting et al., 2012).

5. Proteins degrading extracellular matrix (ECM)

Urokinase-type plasminogen activator (uPA) and its specific receptor (uPAR) regulate renal allograft function. Allogenic renal graft uPAR deficiency, strongly attenuates ischemia reperfusion injury and acute kidney allograft rejection. Deficiency of uPAR in renal graft diminished generation of reactive oxygen species and renal cells apoptosis (Gueler et al., 2008). Therefore serum and urinary uPA may be treated as an early marker of the acute kidney transplant rejection (Alachkar, 2012).

Matrix metalloproteinases (MMPs) are extracellular proteases which depend on bound Ca^{2+} and Zn^{2+} for activity. Urinary panel of metalloproteinases was proposed for the early diagnosis of renal allograft rejection (Metzger et al., 2011; Sánchez-Escuredo et al., 2010; Hu et al., 2010).

Tissue inhibitors of metalloproteinases (TIMP) are extracellular inhibitors protease-specific, which bind tightly to the activated protease, blocking its activity. Presently 2% to 4% of renal allografts are rejected one year after from transplantation, because of chronic allograft injury. Mazanowska et al. (Mazanowska et al., 2011) suggest that determination of TIMP in urine may confirm the process of an active rejection of the transplanted kidney.

6. Immunological mediators of inflammatory state and fibrosis of renal tissue

Urinary chemokines CXCL9 and CXCL10 may be treated as noninvasive screening markers of renal graft rejection in patients with interstitial fibrosis and tubular atrophy (IF/TA), leading to shorter life span of renal graft (Jackson et al., 2011; Schaub et al., 2009). Urinary CXCL10 may be a useful noninvasive screening test for tubulitis in renal graft recipients, and urinary

CXCL10 concentration above 1,97 ng /mmol of creatinine is a threshold for consideration of renal biopsy (Ho et al., 2011).

6.1. Immunological markers of renal inflammatory state

Macrophage inflammatory protein 3alpha (MIP-3alpha), chemokine C-C ligand 20 (CCL20) is a major chemokine expressed by epithelial cells that attracts immature dendritic cells (DC). Graft-infiltrating dendritic cells (DC) and alloreactive T lymphocytes play a critical role in renal allograft rejection. Renal proximal tubular epithelial cells (TEC) are considered as an active players in the attraction of leukocytes during renal inflammatory responses. A significant increase in the excretion of major intrinsic protein MIP-3α/CCL20 to urine was observed in renal graft recipients with symptoms of graft rejection (Woltman et al., 2005; Peng et al., 2008).

Growth-related oncogene-alpha (Gro-alpha) is an analog of the keratinocyte-derived chemokine(KC). An increase in serum and urinary analog of Gro-alpha in the experimental renal damage appears the earliest and persists the longest among the 18 chosen cytokines and chemokines (Molls et al., 2006). Serum and urinary Gro-alpha were the highest 3 hours after ischemia, while histological changes were evident after one hour, whereas serum creatinine increased 24 hours after ischemia. Urinary concentration of Gro-α increased significantly in renal graft recipients who required dialysis in comparison to people with normal renal graft function. Urinary Gro-α is considered as an early marker of diagnosis and prognosis of acute kidney injury (AKI) resulted from ischemia (Molls et al., 2006). It was reported that Gro-alfa, significantly increased in patients who received cadaver kidney with poor function and from living donors with minimal ischemia. Therefore determination of KC and Gro-α may be used as biomarkers in the diagnosis of ischemic acute renal failure (ARF) and in the early diagnosis and prognosis of renal ischemia-reperfusion injury (IRI). IRI is the most frequent cause of acute kidney injury (AKI) and acute renal failure in delayed function graft received from a cadaver (Molls et al., 2006).

Interleukin (IL-18) is a proinflammatory cytokine released to urine by epithelium of renal proximal tubules after stimuli of nephrotoxic factor. Urinary IL-18 concentration >100 pg/mg of urinary creatinine is a good diagnostic marker of the acute renal damage and mortality of patients in intensive care units (Parikh et al., 2005) as well as a predictor of the delayed graft function. It seems that urinary IL-18 helps for a detection of the very early stage of kidney damage caused by ischemia or tubular nephrotoxins and plays a role in detecting prerenal nitrogenemia, chronic renal insufficiency and urinary tract infection (Parikh et al., 2005). Furthermore urinary Il-18 is an early predictive biomarker of the acute kidney injury after cardiac surgery (Parikh et al., 2005). IL-18- proinflammatory cytokine caspase-1 dependent (both derived from ischemic renal proximal tubular cells) is a proinflammatory cytokine activated in damaged renal tubules by caspase -1 and released to urine in a case of the acute kidney injury (AKI). A significant increase in urinary concentration of IL –18 and NGAL after transplantation, however before delay in the renal graft function, was found. IL-18 is also a predictor of the AKI severity preceding the increase in serum creatinine (Dinarello, 1999).

http://dx.doi.org/10.5772/54746

Granzymes (*granule-associated enzymes*) are serine proteases (27-32kDa) of the chymotrypsin family. Granzyme B (GzmB) and Fas-ligand (FAS-L) are cytotoxic molecules involved in the acute renal graft rejection (AR) by the induction of DNA fragmentation of damaged cells (Yannaraki et al., 2006). Granzyme A (GzmA) is a specific noninvasive immunological biomarker for monitoring renal graft condition which facilitate diagnosis and treatment after transplant complications. Granzyme A (GzmA) besides involvement in apoptosis may act as mitogen of B lymphocytes. GzmA is a noninvasive biomarker differentiating patients with subclinical and acute renal graft rejection from patients with renal tubular necrosis or persons with stabile renal graft (van Ham et al., 2010).

6.2. Immunological markers of renal fibrosis

Chemokine regulated upon activation in normal T cells expressed and secreted (RANTES/ CCL5) is a chemokine of the beta subfamily secreted by macrophages and T lymphocytes. RANTES can signal through CCR1, CCR3, CCR5 and US28(cytomegalovirus receptor) receptors. It is chemoattractant towards monocytes, memory T cells(CD4+/CD45RO+), basophils, and neutrophils. RANTES occurs in increased amounts in diseased kidneys and indicate on interstitial inflammatory changes of the tubular cells at the early stages of acute kidney injury, skin or heart graft rejection (Koga et al., 2000; Gwinner, 2007). RANTES expressed in renal different cells (mesanglial cells, endothelium of renal tubules, fibroblasts, lymphocytes) plays an active role in acute and chronic kidney inflammation and development of tubule-interstitial damage. (Baer et al., 2005) reported absence of significant differences in plasma and urinary RANTES in patients with acute renal graft rejection and recipients with normal graft function. Therefore RANTES is not suitable for detection of early kidney graft rejection. However an significant increase in the serum and urinary RANTES was observed immediately after renal transplantation which may reflect an activation of the immunological systems.

Transforming growth factor beta (TGF-β) is responsible for exacerbation of fibrosis, controls growth and differentiation of cells and production of extracellular matrix as well as regulates cellular migration. A participation of TGF-ß1 in lung and kidney fibrosis during chronic allograft rejection was reported by (Awad et al.,1998; Bartnard et al., 1990). Increased excretion of urinary TGF-β was proposed as a marker of the intrarenal production and activity of TGF-ß1 in kidney. An increase in the urinary TGF-ß1 was reported in different nephropathies particularly significant in patients with heavy proteinuria (Schnaper et al., 2003; Böttinger & Bitzer, 2002). The 6-12 month immunosuppression with cyclosporine in renal-transplant recipients caused development of a chronic interstitial nephropathy with decreased GFR. Cyclosporine A (CsA) facilitate the expression of TGF-β in renal tubular cells and cells of renal juxtaglomerular apparatus. Furthermore, CsA stimulates T lymphocytes and endothelial cell to a TGF-β 1 production. Expression of TGF-β 1 is CsA dose dependent. High doses of CsA are risk factors of chronic graft dysfunction, among kidney recipients (Boratyńska et al., 2003).

Vascular endothelial growth factor (VEGF) a dimeric protein containing subunits constituted of 121, 165, 189 or 206 amino acids is a proangiogenic growth factor. In patients with symptoms of acute renal graft rejection high urinary VEGF concentration was found in comparison to people with normal function of renal graft. Therefore monitoring of urinary VEGF was proposed as a marker of detection acute renal graft rejection and the evaluation of the effectiveness of immunotherapy (Peng et al., 2008; Alachkar, 2012).

Hepatocyte growth factor (HGF) induces angiogenesis by stimulation proliferation, migration and adhesion of endothelial cells. Urinary HGF concentration was highest at the first day after transplantation, decreased quickly within next week and later remained on the same level. Determination of the urinary HGF immediately after kidney transplantation may be a quick, noninvasive marker of long lasting renal graft function (Kwiatkowska et al., 2010).

Endothelin-1 (ET-1) is the strongest vasoconstrictory factor produced by endothelium of blood vessels, glomerular mesangium, renal tubular cells, fibroblasts and macrophages. ET-1 regulates fibrosis by joining interstitial fibroblasts, initiation its proliferation and synthesis of extracellular matrix as well as chemotactic action on macrophages. ET-1 is degraded mostly in lungs and kidneys. Urinary ET-1 excretion reflects its renal production. Increase in ET-1 gene expression and urinary excretion correlates positively with proteinuria and negatively with creatinine clearance (Grenda et al., 2007; Saurina et al., 2007). Plasma and urinary ET-1 concentrations are increased in patients treated with Cyclosporine A and FKJ506. Cyclosporine A and FK506 are calcineurine inhibitors broadly applied for immunosuppression in kidney transplant patients. Cyclosporine A and FK506 significantly improve graft survival. However graft recipients may die because of cardiovascular complications as 80% of renal graft recipients reveal vascular hypertension. Increased ET-1 concentration may reflect activation of the ET-1 system in chronic insufficiency of transplanted kidney (Slowinski et al., 2002).

Monocyte chemotactic peptide-1 (MCP-1/CCL2) mediates recruitment of inflammatory cells: monocytes/macrophages and lymphocytes T, to renal tubules damaged by high concentrations of albumin in tubules. A strict relationship between albuminuria, urinary MCP-1/CCL2 and macrophage infiltration in damaged loci, was demonstrated (Urbschat et al., 2011; Viedt & Orth, 2002). In patients with acute renal graft rejection urinary concentration of MPC-1, determined by ELISA, was ten times higher than in patients with stable graft function (Dubiński et al., 2008). Since chronic damage to renal graft as a result of gradual fibrosis and tubular damage (IF/TA) is the most frequent cause of graft loss, urinary CCL2 may be treated as an independent prognostic marker of development of IF/TA during the next 24 months (Ho et al., 2010).

Fractalkine (CX3CL1) is a chemokine from the CX3C group of complement system, stimulated by CX3CR1 receptor connected to G protein. In experimental renal disease induced by albumin overload and proceeding with proteinuria, increased expression of fractalkine gene correlates with applied albumin dose and time of albumin interaction with the renal tubular cells (Donadelli et al., 2003). Fractalkine urinary concentration is a noninvasive method for detection of acute renal graft rejection (Peng et al., 2008).

Angiotensin II (Ang II) is an important intrarenal factor favoring processes of inflammation and fibrosis by an increase in the expression of the proinflammatory genes (IL-6, TNFα, MCP-1, RANTES). According to latest opinions the urinary concentration of angiotensinogen, reflects amounts of produced Ang II inside the kidney better, than immediate evaluation of Ang II in the urine. Improvement of the ELISA method for determination of human urinary angiotensinogen, may allow to disclose influence of Ang II on intrarenal destructive processes (Yamamoto et al., 2007; Katsurada et al., 2007).

Complement is a major mediator system in pathogenesis of various kidney diseases. The presence and localization of complement components in glomerulus and/or the tubule-interstitial area provides diagnostic tools for several human renal diseases (Zoja et al., 2003; Lisowska-Myjak, 2010). Increase in urinary excretion of complement components in patients with proteinuria significantly correlate with urinary excretion of total proteins and decrease in renal function. Therefore increase in urinary C5b-9 in patients with proteinuria may by prognostic marker for the development of kidney insufficiency (Eddy, 2002). Accelerated C3 activation at renal proximal tubules in diseases proceeding with proteinuria are result of increased intratubular protein catabolism, with accompanying increase in ammonia (activator of alternative pathway of complement activation) (Morita et al., 2000; Abbate et al., 2008; Sheerin et al., 2008; Lederer et al., 2003). Everyday urinary determination of C5A and TCC may be a sensitive and reliable marker of the acute insufficiency of the transplanted kidney and predictor of graft rejection (Müller et al., 1997).

Galectin 3 (Gal-3) is a beta-galactoside-binding lectin in diverse fibrotic tissues. Gal 3 plays an important role in fibrosis of transplanted kidney and may be a potential marker of chronic allograft impairment (CAI) (Dang et al., 2012).

7. Tubular enzymes

Currently, in clinical diagnostic practice for renal parenchymal tubular impairment, assessment of urinary enzymes is used. Particular advantage of urinary enzymes determination is its localization in appropriate renal cells (glomeruli, tubules) and their organelles (cytoplasm, lysosomes, membranes), which may deliver detailed information concerning nature and dimension of the renal cells damage and an evaluation of their dysfunction or necrosis (Westhuyzen et al., 2003; Trof et al., 2006). Routine, simple, cheap and broadly available spectrophotometric methods are applied for measurement of urinary enzymes activity. An increase in urinary excretion of enzymes reflects damage of particular renal section (D'Amico & Bazzi, 2003; Jung et al., 1986). Determination of urinary FBP-1,6, NAG, glutathione-S-transferase and pyruvate kinase has recently been recommended for the diagnosis of kidney disease and early detection of transplant rejection (Kotanko et al., 1997; Kotanko et al., 1986).

7.1. Enzymes of brush border membranes

Gamma-glutamyltransferase (GGT) – is connected with cellular membranes of liver, kidney, pancreas and prostatic gland (Kuźniar et al., 2006). Serial determination of urinary enzymes is a reliable proof for nephrotoxicity resulted from long term cyclosporine A treatment. Lack of enzymuria indicates a recovery of renal tubules to normal function (Tataranni et al., 1992).

Alkaline phosphatase (AP) – is present in cellular membranes of many tissues, mainly bonds, liver and intestine where it participates in metabolism of organic phosphates. Frequent cause of deterioration to the renal graft function is nephrotoxicity of immunosuppressive drugs (e.g. cyclosporin A) reflected by increase in activity of urinary enzymes : ALP, LDH, GGT, beta-glucuronidase (Refaie et al., 2000; Takahashi et al., 1989; Simić-Ogrizović et al., 1994).

Alanylaminopeptidase (AAP) – proteolytic enzyme degrading oligopeptides. Increases in urinary concentration of hexosaminidase and AAP accompany acute renal tubular necrosis, renal graft rejection or nephrotoxic action of immunosuppresive drugs (e.g. cyclosporin A) administered to patients after kidney transplantat (Kuźniar et al., 2006; Lisowska-Myjak, 2010; Santos et al., 2010). Increases in urinary excretion of tubular enzymes testifies tubular brush border membrane damage with a loss of microvillus structure (Westhuyzen et al., 2003).

7.2. Cytosolic enzymes

Glutathione S-transferase (alpha-GST, pi-GST) is a specific cytoplasmic enzyme of tubular epithelial cells consisting of two isoenzymes: α-GST with alkaline and πi-GST with acidic pH optimum. GST-α appears in epithelium of proximal tubular cells and GST-π in distal tubules (Branten et al., 2000). Determination in urine α-GST and, π-GST is applied to diagnosis acute renal graft rejection with acute tubular necrosis (Kuźniar et al., 2006; Polak, 1999). Differentiated increase in urinary GST- alpha and GST- pi excretion may point to localization of an nephron damage (Westhuyzen et al., 2003; Trof et al., 2006; Herget-Rosenthal et al., 2004; Branten et al., 2000; Gautier et al., 2010).

Fructose-1,6-bisphosphatase (FBP-1,6) is localized mostly in contorted and to less extend in straight part of proximal renal tubules, similarly to hexosaminidase and GST, points to accurate localization of damaged nephron (Trof et al., 2006; Kotanko et al., 1986). Increase in urinary FBP-1,6 was observed in patients after kidney transplantat. Urinary FBP-1,6 excretion was significantly lower in patients with median of cold ischemia below 22 hours, than above 22 hours. Even in lack of graft dysfunction, in situation where it is a long time of cold ischemia, urinary excretion of FBP-ase correlates with a degree of damage to the renal tubules (Kotanko et al., 1997). It was reported that a panel of urinary enzymes activities: FBP-ase, glutathione S-transferase, N-acetyl-beta-D-glucosaminidase and pyruvate kinase is a good marker of the cyclosporin A nephrotoxicity (Kotanko et al., 1986).

7.3. Renal lysosomal enzymes

N-acetyl-β-D-hexosaminidase (HEX) is one of the most frequently determined urinary markers of renal tubules damage, because its activity increased at early steps of the renal tubules damage, before occurrence of disturbances in renal excretory function. Hexosaminidase localized mainly in renal proximal tubular cells, is a specific marker for proximal tubular cells because its high molecular weight (> 130 kDa) excludes its glomerular filtration. In the course of active kidney disease HEX activity is constantly increased. An increase in urinary activity HEX and its isoenzyme B indicate on damage in the renal tubular cells. Therefore urinary HEX and particularly HEX B activity may be treated as a specific marker of damage in the renal proximal tubules of the transplanted kidney (Liangos et al., 2007; Holdt–Lehmann et al., 2000;).

8. Markers of renal ischemia/reperfusion injury

Leukocyte elastase (LE, neutrophil elastase), is a 30-kDa glycoprotein serine protease released from neutrophils as a mediator of ischemia/reperfusion injury after renal transplantation. Urinary LE is a simple noninvasive marker of the neutrophil activation after renal transplantat (Zynek-Litwin et al., 2010).

9. Biomarkers of dystal renal tubules

In the assessment of distal renal tubule dysfunction it is advised to examine urine osmolarity and/or determination Tamm-Horsfall glycoprotein as well as urinary kallikrein (Bhoola et al., 1992).

Renal kallikrein is a serine protease which releases vasodilatatory peptides: bradykinine and calidine, from kininogen. Renal kallikrein is present in renal collecting tubules and is released to tubular fluid by terminal section of dystal segment of nephron (Manucha & Vallés, 1999; Thongboonkerd & Malasit, 2005). An increase in activity of urinary kallikrein was observed in insufficiency and loss of the renal graft function (Krimkevich, 1990).

AnnexinA11 (**ANXA11**). Annexins are calcium-binding proteins which binds to acidic phospholipid and F-actin. Depending on calcium concentration Annexin A 11 participate in signal transduction, cell proliferation, regulation of vesicular transport and interaction with the cell membranes. Annexin occurs in high quantities in renal distal tubular cells and epithelium of renal glomeruli. Annexin physiologic role seems to be related to cell apoptosis (Rodrigues-Garcia et al., 1996). Significant correlation between urinary Annexin V and other proteins and lack of correlation with urinary urea and creatinine concentration suggests that Annexin V is not an indicator of kidney function, but rather reflects local kidney damage (Matsuda et al., 2000). Annexin A11 may act as an atypical calcium channel and useful marker of acute and chronic renal graft rejection (Srivastava et al., 2011)

Renal papillary antigen-1 (RPA-1) a renal papillary antigen-1, sensitive and specific antigen of renal papillary cells is a sensitive and specific urinary marker of damage renal collecting tubules (Gautier et al., 2010).

Prominin-2 (PROM-2) analog of **CD133 (prominin-1)** is an membrane glycoprotein (112kD) with the highest expression in epithelial cells of matured kidney. Prominin-2 is a cholesterol-binding protein associated with apical and basolateral plasmalemmal protrusions in polarized epithelial cells and released into urine (Florek et al., 2007) and a novel marker of distal tubules and collecting ducts of the human and murine kidney (Jászai et al., 2010).

μ-glutathione-S-transferase (μ-GST) is a conjugating glutathione with electrophilic compounds that occurs in epithelial cells of ascending part of Henle's loop (Gautier et al., 2010; Holmquist & Torffvit, 2008). After nephrotoxic drugs treatment (e.g. cisplatin) μ-GST quickly appear in urine. μ-GST is a more specific marker of nephrotoxicity (AUC 1.000) than α-GST

(AUC 0.984) or albuminuria (AUC 0.984). μ-GST is an early biomarker for Henle's loop and distal tubules damage (Tonomura et al., 2010).

10. The future of biomarkers

Development of new technologies involved in molecular biology, analysis of m-RNA expression, proteomics and metabolomics create a possibility of discovery of new markers for early diagnosis of AKI and IF/TA. Relatively new method of microarrays (microarrays of cDNA and oligonuclotides- DNA chips) are sets of molecular probes attached to solid background in strictly determined order constituting two dimensional system of microscopic areas with defined sequences of nucleic acid. Microarray technology allow for detection of thousands of molecules of nucleic acids due to possibility of performing simultaneously many hybridization experiments (Dean et al., 2012). DNA microarrays technology permit for simultaneous monitoring expression of many genes (Scian et al., 2011). Identification of these genes constitute further step in earlier diagnosis and better prognosis of TA/IF(tubular atrophy/interstitial fibrosis).

Proteomic techniques Recently broadly applied proteomic techniques facilitate discovery of new biomarkers useful in evaluation of transplanted kidney function. Proteomics apply protein analysis using techniques such as MS e.g. (MALDI-TOF-Matrix Assisted Laser Desorption Ionisation - Time of Flight; SELDI-TOF-Surface Enhanced Laser Desorption Ionisation - Time of Flight; ES multielementary I - LTQ – FTICR-Electrospray Ionisation - Linear Trap Quadrupole - Fourier Transform Ion Cyclotron Resonance). Proteomics combine series of techniques for simultaneous analysis of hundreds or thousands of cells proteins. Proteomics objective is not only creation of the list of important proteins, but first of all exploration of differences in protein profiles of healthy and diseased people. Proteomic identification of urinary protein profiles is an noninvasive method for detection of renal proximal tubules dysfunction of transplanted kidney (Srivastava et al., 2011; Gwinner, 2007). Proteomic techniques are alternative for diagnostics based on single markers, because it allows for simultaneous analysis of large numbers of protein and peptide markers creating specific „finger print" of disease. Proteomics determines pattern of expression or secretion taking into account qualitative and quantitative relations between peptides and proteins produced in defined pathophysiological conditions.

Metabolomics based on analysis sets of metabolites connected with proteins, lipids, carbohydrates, hormones, etc. evaluate qualitative and quantitative relations between particular metabolites. Due to metabolomics it is possible to determine definite metabolites characteristic for specific groups of diseases and changes occurring under influence of genetic and pathophysiological stimuli (Wishart, 2006).

New technologies and bioinformatics tools offer tremendous research possibilities which should make possible now and in the future precise monitoring of kidney graft, allow early detection and treatment of renal graft rejection and allow both for preventing and treatment of renal transplant complications as well as to improve number of long term patients survival.

http://dx.doi.org/10.5772/54746

Markers	Acute kidney injury (AKI); Acute graft rejection (AGR); Acute tubular necrosis (ATN)	Chronic allograft nephropathy (CAN/ IFTA); Delayed graft function (DGF)	References
β2M,α1M	+	+	Johnston et al., 2011; Du et al., 2011; Câmara et al., 2009;Kuźniar et al., 2006
Netrin-1	+		Ramesh et al., 2010; Urbschat et al., 2011
NGAL	+		Ramesh et al., 2010; Nauta et al., 2011; Przybyłowski et al., 2011; Halawa, 2011; Devarajan, 2011; Hall&Parikh, 2010; Du et al., 2011;Ting et al., 2012
IL-16,IL-2,IL-6,IL-18,TNF	+	+	Alachkar er al., 2010; Halawa, 2011; Devarajan, 2011; Reinhold et al., 2012; Urbschat et al., 2011
KIM-1	+	+	Nauta et al., 2011; Halawa, 2011; Devarajan,2011; Hall &Parikh, 2010; Du et al., 2011; Ting et al., 2012; Urbschat et al., 2011
NAG		+	Nauta et al. 2011; Câmara et al., 2009; Ting et al., 2012; Kuźniar et al., 2006; Alachkar et al., 2010
H-FABP, L-FABP	+	+	Nauta et al., 2011; Przybylowskiet al., 2011
Cystatin C	+		Przybylowski et al., 2011; Hall &Parikh, 2010
CXCL9,CXCL10	+	+	Ho et al., 2011; Schaub et al., 2009; Jackson et al., 2011; Ting et al., 2012
alpha-GST, pi-GST	+	+	Câmara et al., 2009;Hall &Parikh, 2010; Ting et al., 2012; Kuźniar et al., 2006; Oberbauer , 2008
GzmA,GzmB (granzyme)	+		van Ham et al., 2010; Peng et al., 2008; Oberbauer, 2008
Galectin-3(Gal-3)		+	Dang et al., 2012
Integrin α3, integrinβ2	+	+	Srivastava et al., 2011
ANXA11	+	+	Srivastavaet al., 2011
sVCAM	+		Reinhold et al., 2012
MMP7, MMP-8	+		Metzger et al., 2011; Ling et al., 2010
LDH, ALP, γ-GT, AAP	+		Refaie et al., 2000;Kuźniar et al., 2006

Markers	Acute kidney injury (AKI); Acute graft rejection (AGR); Acute tubular necrosis (ATN)	Chronic allograft nephropathy (CAN/ IFTA); Delayed graft function (DGF)	References
OX40,OX40L,PD-1	+		Afaneh et al., 2010
HLA-DR	+		Ting et al., 2010
CTGF		+	Yue et al., 2010; Bao et al., 2008
uPA	+		Alachkar , 2012
Leukocyte elastase (LE)	+	+	Zynek-Litwin et al., 2010
SERPING1	+		Ling et al., 2010
TIMP1	+		Ling et al., 2010
MIP-1delta,	+	+	Hu et al., 2009
Osteoprotegerin	+	+	Hu et al., 2009
VEGF	+		Peng et al., 2008
fractalkine	+		Peng et al., 2008
MCP-1	+		Dubiński et al., 2008; Urbschat et al., 2011
RBP	+		Kuźniar et al., 2006; Câmara et al., 2009
Perforin	+		Oberbauer, 2008
FOXP3	+		Oberbauer, 2008

Table 1. Urinary biomarkers for the early detection of acute and chronic allograft dysfunction.

11. Conclusion

In this chapter we presented traditional and new biomarkers for diagnostics and monitoring condition of transplant kidneys. Urine is practical, easy to obtain, noninvasive material for diagnosis of kidney diseases. Numerous reports from molecular biology, genetics, proteomics and metabolomics disclosed an array of new markers specifically connected with damage of specific nephron segments in the course of successive steps of disease. Particular expectations are connected with proteins represented particular nephron section, or produced locally in the place of nephron damage. Presence of cytokines and chemokines in urine is an early sign of renal inflammatory state, due to influx of granulocytes to the damaged nephron area. Majority of traditional biomarkers, particularly enzymuria retains diagnostic value in an evaluation of the renal tubules function. Multitude of presented biomarkers suggest their limited diagnostic value. Discovering universal marker seems to be very difficult. However, it is potentially more fruitful to identity the putative biomarker proteins useful in diagnostics of kidney disease.

http://dx.doi.org/10.5772/54746

Scientiscs are still looking for the "kidney troponin". Actually, more than ten promising biomarkers for kidney damage have been identified. The most relevant and the best studied substances are neutrophil gelatinase-associated lipocalin (NGAL), cystatin C, kidney injury molecule-1 (KIM-1), beta-2 microglobulin (β2M), and interleukin-18 (IL- 18). In kidney allograft recipients, urinary KIM-1 expression provides prognostic information in relation to the rate of renal function decline, irrespective of the kidney pathology (Ting et al., 2012; Han et al., 2002; Szeto et al., 2010).

Validation of those kidney markers in various pathologic conditions is actually ongoing. However, the majority of publications reviewed are small cross-sectional studies, and there are only a handful of longitudinal studies. Another important point is that biomarkers only have clinical value if the results are reproducible. However none of the biomarkers reviewed here have been studied in more than 2 longitudinal trials so their clinical applicability needs to be confirmed in good quality, long-term, large longitudinal trials.

Among enzymes which retain high diagnostic value in diagnostics of renal diseases are: hexosaminidase and its isoenzyme B as a marker of the proximal tubular damage as well as AAP or GST as a marker of the tubular brush border membrane. Cytosolic FBP-1,6 is of great diagnostic value for assessment of graft function. It is commonly believed that appropriate panel of urinary proteins and enzymes may by a practical marker for evaluation of the nephron function of transplant kidney and prognosis of the renal allograft fate. In the future, discovery of new biomarkers and research techniques may change practical approach to treating patients with renal grafts. In summary we feel it is necessary for an international body to develop a renal marker utility grading system, to evaluate the usefulness of particular markers of nephron function and to make recommendations for the use of renal transplant markers, similar to those instilled for tumor markers (Hayes et al., 1996; Locker et al., 2006).

Author details

Alina Kępka[1], Napoleon Waszkiewicz[2], Sylwia Chojnowska[3], Beata Zalewska-Szajda[4], Jerzy Robert Ładny[5], Anna Wasilewska[6], Krzysztof Zwierz[7] and Sławomir Dariusz Szajda[5]

1 The Children's Memorial Health Institute, Warsaw, Poland

2 Department of Psychiatry, Medical University, Białystok, Poland

3 Medical Institute, College of Computer Science and Business Administration, Łomża, Poland

4 Department of Radiology, Children Hospital, Medical University of Białystok, Poland

5 Department of Emergency Medicine and Disasters, Medical University, Białystok, Poland

6 Department of Pediatric Nephrology, Medical University of Białystok, Poland

7 Medical College the Universal Education Society, Łomża, Poland

References

[1] Abbate M.; Zoja C.; Corna D.; Rottoli D.; Zanchi C.; Azzollini N.; Tomasoni S.; Berlingeri S.; Noris M.; Morigi M.; Remuzzi G. (2008). Complement – mediated dysfunction of glomerular filtration barrier accelerates progressive renal injury. *J Am Soc Nephrol,* 19, 1158-1167.

[2] Abbate M.; Zoja C.; Remuzzi G. (2006). How does proteinuria cause progressive renal damage? *J Am Soc Nephrol,* 17, 2974-2984.

[3] Afaneh C.; Muthukumar T.; Lubetzky M.; Ding R.; Snopkowski C.; Sharma VK.; Seshan S.; Dadhania D.; Schwartz JE.; Suthanthiran M. (2010). Urinary cell levels of mRNA for OX40, OX40L, PD-1, PD-L1, or PD-L2 and acute rejection of human renal allografts. *Transplantation,* 90, 12, 1381-1387.

[4] Ahmad A.; Roderick P.; Ward M.; Steenkamp R.; Burden R.; O'Donoghue D.; Ansell D.; Feest T. (2006). Current chronic kidney disease practice patterns in the UK: a national survey. *QJM,* 99, 4, 245-51.

[5] Alachkar N.; Rabb H.; Jaar BG. (2010). Urinary biomarkers in acute kidney transplant dysfunction. *Nephron Clin Pract,* 118, 2, c173-c181.

[6] Alachkar N. (2012). Serum and urinary biomarkers in acute kidney transplant rejection. *Nephrol Ther,* 8, 1, 13-19.

[7] Awad MR.; El-Gamel A.; Hasleton P.; Turner DM.; Sinnott PJ.; Huthinson IV. (1998). Genotypic variation in the transforming growth factor-beta1 gene: associacion with transforming growth factor-beta1 production, fibrotic lung disease, and graft fibrosis after lung transplantation. T*ransplantation,* 66, 8, 1014-1020.

[8] Baer PC.; Koziolek M.; Fierlbeck W.; Geiger H. (2005). CC-chemokine RANTES is increased in serum and urine in the early post-transplantation period of human renal allograft recipients. *Kidney Blood Press Res,* 28, 1, 48-54.

[9] Bagshaw SM.; Langenberg Ch.; Haase M.; Wan L.; May CN.; Bellomo R. (2007). Urinary biomarkers in septic acute kidney injury. *Intensive Care Med,* 33, 1285–1296.

[10] Bandukwala F.; Huang M.; Zaltzman JS. (2009). Microalbuminuria post-renal transplantation: relation to cardiovascular risk factors and C-reactive protein. *Clin Transplant,* 23, 3, 313-320.

[11] Bao J.; Tu Z.; Wang J.; Ye F.; Sun H.; Qin M.; Shi Y.; Bu H.; Li YP. (2008). A novel accurate rapid ELISA for detection of urinary connective tissue growth factor, a biomarker of chronic allograft nephropathy. *Transplant Proc,* 40, 7, 2361-2364.

[12] Barnard JA.; Lyons RM.; Moses HL. (1990). The cell biology of transforming growth factor beta. *Bioch Bioph Acta,* 1032, 79-87.

[13] Bhoola KD.; Figueroa CD.; Worthy K. (1992). Bioregulation of kinins: kallikreins, kininogens, and kininases. *Pharmacol Rev*, 44, 1, 1-80.

[14] Boratyńska M;, Radwan-Oczko M.; Falkiewicz K.; Klinger M.; Szyber P. (2003). Gingival overgrowth in kidney transplant recipients treated with Cyclosporine and its relationship with chronic graft nephropathy. *Transplant Proc*, 35, 2238-2240.

[15] Böttinger EP.; Bitzer M. (2002). TGF-β signaling in renal disease. *J Am Soc Nephrol*, 13, 2600-2610.

[16] Branten AJ.; Mulder TP.; Peters WH.; Assmann KJ.; Wetzels JF. (2000). Urinary excretion of glutathione S transferases alpha and pi in patients with proteinuria may reflection the site of tubular injury. *Nephron*, 85, 120–126.

[17] Câmara NO.; Williams WWJr.; Pacheco-Silva A. (2009). Proximal tubular dysfunction as an indicator of chronic graft dysfunction. *Braz J Med Biol Res*, 42, 3, 229-236.

[18] Campo A.; Lanfranco G.; Gramaglia L.; Goia F.; Cottino R.; Giusto V. (2004). Could plasma Cystatin C be useful as a marker of hemodialysis low molecular weight proteins removal. *Nephrol Clin Pract*, 98, 3, c79–c82.

[19] D'Amico G.; Bazzi C. (2003). Urinary protein and enzyme excretion as markers of tubular damage. *Curr Opin Nephrol Hypertens*, 12, 639–643.

[20] Dang Z.; MacKinnon A.; Marson LP.; Sethi T. (2012). Tubular atrophy and interstitial fibrosis after renal transplantation is dependent on galectin-3. *Transplantation*, 93, 5, 477-484.

[21] Dean PG.; Park WD.; Cornell LD.; Gloor JM.; Stegall MD. (2012). Intragraft gene expression in positive crossmatch kidney allografts: ongoing inflammation mediates chronic antibody-mediated injury. *Am J Transplant*, 12, 6, 1551-1563.

[22] Devarajan P. (2010). Neutrophil gelatinase-associated lipocalin: a promising biomarker for human acute kidney injury. *Biomark Med*, 4, 2, 265-280.

[23] Devarajan P. (2011). Biomarkers for the early detection of acute kidney injury. *Curr Opin Pediatr*, 23, 2, 194-200.

[24] Dinarello CA. (1999). IL-18: a TH1-inducing, proinflammatory cytokine and new member of the IL-1 family. *J Allergy Clin Immunol*, 103, 1Pt1, 11-24.

[25] Donadelli R.; Zanchi C.; Morigi M.; Buelli S.; Batani C.; Tomasoni S.; Corna D.; Rottoli D.; Benigni A.; Abbate M.; Remuzzi G.; Zoja C. (2003). Protein overload induces fractalkine upregulation in proximal tubular cells through nuclear factor κB- and p38 mitogen-activated protein kinase-dependent pathways. *J Am Soc Nephrol*, 14, 2436-2446.

[26] Dubiński B.; Boratyńska M.; Kopeć W.; Szyber P.; Patrzałek D.; Klinger M. (2008). Activated cells in urine and monocyte chemotactic peptide-1 (MCP-1)-sensitive rejection markers in renal graft recipients. *Transpl Immunol*, 18, 3, 203-207.

[27] Du Y.; Zappitelli M.; Mian A.; Bennett M.; Ma Q.; Devarajan P.; Mehta R.; Goldstein SL. (2011). Urinary biomarkers to detect acute kidney injury in the pediatric emergency center. *Pediatr Nephrol,* 26, 2, 267-274.

[28] Eddy AA. (2002). Plasminogen activator inhibitor-1 and the kidney. *Am J Physiol Renal Physiol,* 283, F209-F220.

[29] Eddy AA. (2004). Proteinuria and interstitial injury. *Nephrol Dial Transplant,* 19, 277-281.

[30] Einecke G.; Reeve J.; Sis B.; Mengel M.; Hidalgo L.; Famulski KS.; Matas A.; Kasiske B.; Kaplan B.; Halloran PF. (2010). A molecular classifier for predicting future graft loss in late kidney transplant biopsies. *J Clin Invest,* 1, 120, 6, 1862–1872.

[31] Erman A.; Rahamimov R.; Mashraki T.; Levy-Drummer RS.; Winkler J.; David I.; Hirsh Y.; Gafter U.; Chagnac A. (2011). The urine albumin-to-creatinine ratio: assessment of its performance in the renal transplant recipient population. *Clin J Am Soc Nephrol,* 6, 4, 892–897.

[32] Filler G.; Bokenkamp A.; Hofmann W.; Le Bricon T.; Martínez-Brú C.; Grubb A. (2005). Cystatin C as a marker of GFR – history, indications, and future research. *Clin Biochem,* 38, 1, 1–8.

[33] Finney H.; Newman DJ.; Thakker H.; Fell JM.; Price CP. (2000). Adult reference ranges for serum cystatin C and creatinine measurements in premature infants, neonates, and older children. *Arch Dis Child,* 82, 1, 71–75.

[34] Florek M.; Bauer N.; Janich P.; Wilsch-Braeuninger M.; Fargeas ChA.; Marzesco AM.; Ehninger G.; Thiele Ch.; Huttner WB.; Corbeil D. (2007). Prominin-2 is a cholesterol-binding protein associated with apical and basolateral plasmalemmal protrusions in polarized epithelial cells and released into urine. *Cell Tissue Res,* 328, 1, 31-47.

[35] Flower D. (1996). The lipocalin protein family:structure and function. *Biochem J,* 318, 1-14.

[36] Gautier JC.; Riefke B.; Walter J.; Kurth P.; Mylecraine L.; Guilpin V.; Barlow N.; Gury T.; Hoffman D.; Ennulat D.; Schuster K.; Harpur E.; Pettit S. (2010). Evaluation of novel biomarkers of nephrotoxicity in two strains of rat treated with Cisplatin. *Toxicol Pathol,* 38, 6, 943-956.

[37] Giorgio F.; Laviola L.; Cavallo-Perin P.; Solnica B.; Fuller J; Chaturvedi N. (2004). Factors associated with progresion to macroalbuminuria in microalbuminuric type 1 diabetic patients: the EURODIAB Prospective Complications Study. *Diabetologia,* 47, 6, 1020–1028.

[38] Grebe SO.; Mueller TF.; Troeltsch M.; Ebel H.; Lange H. (2004). Effect of mycophenolate mofetil on kidney graft function and body weight in patients with chronic allograft nephropathy. *Transplant Proc,* 36, 10, 2974-2978.

[39] Grenda R.; Wühl E.; Litwin M.; Janas R.; Sladowska J.; Arbeiter K.; Berg U.; Caldas-Afonso A.; Fischbach M.; Mehls O.; Sallay P.; Schaefer F.; ESCAPE Trial group. (2007).

Urinary excretion of endothelin-1 (ET-1), transforming growth factor-β1 (TGF-β1) and vascular endothelial growth factor (VEGF165) in paediatric chronic kidney diseases: results of the ESCAPE trial. *Nephrol Dial Transplant,* 22, 3487-3494.

[40] Guder WG. (2008). Clinical role of urinary low molecular weight proteins: their diagnostic and prognostic implications. *Scand J Clin Lab Invest,* Suppl, 241, 95-98.

[41] Gueler F.; Rong S.; Mengel M.; Park JK.; Kiyan J.; Kirsch T.; Dumler I.; Haller H.; Shushakova N. (2008). Renal urokinase-type plasminogen activator (uPA) receptor but not uPA deficiency strongly attenuates ischemia reperfusion injury and acute kidney allograft rejection. *J Immunol,* 15, 181, 2, 1179-1189.

[42] Gwinner W. (2007). Renal transplant rejection markers. *World J Urol,* 25, 5, 445-455.

[43] Halawa A. (2011). The early diagnosis of acute renal graft dysfunction: a challenge we face. The role of novel biomarkers. *Ann Transplant,* 16, 1, 90-98.

[44] Halbesma N.; Kuiken DS.; Brantsma AH.; Bakker SJ.; Wetzels JF.; De Zeeuw D.; De Jong PE.; Gansevoort RT. (2006). Macroalbuminuria is a better risk marker than low estimated GFR to identify individuals at risk for accelerated GFR loss in population screening. *J Am Soc Nephrol,* 17, 9, 2582-2590.

[45] Hall IE., Parikh CR. (2010). Human models to evaluate urinary biomarkers of kidney injury. *Clin J Am Soc Nephrol,* 5, 12, 2141-2143.

[46] Han WK.; Bailly V.; Abichandani R.; Bailly V.; Abichandani R.; Thadhani R.; Bonventre JV. (2002). Kidney injury molecule-1 (KIM-1): a novel biomarker for human renal proximal tubule injury. *Kidney Int,* 62, 1, 237-244.

[47] Haraldsson B.; Sörensson J. (2004). Why do we not all have proteinuria? An update of our current understanding of the glomerular barrier. *News Physiol Sci,* 19, 7-10.

[48] Hayes DF.; Bast RC.; Desch CE.; Fritsche HJr.; Kemeny NE.; Jessup JM.; Locker GY.; Macdonald, JS.; Mennel RG.; Norton L.; Ravdin P.; Taube S.; Winn RJ. (1996). Tumor marker utility grading system: a framework to evaluate clinical utility of tumor markers. *J Natl Cancer Inst,* 88, 20, 1456-1466.

[49] Herget-Rosenthal S.; Feldkamp T.; Volbracht L.; Kribben A. (2004). Measurement of urinary cystatin C by particle-enhanced nephelometric immunoassay: precision, interferences, stability and reference range. *Ann Clin Biochem,* 41, 111-118.

[50] Ho J.; Rush DN.; Gibson IW.; Karpinski M.; Storsley L.; Bestland J.; Stefura W.; HayGlass KT.; Nickerson PW. (2010). Early urinary CCL2 is associated with the later development of interstitial fibrosis and tubular atrophy in renal allografts. *Transplantation,* 90, 4, 394-400.

[51] Ho J., Rush DN.; Karpinski M.; Storsley L.; Gibson IW., Bestland J.; Gao A.; Stefura W.; HayGlass KT.; Nickerson PW. (2011). Validation of urinary CXCL10 as a marker of borderline, subclinical, and clinical tubulitis. *Transplantation,* 92, 8, 878-882.

[52] Holdt–Lehmann B.; Lehmann A.; Korten G.; Nagel HR.; Nizze H.; Schuff–Werner P. (2000). Diagnostic value of urinary alanine aminopeptidase and N-acetyl- ß –D-glucosaminidase in comparison to α1–microglobulin as a marker in evaluating tubular dysfunction in glomerulonephritis patients. *Clin Chim Acta,* 297, 93–102.

[53] Hollmen ME.; Kyllönen LE.; Inkinen KA.; Lalla ML.; Merenmies J.; Salmela KT. (2011). Deceased donor neutrophil gelatinase-associated lipocalin and delayed graft function after kidney transplantation: a prospective study. *Crit Care,* 15, 3, R121.

[54] Holmquist P & Torffvit O. (2008). Tubular function in diabetic children assessed by Tamm-Horsfall protein and glutathione S-transferase. *Pediatr Nephrol,* 23, 7, 1079–1083.

[55] Hu H.; Kwun J.; Aizenstein BD.; Knechtle SJ. (2009). Noninvasive detection of acute and chronic injuries in human renal transplant by elevation of multiple cytokines/ chemokines in urine. *Transplantation,* 87, 12, 1814-1820.

[56] Hu X.; Ren L.; Yin H.; Zhang X. (2010). Signal transducer and activator of transcription 1 and matrix metalloproteinase 3 genetic expression and clinical significance on urothelial tumors after renal transplantation. *Transplant Proc,* 42, 7, 2534-2537.

[57] Hull RP.; Goldsmith DJ. (2008). Nephrotic syndrome in adults. *BMJ,* 336,7654,1185-1189

[58] Iglesias JH., Richard GA. (1994). Urinary adenosine deaminase binding protein as a predictor of renal transplant rejection in children. *Transplant Proc,* 26, 1, 75-76.

[59] Jackson JA.; Kim EJ.; Begley B.; Cheeseman J.; Harden T.; Perez SD.; Thomas S.; Warshaw B.; Kirk AD. (2011). Urinary chemokines CXCL9 and CXCL10 are noninvasive markers of renal allograft rejection and BK viral infection. *Am J Transplant,* 11, 10, 2228-2234.

[60] Jászai J.; Farkas LM.; Fargeas CA.; Janich P.; Haase M.; Huttner WB.; Corbeil D. (2010). Prominin-2 is a novel marker of distal tubules and collecting ducts of the human and murine kidney. *Histochem Cell Biol,* 133, 5, 527-539.

[61] Johnston O.; Cassidy H.; O'Connell S.; O'Riordan A.; Gallagher W.; Maguire PB.; Wynne K.; Cagney G.; Ryan MP.; Conlon PJ.; McMorrow T. (2011). Identification of β2-microglobulin as a urinary biomarker for chronic allograft nephropathy using proteomic methods. *Proteomics Clin Appl,* 5, 7-8, 422-431.

[62] Jung K.; Diego J.; Strobelt V.; Scholz D.; Schreiber G. (1986). Diagnostic significance of some urinary enzymes for detecting acute rejection crises in renal-transplant recipients: alanine aminopeptidase, alkaline phosphatase, gamma-glutamyltransferase, N-acetyl-β-D-glucosaminidase and lysozyme. *Clin Chem,* 32, 18071811.

[63] Kang NR.; Lee JE.; Huh W.; Kim SJ.; Kim YG.; Kim DJ.; Oh HY. (2009). Minimal proteinuria one year after transplant is a risk factor for graft survival in kidney transplantation. *J Korean Med Sci,* 24,Suppl 1, S129–S134.

[64] Katsurada A.; Hagiwara Y.; Miyashita K.; Satou R.; Miyata K.; Ohashi N.; Navar LG.; Kobori H. (2007). Novel sandwich ELISA for human angiotensinogen. *Am J Physiol Renal Physiol,* 293, F956-F960.

[65] Koga S.; Kapoor A.; Novick A.; Toma H.; Fairchild R. (2000). RANTES is produced by CD8+ T cells during acute rejection of skin grafts. *Transplant Proc,* 32, 4, 796-797.

[66] Kotanko P.; Margreiter R.; Pfaller W. (1997). Graft ischemia correlates with urinary excretion of the proximal marker enzyme fructose-1,6-bisphosphatase in human kidney transplantation. *Nephron,* 77, 1, 62-67.

[67] Kotanko P.; Keiler R.; Knabl L.; Aulitzky W.; Margreiter R.; Gstraunthaler G.; Pfaller W. (1986). Urinary enzyme analysis in renal allograft transplantation. *Clin Chim Acta,* 31, 160, 2, 137-144.

[68] Krimkevich EI. (1990). The kallikrein-kinin system of allogeneic renal transplant. *Fiziol Zh,* 36, 6, 100-104.

[69] Kuźniar J.; Marchewka Z.; Krasnowski R.; Boratyńska M.; Długosz A.; Klinger M. (2006). Enzymuria and low molecular weight protein excretion as the differentiating marker of complications in the early post kidney transplantation period. *Int Urol Nephrol,* 38, 3-4, 753-758.

[70] Kwiatkowska E.; Kędzierska K.; Bober J.; Dołęgowska B.; Dziedziejko V.; Gołembiewska E.; Ciechanowski K.; Wiśniewska M. (2010). Urinary hepatocyte growth factor indicates ischemia/reperfusion injury after kidney transplantation. *Pol Arch Med Wewn,* 120, 11, 437-442.

[71] Lederer SR.; Friedrich N.; Regenbogen C.; Getto R.; Toepfer M.; Sitter T. (2003). Non-invasive monitoring of renal transplant recipients: urinary excretion of soluble adhesion molecules and of the complement-split product C4d. *Nephron Clin Pract,* 94, 1, c19-c26.

[72] Ling XB.; Sigdel TK.; Lau K.; Ying L.; Lau I.; Schilling J.; Sarwal MM. (2010). Integrative urinary peptidomics in renal transplantation identifies biomarkers for acute rejection. *J Am Soc Nephrol,* 21, 4, 646-653.

[73] Liangos O.; Perianayagam MC.; Vaidya VS.; Han WK.; Wald R.; Tighiouart H.; MacKinnon RW.; Li L.; Balakrishnan VS.; Pereira BJ.; Bonventre JV.; Jaber BL. (2007). Urinary N-acetyl-ß-(D)-glucosaminidase activity and kidney injury molecule-1 level are associated with adverse outcomes in acute renal failure. *J Am Soc Nephrol,* 18, 904–912.

[74] Lisowska-Myjak B. (2010). Serum and urinary biomarkers of acute kidney injury. *Blood Purif,* 29, 4, 357-365.

[75] Locker GY.; Hamilton S.; Harris J.; Jessup JM.; Kemeny N.; Mac Donald JS.; Sommerfield MR.; Hayes DF.; Bast RCJr.; ASCO. (2006). ASCO 2006 update of recommenda-

tions for the use of tumor markers in gastrointrestinal cancer. *J Clin Oncol,* 2433, 5319-5327.

[76] Loriga G.; Ciccarese M.; Pala PG.; Satta RP.; Fanelli V.; Manca ML.; Serra G.; Dessole P.; Cossu M. (2010). De novo everolimus-based therapy in renal transplant recipients: effect on proteinuria and renal prognosis. *Transplant Proc,* 42, 4, 1297-1302.

[77] Luke RG. (1999). Hypertensive nephrosclerosis: pathogenesis and prevalence. *Nephrol Dial Transplant,* 14, 2271-2278.

[78] Manucha W.; Vallés P. (1999). Effect of glandular kallikrein on distal bicarbonate transport. Role of basolateral Cl-/HCO3- exchanger and vacuolar H(+)-ATPase. *Biocel,* 23, 3, 1, 61-70.

[79] Matsuda R.; Kaneko N.; Horikawa Y.; Chiwaki F.; Shinozaki M.; Abe S.; Yumura W.; Nihei H.; Ieiri T. (2000). Measurement of urinary annexin V by ELISA and its significance as a new urinary-marker of kidney disease. *Clin Chim Acta,* 2000; 298: 29–43.

[80] Mazanowska O.; Kamińska D.; Krajewska M.; Zabińska M.; Kopeć W.; Boratyńska M.; Chudoba, P.; Patrzalek D.; Klinger M. (2011). Imbalance of metallaproteinase/tissue inhibitors of metalloproteinase system in renal transplant recipients with chronic allograft injury. *Transplant Proc,* 43, 8, 3000-3003.

[81] Melnikov VY.; Molitoris BA. (2008). Improvements in the diagnosis of acute kidney injury. *Saudi J Kidney Dis Transplant,* 19, 537-544.

[82] Metzger J.; Chatzikyrkou C.; Broecker V.; Schiffer E.; Jaensch L.; Iphoefer A.; Mengel M.; Mullen W.; Mischak H.; Haller H.; Gwinner W. (2011). Diagnosis of subclinical and clinical acute T-cell-mediated rejection in renal transplant patients by urinary proteom analysis. *Proteomics Clin App,* 5, 5-6, 322-333.

[83] Metzger J.; Kirsch T.; Schiffer E.; Ulger P.; Mentes E.; Brand K.; Weissinger EM.; Haubitz M.; Mischak H.; Herget-Rosenthal S. (2010). Urinary excretion of twenty peptides forms an early and accurate diagnostic pattern of acute kidney injury. *Kidney Int,* 78, 12, 1252-1262.

[84] Mishra J.; Ma Q.; Prada A.; Mitsnefes M.; Zahedi K.; Yang J.; Barasch J.; Devarajan P. (2003). Identification of neutrophil gelatinase-associated lipocalin as a novel early urinary biomarker for ischemic renal injury. *J Am Soc Nephrol,* 2003, 14, 2534-2543.

[85] Molls RR.; Savransky V.; Liu M.; Bevans S.; Mehta T.; Tuder RM.; King LS.; Rabb H. (2006). Keratinocyte-derived chemokine is an early biomarker of ischemic acute kidney injury. *Am J Physiol Renal Physiol,* 290, F1187-F1193.

[86] Mori K.; Nakao K. (2007). Neutrophil gelatinase-associated lipocalin as the real-time indicator of active kidney damage. *Kidney Int,* 71, 10, 967-970.

[87] Morita Y.; Ikeguchi H.; Nakamura J.; Hotta N.; Yuzawa Y.; Matsuo S. (2000). Complement activation products in the urine from proteinuric patients. *J Am Soc Nephrol,* 11, 700-707.

[88] Müller TF.; Kraus M.; Neumann C.; Lange H. (1997). Detection of renal allograft rejection by complement components C5A and TCC in plasma and urine. *J Lab Clin Med,* 129, 1, 62-71.

[89] Nauta FL.; Bakker SJ.; van Oeveren W.; Navis G.; van der Heide JJ.; van Goor H.; de Jong PE.; Gansevoort RT. (2011). Albuminuria, proteinuria, and novel urine biomarkers as predictors of long-term allograft outcomes in kidney transplant recipients. *Am J Kidney Dis,* 57, 5, 733-743.

[90] Nickolas TL.; Barasch, J.; Devarajan P. (2008). Biomarkers in acute and chronic kidney disease. *Curr Opin Nephrol Hypertens,* 17, 127-132.

[91] Oberbauer R. (2008). Biomarkers-a potential route for improved diagnosis and management of ongoing renal damage. *Transplant Proc,* 40, 10 Suppl, S44-S47.

[92] Ofstad J.; Iversen BM. (2005). Glomerular and tubular damage in normotensive and hypertensive rats. *Am J Physiol Renal Physiol,* 288, F665–F672.

[93] Parikh CR.; Abraham E.; Ancukiewicz M.; Edelstein CL. (2005). Urine Il-18 is an early diagnostic marker for acute kidney injury and predicts mortality in the intensive care unit. *J Am Soc Nephrol,* 16, 10, 3046-3052.

[94] Peng W.; Chen J.; Jiang Y.; Wu J.; Shou Z.; He Q.; Wang Y.; Chen Y.; Wang H. (2008). Urinary fractalkine is a marker of acute rejection. *Kidney Int,* 74, 11, 1454-1460.

[95] Polak WP.; Kosieradzki M.; Kwiatkowski A.; Danielewicz R.; Lisik W.; Michalak G.; Paczek L.; Lao M.; Wałaszewski J.; Rowiński WA. (1999). Activity of glutathione S-transferases in the urine of kidney transplant recipients during the first week after transplantation. *Ann Transplant,* 4, 1, 42-45.

[96] Przybylowski P.; Koc-Zorawska E.; Malyszko JS.; Kozlowska S.; Mysliwiec M.; Malyszko J. (2011). Liver fatty-acid-binding protein in heart and kidney allograft recipients in relation to kidney function. *Transplant Proc,* 43, 8, 3064-3067.

[97] Ramesh G.; Kwon O.; Ahn K. (2010). Netrin-1: a novel universal biomarker of human kidney injury. *Transplant Proc,* 42, 5, 1519-1522.

[98] Refaie MO.; Abo-Zaid H.; Gomma NA.; Aboul-Enein HY. (2000). Determination of urinary and serum beta-glucuronidase and alkaline phosphatase in various renal disease and kidney rejection transplanted patients. *Prep Biochem Biotechnol,* 30, 2, 93-106.

[99] Reinhold SW.; Straub RH.; Krüger B.; Kaess B.; Bergler T.; Weingart C.; Banas MC.; Krämer BK.; Banas B. (2012). Elevated urinary sVCAM-1, IL6, sIL6R and TNFR1 concentrations indicate acute kidney transplant rejection in the first 2weeks after transplantation. *Cytokine,* 57, 3, 379-388.

[100] Remuzzi G.; Benigni A.; Remuzzi A. (2006). Mechanisms of progression and regression of renal lesions of chronic nephropathies and diabetes. *J Clin Invest,* 116, 288–296.

[101] Rodrigues-Garcia MI.; Fernandez JA.; Rodrigues A. (1996). Annexin V autoantibodies in rheumatoid arthritis. *Ann Rheum Dis,* 55, 895-900.

[102] Ruggenenti P.; Remuzzi G. (2006). Time to abandon microalbuminuria? *Kidney Int,* 70, 1214-1222.

[103] Sánchez-Escuredo A.; Pastor MC.; Bayés B.; Morales-Indiano C.; Troya M.; Dolade M.; Jimenez JA.; Romero R.; Lauzurica R. (2010). Inflammation, metalloproteinases, and growth factors in the development of carotid atherosclerosis in renal transplant patients. *Transplant Proc,* 42, 8, 2905-2907.

[104] Sancho Calabuig A.; Pallardó Mateu LM.; Avila Bernabeu AI.; Gavela Martínez E.; Beltrán Catalán S.; Crespo Albiach JF. (2009). Very low-grade proteinuria at 3 months posttransplantation is an earlier marker of graft survival. *Transplant Proc,* 41, 6, 2122-2125.

[105] Santos C.; Marcelino P.; Carvalho T.; Coelho J.; Bispo M.; Mourão L.; Perdigoto R.; Barroso E. (2010). The value of tubular enzymes for early detection of acute kidney injury after liver transplantation: an observational study. *Transplant Proc,* 42, 9, 363936-363943.

[106] Saurina A.; Campistol JM.; Lario S.; Oppenheimer F.; Diekmann F. (2007). Conversion from calcineurin inhibitors to sirolimus in kidney transplant patients reduces the urinary transforming growth factor-beta1 concentration. *Transplant Proc,* 39, 7, 2138-2141.

[107] Schaub S.; Nickerson P.; Rush D.; Mayr M.; Hess C.; Golian M.; Stefura W.; Hayglass K. (2009). Urinary CXCL9 and CXCL10 levels correlate with the extent of subclinical tubulitis. *Am J Transplant,* 9, 6, 1347-1353.

[108] Schnaper HW.; Hayashida T.; Hubchak SC.; Poncelet AC. (2003). TGF-β signal transduction and mesangial cell fibrogenesis. *Am J Physiol Renal Physiol,* 284, F243-F252.

[109] Schuck O.; Teplan V.; Sibova J.; Stollova M. (2004). Predicting the glomerular filtration rate from serum creatinine, serum cystatin C and the Cockcroft and Gault formula with regard to drug dosage adjustment; *Int J Clin Pharmacol Ther,* 42, 2, 93–97.

[110] Scian MJ.; Maluf DG.; David KG.; Archer KJ.; Suh JL.; Wolen AR.; Mba MU.; Massey HD.; King AL.; Gehr T.; Cotterell A.; Posner M.; Mas V. (2011). MicroRNA profiles in allograft tissues and paired urines associate with chronic allograft dysfunction with IF/TA. *Am J Transplant,* 11, 10, 2110-2122.

[111] Sheerin NS.; Risley P.; Abe K.; Tang Z.; Wong W.; Lin T.; Sacks SH. (2008). Synthesis of complement protein C3 in the kidney is an important mediator of local tissue injury. *FASEB J,* 22, 4, 1065-1072.

[112] Simić-Ogrizović S.; Djukanović Lj.; Golubović M.; Dimitrijević Z.; Mimić-Oka J.; Simić T. (1994). Significance of laboratory tests for differential diagnosis of acute renal

allograft rejection and acute cyclosporine nephrotoxicity. *Srp Arh Celok Lek,* 122, 5-6, 133-136.

[113] Slowinski T.; Subkowski T.; Diehr P.; Bachert D.; Fritsche L.; Neumayer HH.; Hocher B. (2002). Interaction of the endothelin system and calcineurin inhibitors after kidney transplantation. *Clin Sci (Lond),* 103, Suppl 48, 396S-398S.

[114] Srivastava M.; Eidelman O.; Torosyan Y.; Jozwik C.; Mannon RB.; Pollard HB. (2011). Elevated expression levels of ANXA11, integrins β3 and α3, and TNF-α contribute to a candidate proteomic signature in urine for kidney allograft rejection. *Proteomics Clin Appl,* 5, 5-6, 311-321.

[115] Szeto CC.; Kwan BC.; Lai KB.; Lai FM.; Chow KM.; Wang G.; Luk CC.; Li PK. (2010). Urinary expression of kidney injury markers in renal transplant recipients. *Clin J Am Soc Nephrol,* 5, 12, 2329-2337.

[116] Takahashi T.; Yoshida K.; Nakame Y.; Saitoh H. (1989). Study on urinary beta-glucuronidase and alkaline phosphatase activities as indicators of CDDP renal toxicity. *Hinyokika Kiyo,* 35, 1, 1-6.

[117] Tataranni G.; Zavagli G.; Farinelli R.; Malacarne F.; Fiocchi O.; Nunzi L.; Scaramuzzo P.; Scorrano R. (1992). Usefulness of the assessment of urinary enzymes and microproteins in monitoring ciclosporin nephrotoxicity. *Nephron,* 60, 3, 314-318.

[118] Teppo AM.; Honkanen E.; Finne P.; Törnroth T.; Grönhagen-Riska CP. (2004). Increased urinary excretion of alpha1-microglobulin at 6 months after transplantation is associated with urinary excretion of transforming growth factor-beta1 and indicates poor long-term renal outcome. *Transplantation,* 15, 78, 5, 719-724.

[119] Thongboonkerd V.; Malasit P. (2005). Renal and urinary proteomics: current applications and challenges. *Proteomics,* 5 ,4, 1033-1042.

[120] Ting YT.; Coates PT.; Walker RJ.; McLellan AD. (2012). Urinary tubular biomarkers as potential early predictors of renal allograft rejection. *Nephrology (Carlton),* 17, 1, 11-16.

[121] Tonomura Y.; Tsuchiya N.; Torii M.; Uehara T. (2010). Evaluation of the usefulness of urinary biomarkers for nephrotoxicity in rats. *Toxicology,* 29, 273, 1-3, 53-59.

[122] Trof RJ.; Di Maggio F.; Leemreis J.; Groeneveld AB. (2006). Biomarkers of acute renal injury and renal failure. *Shock,* 26, 3, 245-253,

[123] Tryggvason K.; Pettersson E. (2003). Causes and consequences of proteinuria: the kidney filtration barrier and progressive renal failure. *J Intern Med,* 254, 216-224.

[124] Uchida K.; Gotoh, A. (2002). Measurement of cystatin –C and creatinine in urine. *Clin Chim Acta,* 323, 1-2, 121-128.

[125] Urbschat A.; Obermüller N.; Haferkamp A. (2011). Biomarkers of kidney injury. *Biomarkers,* 16 Suppl 1, S22-S30.

[126] van Ham SM.; Heutinck KM.; Jorritsma T.; Bemelman FJ.; Strik MC.; Vos W.; Muris, JJ.; Florquin S.; Ten Berge IJ.; Rowshani AT. (2010). Urinary granzyme A mRNA is a

biomarker to diagnose subclinical and acute cellular rejection in kidney transplant recipients. *Kidney Int,* 78, 10, 1033-1040.

[127] van Ree RM.; Oterdoom LH.; de Vries AP.; Homan van der Heide JJ.; van Son WJ.; Navis G.; Gans RO.; Bakker SJ. (2008). Circulating markers of endothelial dysfunction interact with proteinuria in predicting mortality in renal transplant recipients. *Transplantation,* 27, 86, 12, 1713-1719.

[128] Viedt C.; Orth, S. (2002). Monocyte chemoattractant protein-1 (MCP-1) in the kidney: does it more than simply attract monocytes? *Nephrol Dial Transplant,* 17, 2043-2047.

[129] Waanders F.; van Timmeren MM.; Stegeman CA.; Bakker SJ.; van Goor H. (2010). Kidney injury molecule-1 in renal disease. *J Pathol,* 220, 1, 7-16.

[130] Westhuyzen J.; Endre ZH.; Reece G.;Reith DM.; Saltissi D.; Morgan TJ. (2003). Measurement of tubular enzymuria facilitates early detection of acute renal impairment in the intensive care unit. *Nephrol Dial Transplant,* 18, 543–551.

[131] Wishart DS. (2006). Metabolomics in monitoring kidney transplants. *Curr Opin Nephrol Hyperten,* 15, 6, 637-642.

[132] Woltman AM.; de Fijter JW.; van der Kooij SW.; Jie KE.; Massacrier C.; Caux C.; Daha MR.; van Kooten C. (2005). MIP-3alpha/CCL20 in renal transplantation and its possible involvement as dendritic cell chemoattractant in allograft rejection. *Am J Transplant,* 5, 9, 2114-2125.

[133] Yamamoto T.; Nakagawa T.; Suzuki H.; Ohashi N.; Fukasawa H.; Fujigaki Y.; Kato A.; Nakamura, Y.; Suzuki F.; Hishida A. (2007). Urinary angiotensinogen as a marker of intrarenal angiotensin II activity associated with deterioration of renal function in patients with chronic kidney disease. *J Am Soc Nephrol,* 18, 1558-1565.

[134] Yannaraki M.; Rebibou JM.; Ducloux D.; Saas P.; Duperrier A.; Felix S.; Rifle G.; Chalopin JM.; Hervé P.; Tiberghien P.; Ferrand C. (2006). Urinary cytotoxic molecular markers for a noninvasive diagnosis in acute renal transplant rejection. *Transpl Int,* 19, 9, 759-768.

[135] Yue L.; Xia Q.; Luo GH.; Lu YP. (2010). Urinary connective tissue growth factor is a biomarker in a rat model of chronic nephropathy. *Transplant Proc,* 42, 5, 1875-1880.

[136] Zoja C., Morigi M.; Remuzzi G. (2003). Proteinuria and phenotypic change of proximal tubular cells. *J Am Soc Nephrol,* 14, S36–S41.

[137] Zynek-Litwin M.; Kuzniar J.; Marchewka Z.; Kopec W.; Kusztal M.; Patrzalek D.; Biecek P.; Klinger M. (2010). Plasma and urine leukocyte elastase-alpha1protease inhibitor complex as a marker of early and long-term kidney graft function. *Nephrol Dial Transplant,* 25, 7, 2346-2351.

Chapter 4

Non-Invasive Diagnosis of Acute Renal Allograft Rejection – Special Focus on Gamma Scintigraphy and Positron Emission Tomography

Alexander Grabner, Dominik Kentrup,
Uta Schnöckel, Michael Schäfers and Stefan Reuter

Additional information is available at the end of the chapter

http://dx.doi.org/10.5772/54737

1. Introduction

The number of patients treated for end-stage renal failure continuously increases. Because treatment alternatives are limited and transplants are often the first therapeutic choice, the numbers of patients joining the waiting lists in countries world-wide rises. At present transplantation medicine is one of the most progressive fields of medicine. Gradually the "half-life" of renal transplants improved and the five years survival rate ranges now above 80% [1;2]. Despite of the advances made within the last decades, acute rejection (AR) is still a risk for graft survival. The incidence of rejection episodes depends on several factors, e.g., the organ (status), co-morbidities, medication and compliance. Thus, in different situations the incidence of AR varies between 13-53% in the first year after transplantation [3], and, in most cases, cellular and humoral immunity mediated rejections can be distinguished. Usually, AR proceeds substantially as an acute cellular rejection whereas humoral rejection comprises only a smaller proportion of AR [4]. Every single episode of an AR is a negative prognostic factor, increasing the risk for development of chronic allograft deterioration and worsening long-term graft survival [5;6]. Interestingly, the impact of AR on chronic renal allograft failure as the main cause for death-censored graft-loss after kidney transplantation increases, whereas the severity of the episode itself is an independent risk factor [7-9]. Therefore, early detection and rapid and effective treatment of AR are essential to preserve graft`s function. Clinically established screening methods such as elevated serum creatinine, occurrence or aggravation of proteinuria, oliguria, hypertension, graft tenderness, or peripheral edema, often lack the desired sensitivity and specificity for early diagnoses of AR. Hence,a compelling need for high sensitive and specific detection of early AR exists, with core needle biopsy still being the "gold-standard" in rejection diagnostics. However, biopsy as an invasive procedure is cumbersome to the patient, carries the risk of graft injury, and cannot be applied in patients taking anticoagulant drugs. Additionally, the sampling site is small and one might miss AR, i.e., when rejection is focal or patchy. Thus, in diagnostics, non-invasive image-based methods visualizing the whole graft would be superior.

Allograft rejection is the result of interactions between the recipient`s innate and adaptive immune system and the graft antigens serving as a target. Cytotoxic T lymphocytes (CTLs) are central effectors within AR whereas B cells and parts of the congenital immunosystem such as the complement system, monocytes/macrophages, neutrophilic granulocytes, and dendritic cells, have their share, too [4;10]. By recognition of their donor antigen CTLs are activated, undergo clonal expansion and differentiation into effector cells. Subsequently, they migrate into the transplant initiating its destruction [4;10;11]. Before CTLs reach the graft parenchyma, they have to pass the vascular endothelium. This extravasation is mediated by chemoattractant cytokines/chemokines. Chemokines induce the expression of vascular adhesion molecules allowing leukocytes to roll, adhere, and transmigrate into the parenchyma [12]. CTLs destroy their targets through the release of perforin and granzyme or by initiation of the Fas/FasL pathway inducing cell death by triggering the inherent caspase-mediated apoptotic response or caspase-independent cell death [13]. These two cell death-inducing strategies account for almost all contact-dependent target kills. However, activated CTLs can release additional cytokines, such as tumor-necrosis factor and interferon causing apoptosis or necrosis upon secretion [11,13]. Moreover, inflammatory edema and micro thrombi / hemorrhage caused by damaged endothelium add ischemia-dependent hypoxic damage to the graft [11]. All of these single, simplified processes sum up and promote allograft dysfunction. However, if they are characterized at least in part, they can be addressed by different imaging technologies discussed in the following.

2. Ultrasound

Standard care in detection of AR includes (Doppler-) ultrasound examination. Typical ultrasound findings in cases of AR are rejection-related graft enlargement (swelling, more globular shape), reduction of corticomedullary differentiation, increased echogenicity, prominent medullary pyramids, or irregularities in the graft perfusion (reversed plateau of diastolic flow), but its specificity and sensitivity for AR is limited, even when echo enhancers are applied [14;15]. Elevated resistance indices can occur in the presence of acute as well as chronic rejection. However, values lower than 0.8 are expected and usually values above 0.8 indicate increased intrarenal pressure as it occurs for example in acute tubular necrosis (ATN) or AR and is linked to a poor longterm renal allograft function [16-18]. Notably, sensitivity and reliability of this method mainly depend on the investigators experience. A comprehensive overview of "What ultrasound can do and cannot do" in diagnostics of renal transplant pathologies was published by Cosgrove and Chan [16]. Using contrast agent or targeted ultrasound in the future, this method might offer significant potential, whereas at present studies are at best at experimental stage and are completely lacking in patients with renal AR.

3. Computed tomography

Computed tomography (CT) is commonly available, technology and techniques as well as the applied contrast media constantly improve. CT contrast agents allow accurate evaluation of parenchymal, perirenal, renal sinus, pyeloureteral and vascular diseases in renal transplantation in great detail and at lower costs than by magnetic resonance (MR) imaging. Information gathered by CT indicating AR are loss of corticomedullary differentiation, decreased graft enhancement, and delayed or absent contrast excretion [19]. However, this information is rather unspecific and the contrast media used still are nephrotoxic. Thus, at present CT has no role in diagnostics of renal AR.

4. Magnetic resonance imaging

Kalb *et al.* provide a recent overview about MR-based approaches for functional and structural evaluations of renal grafts including a section on diagnostics of AR [20]. Beside exact anatomical information, MR can assess different aspects of renal function. Typical MR findings occurring in AR are enlargement of the graft (due to edema) with loss of corticomedullary differentiation and elevated cortical relative signal. There might be edema of and surrounding the kidney and the ureter. The high spatial and temporal resolution of MR allows perfusion imaging which might be useful to distinguish AR from ATN. 3D gradient echo perfusion imaging might show enhancement of the cortex and markedly delayed excretion of contrast [20]. Recent research with blood-oxygen level-dependent (BOLD) MR was promising for differentiating AR from ATN and a normal functioning kidney [21,22]. Furthermore, MR renography has been applied for diagnosis of the cause of acute dysfunction after kidney transplantation [23,24]. These two studies rely on quantitative evaluation of the shape of the renal enhancement curve to diagnose acute dysfunction. One can observe delayed and lower medullary enhancement in ATN whereas cortical and medullary enhancement curves decrease in AR. However, further studies verifying the results are needed and still some issues about gadolinium-containing contrast agents and nephrogenic systemic fibrosis and gadolinium nephrotoxicity need to be resolved. More recently, Yamamoto *et al.* proposed a new quantitative analysis method of MR renography, including a multicompartmental tracer kinetic renal model for diagnosis of AR and ATN, but state in their paper that findings in patients with normal graft function, AR, and ATN showed a substantial overlap with those of the normal population [25]. Another strategy followed was imaging of macrophage infiltration with ultrasmall superparamagnetic iron oxide particles [26]. Grafts with AR showed significant accumulation of iron particles but only within a time frame of 72 h which is much too late for potential clinical application.

5. Single photon (gamma) imaging and positron emission tomography

Because gamma camera/ single photon emission computer tomography (SPECT) and positron emission tomography (PET) offer high intrinsic activity, excellent tissue penetration (depending on the tracer), cover the whole organ/ body, are relatively independent of the experience of the investigator and provide a huge variety of clinically tested molecular imaging agents/ tracer, SPECT and PET-based approaches for the detection of renal AR are discussed in the following [27;28]. Steps of AR addressed by SPECT or PET-based approaches include recruitment of activated leukocytes into the transplant with consecutive cytokine release, cell death, edema, hypoxia and loss of function.

A comprehensive overview of the studies performed is provided in Table 1.

SPECT				
Target	**Molecular Marker**	**Graft/Organ**	**Species**	**References**
Fibrin thrombi	^{99m}Tc-Sulfur Colloid	Kidney	Human, dog	[64;65]
Proximal tubule uptake	^{99m}Tc-DMSA	Kidney	Human	[66;67]
Renal uptake and excretion	^{99m}Tc-MAG3	Kidney	Human	[68]
Renal perfusion and filtration	^{99m}Tc-pentetate (DTPA)	Kidney	Human	[69;70]
Leukocytes	^{99m}Tc-OKT3	Kidney	Human	[40]
Inflammation	^{99m}Tc- Leukocytes	Kidney	Human	[39]
	^{67}Ga citrate	Kidney	Human	[64;65]
Renal function	^{131}I-OIH	Kidney	Human	[71]
PET				
Metabolism/Inflammation	^{18}F-FDG	Kidney	Rat	[43;44]
Leukocytes	^{18}F-FDG-Leukocytes	Kidney	Rat	*In press*

A Medline literature search by PubMed was performed to select papers in which AR and SPECT/PET play any role. The search period was set from 1970 to July 2012. We used ("Acute renal or kidney rejection" and "positron emission tomography (PET)" or "single photon gamma imaging (SPECT)" or "molecular imaging") as search query. Only papers with an English abstract have been included.

Table 1. Results of literature analysis: SPECT/PET-based diagnosis of renal AR.

5.1. Inflammation

Sterile inflammation is central to the rejection process. Hence, it seems logically to assess inflammatory targets for the diagnosis of AR. In inflammation imaging, one can focus on target mechanisms such as measurement of the metabolic activity (i.e. with the "classical" tracer ^{18}F-fluordesoxyglucose (FDG)), binding to cytokines/chemokines (receptors), assessment of physically trapped tracers in the inflammatory edema, or using leukocytes. Recently, Signore *et al.* published an excellent review on imaging of inflammation discussing different techniques, targets, and approaches [27].

5.2. Vascular adhesion molecules

AR is associated with the expression of cell adhesion molecules like vascular cell adhesion molecule 1 (VCAM-1), intercellular adhesion molecule 1 (ICAM-1), carcinoembryonic antigen-related cell adhesion molecule 1 (CEACAM1), LFA-1 (lymphocyte function-associated antigen-1, and endothelial leukocyte adhesion molecule (E-selectin) on the endothelium of organs undergoing rejection. They are "essentially needed" for the adherence and transmigration of leukocytes into the parenchyma. Because radiolabeled antibodies exist for some of these easily accessible vascular targets, they can be addressed by noninvasive imaging. However, data regarding adhesion markers in SPECT/PET-based imaging are rare and have not been transferred to renal AR imaging yet.

5.3. Imaging using *ex vivo* radiolabeled leukocytes

Because recruitment and activation of inflammatory cells, i.e. lymphocytes, is crucial to AR, efforts have been made to image infiltration by means of labeled leukocytes. Application of *ex vivo* radiolabeled leukocytes is clinically well established particularly in the diagnostic workup of infectious disorders without a focus. Hitherto, white blood cells (WBC) are labeled using for instance ^{99m}Tc-HMPAO or ^{111}In-oxine for SPECT and ^{18}F-FDG or ^{64}Cu for PET analysis, respectively [29]. These cells are considered to accumulate highly specific in inflamed tissues [30-33].

After injection of labeled leukocytes a typical distribution pattern can be observed. First, cells shortly accumulate in the lungs and then continuously migrate from the blood pool into spleen, liver, and bonemarrow, the so called reticulo-endothelial system, and certainly in inflamed sites [34-36]. After endothelial adhesion, labeled leukocytes migrate through the vessel`s wall to the focus of inflammation providing a typical radioactivity pattern indicating infiltration. For instance, Forstrom *et al.* have shown that ^{18}F-FDG labeled leukocytes exhibit comparable distribution patterns in normal human subjects compared with ^{111}In or ^{99m}Tc-labeled WBC [37]. Although ^{18}F-FDG seems to exhibit the lowest labeling stability when compared to ^{111}In and ^{64}Cu only neglectible free ^{18}F-FDG uptake can be observed [37]. However, labeling stability is relevant in order to assure that assessed activity refers to accumulation of labeled leukocytes and not to the unlabeled tracer only. Since half-life time of ^{18}F-FDG is 109 min, longtime stability of ^{18}F-FDG labeled leukocytes for clinical analysis is not of interest. However, if longtime stability is of interest this could be addressed using other tracers like ^{99m}Tc with a half life of approximately 66h.

Successful imaging using labeled leukocytes depends on viability of labeled cells. Several studies assessed cell viability after labeling concluding satisfactory and comparable viability rates for ^{111}In, ^{99m}Tc, ^{18}F-FDG and ^{64}Cu in the first 4h after labeling [38]. However, cell viability significantly decreases within one day limiting long term monitoring of AR using a single shot approach.

At present only a few preclinical and clinical studies are published dealing with labeled leukocytes and detection of AR in intestine, hearts, pancreas islets and skin. Only one study performed in a small cohort of kidney transplant recipients evaluated ^{99m}Tc-mononuclear cell scintigraphy for diagnosis of AR. In this study, the authors were able to show that AR was diagnosed correctly and successfully discriminated from ATN [39]. In a further development of their approach, we established leukocyte PET imaging using very low amounts of ^{18}F-FDG for the diagnosis of AR in a rat kidney transplant model. *Ex vivo* ^{18}F-FDG labeled human CTLs were able to diagnose renal AR within a time frame of 1 h after application and discriminate AR from important differential diagnoses such as acute cyclosporine toxicity or ATN (*Grabner et al. in press*) (Fig. 1).

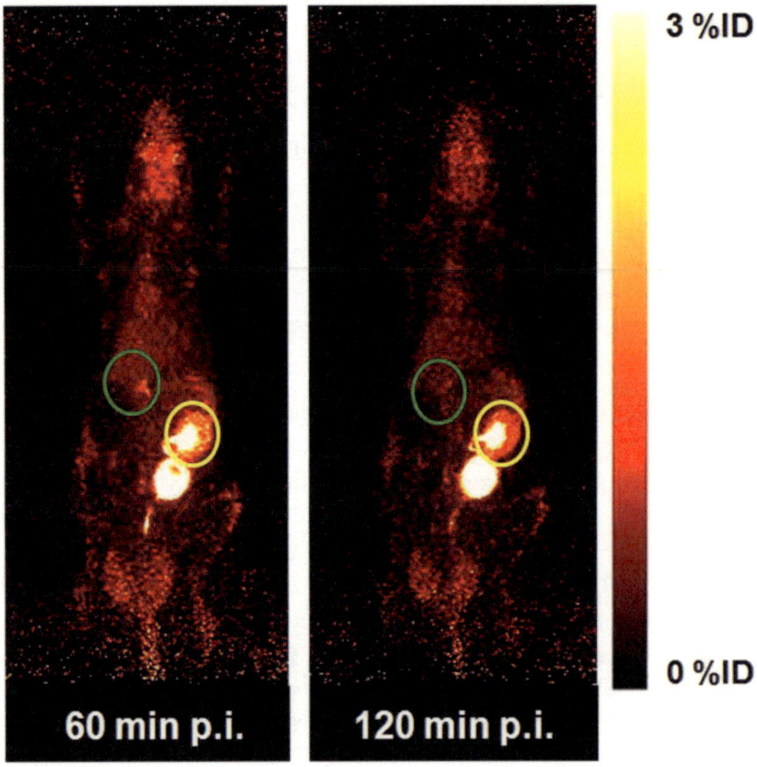

Figure 1. Representative PET-images of dynamic whole body acquisitions of a series of an allogeneically kidney transplanted rat on postoperative day 4 60 min and 120 min after tail vein injection of 30 x 10^{6} ^{18}F-FDG labeled CTL. While the parenchyma (yellow circle) of renal allograft developing AR accumulates ^{18}F-FDG-CTLs, the native kidney (green circle) does not show any accumulation at any time. Please note that the renal pelvis can contain eliminated ^{18}F-FDG/ ^{18}F-fluoride. Therefore, it has to be excluded from the measurements. ID: injected dose

Since infiltration of leukocytes, especially CTLs, in allografts appears before physiologic or mechanical manifestations of organ dysfunction is apparent, nuclear imaging employing leukocytes might be a promising tool for specific, sensitive and early detection of AR.

5.4. Imaging using *in vivo* radiolabeled leukocytes

Instead of employing *ex vivo* labeled leukocytes, radiolabeled monoclonal antibodies (fragments) (mAbs) have been established for detection of leukocyte (related) antigens. Their advantages include standardized production, easier storage and handling, while they are highly specific for their target leading to a good background/target ration. However, limitations might be the targeting of extravascular antigens and potential but rare allergic complications, when using the antibodies in a patient.

As discussed, CTLs are the major cell type involved in AR. Martins *et al.* used ^{99m}Tc-OKT3 targeting CTLs in recipients of renal transplants [40]. In their preliminary results they state that out of 22 patients they successfully identified 3 patients with AR using ^{99m}Tc-OKT3 scans. Apparently, their results published in 2004 have to be confirmed in further studies. A recently published attractive, being somehow better biocompatible, alternative might be CD3 targeting ^{99m}Tc-SHNH-visilizumab which needs to be evaluated in the future [41].

5.5. Metabolic activity (^{18}F-FDG)

^{18}F-FDG is a daily routine tracer to assess regional glucose metabolism as a surrogate for metabolic activity widely used for the PET-based routine detection of tumors, infection and inflammation. The major energy source in leukocytes during the metabolic burst is glucose. Analogously, activated leukocytes highly accumulate ^{18}F-FDG (in the same way they take up glucose but without further processing) which can be quantified by PET [42]. A clear limitation when using free ^{18}F-FDG is that an increased uptake can be observed in any kind of cellular activation (high glycolytic activity). Hence, ^{18}F-FDG is not a disease or target specific tracer.

Nevertheless, ^{18}F-FDG is one of the few tracers successfully applied for the non-invasive detection of AR. Others have applied ^{18}F-FDG in settings of lung, heart and liver transplantations. We have demonstrated very promising results for ^{18}F-FDG-PET in diagnostics of renal AR [43;44]. Using a rat model of renal AR, ^{18}F-FDG-PET performed well in terms of early, accurate detection and follow-up of AR [43] (Fig. 2). Using ^{18}F-FDG, we discriminated AR non-invasively from important differential diagnoses like ATN or acute cyclosporine toxicity. Moreover, therapy response monitoring by ^{18}F-FDG might be useful to identify treatment unresponsive AR for earlier escalation of immunosuppressive regimen [44]. This might reduce graft damage by shortening AR episodes because at present (steroid) resistant rejection is diagnosed lately [45].

One important issue of imaging of kidney AR with ^{18}F-FDG is that it is eliminated with the urine in contrast to normal glucose. Thus, drainage of ^{18}F-FDG into the renal pelvis must be taken care of when assessing ^{18}F-FDG-uptake in the renal parenchyma. We avoided this problem by using late acquisitions after ^{18}F-FDG injection to reduce the instantaneous amount of tracer in the urine during the PET scan. Moreover, an impact of renal function on ^{18}F-FDG-uptake has to be excluded e.g. by renal fluoride clearance (a non-invasive measure of renal function) [46].

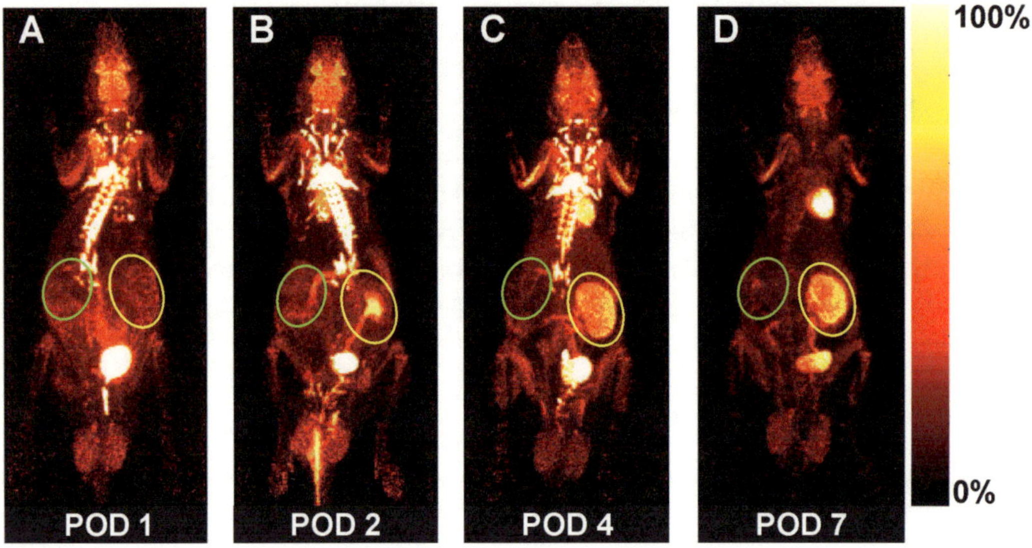

Figure 2. Representative PET-images of dynamic whole body acquisitions of a series of an allogeneically kidney transplanted rat (POD 1 (A), 2 (B), 4 (C), and 7 (D), after tail vein injection of ^{18}F-FDG. While the parenchyma (yellow circle) of renal allograft developing AR accumulates ^{18}F-FDG with a maximum on post operative day (POD) 4, the native kidney (green circle) does not show any accumulation at any time. Please note that the renal pelvis can contain eliminated ^{18}F-FDG/^{18}F-fluoride. Therefore, it has to be excluded from the measurements. Figure taken from [43]. Scale bar: percent injected dose

5.6. Matrix metalloproteinases

One step further, one cannot assess infiltrating leukocytes only but rather their tissue damaging activity by detection of activated matrix metalloproteinases (MMPs). Leukocyte-derived MMPs, like MMP-2 or MMP-9, were found to be active in AR [47;48]. Since MMP activity can be assessed using radiolabeled MMP-inhibitors in SPECT or PET this approach for detection of AR might be evaluated in future studies [49-52]. Maybe one can gather additional information regarding graft`s prognosis because MMPs are involved in tissue remodelling, too.

5.7. Hypoxia

Acute tissue inflammations regardless of their origin present with a unique and challenging microenvironment including hypoxia (low oxygen), anoxia (complete lack of oxygen), hypoglycemia (low blood glucose), acidosis (high H^+ concentration) and abundant free oxygen radicals. These conditions are characteristic features of inflamed tissues, along with the influx of leukocytes. In renal allografts, hypoxia and hypoxic adaptation are common within 2 weeks after surgery whereas graft hypoxia assessed in the long run is associated with clinical/subclinical rejection [53]. Therefore, assessment of hypoxia by targeting hypoxia (related gene products), i.e. hypoxia inducible factors (HIF), might offer additional diagnostic information in subclinical or ambiguous cases of AR.

Two major classes of hypoxia tracer, nitroimidazoles and *bis*(thiosemicarbazonato)copper(II) complexes, have been extensively investigated for measuring hypoxia. The applications of both tracer as well as several alternative reagents tested e.g., ^{18}F-fluoroerythronitroimidazole (^{18}F-FETNIM) and ^{18}F-fluoroazomycin-arabinofuranoside (^{18}F-FAZA), are summarized in a review recently published by Krohn *et al.* [54]. Until present and to the best of our knowledge, no study has been performed assessing hypoxia in renal AR by SPECT or PET so far. At least one has to evaluate if the SPECT and PET-based approaches are advantageous when compared to BOLD MR.

5.8. Apoptosis

Apoptosis in AR is probably the result of different events occurring in AR. It may be a direct consequence of different cytokines discharged by leukocytes or directly provoked e.g. by CTLs. Within the inflammatory milieu of AR apoptosis might, among other factors, also be related to hypoxia, acidosis, or reactive oxygen species. Non-invasive detection of apoptosis in AR might be attractive because it may not serve for early detection of AR only, but also for monitoring of rejection kinetics and therapy response. Especially, early assessment of therapeutic success or failure is interesting to promptly adjust the therapeutic regimen. Likewise, quantification of apoptosis might provide information regarding the extent of graft damage and therefore for its prognosis. However, small studies with different tracers targeting different steps in apoptosis have been performed in both, animal and man. A comprehensive review on detecting cell death *in vivo* has been recently published by us [55]. Two main operational strategies are followed. While imaging of caspases` activity using substrate-derived agents offers high selectivity, the detection of membrane phospholipid redistribution using extracellular agents has the advantage of high target density and accessibility [56]. We and others recently proposed different isatin analogues for ^{18}F-labeling and detection of apoptosis [55]. However, studies detecting apoptosis in renal grafts using radiotracers for evaluation of their potential clinical value in AR have not been performed yet.

5.9. Imaging allograft function

A rather unspecific but reasonable approach is to simply determine graft function as a surrogate for stable function or (acute) graft affection.

Especially scintigraphic methods have been established for the assessment of renal function. Primarily, two types of imaging are common: static and dynamic. ^{99m}Tc-dimercaptosuccinic acid (DMSA) is the tracer used in static imaging allowing on the one hand identification of pathological conditions such as anatomical abnormalities or scarring, on the other hand accurate assessment of the differential function of the kidneys [57]. DMSA uptake correlates with the effective renal plasma flow, glomerular filtration rate, and creatinine clearance. Therefore,

DMSA has been successfully applied in the evaluation of renal function in living donors (before and after transplantation) and in kidney recipients [58]. For dynamic imaging ^{99m}Tc-mercaptoacetyltriglycine (MAG-3) and diethylenetriaminepentaacetic acid (DTPA) are the most commonly used tracers, whereas MAG-3 is going to replace DTPA because of superior extraction efficiency. It was proposed that MAG-3 scintigraphy can be useful for discrimination of AR from ATN [59]. Despite a reasonable perfusion and tracer extraction in ATN as assessed in these studies, tracer excretion rate is low, whereas one of the typical findings in AR is impaired perfusion. This fact was already taken into account by Hilson *et al.* in the seventies who developed a DTPA-based perfusion index which allows separation of rejection from ATN and, particularly, rejection from healthy kidneys [60]. These findings are somehow discrepant to typical findings in ultrasound when assessing RI which reflects renal perfusion as well. High RIs can be observed in ATN as well as in AR denying a differentiation of these entities by ultrasound-based measure of renal perfusion. Potentially, the modified renal perfusion index using ^{18}F-fluoride developed by us can be used for further clarification [61]. Aside from this recent studies using PET for the evaluation of renal function other approaches have been emerged. Renal blood flow for instance was successfully measured with $H_2{}^{15}O$ in rats and man [62,63]. Furthermore, we established ^{18}F-fluoride clearance for assessment of renal function in different renal failure models including AR [43,46]. As said before, decreased renal function is not disease specific but can assist in the differential diagnoses of AR.

6. Conclusion

The diagnosis and therapy follow-up of AR in transplant recipients demands for non-invasive and serial imaging approaches *in vivo.* Molecular and cellular imaging has significant potential for transplantation medicine as it may serve for monitoring the graft. With more optimal tracers as they are numerously being developed, PET (and other devices) may serve as valuable tools for the diagnosis and management of renal AR. In this term, these techniques will find their share to impact on detection of AR, graft function, assessment of therapy response as well as of the progression of lesions and therefore on graft´s prognosis.

Taken the new developments in molecular imaging into account, non-invasive methods including ultrasound, magnetic resonance, as well as SPECT and PET get increasingly helpful for research. Currently, nearly all of these promising new approaches are still at an experimental stage and have to evidence their potential in humans in daily routine in the future.

Acknowledgements

This work was supported by the Deutsche Forschungsgemeinschaft (DFG), Sonderforschungsbereich 656, Münster, Germany (SFB 656 C7).

http://dx.doi.org/10.5772/54737

Author details

Alexander Grabner[1], Dominik Kentrup[1], Uta Schnöckel[2], Michael Schäfers[3] and Stefan Reuter[1*]

*Address all correspondence to: sreuter@uni-muenster.de

1 Department of Internal Medicine D, Experimental Nephrology, University of Münster, Münster,, Germany

2 Department of Nuclear Medicine, University of Münster, Münster,, Germany

3 European Institute for Molecular Imaging, University of Münster, Münster, Germany

References

[1] Lamb, K. E, Lodhi, S, & Meier-Kriesche, H. U. Long-term renal allograft survival in the United States: a critical reappraisal. Am J Transplant (2011). Mar;, 11(3), 450-62.

[2] Lemy, A, Andrien, M, Lionet, A, Labalette, M, Noel, C, Hiesse, C, et al. Posttransplant Major Histocompatibility Complex Class I Chain-Related Gene A Antibodies and Long-Term Graft Outcomes in a Multicenter Cohort of 779 Kidney Transplant Recipients. Transplantation (2012). Mar 29.

[3] Cohen, D. J, St, M. L, Christensen, L. L, Bloom, R. D, & Sung, R. S. Kidney and pancreas transplantation in the United States, Am J Transplant 2006;6(5 Pt 2):1153-69., 1995-2004.

[4] Cornell, L. D, Smith, R. N, & Colvin, R. B. Kidney transplantation: mechanisms of rejection and acceptance. Annu Rev Pathol (2008). , 3, 189-220.

[5] Matas, A. J, Gillingham, K. J, Payne, W. D, & Najarian, J. S. The impact of an acute rejection episode on long-term renal allograft survival (t1/2). Transplantation (1994). Mar 27;, 57(6), 857-9.

[6] Wu, O, Levy, A. R, Briggs, A, Lewis, G, & Jardine, A. Acute rejection and chronic nephropathy: a systematic review of the literature. Transplantation (2009). May 15;, 87(9), 1330-9.

[7] Meier-kriesche, H. U, Ojo, A. O, Hanson, J. A, Cibrik, D. M, Punch, J. D, Leichtman, A. B, et al. Increased impact of acute rejection on chronic allograft failure in recent era. Transplantation (2000). Oct 15;, 70(7), 1098-100.

[8] Chapman, J. R, Connell, O, & Nankivell, P. J. BJ. Chronic renal allograft dysfunction. J Am Soc Nephrol (2005). Oct;, 16(10), 3015-26.

[9] Massy, Z. A, Guijarro, C, Wiederkehr, M. R, Ma, J. Z, & Kasiske, B. L. Chronic renal allograft rejection: immunologic and nonimmunologic risk factors. Kidney Int (1996). Feb;, 49(2), 518-24.

[10] Nickeleit, V, & Andreoni, K. Inflammatory cells in renal allografts. Front Biosci (2008)., 13, 6202-13.

[11] Ingulli, E. Mechanism of cellular rejection in transplantation. Pediatr Nephrol (2010). Jan;, 25(1), 61-74.

[12] Dedrick, R. L, Bodary, S, & Garovoy, M. R. Adhesion molecules as therapeutic targets for autoimmune diseases and transplant rejection. Expert Opin Biol Ther (2003). Feb;, 3(1), 85-95.

[13] Barry, M, & Bleackley, R. C. Cytotoxic T lymphocytes: all roads lead to death. Nat Rev Immunol (2002). Jun;, 2(6), 401-9.

[14] Fischer, T, Filimonow, S, Dieckhofer, J, Slowinski, T, Muhler, M, Lembcke, A, et al. Improved diagnosis of early kidney allograft dysfunction by ultrasound with echo enhancer--a new method for the diagnosis of renal perfusion. Nephrol Dial Transplant (2006). Oct;, 21(10), 2921-9.

[15] Kirkpantur, A, Yilmaz, R, Baydar, D. E, Aki, T, Cil, B, Arici, M, et al. Utility of the Doppler ultrasound parameter, resistive index, in renal transplant histopathology. Transplant Proc (2008). Jan;, 40(1), 104-6.

[16] Cosgrove, D. O, & Chan, K. E. Renal transplants: what ultrasound can and cannot do. Ultrasound Q (2008). Jun;, 24(2), 77-87.

[17] Radermacher, J, Mengel, M, Ellis, S, Stuht, S, Hiss, M, Schwarz, A, et al. The renal arterial resistance index and renal allograft survival. N Engl J Med (2003). Jul 10;, 349(2), 115-24.

[18] Kramann, R, Frank, D, Brandenburg, V. M, Heussen, N, Takahama, J, Kruger, T, et al. Prognostic impact of renal arterial resistance index upon renal allograft survival: the time point matters. Nephrol Dial Transplant (2012). Jan 13.

[19] Sebastia, C, Quiroga, S, Boye, R, Cantarell, C, Fernandez-planas, M, & Alvarez, A. Helical CT in renal transplantation: normal findings and early and late complications. Radiographics (2001). Sep;, 21(5), 1103-17.

[20] Kalb, B, Martin, D. R, Salman, K, Sharma, P, Votaw, J, & Larsen, C. Kidney transplantation: structural and functional evaluation using MR Nephro-Urography. J Magn Reson Imaging (2008). Oct;, 28(4), 805-22.

[21] Sadowski, E. A, Fain, S. B, Alford, S. K, Korosec, F. R, Fine, J, Muehrer, R, et al. Assessment of acute renal transplant rejection with blood oxygen level-dependent MR imaging: initial experience. Radiology (2005). Sep;, 236(3), 911-9.

[22] Sadowski, E. A, Djamali, A, Wentland, A. L, Muehrer, R, Becker, B. N, Grist, T. M, et al. Blood oxygen level-dependent and perfusion magnetic resonance imaging: detect-

ing differences in oxygen bioavailability and blood flow in transplanted kidneys. Magn Reson Imaging (2010). Jan;, 28(1), 56-64.

[23] Wentland, A. L, Sadowski, E. A, Djamali, A, Grist, T. M, Becker, B. N, & Fain, S. B. Quantitative MR measures of intrarenal perfusion in the assessment of transplanted kidneys: initial experience. Acad Radiol (2009). Sep;, 16(9), 1077-85.

[24] De Priester, J. A. den Boer JA, Christiaans MH, Kessels AG, Giele EL, Hasman A, et al. Automated quantitative evaluation of diseased and nondiseased renal transplants with MR renography. J Magn Reson Imaging (2003). Jan;, 17(1), 95-103.

[25] Yamamoto, A, Zhang, J. L, Rusinek, H, Chandarana, H, Vivier, P. H, Babb, J. S, et al. Quantitative evaluation of acute renal transplant dysfunction with low-dose three-dimensional MR renography. Radiology (2011). Sep;, 260(3), 781-9.

[26] Hauger, O, Grenier, N, Deminere, C, Lasseur, C, Delmas, Y, Merville, P, et al. USPIO-enhanced MR imaging of macrophage infiltration in native and transplanted kidneys: initial results in humans. Eur Radiol (2007). Nov;, 17(11), 2898-907.

[27] Signore, A, Mather, S. J, Piaggio, G, Malviya, G, & Dierckx, R. A. Molecular imaging of inflammation/infection: nuclear medicine and optical imaging agents and methods. Chem Rev (2010). May 12;, 110(5), 3112-45.

[28] Hall, L. T, Struck, A. F, & Perlman, S. B. Clinical Molecular Imaging with PET Agents other than (18)F-FDG. Curr Pharm Biotechnol (2010). Apr 26.

[29] Dumarey, N, Egrise, D, Blocklet, D, Stallenberg, B, Remmelink, M, Del, M, et al. Imaging infection with 18F-FDG-labeled leukocyte PET/CT: initial experience in 21 patients. J Nucl Med (2006). Apr;, 47(4), 625-32.

[30] Datz, F. L. Indium-111-labeled leukocytes for the detection of infection: current status. Semin Nucl Med (1994). Apr;, 24(2), 92-109.

[31] Peters, A. M. The utility of [99mTc]HMPAO-leukocytes for imaging infection. Semin Nucl Med (1994). Apr;, 24(2), 110-27.

[32] Peters, A. M, Danpure, H. J, Osman, S, Hawker, R. J, Henderson, B. L, Hodgson, H. J, et al. Clinical experience with 99mTc-hexamethylpropylene-amineoxime for labelling leucocytes and imaging inflammation. Lancet (1986). Oct 25;, 2(8513), 946-9.

[33] Mcafee, J. G, & Thakur, M. L. Survey of radioactive agents for in vitro labeling of phagocytic leukocytes. I. Soluble agents. J Nucl Med (1976). Jun;, 17(6), 480-7.

[34] Isobe, M, Haber, E, & Khaw, B. A. Early detection of rejection and assessment of cyclosporine therapy by 111In antimyosin imaging in mouse heart allografts. Circulation (1991). Sep;, 84(3), 1246-55.

[35] Forstrom, L. A, Dunn, W. L, Rowe, F. A, & Camilleri, M. In-oxine-labelled granulocyte dosimetry in normal subjects. Nucl Med Commun (1995). May;, 16(5), 349-56.

[36] Eisen, H. J, Eisenberg, S. B, Saffitz, J. E, & Bolman, R. M. III, Sobel BE, Bergmann SR. Noninvasive detection of rejection of transplanted hearts with indium-111-labeled lymphocytes. Circulation (1987). Apr;, 75(4), 868-76.

[37] Forstrom, L. A, Dunn, W. L, Mullan, B. P, Hung, J. C, Lowe, V. J, & Thorson, L. M. Biodistribution and dosimetry of [(18)F]fluorodeoxyglucose labelled leukocytes in normal human subjects. Nucl Med Commun (2002). Aug;, 23(8), 721-5.

[38] Bhargava, K. K, Gupta, R. K, Nichols, K. J, & Palestro, C. J. In vitro human leukocyte labeling with (64)Cu: an intraindividual comparison with (111)In-oxine and (18)F-FDG. Nucl Med Biol (2009). Jul;, 36(5), 545-9.

[39] Lopes de Souza SABarbosa da Fonseca LM, Torres GR, Salomao PD, Holzer TJ, Proenca Martins FP, et al. Diagnosis of renal allograft rejection and acute tubular necrosis by 99mTc-mononuclear leukocyte imaging. Transplant Proc (2004). Dec;, 36(10), 2997-3001.

[40] Martins, F. P, Souza, S. A, Goncalves, R. T, Fonseca, L. M, & Gutfilen, B. Preliminary results of [99mTc]OKT3 scintigraphy to evaluate acute rejection in renal transplants. Transplant Proc (2004). Nov;, 36(9), 2664-7.

[41] Shan, L, & Tc-labeled, m. succinimidyl-hydrazinonicotinate hydrochloride (SHNH)-conjugated visilizumab. (2004)., 6.

[42] Pellegrino, D, Bonab, A. A, Dragotakes, S. C, Pitman, J. T, Mariani, G, & Carter, E. A. Inflammation and infection: imaging properties of 18F-FDG-labeled white blood cells versus 18F-FDG. J Nucl Med (2005). Sep;, 46(9), 1522-30.

[43] Reuter, S, Schnockel, U, Schroter, R, Schober, O, Pavenstadt, H, Schafers, M, et al. Noninvasive imaging of acute renal allograft rejection in rats using small animal F-FDG-PET. PLoS One (2009). e5296.

[44] Reuter, S, Schnockel, U, Edemir, B, Schroter, R, Kentrup, D, Pavenstadt, H, et al. Potential of noninvasive serial assessment of acute renal allograft rejection by 18F-FDG PET to monitor treatment efficiency. J Nucl Med (2010). Oct;, 51(10), 1644-52.

[45] Guttmann, R. D, Soulillou, J. P, Moore, L. W, First, M. R, Gaber, A. O, Pouletty, P, et al. Proposed consensus for definitions and endpoints for clinical trials of acute kidney transplant rejection. Am J Kidney Dis (1998). Jun;31(6 Suppl 1):SS46., 40.

[46] Schnockel, U, Reuter, S, Stegger, L, Schlatter, E, Schafers, K. P, Hermann, S, et al. Dynamic 18F-fluoride small animal PET to noninvasively assess renal function in rats. Eur J Nucl Med Mol Imaging (2008). Dec;, 35(12), 2267-74.

[47] Edemir, B, Kurian, S. M, Eisenacher, M, Lang, D, Muller-tidow, C, Gabriels, G, et al. Activation of counter-regulatory mechanisms in a rat renal acute rejection model. BMC Genomics (2008).

[48] Einecke, G, Reeve, J, Sis, B, Mengel, M, Hidalgo, L, Famulski, K. S, et al. A molecular classifier for predicting future graft loss in late kidney transplant biopsies. J Clin Invest (2010). Jun;, 120(6), 1862-72.

[49] Wagner, S, Breyholz, H. J, Holtke, C, Faust, A, Schober, O, Schafers, M, et al. A new 18F-labelled derivative of the MMP inhibitor CGS 27023A for PET: radiosynthesis and initial small-animal PET studies. Appl Radiat Isot (2009). Apr;, 67(4), 606-10.

[50] Breyholz, H. J, Wagner, S, Faust, A, Riemann, B, Holtke, C, Hermann, S, et al. Radiofluorinated pyrimidine-2,4,6-triones as molecular probes for noninvasive MMP-targeted imaging. ChemMedChem (2010). May 3;, 5(5), 777-89.

[51] Hugenberg, V, Breyholz, H. J, Riemann, B, Hermann, S, Schober, O, Schafers, M, et al. A new class of highly potent matrix metalloproteinase inhibitors based on triazole-substituted hydroxamates: (radio)synthesis and in vitro and first in vivo evaluation. J Med Chem (2012). May 24;, 55(10), 4714-27.

[52] Schrigten, D, Breyholz, H. J, Wagner, S, Hermann, S, Schober, O, Schafers, M, et al. A new generation of radiofluorinated pyrimidine-2,4,6-triones as MMP-targeted radiotracers for positron emission tomography. J Med Chem (2012). Jan 12;, 55(1), 223-32.

[53] Rosenberger, C, Pratschke, J, Rudolph, B, Heyman, S. N, Schindler, R, Babel, N, et al. Immunohistochemical detection of hypoxia-inducible factor-1alpha in human renal allograft biopsies. J Am Soc Nephrol (2007). Jan;, 18(1), 343-51.

[54] Krohn, K. A, Link, J. M, & Mason, R. P. Molecular imaging of hypoxia. J Nucl Med (2008). Jun;49 Suppl 2:129S-48S.

[55] Faust, A, Hermann, S, Wagner, S, Haufe, G, Schober, O, Schafers, M, et al. Molecular imaging of apoptosis in vivo with scintigraphic and optical biomarkers--a status report. Anticancer Agents Med Chem (2009). Nov;, 9(9), 968-85.

[56] Zhao, M. Molecular Recognition Mechanisms for Detecting Cell Death In Vivo. Curr Pharm Biotechnol (2010). May 24.

[57] Hain, S. F. Renal imaging. Clin Med (2006). May;, 6(3), 244-8.

[58] Even-sapir, E, Weinbroum, A, Merhav, H, Lerman, H, Livshitz, G, & Nakache, R. Renal allograft function prior to and following living related transplantation: assessment by quantitative Tc99m DMSA SPECT. Transplant Proc (2001). Sep;, 33(6), 2924-5.

[59] Sfakianakis, G. N, Sfakianaki, E, Georgiou, M, Serafini, A, Ezuddin, S, Kuker, R, et al. A renal protocol for all ages and all indications: mercapto-acetyl-triglycine (MAG3) with simultaneous injection of furosemide (MAG3-F0): a 17-year experience. Semin Nucl Med (2009). May;, 39(3), 156-73.

[60] Hilson, A. J, Maisey, M. N, Brown, C. B, Ogg, C. S, & Bewick, M. S. Dynamic renal transplant imaging with Tc-99m DTPA (Sn) supplemented by a transplant perfusion index in the management of renal transplants. J Nucl Med (1978). Sep;, 19(9), 994-1000.

[61] Kentrup, D, Reuter, S, Schnockel, U, Grabner, A, Edemir, B, Pavenstadt, H, et al. Hydroxyfasudil-mediated inhibition of ROCK1 and ROCK2 improves kidney function in rat renal acute ischemia-reperfusion injury. PLoS One (2011). e26419.

[62] Kudomi, N, Koivuviita, N, Liukko, K. E, Oikonen, V. J, Tolvanen, T, Iida, H, et al. Parametric renal blood flow imaging using [15O]H2O and PET. Eur J Nucl Med Mol Imaging (2009). Apr;, 36(4), 683-91.

[63] Juillard, L, Janier, M. F, Fouque, D, Cinotti, L, Maakel, N, Le, B. D, et al. Dynamic renal blood flow measurement by positron emission tomography in patients with CRF. Am J Kidney Dis (2002). Nov;, 40(5), 947-54.

[64] George, E. A, Codd, J. E, Newton, W. T, Haibach, H, & Donati, R. M. Comparative evaluation of renal transplant rejection with radioiodinated fibrinogen 99mTc-sulfur collid, and 67Ga-citrate. J Nucl Med (1976). Mar;, 17(3), 175-80.

[65] George, E. A, Codd, J. E, Newton, W. T, & Donati, R. M. Ga citrate in renal allograft rejection. Radiology (1975). Dec;117(3 Pt 1):731-3.

[66] Even-sapir, E, Gutman, M, Lerman, H, Kaplan, E, Ravid, A, Livshitz, G, et al. Kidney allografts and remaining contralateral donor kidneys before and after transplantation: assessment by quantitative (99m)Tc-DMSA SPECT. J Nucl Med (2002). May;, 43(5), 584-8.

[67] Budihna, N. V, Milcinski, M, Kajtna-koselj, M, & Malovrh, M. Relevance of Tc-99m DMSA scintigraphy in renal transplant parenchymal imaging. Clin Nucl Med (1994). Sep;, 19(9), 782-4.

[68] Bajen, M. T, Mora, J, Grinyo, J. M, Castelao, A, Roca, M, Puchal, R, et al. Study of renal transplant by deconvoluted renogram with 99m Tc-mercaptoacetyltriglycine (Mag3)]. Rev Esp Med Nucl (2001). Oct;, 20(6), 453-61.

[69] Dubovsky, E. V, Russell, C. D, Bischof-delaloye, A, Bubeck, B, Chaiwatanarat, T, Hilson, A. J, et al. Report of the Radionuclides in Nephrourology Committee for evaluation of transplanted kidney (review of techniques). Semin Nucl Med (1999). Apr;, 29(2), 175-88.

[70] Sundaraiya, S, Mendichovszky, I, Biassoni, L, Sebire, N, Trompeter, R. S, & Gordon, I. Tc-99m DTPA renography in children following renal transplantation: its value in the evaluation of rejection. Pediatr Transplant (2007). Nov;, 11(7), 771-6.

[71] Salvatierra, O. Jr., Powell MR, Price DC, Kountz SL, Belzer FO. The advantages of 131I-orthoiodohippurate scintiphotography in the management of patients after renal transplantation. Ann Surg (1974). Sep;, 180(3), 336-42.

Chapter 5

Detection of Antibody-Mediated Rejection in Kidney Transplantation and the Management of Highly Sensitised Kidney Transplant Recipients

Shyam Dheda, Siew Chong, Rebecca Lucy Williams,
Germaine Wong and Wai Hon Lim

Additional information is available at the end of the chapter

http://dx.doi.org/10.5772/54735

1. Introduction

With the evolution in our understanding of the human leukocyte antigen (HLA) system, there have been substantial improvements in the HLA-typing techniques and the ability to detect anti-HLA antibodies, allowing accurate assessment of immunological risk among potential renal transplant candidates. Specifically, flow cytometry and the solid phase assay such as the enzyme-linked immunosorbent assay (ELISA) and Luminex technology have improved the sensitivity of detecting low levels class I and II donor-specific anti-HLA antibodies (DSA). Although there is now established evidence showing the presence of DSA is associated with a greater risk of antibody-mediated rejection (AMR) and early graft loss, the clinical significance of low levels DSA remains unclear. As a result of prior sensitizing events, there has been an expansion in the number of highly sensitized transplant candidates with multiple anti-HLA antibodies. Management of these candidates for the preparation of transplantation continues to be a subject of intense debate. In this chapter, we will discuss the identification of potential clinically relevant DSA detected by the different assays including the 'acceptable' level of clinically significant DSA and the advantage of C1q-positive DSA in further stratifying the immunological risk of transplant candidates. The association between DSA and non-DSA with graft and patient outcomes following kidney transplantation will be discussed in greater detail. Furthermore, we will examine the transplant outcomes of highly sensitized patients undergoing desensitization regimens and to determine the optimal desensitization regimens along with their risks and benefits.

2. Evolution of techniques to detect donor-specific anti-HLA antibodies (Figure 1)

HLA forms part of the major histocompatibility complex (MHC) in humans and MHC antigens are an integral component of the normal functioning of the human immune system. HLA antigens play a crucial role in the recognition of self-antigens and are therefore crucial in the defence of foreign antigens, including donor antigens in solid organ transplantation. HLA antigens are comprised of both class I and II antigens, with class I antigens being expressed on all nucleated cells, whereas class II antigens are being expressed on antigen presenting cells, B cells and endothelial cells [1]. The evolution in our understanding of the HLA system is closely linked to advancements in technology. Traditional serological-based (i.e. antibody-based) low-resolution techniques have been the standard method for HLA typing, enabling efficient and effective anti-HLA antibody detection. However, these techniques are dependent on the availability of specific cell types, cell viability and appropriate anti-sera that are capable of recognising HLA antigens. The emergence of molecular HLA typing techniques over the past two decades has allowed for a more specific and robust method of high resolution HLA typing. In 1982, *Wake et al* described restriction fragment length polymorphism (RFLP), which eventually highlighted the shortcomings of serology-based methods ensuing the establishment of molecular-based HLA-typing for routine detection of anti-HLA antibodies pre-transplantation [2]. Data generated via the genome project and the initiation of polymerase chain reaction (PCR) techniques through the 1980s further refined DNA-based techniques for HLA-typing, which has led to the development of a number of PCR-based techniques still in use to the present day.

Alongside with the advances in the typing of HLA alleles, the techniques used to detect anti-HLA antibodies has evolved from CDC assays to the more sensitive techniques including flow-cytometry and solid-phase assays (e.g. enzyme-linked immunosorbent assay [ELISA] or Luminex), allowing for accurate assessment of pre-transplant immunological risk (e.g. calculated panel reactive antibodies to determine level of sensitization and application of virtual cross-match to determine transplant suitability) [3] (Figure 4).

Since the recognition of the clinical importance of CDC assay in kidney transplantation in the 1960s, CDC cross-match has become the foundation of determining transplant suitability in kidney transplantation [4]. CDC cross-match can detect donor-specific anti-HLA antibodies that may have the potential to induce an anti-HLA antibody-associated hyperacute rejection following transplantation. Donor T and B cells are isolated from peripheral blood mononuclear cells using density gradient separation and incubated in the presence of recipients' sera and complements. If donor-specific anti-HLA antibodies are present, these will bind to specific antigen(s) expressed on donor cells, and with the addition of rabbit serum as a source of exogenous complement, will result in the initiation of the classical complement cascade causing direct damage to the donor cell membrane and therefore making these cells permeable to an important dye. The percentage of cell lysis is quantified and forms the basis of determining transplant candidate's suitability for transplantation with a lysis score of 20% generally considered a contraindication for transplantation. Many laboratories perform CDC assays in

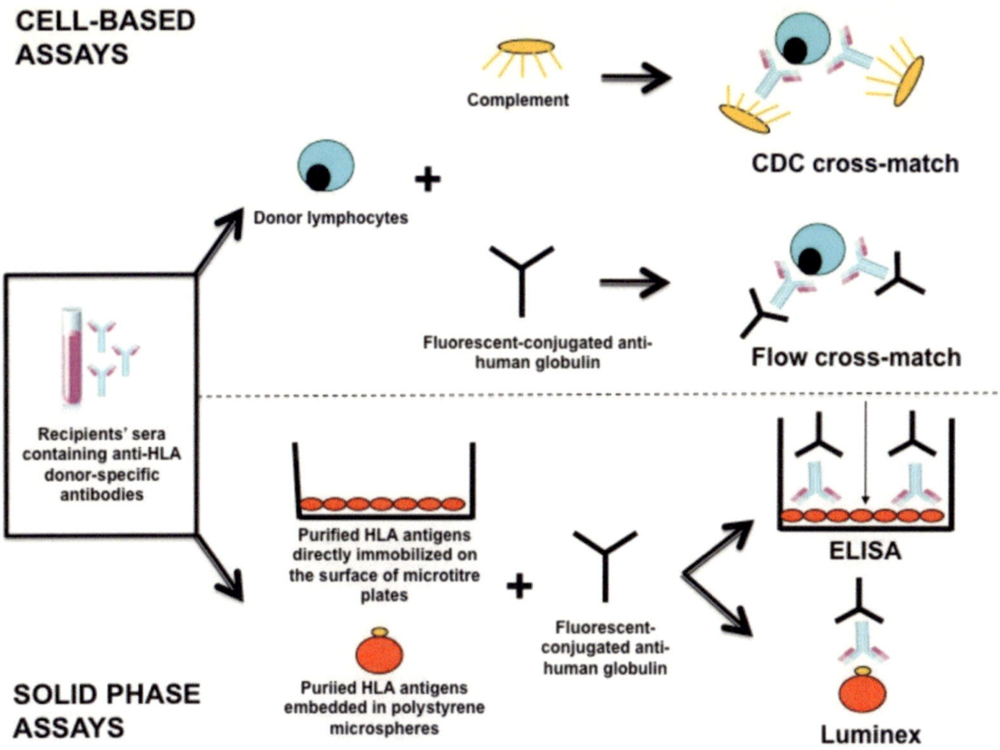

Assays	Complement fixing vs non-complement fixing antibodies	Identify specific HLA antigens	Quantify anti-HLA antibodies	Problems
CDC-XM	Complement fixing antibodies	No	No	No cell targets that expressed only class II antigens
FCXM	Complement and non-complement-fixing antibodies	Yes (class I and II)	Yes	Too sensitive Costly
ELISA	Complement and non-complement-fixing antibodies	Yes (class I and II)	Yes	Too sensitive Costly
Luminex	Complement and non-complement-fixing antibodies	Yes (class I and II)	Yes	Too sensitive Costly

HLA – human leukocyte antigen, CDC-XM – complement-dependent cytotoxicity cross-match, FCXM – flow cytometric cross-match, ELISA – enzyme-linked immunosorbent assay.

Figure 1. Detection of anti-HLA antibodies – differences between cell-based and solid-phase assays.

the presence of anti-human globulin, which augments the sensitivity of this assay by increasing the number of Fc receptors available to bind complements, and/or dithiothreitol (which breaks down the disulfide bonds in IgM antibodies believed to be of no clinical significance) to reduce the false positivity of these assays [5, 6]. Initial studies evaluating the clinical validity of CDC assays demonstrated that 80% of CDC cross-match–positive kidney transplants and 4% of cross-match–negative kidney transplants were associated with early graft loss, thereby verifying the clinical significance of anti-HLA antibodies in renal transplantation. It is noteworthy that 20% of patients transplanted across a positive cross-match did not lose their grafts [3]. Given that T cells express class I antigens and B cells express both class I and II antigens, the interpretation of T cell together with B cell cross-match will assist in establishing whether class I and/or II anti-HLA antibodies are present. A positive B cell CDC cross-match invariably accompanies a positive T cell CDC cross-match but this may reflect either anti-HLA antibodies to class I antigens and/or multiple antibodies to class I and/or II antigens. However, a positive B cell CDC cross-match may occur in the absence of a positive T cell CDC cross-match and suggest the presence of class II antigens or low levels class I antigens. The presence of a positive T cell CDC cross-match is an absolute contraindication for transplantation whereas a positive B cell cross-match is a relative contraindication because of the uncertainty regarding the clinical significance and the chance of false-positive results [7, 8]. The presence of a positive T cell cross-match is an absolute contraindication for transplantation within the deceased donor kidney allocation algorithm in Australia and New Zealand. \On the contrary, B cell cross-match is not routinely performed and therefore not utilized in the decision-making process for transplantation. With the increasing recognition of the potential importance of a positive CDC B cell cross-match, these results are now often interpreted in the context of solid phase assays. The immunological risk of potential renal transplant candidates are established by regular monitoring and storage of their sera to establish peak and current immune reactivity against a panel of donor cells, termed peak and current panel reactive antibodies. When a potential donor becomes available, donor cells are incubated in the presence of both peak and current sera. The presence of a positive CDC cross-match with peak sera even in the presence of a negative CDC cross-match with current sera poses a contraindication to transplantation, as this suggests suggest immunological memory to donor antigens from prior sensitizing events.

The inability to correlate all graft losses to anti-HLA antibodies detected using CDC assays (i.e. an inability of CDC assays to detect low levels of clinically significant anti-HLA antibodies) has led to the development of the more sensitive cell-based flow cytometric cross-match assays. The fundamental principle that forms the basis of the flow cytometric cross-match assay is similar to that of the CDC assay. Since the description of this assay in the early 1980s, this technique has been widely adopted to determine transplant suitability in many countries [9]. Similar to the CDC assay, flow cytometric cross-match assays require the addition of donor cells to recipients' sera, followed by the addition of a fluorescein-labelled secondary antibody allowing for the detection and quantification of anti-HLA antibodies by flow cytometer expressed as mean channel shifts. Unlike CDC cross-match, flow cross-match identifies both complement-fixing and non-complement-fixing anti-HLA donor-specific antibodies. However, the availability of different subtypes of detection antibodies has allowed clinicians to differentiation between complement-fixing versus non-complement-fixing anti-HLA antibodies [10]. Although an universal mean channel shifts cut-off value corresponding to positive flow cross-match has not been determined, it is generally accepted that the use of a low cut-

http://dx.doi.org/10.5772/54735

off value may disadvantage many transplant candidates as it may detect anti-HLA donor specific antibodies of no clinical significance, especially in the presence of negative CDC cross-match. Nevertheless, several studies have shown that the presence of a positive flow cytometric cross-match with a negative CDC cross-match is associated with a significantly greater risk of AMR and early graft loss with a positive predictive value for predicting AMR of 83% [10, 11].

To avoid problems associated with the availability and viability of donor cells that could affect the accuracy of cell-based assays, solid-phase assays were introduced which have largely circumvented these problems and improved the sensitivity of detection of anti-HLA antibodies [12]. The identification of anti-HLA antibodies using ELISA was first described in 1993 where purified HLA antigens were directly immobilized on the surface of microtitre plates but the basic principle of antibody detection was similar to cell-based assays [13]. The Luminex platform is a solid-phase assay that utilizes polystyrene microspheres (beads), each embedded with fluorochromes of differing intensity attached to one (single-antigen beads) or several HLA molecules (screening beads) to determine anti-HLA antibody specificity. The Luminex assay has been used in many transplant centres to select the appropriate desensitization regimen according to DSA strength and to establish an acceptable DSA cut-off that may allow kidney transplantation to proceed following desensitization [14, 15]. Similar to other assays, the addition of recipients' sera containing anti-HLA antibodies are added to the bead mix, these antibodies will bind to the appropriate beads expressing single or multiple specific antigen(s). A phycoerytherin-labelled secondary anti-human IgG is then added to this mixture and these antibodies will bind to the primary anti-HLA antibody already attached to the beads expressing the antigens. The sample is then passed through lasers, which would independently excite the beads and the phycoerytherin, therefore allowing the laser detector to define antibody specificity [16, 17]. Unlike the CDC assays, Luminex assay detect both complement-fixing and non-complement-fixing anti-HLA antibodies but does not detect IgM autoantibodies or non-HLA antibodies. The concept of virtual cross-match using solid phase assays relies on accurate HLA typing accompanied by evaluation of anti-HLA antibodies. The presence of a negative solid phase virtual cross-match reliably excludes the presence of donor-specific anti-HLA antibodies and is capable of predicting a negative flow cytometric cross-match in >90% of cases and CDC cross-match in 75% of cases. With the continued reliance on using cell-based cross-match assays, especially CDC cross-match assays to determine transplant suitability, a potential disadvantage of virtual cross-match is that transplants may be excluded based on antibody results with unknown clinical relevance [18]. It is generally accepted that solid phase virtual cross-match to identify anti-HLA donor specific antibodies complements the results of cell-based assays to help inform decision-making process with regards to transplant suitability.

3. Association between anti-HLA donor-specific antibodies and transplant outcomes (Table 1)

Despite technological advances in detecting pre-transplant DSA, the incidence of acute and chronic AMR appears to increase over time. However, the true incidence of AMR remains

Study	Cohort	Rejection	Graft survival
Eng H et al [24]	N=471 DD renal transplant recipients 83 T-B+ XM vs 386 T-B- XM IgG DSA in 33% of T-B+ XM patients	Vascular: 19% T-B- XM vs 32% T-B+ XM (p=0.01) DSA+ significantly predict vascular or glomerular rejection	Graft loss: T-B+ 44% vs T-B- 27%
Lefaucheur C et al [25]	N=402 DD renal transplant recipients Peak sera: positive DSA 21% (Luminex) Current sera: positive DSA 19%	PPV for AMR with peak DSA 35% vs current DSA 32% Prevalence of AMR categorized by MFI: MFI <465 – prevalence 1% MFI 466 to 3000 – prevalence 19% MFI 3001 to 6000 – prevalence 36% MFI >6000 – prevalence 51% Peak DSA MFI predicted AMR better than current DSA MFI	5 and 8-year DCGS: Non-sensitized - 89% and 84% Sensitized with no DSA - 92% and 92% DSA-positive - 71% and 61 Relative risk for graft loss if AMR 4.1 (95% CI 2.2 to 7.7) vs no AMR
Lefaucheur C et al [26]	N=237 LD/DD renal transplant recipients All negative T and B-cell CDC-XM 27% class I or II anti-HLA antibody with 52% anti-HLA antibody being DSA	Incidence of AMR: preformed DSA 35% vs no DSA 3% (p < 0.001)	Overall graft survival at 8 years: DSA-positive 68% DSA-negative 77% Graft survival lower in patients with DSA and AMR compared to DSA and no AMR and in non-DSA patients
Mujtaba M et al [34]	N=44 desensitized LD transplant recipients Negative CDC T-cell XM Sensitization = CDC B+ & T+ ± B+ flow XM	Incidence AMR 31% Total MFI and AMR: <9500 7% vs >9500 36% Class II DSA but not class I DSA greater risk of AMR	3-year graft survival was 100% for total MFI <9500 vs 76% for total MFI >9500.
Amico P et al [94]	N=334 LD and DD renal transplant recipients 332 negative T and B cell CDC-XM 67 DSA vs 267 no DSA (Luminex)	Overall incidence of clinical/subclinical rejection including AMR and/or acute T-cell mediated rejection at day 200 post-transplant: DSA-positive 71% vs DSA-negative 35%	5-year DCGS: No DSA 89% vs DSA without AMR 87% vs DSA with AMR 68%
Song EY et al [95]	N=28 LD and DD renal transplant recipients Positive flow XM but negative CDC-T cell XM, 57% positive DSA	BPAR: DSA-positive 56% vs DSA-negative 0% Class II > class I DSA higher incidence of AMR: 100% vs 22% Class II DSA MFI of 4487 predicted AMR with sensitivity of 100% and specificity of 87%.	No difference in graft survival

HLA – human leukocyte antigen, DD – deceased donor, LD – live-donor, CDC-XM – complement dependent cytotoxicity cross-match, DSA – donor-specific antibodies, SAB – single antigen bead, AMR – antibody mediated rejection, DCGS – death-censored graft survival, MFI – mean fluorescent intensity, BPAR – biopsy-proven acute rejection, PPV – positive predictive value.

Table 1. Association between pre-transplant donor-specific antibodies and graft outcomes.

unclear with suggestions that acute AMR may account for up to 7% of all acute rejections (and up to 50% of acute rejection episodes experienced by pre-sensitized patients with positive cross-match); whereas the prevalence of chronic AMR manifesting as transplant glomerulopathy may be as high as 20% at 5 years post-transplant [19, 20]. The growing incidence may be attributed to a number of plausible reasons including: greater acceptance of highly-sensitized candidates for transplantation, the use of non-calcineurin-inhibitor-based immunosuppressive regimen such as mammalian target of rapamycin inhibitors, better detection techniques for DSA, availability of markers of antibody injury such as C4d staining and a greater understanding of AMR, which may have been misinterpreted as chronic allograft nephropathy or undefined rejection in the past [21].

In most countries, a large proportion of renal transplant candidates on the transplant wait-list are sensitized with high PRA levels and have multiple anti-HLA antibodies, which often result in protracted wait-list time [22]. In Australia, 23% of transplant candidates have a peak class I PRA of >20% and these sensitized transplant candidates often have twice as long a waiting time as unsensitized candidates [23]. Pre-transplant DSA is a major immunological hurdle for successful kidney transplantation. The clinical importance of pre-transplant DSA has been clearly established over the past decade and the presence of high levels of pre-transplant class I (HLA-A and B) ± II (HLA-DR) DSA, typically occurring as a result of prior sensitizing events including previous blood transfusions, HLA-mismatched transplants and/or pregnancy, is associated with inferior graft outcomes, including an increased risk of developing acute and chronic antibody-mediated rejection (AMR), transplant glomerulopathy and late graft loss (Table 1) [24-27]. However, few studies have suggested that the association between pre-transplant DSA and graft survival was restricted to recipients who had developed early AMR or those with high levels of DSA as determined by peak HLA-DSA strength expressed as mean fluorescent intensity (MFI) using Luminex technology and that pre-transplant screening for preformed DSA may not be cost-effective [28, 29]. *Lefaucheur C et al* demonstrated in a large single centre study that renal transplant recipients with a peak pre-transplant DSA >465 MFI determined by Luminex have a significantly higher risk of developing AMR and that recipients with peak DSA >3000 have almost a four-fold increase in the risk of graft loss compared to recipients with peak DSA MFI of <3000 highlighting the importance of using DSA strength to more accurately assess the immunological risk of transplant recipients [29]. There is also increasing evidence demonstrating that the development of *de novo* DSA may occur in over 50% of renal transplant recipients at 2-years post-transplant suggesting that regular monitoring of de novo DSA post-transplant may help identify those at risk of developing poorer graft outcome [30]. Several studies have shown that the development of *de novo* DSA (occurring post-transplantation), especially DSA directed against HLA-DQ graft molecules in HLA-class II incompatible graft transplantations, are both associated with acute and subclinical AMR and graft loss in kidney transplant only and/or simultaneous pancreas-kidney transplant recipients and post-transplant monitoring of DSA could potentially help clinicians to individualize the amount of immunosuppression to better assess immune reactivity [25, 30-33]. Although there is no current consensus on the level of clinically significant DSA identified by flow cytometric or Luminex assays, most studies have demonstrated that increasing single, peak or total DSA levels were associated with an incremental risk of rejection and/or graft loss [29, 34]. Recent studies have suggested that the detection of C1q-fixing DSA (i.e. the potential to identify DSA that can activate complements by binding C1q) may be more accurate in predicting acute rejection, biopsy C4d-deposition, transplant glomerulopathy and late graft failure following kidney transplantation and the authors suggested that the absence of C1q-positive de novo DSA has a high negative predictive value for transplant glomerulopathy (100%) and graft failure (88%) [35]. However, a recent retrospective study showed that the identification of strong complement-activating DSA (of IgG subclasses 1 and 3) pre-transplant was unlikely to improve AMR risk stratification compared to patients with a combination of both strong and weak/no complement-activating DSA (of IgG subclasses 2 and 4) [36]. The clinical importance of C1q-specific DSA in predicting graft outcome remains controversial and not routinely performed in many transplanting centres [35, 37]. With the greater understanding of HLA antigens and anti-HLA antibodies, innovative techniques have been established to allow transplantation across positive CDC and/or flow cross-match barriers by removing circulating DSA and/or B or plasma cells and the success and outcomes of these initiatives will be discussed later in this chapter.

4. Clinical relevance of non-anti-HLA donor-specific antibodies (Table 2)

Although it is well established that AMR is attributed to the presence of class I and/or II DSA, non-donor HLA-antibodies and other non-HLA antibodies have been implicated in the development of acute and chronic AMR following kidney transplantation. *Opelz G et al* and others have demonstrated that increasing panel reactive antibodies (PRA) in HLA-identical sibling transplants was associated with a greater risk of rejection (defined as functional graft survival) and poorer graft survival (PRA 0% 10-year graft survival 72%, PRA 1-50% 63%, PRA >50% 55%; o<0.01) suggesting that immune response against non-HLA targets may be important in kidney transplantation, especially in the prediction of chronic graft loss [38]. Alloantigenic and tissue-specific autoantigenic targets of non-HLA-DSA and non-HLA antibodies may include various minor histocompatibility antigens, major histocompatibility complex (MHC) class I chain-related gene A (MICA) antigens, endothelial cell, vimentin, collagen V, glutathione-S-transferase T1, agrin, and angiotensin II receptor type I. Table 2 provides an up-to-date summary of the significance of these non-HLA-DSA and non-HLA antibodies in kidney transplantation and discuss the interplay between alloimmunity and autoreactivity in renal allograft rejection [39, 40].

Antibodies	HLA-antigen (Yes/No)	Target antigen	Location	Transplant outcomes
Anti-angiotensin type 1–receptor antibody [96,97]	No	Angiotensin type I receptor (cell-based ELISA)	Endothelial cells	Increased risk of ACR, vascular rejection and AMR ± malignant hypertension
MICA antibody [98]	Yes	Major histocompatibility-complex class I related chain A antigens (Luminex)	Endothelial cells (also fibroblasts, epithelial cells)	Increased risk of rejection and graft failure, remains debatable
Anti-endothelial cell antibody [39,99]	No	Endothelial cell precursors (flow cytometry)	Endothelial cells	Increased risk of acute and chronic rejections
Vimentin antibody [100]	No	Intermediate filament protein (flow cytometry)	Endothelial cells	Increased risk of rejection
Agrin antibody [101]	No	Highly purified GBM heparan sulphate proteoglycans (ELISA)	GBM	Increased risk of transplant glomerulopathy
Glutathione-S-transferase T1 antibody [40]	No	Glutathione-S-transferase T1 enzyme (ELISA)	Endothelial cells	Increased risk of C4d-negative acute and chronic AMR
Anti-GBM antibody [102]	No	Alpha-3 chain (the Goodpasture antigen) and alpha-5 chain of type IV collagen (ELISA)	GBM	Increased risk of vascular rejection (Alport patients)
Antibodies to MIG (also called CXCL9), ITAC (also called CXCL11), IFN-γ, and glial-derived neurotrophic factor [103]	No	Chemokine or cytokine (ELISA)	Circulating proteins	Association with chronic renal allograft injury
Protein kinase Czeta antibody [104]	No	Protein kinase (microarray)	Kidney and lymphocytes	Increased risk of graft loss
Anti-HLA-Ia antibody [105]	Yes	HLA-Ia alleles	Endothelial cells	Correlate with poorer graft survival, possibly mediated via anti-HLA-E IgG antibody

Abbreviations: MICA – major histocompatibility complex class I chain-related gene A, ACR – acute cellular rejection, AMR – antibody mediated rejection, GBM – glomerular basement membrane, ELISA – enzyme-linked immunosorbent assay, HLA – human leukocyte antigen

Table 2. Association between non-HLA-DSA and non-HLA antibodies and renal transplant outcomes.

5. Complexities in the diagnosis of antibody mediated rejection (Table 3)

The diagnosis of AMR has improved dramatically with the advent of C4d staining and the ability to detect DSA [41]. The diagnosis of acute AMR according to BANFF criteria requires a triad of [1] histological evidence of graft damage including acute-tubular necrosis-like minimal inflammation, capillaritis and/or glomerulitis and/or thromboses and arteritis, [2] immunological evidence of complement activation inferred by C4d positivity in the peritubular capillaries (PTC), and [3] presence of DSA; whereas the diagnostic criteria for chronic AMR requires [1] morphological evidence of chronic damage of the allograft including duplication of glomerular basement membrane, lamination of peritubular capillaries, arterial intimal fibrosis or interstitial fibrosis/tubular atrophy, [2] diffuse C4d deposition in PTC, and [3] presence of DSA [42]. C4d, a complement split product, is formed by the binding and activation of the classical complement pathway by DSA, which then binds covalently to specific target molecules on the endothelium of PTC and is therefore considered a footprint of AMR [43]. The sensitivity and specificity of diffuse PTC C4d staining for the presence of DSA is >95% [44].

Acute antibody-mediated rejection Peritubular capillary C4d deposition Circulating anti-HLA donor specific antibody Morphological evidence of acute tissue injury (e.g. capillaritis, glomerulitis)	Chronic antibody-mediated rejection Peritubular capillary C4d deposition Circulating anti-HLA donor specific antibody Morphological evidence of chronic tissue injury (e.g. transplant glomerulopathy, interstitial fibrosis, tubular atrophy)
Controversies of C4d staining Peritubular capillary C4d deposition Glomerular C4d deposition Arteriolar C4d deposition AMR Erythrocyte C4d deposition better PPV in peritubular capillary	Useful to detect AMR, diffuse > focal, PTC C4d negative in 60% AMR Correlates with AMR and graft survival No association with graft survival or Similar sensitivity and specificity but detecting AMR compared with C4d deposition
Abbreviation: AMR – antibody mediated rejection, HLA – human leukocyte antigen	

Table 3. Histological criteria for acute and chronic antibody mediated rejection and corresponding table of controversies of relying on peritubular capillary C4d deposition as a marker for antibody mediated rejection.

However, there are concerns regarding whether the presence of C4d within peritubular capillaries is essential for the diagnosis of AMR with reports of C4d-negative AMR being identified. There have been a few studies that have demonstrated an association between glomerular or erythrocyte C4d deposition and the presence of acute and chronic AMR but the clinical significance of these deposits remain debatable.

Problems with C4d staining:

i. Accomodation

The presence of C4d deposition in PTC does not always denote the presence of AMR or tissue injury. In ABO-incompatible renal transplant, the presence of PTC C4d staining often occurs in the absence of tissue injury or AMR, a process known as accommodation and may be observed in >70% of ABO-incompatible transplants; whereas the presence of PTC C4d staining in HLA-incompatible grafts correlates strongly with the presence of AMR [45].

ii. C4d negative AMR

AMR in the absence of PTC C4d staining has been reported more frequently. In an analysis of 173 indication kidney biopsies, *Sis et al* demonstrated that a combination of high expression of endothelial-associated transcripts (ENDAT) detected using microarray on tissue biopsy, suggesting endothelial damage from alloantibody, plus the presence of DSA was strongly associated with morphological evidence of AMR but only 38% of these biopsies had evidence of PTC C4d positivity [46]. Other studies have corroborated this initial finding suggesting that over reliance of C4d positivity to diagnose acute or chronic AMR could miss up to 60% of patients with morphological evidence of AMR and C4d staining should always be interpreted in the context of tissue morphology [47, 48]

iii. Focal versus diffuse C4d staining

It is generally accepted that the detection of C4d in renal allograft biopsies using immunofluorescence staining is more sensitive than immunohistochemical staining [42, 49]. The level of C4d staining appears to have prognostic significance and it is widely accepted that diffuse C4d staining involving >50% of PTC by either technique is considered positive and correlates much more strongly with adverse graft outcome compared to focal C4d staining involving <50% of PTC, but this remains controversial [50]. However, there are other studies suggesting that focal C4d staining is also associated with histological evidence of AMR including glomerulitis and/or peritubular dilatation [51].

iv. Non-PTC C4d staining

Glomerular, arteriolar and/or erythrocyte C4d positivity often occurs in the absence of PTC C4d staining but the clinical significance of these patterns remains unclear. In a retrospective study of 539 indication renal allograft biopsies, *Kikic et al* demonstrated a poor correlation between arteriolar C4d staining and graft survival, whereas linear glomerular C4d staining was strongly associated with graft failure [52]. There has been considerable interest in the detection of erythrocyte C4d deposition (eC4d) by indirect immunofluorescence as a potential surrogate marker of disease activity in patients with systemic lupus erythematosus and may be useful for the monitoring of disease activity and/or response to treatment in these patients [53, 54]. In kidney transplantation, *Haidar et al* showed a greater amount of eC4d in PTC C4d positive samples compared to PTC C4d negative samples. The authors reported that the positive (PPV) and negative predictive value (NPV) of PTC C4d and eC4d for peritubular capillaritis were 28% and 46% for PPV and 93% and 94% for NPV respectively suggesting that monitoring of eC4d may be an useful non-invasive marker of AMR [55].

6. Management of highly sensitized renal transplant candidates with anti-HLA antibodies

The complexity of transplantation has evolved over the years such that many transplanting centres are performing ABO-incompatible transplants and desensitizing highly allo-sensitized transplant candidates to improve their transplant potential. There is an increasing number of transplant candidates who are allo-sensitised to HLA as a result of previous exposure to HLA antigens, typically following blood transfusion, prior transplantation and pregnancy. It is well known that the presence of high levels of pre-transplant DSA is associated with poorer graft outcomes, including the development of acute and chronic AMR resulting in late graft loss [26, 56]. Finding a compatible donor for potential transplant candidates with multiple anti-HLA antibodies is often difficult and these patients may remain on the deceased donor transplant wait-list for a much longer period compared to unsensitized transplant candidates. Paired kidney exchange program is a potential and proven option for highly sensitized patients who have a positive cross-match with their potential live donors to receive a compatible cross-match negative donors [57]. With the greater understanding of HLA antigens and anti-HLA antibodies, innovative techniques have been established to allow transplantation across a 'positive CDC and/or flow cytometric cross-match' barrier resulting from anti-HLA antibodies directed against the donor. Nevertheless, graft outcomes of highly sensitized transplant recipients are poorer compared to compatible transplant recipients, particularly a much greater risk of acute AMR (Table 4).

	Number of patients	AMR incidence (%)	1-year graft survival (%)	2-year graft survival (%)
Lefaucheur et al ^ [26]	43	35	89	89
Thielke et al$^{\theta}$ [70]	51	32	93	81
Magee et al [71]	28	39	92	89
Gloor et al [106]	119	41	89	89
Haririan et al [106]	41	12	90	85
Vo et al [72]	16	30	94	Not reported
Vo et al$^{\#}$ [62]	76	29	87	84
ANZDATA 2010* [107] Primary DD grafts Primary LD grafts	550 296	<5% <5%	95 96	93 96

*ANZDATA 2010 – graft failure secondary to AR 2%; #Stratified by donor type – death-censored graft survival at 1 and 2 years for LD 90% and 90%; for DD 82% and 80%. [Note: Of the total 374 recipients, only 51 [13.6%) were DD transplants].

Acute AMR is a strong predictor of inferior graft survival: 1] ^AMR vs no AMR – 1y GS 60% vs 89% (Lefaucheur et al); 2] $^{\theta}$AMR vs no AMR – development of transplant glomerulopathy 44% and 12% (Gloor et al).

Abbreviations: ANZDATA – Australia and New Zealand Dialysis and Transplant registry, AMR – antibody mediated rejection, DD – deceased donor, LD – live-donor.

Table 4. Incidence of antibody mediated rejection and graft survival following positive crossmatch kidney transplantation.

http://dx.doi.org/10.5772/54735

	Number	Technique	Outcomes	Complications
Vo A et al [72]	• 10/11 LD and 6/9 DD with CDC-XM or FCMX+ (Note: 13/16 had persistently positive XM at time of transplant)	• IVIg 2g/kg day 0 and 30 + rituximab 1g day 7 and 22 (5/16 CDC-XM+)	• Wait-time pre-transplant 144±89m, additional 5±6m (range 2-18) post-desensitisation • 12mGS 94% • 12mPS 100% • 50% AR (30%AMR)	• 44% asymptomatic UTI
Vo A et al [62]	• 76 (31 LD & 45 DD) with T cells FCMX+ F/up 18m	• IVIg 2g/kg day 1 and 30 + rituximab 1g day 15	• Wait-time for DD pre-transplant 95±46m, additional 4.2±4.5 post-desensitisation • AMR 29% (11DD/11LD) • 2yGS 84%, PS 95% (LD 90%/100%, DD 80%/91%) • 2yCr - 143µmol/L	• 11% infections, 8% CMV/BKV • 5% mortality (2.5% infections)
Rogers N et al [108]	• 10/13 LD with CDCXM+ and DSA+ successful(DSA up to 18,000 MFI)	• Rituximab 375mg/m2 day -14 + 5PP with 0.1g/kg post-4PP + 2g/kg IVIg post-final PP • Induction basiliximab	• 80% Cr <160 • 30% AR (cellular) <3m (Pre-Tx DSA <5000)	• 10% PNF • 10% mortality (sepsis) • 70% transfusions ≥5 units • 30% sepsis • 21% CMV
Haririan A et al [69]	• 41 LD with FCMX+ with 27 B/T cell+ (vs historical controls)	• Alternate day PP (mean 4) + post-PP 0.1g/kg IVIg + induction T cell depletion	• 1y GS – 90% vs 98% (historical controls) • 5y GS – 69% vs 81% • Graft half-life 6.8y • 12% AMR	• Infection rates similar
Gloor J et al [106]	• 119 LD +CM (52 CDC-XM+) vs 70 controls	• Daily PP with post-PP 0.1g/kg IVIg ± splenectomy or rituximab (d-7) + rATG induction	• 50% AMR and 54$ TG in CDC-XM+ (vs 1% and 0% controls) • DCGF 46% vs 0% at 2y	• Not reported
Thielke J et al [109]	• 49/57 LD FCMX+ successfully desensitised to XM-	• 3-5 PP with post-PP 0.1g/kg IVIg ± rituximab (1-2 doses 375mg/m2)	• 1y DCGS 93% • 1y PS 95% • AR 43% 1y (24% AMR)	• Infection risk with rituximab • 7% CMV
Magee C et al [110]	• 29 LD CDC-XM T or B-cell +	• 3x/week PP with 10g IVIg post-PP ± rituximab pre-transplant (375mg/m2)	• 42% ACR and 39% AMR (no difference with rituximab)	• Not significant

	Number	Technique	Outcomes	Complications
Jordan S et al [61]	• 98 PRA ≥50% randomised 1:1 to IVIg or placebo (LD and DD)	• IVIg 2g/kg monthly for 4 months or placebo	• Improved DD transplant rate in IVIg group compared to placebo (31% vs 12%, p=0.01) • Estimated projected mean time to transplantation is 4.8y for IVIG vs 10.3y for placebo • GS and PS similar	• More headaches in IVIg group
Jordan S et al [111]	• N=42 (62% LD)	• LD 1x 2g/kg IVIg • DD monthly 2g/kg IVIg x 4 + pre-Tx 2g/kg IVIg	• 31% AR (<1m), 38% ATG and 23% graft loss from AR • 2y GS 89%, PS 98%	• Not reported

Abbreviations: LD = live-donor, DD – deceased donor, CDC – complement dependent cytotoxicity, FCMX – flow cytometric cross-match, DSA – donor specific antibody, PP – plasmapheresis, AR – acute rejection, rATG – rabbit antithymocyte globulin, GS – graft survival, DCGF – death-censored graft failure, PS – patient survival, AR – acute rejection, AMR – antibody mediated rejection, ACR – acute cellular rejection, TG – transplant glomerulopathy, IVIg – intravenous immunoglobulin, PNF – primary non-function, CMV – cytomegalovirus

Table 5. Relevant studies of desensitization in live and deceased-donor transplantation.

Studies reporting the utilization of desensitisation techniques to allow transplantation in highly sensitized transplant candidates have focussed predominantly on live-donor transplantation, which allows early planning and implementation of treatment at a suitable time (Table 5). A recent paper by *Montgomery R et al* had demonstrated that desensitization of highly sensitized patients for live-donor transplantation was associated with a significant survival benefit compared with waiting for a compatible deceased donor organ. By 8 years, this survival advantage more than doubled suggesting that desensitization protocols to overcome incompatibility barriers in live-donor renal transplantation may be justified [58]. However, the benefit of desensitization of highly sensitized patients on the deceased donor transplant wait-list remains debatable due to the uncertainty of kidney availability [59, 60]. The only randomized study evaluating the benefit of IVIg to improve transplant potential in highly sensitized transplant candidates on the deceased donor transplant wait-list was a double-blind, placebo-controlled, multicentre study whereby 101 patients with PRA >50% who have been waiting for >5 years on the transplant wait-list were randomized to receive IVIg (2g/kg monthly for 4 months) or placebo. The administration of high-dose IVIg was associated with a reduction in PRA levels with 35% of IVIg-treated patients being transplanted compared with 17% of patients receiving placebo suggesting that this regimen was associated with improved transplant potential for highly sensitized patients [61]. This same group modified this initial regimen by adding rituximab and subsequently reported that desensitization of highly sensitized patients with PRA >30% using high dose IVIg (2 doses of of 2 g/kg days 1 and 30) and a 1g dose of rituximab (day 15) reduced the deceased donor transplant wait-list time from 95±46 months to 4.2±4.5 months achieving acceptable rejection rates and graft survival at 24 months [62]. In contrast, a recent prospective cohort study evaluating pre-transplant desensitization with two doses of IVIg (2 g/kg up to a maximum of 120g per dose) plus a single dose of rituximab (375 mg/m^2) in highly sensitized kidney transplant candidates with a calculated panel reactive antibody (cPRA) of >90% and had spent >5 years on the deceased donor wait-list did not improve their transplant potential or reduced class I and II cPRA levels. This finding has been corroborated by other studies that have demonstrated that treatment with high dose IVIg in highly sensitized patients (flow cytometric calculated PRA of 100%) on the deceased donor transplant wait-list did not significantly alter their cPRA levels or improved their transplant potential highlighting that the potential benefit of desensitization of highly sensitized transplant candidates on the deceased donor wait-list remain uncertain [63-65].

The optimal desensitization regimen for highly sensitized renal transplant candidates in the context of living related and unrelated donation remains unclear. Most of the current desensitization protocols are modifications of plasmapheresis and intravenous immunoglobulin (IVIg) ± rituximab and have been used successfully to desensitize highly allo-sensitized transplant candidates, therefore allowing transplantation to occur [61, 66-73] (Table 2). However, desensitization of positive CDC or flow cytometric cross-match patients using immunoadsorption with rituximab followed by ongoing immunoadsorption post-transplant appears promising achieving rapid elimination of DSA and excellent short-term graft outcomes [74]. Immunoadsorption appears to be more effective than plasmapheresis in removing circulating DSA and studies have shown that a single pre-transplant immunoadsorption could render a positive cross-match to become negative [75, 76]. Encouraging results have been obtained with the use of bortezomib and/or eculizumab in desensitization protocols to achieve successful transplantation across a positive CDC and/or flow cytometric cross-match barrier but the use of these agents are usually considered adjunctive treatments to standard protocol [77]. Although splenectomy has historically been used in the desensitization protocols for ABO-incompatible transplants and treatment of refractory AMR by removing an essential source of B lymphocytes, this has largely been superseded by B cell depleting agents [78]. These techniques aim to lower the DSA to an 'acceptable' level pre-transplant to allow transplantation to proceed and preventing immediate acute renal allograft injury. Most published studies of desensitization protocols are non-randomized and observational with varying techniques and threshold of detecting pre-transplant DSA, thereby making comparisons between studies difficult. Plasmapheresis with low dose IVIg (0.1g/kg following each plasmapheresis) for 2-3 weeks pre-transplant followed by interleukin-2 receptor antibody or CD3-T cell depletive agent induction is the most common desensitization protocol utilized in many transplanting centres although the duration of treatment pre- and post-transplant would depend on achieving a negative cross-match pre-transplant and on the DSA titres. Studies utilizing this protocol have reported high risk of AMR (between 12-100%) with a reduction in longer-term graft survival (66% at 4 years) despite acceptable short-term graft survival [69, 79, 80]. Although high-dose IVIg (2g/kg) was initially considered for deceased donor kidney transplant candidates, it has been implemented with and without rituximab in positive CDC and/or flow cytometric cross-match live-donor transplant candidates with similar risk of rejection and graft survival to studies using plasmapheresis and low-dose IVIg [62, 80-82]. A retrospective study by *Stegall et al* showed that CDC T cell cross-match positive renal transplant recipients receiving high dose IVIg alone had a higher rate of AMR [80%) compared to recipients receiving plasmapheresis, low-dose IVIg with rituximab (37%) or plasmapheresis, low-dose IVIg, rituximab and pre-transplant anti-thymocyte globulin (29%) suggesting that high dose IVIg may be inferior to the combination of plasmapheresis and IVIg but it is difficult to draw any firm conclusion from an uncontrolled study [73]. Furthermore, there are suggestions that pre-transplant treatment to lower DSA MFI to <6000 using Luminex is recommended for successful transplantation and is associated with lower risk of AMR but again, this remains debatable [14].

Following successful transplantation, ongoing monitoring of DSA and early recognition of AMR is crucial to avoid early graft loss. On re-exposure to donor antigens against which the recipient is sensitized, memory B lymphocytes in their spleen, bone marrow and lymph nodes undergo an anamnestic reaction leading to the development of antibody-producing cells, which can produce high levels of DSA within days or weeks and therefore, positive cross-match kidney transplantation requires both pre- and post-transplant interventions to continually suppress DSA levels. Although continuing plasmapheresis and/or IVIg post-transplant following successful desensitization of highly sensitized recipients with positive cross-match against the donor is generally accepted, there has been no study addressing the type, amount, duration and cost-effectiveness of such approach [70]. Nevertheless, studies have demonstrated a strong association between the development of *de novo* DSA (especially DQ-DSA or when there is a rise of DSA >500 MFI) and AMR and graft loss suggesting that that long-term monitoring of DSA in highly sensitized patients may be appropriate, especially those receiving class II-incompatible grafts [83-85]. A recent single centre study suggested that post-transplant DSA surveillance followed by pre-emptive initiation of IVIg and plasmapheresis with rising DSA titres have successfully improved long-term graft survival [86].

Intravenous gammaglobulins (IVIG) are effective in the successful management of a number of autoimmune and inflammatory disorders attributed to their immunomodulatory and immunoregulatory properties. IVIG has been suggested in the management of highly sensitized renal transplant patients because it eliminates eliminate circulating anti-HLA antibodies, suppresses the production of these antibodies by inducing B cell apoptosis (and also T cells and monocytes *in vitro*) and is a modifier of complement activation and injury [87, 88]. There is now considerable debate among the transplant community regarding the balance between the benefits and harms associated with IVIG desensitising patients with high immunological risks. t[89, 90]. One small but significant side effect associated with the use of high dose IVIg is the risk of thrombosis, which may be mitigated by slowing infusion rate (maximum infusion rate of 100mg/kg/hour), aspirin, enoxaparin and intravenous hydration pre- and post-infusion [91]. The important side effects of IVIg along with other agents commonly used in the desensitization protocol are summarized in Table 6. However, it is important to note that many of the side effects associated with desensitization treatment have been reported in non-transplant population but should be recognized and advised to patients receiving these treatments.

http://dx.doi.org/10.5772/54735

Treatment	Actions	Complications	Cost	Comments
Intravenous immuno-globulin [112]	Neutralize circulating anti-HLA antibodies Enhance clearance of anti-HLA antibodies Inhibit complement activation Induce B cell apoptosis Inhibitory effects on other immune cells such as macrophages and natural killer cells by binding to their Fcγ receptors	Thrombotic events Acute renal failure Haemolytic anaemia Aseptic meningitis Anaphylactoid reactions	US$8700 for 120g	Infusion related adverse events related to osmolality, minimized by slowing infusion rate Reduce thrombotic events by using aspirin, heparin/ enoxaparin, intravenous fluids Newer preparation, iso-osmolar products have higher titres of antiA±B, resulting in higher rates of haemolysis
Plasmapheresis [113]	Removal of circulating anti-HLA antibodies	Hypotension Bleeding diathesis Potential blood-borne pathogen transmission if replacement with fresh frozen plasma is required (rare)	US$2000 per session	Non-selective removal of antibodies
Immuno-adsorption [74, 114]	Removal of circulating anti-HLA antibodies	Similar complications as plasmapheresis	US1600 per session	Higher plasma volume exchange resulting in higher antibody removal rate may be achieved over plasmapheresis. More selective IgG removal compared to plasmapheresis
Rituximab [115]	Chimeric murine/human monoclonal antibody that binds to CD20 on pre-B and mature B lymphocytes	Infection (fungal and other opportunistic) Progressive multifocal leukoencephalopathy	US$3900 for 700mg	Similar effectiveness using smaller dose
Bortezomib [116, 117]	Proteasomal inhibitor causing apoptosis of plasma cells	Fatigue, weakness Gastrointestinal disturbances (common, mild) Anaemia, thrombocytopenia (mild, transient) Peripheral neuropathy (mild, transient)	US$1322 for 3.5mg	Role in desensitization unclear
Eculizumab [118, 119]	Humanized monoclonal antibody against C5 preventing the formation of membrane attack complex (C5b-9)	Meningococcal infections (rare, severe) Other infections especially with encapsulated bacteria Anaemia (rarely serious), leukopenia Hypertension, headache, gastrointestinal upset (common, mild)	US$5990 per 300mg	Role in desensitization unclear Requires meningococcal vaccination at least 2 weeks prior to transplant

Abbreviation: HLA – human leukocyte antigens.

Table 6. Complications and cost of desensitization treatment.

In the absence of large randomized controlled trials, the optimal desensitization protocol is unclear. Observational data have reported desensitization protocols comprising of high or low-dose IVIg and plasmapheresis with or without rituximab and othetr newer agents such as bortezomib and eculizumab may be beneficial in selected patients, the rate of AMR remains extremely high (up to 50% in pre-sensitized positive cross-match patients undergoing desensitization) and may not be justified in circumstances such as in patients with very strong pre-transplant DSA levels [19]. The lack of treatment effectiveness among highly sensitised individuals is not unexpected, because most recommended treatment options such as plasmapheresis, IVIg and rituximab have minimal effects on plasma cells, the critical element of anti-HLA antibodies production, and AMR. Clinicians should discuss with their patients about the complexities and the potential side effects associated with any desensitisation protocols, taking into considerations the underlying immunological risks of the potential transplant candidates, the potential benefits against the short and longer-term harms such as infection and cancer risks. Specifically transplant candidates with prior sensitizing events and have DSA (even at low levels) against potential donor (e.g. husband to wife transplant) are at significant risk of AMR after transplantation despite r adequate desensitization. If desensitization is undertaken, this should be initiated 2-3 weeks post-transplant to ensure adequate removal of anti-HLA DSA pre-transplant with at least a negative CDC cross-match (or reduction in flow cytometric cross-match results) and persistent reduction in DSA MFI below 2000-5000. Transplantation should be abandoned if there is rebound of high titres DSA and/or the crossmatches remained unchanged/positive following desensitisation protocols. Although the benefit or cost-effectiveness of post-transplant DSA monitoring ± protocol biopsies in improving post-transplant graft outcomes remains unclear, it is well established that *de novo* DSA and rising pre-transplant DSA are associated with a greater risk of rejection and poorer graft survival [32, 92, 93]. However, there is no data suggesting that early interventions in renal transplant recipients who develop *de novo* DSA or rising DSA would result in an improvement in graft outcomes. Nevertheless, prospective monitoring of pre-existing DSA or for *de novo* DSA ± protocol biopsies should be considered and appropriate treatment instituted in those who develop histological evidence of rejection. Several proposed desensitization and post-transplant follow-up algorithms for positive cross-match highly sensitized recipients are available but the cost-effectiveness and outcomes of these programs remains unknown [80].

7. Conclusion

Despite the availability of more potent immunosuppression, the incidence of AMR continues to be an important cause of graft loss. Nevertheless, with the evolution of more sensitive molecular-based HLA-typing and the ability to detect DSA, clinicians have the necessary facts to critically appraise the immunological risk of each transplant candidate. However, there continues to be debate on several major issues including the role of non-DSA in transplantation, the appropriate DSA threshold, complexity in the diagnosis of acute and chronic AMR and the optimal desensitization protocol for highly sensitized patients. As there continues to be an increase in the number of highly sensitized renal transplant candidates on the transplant wait-

http://dx.doi.org/10.5772/54735

list as a result of prior sensitizing events, future studies addressing all these unanswered issues are critical.

Author details

Shyam Dheda[1,2], Siew Chong[1], Rebecca Lucy Williams[1], Germaine Wong[3] and Wai Hon Lim[1,2*]

*Address all correspondence to: wai.lim@health.wa.gov.au

1 Department of Renal Medicine, Sir Charles Gairdner Hospital, Perth, Australia

2 School of Medicine and Pharmacology, University of Western Australia, Perth, Australia

3 Sydney School of Public Health, University of Sydney; Centre for Kidney Research, The Children's Hospital at Westmead; Centre for Transplant and Renal Research, Westmead Hospital, Sydney, Australia

References

[1] Hawkins B. The HLA system and transplantation matching in the 1990s. J Hong Kong Med Assoc 1993; 45 (2): 77.

[2] Wake C, Long E. Allelic polymorphism and complexity of the genes for HLA-DR β-chains—direct analysis by DNA–DNA hybridization. 1982.

[3] Gebel H, Bray R. Laboratory assessment of HLA antibodies circa 2006: making sense of sensitivity. Transplant Revs 2006; 20 (4): 189.

[4] Patel R, Terasaki P. Significance of the positive crossmatch test in kidney transplantation. N Engl J Med 1969; 280 (14): 735.

[5] Bryan C, Martinez J, Muruve N, et al. IgM antibodies identified by a DTT-ameliorated positive crossmatch do not influence renal graft outcome but the strength of the IgM lymphocytotoxicity is associated with DR phenotype. Clin Transplant 2001; 15 (Suppl 6): 28.

[6] Mulley W, Kanellis J. Understanding crossmatch testing in organ transplantation: A case-based guide for the general nephrologist. Nephrology 2011; 16: 125.

[7] Eng H, Bennett G, Chang S, et al. Donor HLA Specific Antibodies Predict Development and Define Prognosis in Transplant Glomerulopathy. Hum Immunol 2011.

[8] Le Bas-Bernardet S, Hourmant M, Valentin N, et al. Identification of the antibodies involved in B-cell crossmatch positivity in renal transplantation. Transplantation 2003; 75 (4): 477.

[9] Garovoy M, Bigos M, Perkins H, Colombe B, Salvatierra O. A high technology crossmatch technique facilitating transplantation. Transplant Proc 1983; XV: 1939.

[10] Limaye S, O'Kelly P, Harmon G, et al. Improved graft survival in highly sensitized patients undergoing renal transplantation after the introduction of a clinically validated flow cytometry crossmatch. Transplantation 2009; 87 (7): 1052.

[11] Karpinski M, Rush D, Jeffery J, et al. Flow cytometric crossmatching in primary renal transplant recipients with a negative anti-human globulin enhanced cytotoxicity crossmatch. J Am Soc Nephrol 2001; 12 (12): 2807.

[12] Schlaf G, Pollok-Kopp B, Manzke T, Schurat O, Altermann W. Novel solid phase-based ELISA assays contribute to an improved detection of anti-HLA antibodies and to an increased reliability of pre- and post-transplant crossmatching. NDT Plus 2010; 3: 527.

[13] Kao K, Scornik J, Small S. Enzyme-linked immunoassay for anti-HLA antibodies-an alternative to panel studies by lymphocytotoxicity. Transplantation 1993; 55: 192.

[14] Akalin E, Dinavahi R, Friedlander R, et al. Addition of plasmapheresis decreases the incidence of acute antibody-mediated rejection in sensitized patients with strong donor-specific antibodies. Clin J Am Soc Nephrol 2008; 3: 1160.

[15] Reinsmoen N, Lai C, Vo A, et al. Acceptable donor-specific antibody levels allowing for successful deceased and living donor kidney transplantation after desensitization therapy. Transplantation 2008; 86: 820.

[16] Gibney E, Cagle L, Freed B, Warnell S, Chan L, Wiseman A. Detection of donor-specific antibodies using HLA-coated microspheres: another tool for kidney transplant risk stratification. Nephrol Dial Transplant 2006; 21 (9): 2625.

[17] Muro M, Llorente S, Gónzalez-Soriano M, Minguela A, Gimeno L, Alvarez-López M. Pre-formed donor-specific alloantibodies (DSA) detected only by luminex technology using HLA-coated microspheres and causing acute humoral rejection and kidney graft dysfunction. Clin Transpl 2006: 379.

[18] Lee P, Ozawa M. Reappraisal of HLA antibody analysis and crossmatching in kidney transplantation. Clin Transplant 2007: 219.

[19] Colvin R, Smith R. Antibody-mediated organ-allograft rejection. Nat Rev Immunol 2005; 5 (10): 807.

[20] Cosio F, Gloor J, Sethi S, Stegall M. Transplant glomerulopathy. Am J Transplant 2008; 8 (3): 492.

[21] Liefeldt L, Brakemeier S, Glander P, et al. Donor-Specific HLA Antibodies in a Cohort Comparing Everolimus with Cyclosporine After Kidney Transplantation. Am J Transplant 2012; 12 (5): 1192.

[22] Recipients OPaTNOaSRoT. Organ Procurement and Transplantation Network and Scientific Registry of Transplant Recipients 2010 Data Report. Am J Transplant 2010; 12 (Supp 1).

[23] McDonald S. Transplant waiting list. In: McDonald S, Hurst K, eds. ANZDATA Registry Report 2011. Adelaide: Australia and New Zealand Dialysis and Transplant Registry, 2011.

[24] Eng H, Bennett G, Tsiopelas E, et al. Anti-HLA donor-specific antibodies detected in positive B-cell crossmatches by Luminex predict late graft loss. Am J Transplant 2008; 8 (11): 2335.

[25] Lefaucheur C, Loupy A, Hill G, et al. Preexisting donor-specific HLA-antibodies predict outcome in kidney transplantation. J Am Soc Nephrol 2010; 21: 1398.

[26] Lefaucheur C, Suberbielle-Boissel C, Hill G, et al. Clinical relevance of preformed HLA donor-specific antibodies in kidney transplantation. Am J Transplant 2008; 8 (2): 324.

[27] Amico P, Honger G, Mayr M, Steiger J, Hopfer H, Schaub S. Clinical Relevance of Pretransplant Donor-Specific HLA Antibodies Detected by Single-Antigen Flow-Beads. Transplantation 2009; 87 (11): 1681.

[28] Ziemann M, Schonemann C, Bern C, et al. Prognostic value and cost-effectiveness of different screening strategies for HLA antibodies prior to kidney transplantation. Clin Transplant 2012; e-pub.

[29] Lefaucheur C, Loupy A, Hill G, et al. Preexisting donor-specific HLA antibodies predict outcome in kidney transplantation. J Am Soc Nephrol 2010; 21 (8): 1398.

[30] Hoshino J, Kaneku H, Everly M, Greenland S, Terasaki P. Using donor-specific antibodies to monitor the need for immunosuppression. Transplantation 2012; 93: 1173.

[31] Cantarovich D, De Amicis S, Aki A, et al. Posttransplant donor-specific anti-HLA antibodies negatively impact pancreas transplantation outcome. Am J Transplant 2011; 11: 2737.

[32] Ntokou I-SA, Iniotaki A, Kontou E, et al. Long-term follow up for anti-HLA donor specific antibodies postrenal transplantation: high immunogenicity of HLA class II graft molecules. Transplant Int 2011; 24: 1084.

[33] Wiebe C, Gibson I, Blydt-Hansen T, et al. Evolution and clinical pathologic correlations of de novo donor-specific HLA antibody post kidney transplant. Am J Transplant 2012; 12: 1157.

[34] Mujtaba M, Goggins W, Lobashevsky A, et al. The strength of donor-specific antibody is a more reliable predictor of antibody-mediated rejection than flow cytometry crossmatch analysis in desensitized kidney recipients. Clin Transplant 2011; 25 (1): E96.

[35] Yabu J, Higgins J, Chen G, Sequeira F, Busque S, Tyan D. C1q-fixing human leukocyte antigen antibodies are specific for predicting transplant glomerulopathy and late graft failure after kidney transplantation. Transplantation 2011; 91 (3): 342.

[36] Hönger G, Hopfer H, Arnold M, Spriewald B, Schaub S, Amico P. Pretransplant IgG subclasses of donor-specific human leukocyte antigen antibodies and development of antibody-mediated rejection. Transplantation 2011; 92 (1): 41.

[37] Sutherland S, Chen G, Sequeira F, Lou C, Alexander S, Tyan D. Complement-fixing donor-specific antibodies identified by a novel C1q assay are associated with allograft loss. Pediatr Transplantation 2012; 16: 12.

[38] Opelz G. Non-HLA transplantation immunity revealed by lymphocytotoxic antibodies. Lancet 2005; 365: 1570.

[39] Jackson A, Lucas D, Melancon J, Desai N. Clinical Relevance and IgG Subclass Determination of Non-HLA Antibodies Identified Using Endothelial Cell Precursors Isolated From Donor Blood. Transplantation 2011; 92 (1): 54.

[40] Alvarez-Márquez A, Aguilera I, Gentil M, et al. Donor-specific antibodies against HLA, MICA, and GSTT1 in patients with allograft rejection and C4d deposition in renal biopsies. Transplantation 2009; 87 (1): 94.

[41] Racusen LC, Colvin RB, Solez K, et al. Antibody-mediated rejection criteria - an addition to the Banff 97 classification of renal allograft rejection. Am J transplant 2003; 3 (6): 708.

[42] Solez K, Colvin RB, Racusen LC, et al. Banff 07 classification of renal allograft pathology: updates and future directions. Am J Transplant 2008; 8 (4): 753.

[43] Racusen L, Colvin R, Solez K, et al. Antibody-mediated rejection criteria - an addition to the Banff 97 classification of renal allograft rejection. Am J Transplant 2003; 3 (6): 708.

[44] Mauiyyedi S, Crespo M, Collins A, et al. Acute humoral rejection in kidney transplantation: II. Morphology, immunopathology, and pathologic classification. J Am Soc Nephrol 2002; 13 (3): 779.

[45] Haas M, Rahman MH, Racusen LC, et al. C4d and C3d staining in biopsies of ABO- and HLA-incompatible renal allografts: correlation with histologic findings. Am J Transplant 2006; 6 (8): 1829.

[46] Sis B, Jhangri GS, Bunnag S, Allanach K, Kaplan B, Halloran PF. Endothelial gene expression in kidney transplants with alloantibody indicates antibody-mediated damage despite lack of C4d staining. Am J Transplant 2009; 9 (10): 2312.

[47] Loupy A, Suberbielle-Boissel C, Hill GS, et al. Outcome of subclinical antibody-mediated rejection in kidney transplant recipients with preformed donor-specific antibodies. Am J Transplant 2009; 9 (11): 2561.

[48] Sis B, Campbell P, Mueller T, et al. Transplant glomerulopathy, late antibody-mediated rejection and the ABCD tetrad in kidney allograft biopsies for cause. Am J Transplant 2007; 7 (7): 1743.

[49] Seemayer CA, Gaspert A, Nickeleit V, Mihatsch MJ. C4d staining of renal allograft biopsies: a comparative analysis of different staining techniques. Nephrol Dial Transplant 2007; 22 (2): 568.

[50] Botermans J, de Kort H, Eikmans M, et al. C4d staining in renal allograft biopsies with early acute rejection and subsequent clinical outcome. Clin J Am Soc Nephrol 2011; 6 (5): 1207.

[51] Magil AB, Tinckam KJ. Focal peritubular capillary C4d deposition in acute rejection. Nephrol Dial Transplant 2006; 21 (5): 1382.

[52] Kikic Z, Regele H, Nordmeyer V, et al. Significance of peritubular capillary, glomerular, and arteriolar C4d staining patterns in paraffin sections of early kidney transplant biopsies. Transplantation 2011; 91 (4): 440.

[53] Singh V, Mahoney JA, Petri M. Erythrocyte C4d and complement receptor 1 in systemic lupus erythematosus. J Rheumatol 2008; 35 (10): 1989.

[54] Kao A, Navratil J, Ruffing M, et al. Erythrocyte C3d and C4d for monitoring disease activity in systemic lupus erythematosus. Arthritis Rheum 2010; 62 (3): 837.

[55] Haidar F, Kisserli A, Tabary T, et al. Comparison of C4d detection on erythrocytes and PTC-C4d to histological signs of antibody-mediated rejection in kidney transplantation. Am J Transplant 2012; 12 (6): 1564.

[56] Gloor J, Winters J, Cornell L, et al. Baseline donor-specific antibody levels and outcomes in positive crossmatch kidney transplantation. Am J Transplant 2010; 10 (3): 582.

[57] Gentry S, Segev D, Simmerling M, Montgomery R. Expanding kidney paired donation through participation by compatible pairs. Am J Transplant 2007; 10: 2361.

[58] Montgomery RA, Lonze BE, King KE, et al. Desensitization in HLA-incompatible kidney recipients and survival. N Engl J Med 2011; 365 (4): 318.

[59] Jordan SC, Reinsmoen N, Lai CH, et al. Desensitizing the broadly human leukocyte antigen-sensitized patient awaiting deceased donor kidney transplantation. Transplant Proc 2012; 44 (1): 60.

[60] Vo A, Peng A, Toyoda M, et al. Use of intravenous immune globulin and rituximab for desensitization of highly HLA-sensitized patients awaiting kidney transplantation. Transplantation 2010; 89: 1095.

[61] Jordan SC, Tyan D, Stablein D, et al. Evaluation of intravenous immunoglobulin as an agent to lower allosensitization and improve transplantation in highly sensitized adult patients with end-stage renal disease: report of the NIH IG02 trial. J Am Soc Nephrol 2004; 15 (12): 3256.

[62] Vo AA, Peng A, Toyoda M, et al. Use of intravenous immune globulin and rituximab for desensitization of highly HLA-sensitized patients awaiting kidney transplantation. Transplantation 2010; 89 (9): 1095.

[63] Marfo K, Ling M, Bao Y, et al. Lack of Effect in Desensitization With Intravenous Immunoglobulin and Rituximab in Highly Sensitized Patients. Transplantation 2012; Epub Jul 19.

[64] Alachkar N, Lonze BE, Zachary AA, et al. Infusion of high-dose intravenous immunoglobulin fails to lower the strength of human leukocyte antigen antibodies in highly sensitized patients. Transplantation 2012; 94 (2): 165.

[65] Gozdowska J, Urbanowicz A, Perkowska-Ptasinska A, et al. Use of high-dose human immune globulin in highly sensitized patients on the kidney transplant waiting list: one center's experience. Transplant Proc 2009; 41 (8): 2997.

[66] Zachary A, Montgomery R, Ratner L, et al. Specific and durable elimination of antibody to donor HLA antigens in renal-transplant patients. Transplantation 2003; 76 (10): 1519.

[67] Jordan S, Vo A, Bunnapradist S, et al. Intravenous immune globulin treatment inhibits crossmatch positivity and allows for successful transplantation of incompatible organs in living-donor and cadaver recipients. Transplantation 2003; 76 (4): 631.

[68] Rogers N, Eng H, Yu R, et al. Desensitization for renal transplantation: depletion of donor-specific anti-HLA antibodies, preservation of memory antibodies, and clinical risks. Transpl Int 2010; 24 (1): 21.

[69] Haririan A, Nogueira J, Kukuruga D, et al. Positive cross-match living donor kidney transplantation: longer-term outcomes. Am J Transplant 2009; 9 (3): 536.

[70] Thielke J, West-Thielke P, Herren H, et al. Living donor kidney transplantation across positive crossmatch: the University of Illinois at Chicago experience. Transplantation 2009; 87 (2): 268.

[71] Magee C, Felgueiras J, Tinckam K, Malek S, Mah H, Tullius S. Renal transplantation in patients with positive lymphocytotoxicity crossmatches: one center's experience. Transplantation 2008; 86 (1): 96.

[72] Vo A, Lukovsky M, Toyoda M, et al. Rituximab and intravenous immune globulin for desensitization during renal transplantation. N Engl J Med 2008; 359: 242.

[73] Stegall MD, Gloor J, Winters JL, Moore SB, Degoey S. A comparison of plasmapheresis versus high-dose IVIG desensitization in renal allograft recipients with high levels of donor specific alloantibody. Am J Transplant 2006; 6 (2): 346.

[74] Morath C, Beimler J, Opelz G, et al. Living donor kidney transplantation in crossmatch-positive patients enabled by peritransplant immunoadsorption and anti-CD20 therapy. Transpl Int 2012; 25 (5): 506.

[75] Lorenz M, Regele H, Schillinger M, et al. A strategy enabling transplantation in highly sensitized crossmatch-positive cadaveric kidney allograft recipients. Transplantation 2005; 79: 696.

[76] Higgins R, Bevan D, Carey B, et al. Prevention of hyperacute rejection by removal of antibodies to HLA immediately before renal transplantation. Lancet 1996; 348: 1208.

[77] Lonze B, Dagher N, Simpkins C, et al. Eculizumab, bortezomib and kidney paired donation facilitate transplantation of a highly sensitized patient without vascular access. Am J Transplant 2010; 10 (9): 2154.

[78] Locke J, Zachary A, Haas M, et al. The utility of splenectomy as rescue treatment for severe acute antibody mediated rejection. Am J Transplant 2007; 7: 842.

[79] Schweitzer E, Wilson J, Fernandez-Vina M, et al. A high panel-reactive antibody rescue protocol for cross-match-positive live donor kidney transplants. Transplantation 2000; 70: 1531.

[80] Marfo K, Lu A, Ling M, Akalin E. Desensitization protocols and their outcome. Clin J Am Soc Nephrol 2011; 6: 922.

[81] Jordan S, Vo A, Bunnapradist S, et al. Intravenous immune globulin treatment inhibits crossmatch positivity and allows for successful transplantation of incompatible organs in living-donor and cadaver recipients. Transplantation 2003; 76: 631.

[82] Glotz D, Antoine C, Julia P, et al. Desensitization and subsequent kidney transplantation of patients using intravenous immunoglobulins (IVIg). Am J Transplant 2002; 2: 758.

[83] Ntokou I, Boletis J, Apostolaki M, Vrani V, Kostakis A, Iniotaki A. Long-term post transplant alloantibody monitoring: a single center experience. Clin Transpl 2011: 341.

[84] DeVos J, Patel S, Burns K, et al. De novo donor specific antibodies and patient outcomes in renal transplantation. Clin Transpl 2011: 351.

[85] Mohamed M, Muth B, Vidyasagar V, et al. Post-transplant DSA monitoring may predict antibody-mediated rejection in sensitized kidney transplant recipients. Clin Transpl 2011: 389.

[86] Kimball P, King A. A novel post-transplant alloantibody surveillance and intervention strategy that improves graft outcomes in sensitized renal transplant recipients. Clin Transpl 2011: 369.

[87] Jordan S, Toyoda M, Vo A. Intravenous immunoglobulin a natural regulator of immunity and inflammation. Transplantation 2009; 88 (1): 1.

[88] Toyoda M, Pao A, Petrosian A, Jordan S. Pooled human gammaglobulin modulates surface molecule expression and induces apoptosis in human B cells. Am J Transplant 2003; 3 (2): 156.

[89] Jordan S, Cunningham-Rundles C, McEwan R. Utility of intravenous immune globulin in kidney transplantation: efficacy, safety, and cost implications. Am J Transplant 2003; 3 (6): 653.

[90] Dwyer J. Manipulating the immune system with immune globulin. N Engl J Med 1992; 326 (2): 107.

[91] Huang L, Kanellis J, Mulley W. Slow and steady. Reducing thrombotic events in renal transplant recipients treated with IVIg for antibody-mediated rejection. Nephrology 2011; 16 (2): 239.

[92] Kimball P, King A. A novel post-transplant alloantibody surveillance and intervention strategy that improves graft outcomes in sensitized renal transplant recipients. Clin Transplant 2011: 369.

[93] Almeshari K, Pall A, Chaballout A, et al. Targeted monitoring of donor-specific HLA antibodies following renal transplantation. Clin Transplant 2011: 395.

[94] Amico P, Hönger G, Mayr M, Steiger J, Hopfer H, Schaub S. Clinical relevance of pretransplant donor-specific HLA antibodies detected by single-antigen flow-beads. Transplantation 2009; 87 (11): 1681.

[95] Song E, Lee Y, Hyun J, et al. Clinical relevance of pretransplant HLA class II donor-specific antibodies in renal transplantation patients with negative T-cell cytotoxicity crossmatches. Ann Lab Med 2012; 32 (2): 139.

[96] Reinsmoen N, Lai C, Heidecke H, et al. Anti-angiotensin type 1 receptor antibodies associated with antibody mediated rejection in donor HLA antibody negative patients. Transplantation 2010; 90 (12): 1473.

[97] Dragun D, Müller D, Bräsen J, et al. Angiotensin II type 1-receptor activating antibodies in renal-allograft rejection. N Engl J Med 2005; 352 (6): 558.

[98] Lemy A, Andrien M, Lionet A, et al. Posttransplant Major Histocompatibility Complex Class I Chain-Related Gene A Antibodies and Long-Term Graft Outcomes in a Multicenter Cohort of 779 Kidney Transplant Recipients. Transplantation 2012; Epub.

[99] Sun Q, Liu Z, Chen J, et al. Circulating anti-endothelial cell antibodies are associated with poor outcome in renal allograft recipients with acute rejection. Clin J Am Soc Nephrol 2008; 3 (5): 1479.

[100] Carter V, Shenton B, Jaques B, et al. Vimentin antibodies: a non-HLA antibody as a potential risk factor in renal transplantation. Transplant Proc 2005; 37 (2): 654.

[101] Joosten S, Sijpkens Y, van Ham V, et al. Antibody response against the glomerular basement membrane protein agrin in patients with transplant glomerulopathy. Am J Transplant 2005; 5 (2): 383.

[102] Charytan D, Torre A, Khurana M, Nicastri A, Stillman I, Kalluri R. Allograft rejection and glomerular basement membrane antibodies in Alport's syndrome. J Nephrol 2004; 17 (3): 431.

[103] Sigdel T, Li L, Tran T, et al. Non-HLA antibodies to immunogenic epitopes predict the evolution of chronic renal allograft injury. J Am Soc Nephrol 2012; 23 (4): 750.

[104] Sutherland S, Li L, Sigdel T, et al. Protein microarrays identify antibodies to protein kinase Czeta that are associated with a greater risk of allograft loss in pediatric renal transplant recipients. Kidney Int 2009; 76 (12): 1277.

[105] Ravindranath M, Pham T, Ozawa M, Terasaki P. Antibodies to HLA-E may account for the non-donor-specific anti-HLA class-Ia antibodies in renal and liver transplant recipients. Int Immunol 2012; 24 (1): 43.

[106] Gloor J, Stegall MD. Sensitized renal transplant recipients: current protocols and future directions. Nat Rev Nephrol 2010; 6 (5): 297.

[107] Clayton P, Campbell S, Hurst K, McDonald S, Chadban S. Transplantation. In: McDonald S, Excell L, Livingston B, eds. The Thirty Fourth Report Australia and New Zealand Dialysis and Transplant Registry. Adelaide, 2011.

[108] Rogers NM, Eng HS, Yu R, et al. Desensitization for renal transplantation: depletion of donor-specific anti-HLA antibodies, preservation of memory antibodies, and clinical risks. Transpl Int 2011; 24 (1): 21.

[109] Thielke JJ, West-Thielke PM, Herren HL, et al. Living donor kidney transplantation across positive crossmatch: the University of Illinois at Chicago experience. Transplantation 2009; 87 (2): 268.

[110] Magee CC, Felgueiras J, Tinckam K, Malek S, Mah H, Tullius S. Renal transplantation in patients with positive lymphocytotoxicity crossmatches: one center's experience. Transplantation 2008; 86 (1): 96.

[111] Jordan SC, Vo A, Bunnapradist S, et al. Intravenous immune globulin treatment inhibits crossmatch positivity and allows for successful transplantation of incompatible organs in living-donor and cadaver recipients. Transplantation 2003; 76 (4): 631.

[112] Jordan SC, Toyoda M, Kahwaji J, Vo AA. Clinical aspects of intravenous immunoglobulin use in solid organ transplant recipients. Am J Transplant 2011; 11 (2): 196.

[113] Ahmed T, Senzel L. The role of therapeutic apheresis in the treatment of acute antibody-mediated kidney rejection. J Clin Apher 2012; 27 (4): 173.

[114] Morath C, Opelz G, Zeier M, Susal C. Recent Developments in Desensitization of Crossmatch-positive Kidney Transplant Recipients. Transplant Proc 2012; 44 (6): 1648.

[115] Gurcan H, Keskin D, Stern J, Nitzberg M, Shekhani H, Razzaque Ahmed A. A review of the current use of rituximab in autoimmune diseases. Int Immunopharmacol 2009; 9 (1): 10.

[116] Kolesar J, Utecht KN. Bortezomib: a novel chemotherapeutic agent for hematologic malignancies. American Journal of Health-System Pharmacy 2008; 65 (13): 1221+.

[117] Schmidt N, Alloway R, Walsh R, et al. Prospective Evaluation of the Toxicity Profile of Proteasome Inhibitor-Based Therapy in Renal Transplant Candidates and Recipients. Transplantation 2012; epub.

[118] McKeage K. Eculizumab: a review of its use in paroxysmal nocturnal haemoglobinuria. Drugs 2011; 71 (17): 2327.

[119] Davis J. Eculizumab. American Journal of Health-System Pharmacy 2008; 65 (17): 1609+.

Section 2

Clinical Aspects of Renal Transplantation

Chapter 6

Policies and Methods to Enhance the Donation Rates

Lucan Mihai, Lucan Valerian Ciprian and Iacob Gheorghiță

Additional information is available at the end of the chapter

http://dx.doi.org/10.5772/55245

1. Introduction

The therapeutic promise of transplanting organs from cadaveric donors, as envisioned by the pioneers of transplantation, has never been kept because the demand for cadaveric organs has by far exceeded the supply.

Besides the fact that renal transplantation is the optimal treatment for patients with end stage renal disease, it provides benefits to the society as a whole as well as to the recipients. Yet, the donor shortage poses a significant challenge to the transplant community and bare unfavorable consequences: prolonged waiting time and compromise patient survival. Sustained efforts were done during times to increase both the deceased donor and living donor pool.

The expanded criteria donors also known as non-traditional donors has been credited to lessen the current shortage of grafts available for transplantation by providing more grafts. Any such attempt is a two-edged sword since it increases the outcome risk of the suboptimal grafts.

Criteria for living donation were more restrictive compared with cadaver donation but such reluctance to use living donor marginal grafts is declining since transplantation is a better option than dialysis.

Expansion criteria allows transplantation of grafts from deceased donors at the extreme age (above 60 and below 16), with history of hypertension, diabetes or malignancy, hemodynamically unstable, non-heartbeating, seropositive for hepatitis B or C, with systemic infections, at high-risk for HIV infection, reduced renal function, anatomic anomalies, or injuries [1].

The waiting list for transplant organs continues to grow and many patients continues to die while waiting or become unsuitable for organ transplantation. Consequently, many patients with end stage organ failure are no longer relaying on the waiting list for cadaver transplantation. There is a trend not only to reconsider the living donor but also to turn the attention toward spouses, friends or even strangers as possible donors. From medical point of view, all these are acceptable alternatives due to advances in immunosuppression which have eliminated the requirement for a perfect genetic match for a successful organ transplantation. In many US transplant centers, the number of kidneys obtained from living donors has exceeded the number of kidneys obtained from cadaver [2].

Although organs from living donors can be transplanted safely, concerns about the protection of well-being of such donors has prompted the transplantation community to develop a consensus statement, emphasizing that a living donor should be competent, willing to donate an organ, and free of coercion.

Regardless of donor type and graft quality, one should keep in mind that never should be transplanted grafts with a heightened potential for the development of a progressive disease.

Since the rules are continuously evolving, the approach to use of each graft and recipient selection should be done with caution in order to obtain acceptable results.

2. The living donor

The use of living donors for renal transplantation was critical for the early development of the field, and in fact, preceded the use of cadaveric donors. At the moment, 20-22% of all kidney transplants performed in the world were done with grafts from living donors. Most donors are related genetically to the recipient, but there is an increasing percentage of cases, where donors are genetically unrelated and includes spouses, friends, or other emotionally related individuals. As it is known, ethical guidelines mandate that the living donors should not be coerced and there will be no evidence of financial profit for the donor. As a consequence, the donation should be considered "a gift of extraordinary value". It is known that the use of living donors has been associated with a higher success rate than that seen with cadaveric donation. Due to a higher demand for transplantation and the lack of a parallel increase in the number of available cadaveric organs, living donation is the only solution for some patients to avoid long times on waiting list, and occasionally, even the need of dialysis (1).

Better results (both long and short-term)
Consistent early function and easier management
Avoidance of long waiting time for transplantation
Less aggressive immunosuppressive regimens
Emotional gain to donor

Table 1. Advantages of living donation

There is a remote risk of catastrophic outcome of the living donor (1 in 3200 patients), but most transplant centers and surgeons accept this. Some centers accept only living related donors; others accept related as well as unrelated donors. These centers come to turns with the possibility of harming living donors by being highly selective in their acceptance of donors. While surgically

http://dx.doi.org/10.5772/55245

pragmatic, there is a philosophic fallacy in this approach. The important issues regarding the donor, in addition to medical suitability, are whether the donor understands the risk of nephrectomy and whether the donor freely consents. The risk for the donor is the same regardless of the donor's relationship to the recipient and regardless of the recipient's outcome. The risk for the surgeon, that is the death of the donor, is no less devastating for the surgeon if the patient is a close relative to the recipient than if the donor is a stranger.

2.1. Evaluation of the living donor

Usually, the potential living donor is the one who initiates the discussion about donation, although the recipient or the physician can also rise the issue. The donor than meets with the nephrologist, transplant surgeon, social worker, and transplant coordinator. All donors are informed of the risks and benefits of the transplantation compared with the dialysis and the risks to themselves by donating a kidney, on both short and long term [3, 4]. 1995 data of US practices founded that reported mortality rate for living donors to be 0.03% and the morbidity rate to be 0.23%. It is important to screen any relative of a patient with familial renal disease (polycystic kidney disease, hereditary nephritis) for evidence of occult signs and symptoms, in order to exclude such donors [5]. On the other hand, kidneys with minor renal abnormalities can be used safely, once it is determined that function of the such kidneys could not be impaired after transplantation [6].

Initial evaluation of all potential donors consists of blood and tissue typing. Usually, those with ABO incompatibility are excluded; compatibility with the Rh factor is unnecessary. All blood group compatible donors are then tested with the T lymphocyte cross-match. A negative cross-match will allow further consideration for donation. In the case of multiple potential donors, the better the antigen match, the grater is the likelihood of being selected for donation, if all other testing are within normal limits. In general, as long as the donor and the recipient have a negative T cell cross-match, the operation can be cared out. This is true for both related and non-related donors who are ABO compatible. Many centers perform a mixed lymphocyte reaction (MLR) as part of the routine evaluation, but the importance of this test has decreased with the introduction of better immunosuppression.

Further evaluation for a potential donor consist of a complete medical history and a complete physical examination, routine laboratory, testing, and serologic evaluation for EBV, herpes virus, CMV, HIV, and hepatitis B and C viruses. Urinalysis and culture along with 24 hour urine collection for creatinine clearance and protein excretion, are included as part of the routine evaluation. If there is any concern regarding a borderline hypertensive pressure reading, the blood pressure should be measured on the least three and as many as ten separate occasions. Once all laboratory testing has been performed, the next step is renal arteriography with an excretion faze to visualize the collecting system. This eliminate the need for intravenous pyelography. Such testing can be performed on an outpatient basis. Nowadays spiral CT scan has been used routinely instead of conventional angiography in all centers. The use of magnetic resonance (MR) angiography is also growing in importance. Donors are judged unsuitably for a variety of reasons (2).

Absolute
Lack of discernment
Alcohol or drug addiction
Age less than 18 years
Hypertension: blood pressure over 140/90 mm Hg requiring medication
Diabetes: abnormal glucose tolerance test or HbA1c
Proteinuria: over 300 mg/24 hours
Abnormal glomerular filtration rate: creatinine clearance less than 75 mL/min.
Microscopic hematuria of unexplained cause
History of thrombosis or thrombembolism
Medical significant illness: chronic lung disease, recent malignant tumor, heart disease, vascular collagen disease,
History of bilateral kidney stones
Family history of autosomal dominant polycystic kidney disease (ADPKD), unless ultrasound or CT scan is normal and age is over 30 years
Familial history of renal cancer
Bilateral fibromuscular arterial dysplasia
Long-term use of nephrotoxic drugs
HIV positive
Hepatitis B antigen-positive to a negative recipient or unprotected
Other severe infections
Relative
Anatomic abnormalities of the donor's kidney: vascular or urological
Obesity: 30% or more above ideal weight
Young donor with a first degree relative with type I diabetes or renal disease
Significant previous abdominal surgery
Single history of unilateral renal stone disease
ABO incompatible
Positive cross-match
Smoking
Psychiatric disorders

Table 2. Exclusion criteria for living donors

Anyone at risk for the development of acquired renal disease should be excluded.This includes individuals with diastolic blood pressure constantly above 90 mm Hg, or who required hypertensive medication to control their blood pressure.

History of hypertension is not by itself a reason for exclusion if the donor is normotensive and off medication, but the donor should be carefully examined for preexisting renal disease or for the risk of development of renal disease later in life.

Potential donors for siblings with diabetes routinely undergo a five hours glucose tolerance test, and 24 hour urine specimen must be free of proteinuria. Some centers require that the

http://dx.doi.org/10.5772/55245

donor be at least 10 years older than the age of the recipient at the time of diagnosis of the diabetes. The measurement of the haemoglobin A1c and anti-islet antibodies also can be included in the evaluation of any potential related living donor for a recipient with diabetes. Unexplained microscopic hematuria may be an indication of an underlying renal disease such as glomerulonephritis, but it may not be detected before donation. Finding as few as three red cells per high power field may appear unimportant at first but may be an indicator of potential future problems.

History of thrombembolism or thromboflebitis places the potential donor at increased risk of pulmonary embolism and therefore it precludes donation. This is also true for patients with heart disease, or history of malignant neoplasia. Obesity may be a relative contraindication for any potential donor, if it is more than 30% above ideal body weight. These individuals should be advised to loose the excess body weight before the transplant is scheduled, to decrease the risk of pulmonary embolism or cardiac complications.

Patients with clinically significant psychiatric disorders should be fully evaluated by a psychiatrist to established that the donor understands and agrees to the proposed procedure.

Once a full evaluation has been performed, if examination of the donor's kidney vascular supply and drainage system reveals an abnormality, it must be decided whether the risk imposed on the donor or the recipient are too great. With regard to vascular abnormalities we tend to use donor kidneys with three or more arteries if there is a good immunological correspondence and a strong determination for donation and if dialysis tolerance of the recipient is bad [7,8]. Abnormalities such as aneurisms, renal artery stenosis, fibro-muscular dysplasia, if limited in sized and area, can often be resected, repaired, or excised on the back table. Such pathological addition should bee limited to one kidney, living as a rule, the normal kidney in place. Given this caveats, it may be possible to use such donors [9].

Excision and reconstruction of such abnormalities is, in a sense, a of form of treatment of this donors, although care must be taken to avoid living either the donor or the recipient with less than a perfect outcome.

2.2. Preoperative management

Once the evaluation has demonstrated that there are no abnormalities serious enough to exclude donation, the donor can be admitted to the hospital after a spiral CT scan was performed. Many insurance companies are now restricting admissions to the day of the operation. In such cases intravenous hydration can be given overnight on an outpatient basis, or started on arrival at the hospital. Such hydration is important to help ensure adequate diuresis during the donor operation. Preoperative assessment by the anesthesiologist and the pain management team can make for a more comfortable postoperative recovery.

The donor is instructed preoperatively on the use of spirometer, and on the use of leg support stockings and the sequential compression device system to prevent venous stasis. After entering the operating room and before the incision, the patient should receive a dose of intravenous antibiotic. Although preoperative skin cleaning is recommended; hair clipping is avoid until just before incision.

2.3. Surgical alternatives in life donor nephrectomy

Regarding the surgical habits and the existing experience, there are several ways of harvesting kidneys from living donors [10-12].

- Classic transperitoneal approach, either throw midline, or throw a left or right subcostal incision.
- Subcostal extraperitoneal approach (left or wright).
- Dorsal lumbotomy approach. The incision can be performed either underneath the XIIth rib, resecting the XIIth rib, or above the XIIth rib (extraperitoneal, extrapleural).
- Laparoscopic approach either transperitoneal or retroperitoneoscopic.

2.4. Laparoscopic approach for living donor nephrectomy

The introduction of laparoscopic living kidney donation has been a major advance in organ donation. First introduced with some reticence only in selected centers, this procedures are now the preferred surgical approach in almost all transplant programs in United States and Europe. Usually, the program that offers this kind of procedure have a high rates of living kidney donation. The major benefit of laparoscopic technique includes significant reduction of surgical pain, postoperative convalescence, and recovery time. As a result, the laparoscopic donor nephrectomy has been responsible for expanding the pool of living donors and may account for the increased popularity and frequency of living donation. Long term renal function is not different between open nephrectomy and laparoscopic nephrectomy. About 75% of living donor transplant nephrectomies world wide employ laparoscopic technique, either transperitoneal or retroperitoneal.

2.5. Open living donor nephrectomy

The traditional method for removing kidney from a living donor has been open surgical technique, in majority of cases using a flank incision. In selected cases in which the donor has motivation which precluded laparoscopic access (e.g. significant prior abdominal surgery), or in some cases of complex vascular anatomy, an open surgical approach is preferred. Some centers advocate the use of open surgery for pediatric patients, although the age of recipient is not universally considered an indication for open renal procurement. Most donor surgeon use a donor flank incision, extra pleural and extra peritoneal above or below the XIIth rib.

As it is in any surgical approach, the kidney must be very carefully dissected to preserve renal veins and periureteral blood supply. Excessive pressure on the renal artery is avoided to prevent a vasospasm. After the renal vessels are securely ligated and divided the kidney is removed and placed in a basin of frozen saline slush to decrease the renal metabolism and after that the vessels are un-ligated and flushed with heparinized solution for both procedures, either laparoscopic harvesting or classic surgery.

2.6. Postoperative care

Postoperative care of a living donor is fairly standard. Adequate postoperative analgesia is a key factor including postoperative complications such atelectasia and pneumonia [15]. Infections should not occur with appropriate antibiotic prophylaxis. The continuous use of leg stoching and sequential compression devices are essential to prevent deep venous thrombosis of the lower limb. Most patients are often ambulatory by postoperative day 1 or 2 and tolerating oral feedings by postoperative day 2 or 3. The donor can be discharged by postoperative day 2 to 6. The renal function of the donor should be assessed periodically after the operation, as some patients experience a 25% increase in serum creatinine level; this should return near baseline by 3 months after the operation. In fact there are no convincing data to suggest that living donors are at any increased long term risk as a result as having donating the kidney.

2.7. Long term complications

The immediate operative risk to the donor can be stated with some certainty but the long terms effects are not completely understood. Follow-up, in general, is reassuringly but incomplete. Most folow-up studies of living kidney donors find no decrease in long term survival. All existing follow-up found an at least 85% survival up to 31 year after donation, compared to a predicted 66% in general population of similar age. The survival advantage at the living donors was attributed to the selection bias of only healthy individual as renal donors and at better follow up for them. Concerns regarding the possibility that donors will develop end stage renal disease (ESRD) is:

- hyper filtration in the remaining kidney will lead to focal segmental glomerulosclerosis and renal failure, that is donation per se will cause renal failure,
- the second concern is that donor will develop primary renal disease. The donors who develop primary renal disease will progress to renal failure more quickly because they have a lower than normal renal mass at onset of a primary renal disease. The later concern applies to a family with a history that put them for a risk of renal disease, for example: patient with type II diabetes.

Many follow-up studies have noted an increase in hypertension and proteinuria as well as a statistically but not clinically significant increase in serum creatinine. There are studies which found an increase in 20% of patients with blood pressure (15%-48%) [16] but it is not clear if hypertension is more common to this group than in general population.

Another study is finding that 35% of patients are taking anti-hypertensive medications and 23% are having proteinuria compared with 44% and 22% respectively for controls [17]. On the other side, even if the donor has a normal renal function, the glomerular filtration rate is in fact maintained by hyper filtration.

One thing is for sure, that in all follow-up studies, majority of the donors which are altruistic donors, drive a tremendous degree of satisfaction and an increased of self esteem for their donation. As a consequence, donors interviewed considered their donation as an act of heroism and generosity with which nothing else in their life can be compared [18]. More than 90% said that they would donate if they have it to do over again, and fewer than 10% expressed any regret about donating [19].

2.8. Policies to enhance living donation

The therapeutic promise of transplanting organs from cadaveric donors has never been kept because the demand for transplantation has by far exceeded the possibilities. The waiting list for transplants continues to grow and in 2005 nearly 5000 patients were removed from the waiting list because of the death. Consequently many patients with end stage organ failure are no longer relaying on waiting list. Than the attention was turning toward living donors others than they have been classically admitted i.e. toward spouses, friends, or even strangers, as possible donors. From medical point of view, these are acceptable alternatives, due to the fact that immunosuppression has eliminated the requirement for a perfect genetic match in order to have a successful transplantation [20]. In many centers world wide, specially US transplantation centers and scandinavian transplant centers, the number of kidneys transplanted from living donors has exceeded the number of kidneys obtained from cadaver donors (over 35%) [21].

Although donors from living donors can be transplanted safely, concerns about the protection of well being of donors has prompted the transplantation community to develop a consensus statement emphasizing that a living donor should be competent, willing to donate an organ, and free of any kind of coercion [22]. More than that, the new reliance on organs from living donor has increased the risk of donation for financial reasons, especially in the case of unrelated donor. It is world-wide admitted that organ donation has to rely on the voluntarism and altruism, and uncompensated family members of the donor.

Donor type	1990	2000	2010	relative ratio
Cadaveric	4306	5489	7241	+ 1,68
Biologically related living donors	1831	4030	3046	+ 1,66
Emotionally related living donors	59	667	715	+ 12,11
Unrelated living donors	204	804	2516	+ 12,33
Total transplants	6400	10990	13518	+ 2,11

Table 3. Reported kidney transplants performed in USA [OPTN data]

The purchase of organs is explicitly unlawful in Europe, US, as virtually all other countries but the shortage of cadaveric organs has led to a world-wide black market for organs from living donors. That's why patients with sufficient means can travel to distant locations in order to purchase kidneys for transplantation [23, 24].

This is a dramatic situation which is generated by continuous shortage of organs for transplantation and by the increasingly donation rate from unrelated living donors. Such a situation require significant changes in the transplantation laws which should permit the increase of living donors and in the same time to stop the organ trade. Very difficult task.

The rate of living donation can be increased by two methods:

- organizing and ethic alternatives,
- medical methods are represented by: laparoscopic harvesting, paired kidney exchange, transplantation of grafts with anatomic abnormalities (vascular, urinary tract or fusion), acceptance of patients with low compatibility after a treatment with plasmapheresis and iv Ig.

2.8.1. Organizing and ethic alternatives to increase the rate of living donation

The motives of living donors and the motives of families of deceased donors, are complex and not necessarily always pure altruistic [25]. Spouses and siblings, who act as a living donor, experience a personal reward seeing that the recipient well being is restored. Because the organ donation is a voluntary and valuable act it should be considered as a charitable gift. Society could explicitly thank the organ donors for their gift, as it is done with other charitable contributions, without jeopardizing its altruistic basis. New legislations should embrace ethically acceptable ways to encourage such charitable donation of organs.

2.8.1.1. Incentives for organ donation

The issue of public incentives to enhance donation is more than just complex but mainly sensitive. From a philosophical point of view, the body is a part of our personality, thus in respect with human dignity it would be wrong to use parts of our body as means only [26]. On the other hand, one may assert that everyone is the rightful owner of his person supporting the idea that the self can decide over its body like any kind of property [27].

Most frequently, the background attitude of general population is to reject incentives for donation but there might be circumstances under which attitudes may change [28]. For instance, when the process became transparent: the amount of compensations are specified or there might be some ethical reasons to do so. The main risk is exploitation of those severe impoverished on a black market [29].

The valuable exchange of organs is prohibited worldwide, yet there exists national law or regulations which allows incentives for deceased or living donation [30]. Such incentives including financial reimbursement, health care-related reimbursement or other recognition for living donors or deceased donors' families have been widely debated [31].

Donor medal of honor. Organ procurement organizations must have ceremonies which recognize and appreciate organ donation. A donor medal of honor enacted by a top official of the country expresses the appreciation and gratitude on behalf of the whole community to the living donors and even to the families of the deceased donor [32, 33].

Medical leave for organ donation. Currently organ donors risk loss of wages or even loss of employment because the time away from the work that is required for donation [34,35]. In many countries there are legislations that provide a 30 day medical leave for all employees who donate an organ for transplantation [36]. However, no one should have to incur a personal expense for donating an organ. Many national organizations are doing an effort to encourage hospitals with transplantation services to provide paid medical leave for employees who become organ donors. Even if legislation emphasizing that enrichment should not be the reason for the donation, paid medical leave has to be available to a larger number of would-be donors [37].

Ensuring access to organs for previous donors. As you have seen up to now, the majority of living donors are doing well after donation. However, it has been established that at 10 years after donation, under 5% of those who donated the kidney developed ESRD; this donors are being placed on waiting list for cadaver organs [38]. Despite the additional allocation priority points, these donors have to wait for a cadaveric kidney, some of them for a long period of time. The health and well being of living donor should be monitored in a follow-up register in order to document medical problems associated with donation that occur over ensuing years [22]. The need for a transplant in a previous kidney donor should be considered a high priority in the allocation of the organs.

Donor insurance. The fact that there are being cases in which a kidney donor died immediately after donation or needed a kidney transplant at a later date, serves as a reminder that a nephrectomy (any kind of nephrectomy) is not a risk free procedure. A survey at some centers of transplantation show that at least two kidney donors had died from perioperative complications after a kidney donation and some of them had a persistent complication [39].

As a consequence, it should be enacted national plans to provide life and disability ensures for all living donors including a mechanism to ensure that they do not incur catastrophic medical expenses as a result of a donation.

2.8.1.2. Organ exchanges

Since the report of Rapaport which introduced the concept of paired kidney exchange as a method to enhance the number of living donors, these techniques have been applied in several countries with lower cadaver donation rates like Mexico, South Korea, Japan, and Europe (Holland and Romania).

Many persons who wished to donate an organ to a spouse or another family member where unable to help them due to incompatible blood type or other immunological barriers (positive cross-match). A program of paired kidney exchange addresses this problem by permitting an exchange of organs from two living donors [34] or from one living donor to one deceased donor. In the later approach, recently introduced in New England and Holland, a living donor incompatible with his intending recipient, donates an organ to a compatible patient on the waiting list for cadaveric organs in exchange for a priority allocation of a cadaveric organ to the donor's intended recipient. Thus, two transplantations are performed in circumstances that otherwise had permitted neither. Because such exchange could open the door to a paid donorship, the same prohibition against the payment donor should be applied to organ exchanges.

Legal issues. Initially, most countries limited traditional transplantation to genetically of strong emotionally related pairs. With extend of paired kidney donation, such limitations were removed to allow both altruistic non-directed donation and paired donation. Although, any exchange in paired donation represent in fact a transaction between parts, it do not involve financial values. It is advisable that such a issue should be explicitly addressed by the legal framework of every country.

Allocation algorithm. Grafts allocation in paired kidney donation is one of the domain who largely benefits from theories derived from economics regarding stable allocation and the practice of market design [40]. The main goal is to maximize the number of matched pairs. Any such program should overcome the disadvantage of O recipients by increasing the likelihood to receive a compatible graft. The risk of a positive cross-match with a from the donor pool might be assessed by considering the HLA antibody profile of the recipients and the HLA profile of the donors [41, 42]. When done on a national scale, such a matching should include distance between transplant centers, matching the virusologic profile of the recipient and donor, donor's age and size. Recipients from such pairs will be suspended from the waiting list until either they will be transplanted or a incompatibility test will reveal that the exchange is not possible. List paired donation may increase the rate of transplants by expanding the donor pool. In such an exchange, an incompatible donor who will donate to a recipient from the waiting list while his recipient will receive a high priority for the allocation for a deceased donor kidney [43, 44]. There are several concerns regarding ethical and legal issues. Such a transplant is designed to give an alternative to O blood type recipients with a non-O incompatible donor. The immediate consequence is the transplantation of a non-O blood group recipient from the waiting list and the addition of a O blood group recipient. This way, there will be an increased pressure over the O blood group recipients [43, 44].

Matching algorithms. Different matching algorithms were designed to maximize the number of recipients with an incompatible living donor will undergo renal transplantation. After an initial experience with two pairs, the number of pairs involved in a paired kidney transplantation increases to three, four and even more and the procedure gain worldwide acceptance. Involving of more than two pairs increases the chances to get a renal transplant but in order to avoid the withdrawal risk requires six or more operations to be done at the same time. Designed for O blood group recipients, exchanging of an incompatible kidney for a preferential position on the waiting list increases the recipient's chances for a renal transplantation but decreases the chances of other O blood group recipients from the waiting list [45-48]. This situation creates ethic dilemmas. Generalizing such list exchanges to any blood group recipient with a living donor available but incompatible, may overcome this issue.

Altruistic donation or non-directed donation is more ethical and legal challenging. It is difficult to believe and understand that a good Samaritan really exists and even when exists, national law framework should allow transplantation from unrelated living donor. Altruistic donors may be allocated to a waiting list or to initiate an open chain of paired transplantations [46,49].

Utilizing living donors may decrease the pressure for renal transplantation. Moreover, implementing of different types of kidney exchange could give further solutions to increase the transplantation rates. Combining different approaches to kidney exchange may create complex and versatile solutions to the incompatibility issue, even finding a better match for compatible pairs.

2.8.2. Medical methods to increase the number of living donation

2.8.2.1. Acceptance of grafts with anatomic anomalies

The number of donations can be increased by accepting donors with anatomic anomalies (multiples arteries, multiple veins, moderate dysfunction of the UPJ, renal cyst, complete duplicate ureteral system, solitary stone) which can be corrected in bench surgery.

Anatomical anomalies of the kidney have been considered for a long time as an absolute contraindication for living donation. Even now, many nephrological centers are including in their exclusion criteria for live related or unrelated donation items like urological abnormalities in donors or history or presence of any kidney stones.

But in our days, the majority of transplant centers with experience in the field, due to the shortage of the living donors pool, are considering the contraindication for using grafts with anatomical anomalies just a relative contraindication. Occasionally, the donor has minor unilateral abnormalities such as a renal cyst, ureteropelvic junction obstruction, solitary stones, duplex ureteral system, etc. If the related donor with a good immunological correspondence with the recipient has an abnormal kidney and is the only one available and the evolution of the recipient on hemodialysis is unacceptable, it is advisable to transplant the abnormal kidney, living the donor with the best one.

2.8.2.2. Acceptance of donors with multiple arteries and veins

The management of multiple renal arteries (MRA) are considered technically demanding in renal transplantation programs with kidneys from related or unrelated living donors. Some programs consider the use of multiple arteries and veins as a relative contraindication, because of increased risk of vascular and urological complications.

In addition, the rapidly increasing laparoscopic kidney donation has been accompanied by a significant shift in surgical practice [50,51]. Many centers which are performing laparoscopic harvesting restrict it to the left kidney [52-54]. The limitation to the left kidney leads to a higher utilization rate of kidneys with multiple arteries; in the literature, incidence of unilateral multiple renal arteries is between 18% and 30%, unless one limits laparoscopic nephrectomy only to the kidney with normal anatomy which is precluding 30% of all donors.

By accepting grafts with multiple renal arteries, one may theoretically accept an adverse effect on the outcome of those grafts. Previous authors [55,56], stated that MRA in their reconstruction were associated with several post-transplant complications. This is the motivation why such anatomy was considered to be a transplant contraindication. The most frequent vascular

http://dx.doi.org/10.5772/55245

complications which were encountered in reconstruction of multiple arteries were graft thrombosis, stenosis of the renal artery, and an increased risk of reno-vascular hypertension [55-57]. The most frequently ureteral complication encountered [58] were ureteral necrosis and pelvi-caliceal fistulas.

Smaller arteries are more prone to develop premature atherosclerotic occlusion. If that happens with a small accessory lower pole artery it would lead to ischemic distal ureteral stricture.

Any way, recent data collected from the centers and program of renal transplantation with experience in the field, display above any doubt that procurement of kidneys with multiple renal arteries can be accomplished safely and not impose additional medical, social, economical or postoperative clinical evolution burden, on the donor and the recipient.

Overall intraoperative and early postoperative complications of the recipients are not significantly different from the evolution of the recipients who received grafts with single arteries. A low rate of vascular complications is achieved using standard microvascular reconstruction technique with or without autologous vein patches [59-61] or extension graft. More than that, early graft function assessed by urine output and serum creatinine measurements were not significantly different among grafts with single arteries or grafts with multiple reconstructed arteries. In addition, long term quality of function, rejection, graft loss rates and graft survival were also similar. More than that, overall graft survival rates of this patients is exceeding 90% at 3 years.

In summary, the introduction of laparoscopic donor nephrectomy has significantly increased the number of grafts with multiple renal artery. Utilization of this donors, increase the rate of donation with 30% in specific centers. Modern techniques based on microsurgery have reduced dramatically incidence of above mentioned complications. From a patient outcome based perspective, this change in practice showed to be safe for both donors and recipients.

2.8.2.3. Laparoscopic donor nephrectomy - alternative to increase the rate of living donation

One great potential means for obtaining more kidneys is throw live donation. When compared with cadaveric renal transplantation, living donor transplantation has several advantages, in fact well known, which includes better graft survival, more rapid renal function after transplantation, shorter hospitalization and finally lower cost. However, several barriers exists for potential living donors. Significant time is involved when one donates a kidney. Many individuals do not have adequate financial and social support available that would allow them to make a personal sacrifice and a time commitment necessary for kidney donation. Moreover, the relatively prolonged convalescence can have significant financial impact on donor. Finally, fear of pain as well cosmetic concerns, associated with flank incision, can militate against kidney donation.

Laparoscopic living donor nephrectomy (LLDN) with all its alternatives (transperitoneal approach, retroperitoneal approach, hand assisted laparoscopic nephrectomy) was introduced in 1995 by Ratner and Kavoussi [62].

Laparoscopic nephrectomy is more technically demanding than other standard abdominal laparoscopic procedures. The surgeon experience is crucial for minimizing potential morbidity. Significant operative differences are between open and laparoscopic donor nephrectomy. The later approach requires a different set of technical skills than that associated with traditional open surgery. The endoscopic video image is only two dimensional and much narrower when compared with direct vision afforded by open surgery. The types of instrumentation available for working throw the small incision afford only restricted degrees of freedom when compared to the human hand. Moreover, the tactile sensation, currently can not be transmitted through the instrument. The differences are giving a longer operative time with one or even two hours when compared with open donation. All these drawbacks are only partially eliminated by robotic surgery, even if now there is a three dimensional vision of operative field and the mobility of the working instruments is better than that of human hand.

Even so, laparosccopic renal donation and robotic laparoscopic harvesting offers both introperatively and postoperatively great benefits to the donor.

Due to magnification provided by the optical system and the video camera, in experienced hands, the dissection of the renal pedicle is more accurate and if it is realized through retroperitoneal approach it is much more direct and quicker than classical approach.

The decreased size of the incision for extracting kidney and placement of that incision in the lower abdomen, significantly reduce postoperative pain when compared with traditional opened surgery; it also reduce traumatism of the abdominal wall, which is followed by a quicker and better healing and mobilization postoperatively and quicker reintegration of the patient in society.

Usually, these patients resume their oral intake in the first postoperative day and normal alimentation in maximum two days after surgery.

All retrospective comparations between open and laparoscopic kidney donation show that analgesic requirements for LLDN and robotic LDN, were 30% lower than those for open procedures. Need for oral pain medication is also reduced.

Return to physical demanding work also occurs, on average, 17th days sooner for the laparoscopic group compared with classic operation.

Recipient and graft survival. All retrospective review of the recipient who received a kidney through laparoscopic or robotic laparoscopic donation compared with those who received kidney via standard open nephrectomy shows no statistical differences if the groups are matched in regard with the number of HLA mismatches, donor relationship, diabetes, previous transplant, gender, or race.

Allograft function. The majority experience in the field attest that all grafts functioned intraoperatively and no clinical significant injury occurred to the graft.

	Laparoscopic	Open	P value
Estimated blood loss (mL)	266+/-174	393+/-335	0.027
Operative time (min.)	232+/-33	183+/-27	<0.001
Hospital stay (days)	3.0+/-0.9	5.7+/-1.7	<0.001
Analgesia (days of use)			
Oral narcotics	4	12	<0.001
Acetaminophen	3	17	<0.001
Resumed oral intake (days)	0.8+/-0.5	2.6+/-1.0	<0.001
Returned to work (weeks)	4.0+/-2.3	6.4+/-3.1	0.003

Table 4. Open versus laparoscopic donor nephrectomy

Allograft rejection. The pneumoperitoneum and retropneumoperitoneum reduces renal blood flow and urine output. The potential for ischemia can make the donor kidney more allogenic by inducing MHC class II expression. This problem could be avoided giving donors intraoperatively a 6-8 liters of crystalloid to promote brisk diuresis, and having an accurate dissection of the renal pedicle and harvesting the kidney only in full diuresis. Biopsy proved rejection in laparoscopically obtained kidney occurred in 30% of cases compared with 35.4% of cases of kidneys harvested by open procedure. At 12 months, creatinine clearance in recipient of kidney from laparoscopic and open procedure were both 66 mL/min. (p = not significant).

Laparoscopic nephrectomy gives less postoperative pain, quicker convalescence, better cosmetic results when compared with traditional open operation. In experienced hands, this procedure is accomplished without increasing the risks to donor safety and allograft function. Complications are comparable to those reported in historic series using open surgery. Longer operative time and the need of disposable equipment result in greater hospital costs. However, quicker convalescence permit patients to resume activities sooner and produce market cost savings both for patients and employer.

2.8.2.4. HLA sensitized and ABO incompatible donor and recipient

During the past decade, several innovative protocols have been adopted to overcome transplantation across a positive cross-match or an ABO blood group barrier. Protein A immunoadsorbtion, high dose intravenous immunoglobuline (IVIG), low dose iv Ig in combination with plasmapheresis, rituximab, splenectomy, all of them alone or in combination, can abrogate a positive cross-match and enhance the chance of a highly sensitized patients to receive a cross-match negative organ. Similar strategies can be used for ABO incompatible donors and are particularly effective when the titter of blood group antigen is low.

Plasmapheresis and intravenous immunoglobuline as a rescue therapy for a positive cross-match live donor kidney transplants. The positive cross-match can present a virtually an insurmountable barrier to kidney transplantation. Anti HLA antibodies have been identified as the predominant cause of early graft failure from hyperacute rejection and acute humoral rejection.

Once the consequence of performing a transplant, in the face of a circulating donor specific alloantibody were fully appreciated and routine pre-transplant cross-matching emerged as a standard, hyperacute rejection became rare, but a large population of a highly sensitized patients who have a little hope of receiving transplant has been subsequently identified.

Some of the longest waiting times for a kidney transplant are observed in patients who are allo-sensitized because of a prior transplant, blood transfusions or pregnancy. Some of these recipients have live donor, meet standards criteria for living donor transplantation, but have a positive cross-match with their donor. A combination of plasmapheresis and IVIG under the cover of standard doses of calcineurin inhibitors or rituximab, together with mycophenolate mofetil and steroids, can effectively and durably remove donor specific anti-HLA antibody, preemptively desensitize the recipient who had positive cross-matches with a potential live donor, allowing the transplantation of this patients using a live donor without cases of hyperacute rejection [63].

This preemptive therapy is initiated several weeks before a planned live donor transplant. Our standard protocol was designed to include oral immunosuppressants before first plasmapheresis treatment followed by a maximum six plasmapheresis on alternate days. The recipients, also received seven days of IVIG (100 mg/kg/day).

Cross-over transplantation and paired kidney exchange as a method to fill the gap of positive cross-match and ABO incompatibility. The gap between the number of donors and number of patients waiting for a kidney transplant continues to widen. Fewer patients get transplants every year because of the organ shortage. This patients can receive a donor from a living donor such a family member, a friend, or even a foreign individual.

The pool of such kidneys has not been fully utilized because not all living donors are compatible with their recipient. Patients with available living donor continue dialysis and many of them die because of ABO incompatibility, cross-match positive, low HLA-matching. Since the report made by Rapaport, when was set the bases of kidney exchange between two donor-recipient pairs in order to obtain a better compatibility, things have changed [64-66]. A spouse donor would give her kidney to an unrelated recipient who matched her blood type. That recipient's mate would provide a kidney for the donor's ill spouse. This swap would imply more than two pairs in order to obtain best compatibility. A cross-over renal transplantation or a paired kidney exchange transplantation is defined by a living kidney donation or a living kidney cadaver pool donation and exchange between two or more such couples who are hindered by ABO incompatibility or positive cross-match to give the kidneys not to the own recipients but solve the problem by cross-exchange the kidney between the pairs to make more matches.

The most frequent reason for ABO incompatibility, preventing living donors from donating is a blood group A or B donor and a blood group O recipient. There are many vice-versa pairs but the problem is that the blood group O donors are universal donors for all blood groups. They can give the kidney directly to their recipients than rather to a stranger. When the cross-match is positive with own one's recipient, but this recipient has a negative cross-match with blood group A or B donor from another couple, the problem is solved by exchanging the kidneys between these pairs. Another reason for kidney exchange is when the O to A or B pair get a better HLA matching from 6 miss-matches to 0-3 miss-matches by swapping the kidney with a A or B to O pair.

The pairs involved in a paired exchange program are interviewed to exclude any coercion of the donor, they are informed about the advantage and the risk of the living donation and the informed consent is obtained. Beside that, all donors undergo psychological evaluation.

The inclusion criteria pursued the goal of exchanging equivalent kidneys with equivalent size, anatomy, similar renal function and similar age. The donor are assessed preoperatively by high resolution iv pyelograms, quantitative renal scan and spiral CT scan or MRI. As a general rule, the donors accept to join this program as this is the only way to help their relatives or friends. The transplants involving two or three pairs can be performed simultaneously excepting the session with more than three pairs when the transplants are performed successively. All the transplants are performed by the same surgical team in respect to the principle to equivalent quality of the surgical act.

The basic principle of kidney exchange is the equivalent exchange. To accomplished this, high resolution preoperative work-ups required and unpredicted situation which can hinder harvesting are avoided. This way, simultaneously harvesting is not mandatory.

By using kidney exchange, the recipient benefit from the better matching as well as the known advantages of living donation. Paired kidney exchange reduce the duration of dialysis before transplantation and expand the pool of living donors.

In the countries where the living donation is the main source of organs, cross-over transplantation may become more popular as it increase the number of transplants. The kidney exchange program has to be promoted as it offers solutions where apparently there is none.

Transplantation of ABO incompatible pairs. Developed initially in countries with predominant living donation, transplantation of a ABO incompatible kidney is a demanding task but it was possible mainly due to development of more potent immunosuppressive drugs which reduces the risk of hyperacute rejection [67]. In japan, transplantation of a ABO incompatible kidney from a living donor is preferred to a deceased donor graft but the experience already acquired was extended in many other countries for recipients having only a ABO incompatible donor willing to donate [68].

The procedure involves a pretransplant treatment in order to remove the ABO antibody and to prevent furture production. Thus, Rrituximab is administred one month before transplantation followed by plasmapheresis 7 to 14 days before transplantation. With Rituximab there is no need for splenectomy and plasmapheresis is done in alternate days or even daily in order to reduce the ABO antibody titer under 8. The plasma removed is replaced with albumin solution and a combination of albumin and fresh frozen solution just immediately before transplantation to correct the coagulation. A key point is the administration of IVIG immediately after each plasmapheresis. The plasmapheresis is continued in the first two weeks after transplantation if ABO antibody titer was over 256 before Rituximab, if there is an increase of ABO antibody more than three times after transplantation, and if the serum creatinine increases more than 15% in two weeks after transplantation. The immunosuppression includes Tacrolimus, mycophenolate mofetil and steroids. In the first three weeks, the patient is at high risk of developing hyperacute humoral rejection, thus a graft biopsy is warranted whenever the serum creatinine increase over 15% in two weeks [69].

The use of specific immunoadsorbtion instead of plasmapheresis is not only less aggressive but also more effective since it allows more than two plasma exchange equivalent per one session [70].

Even if renal transplantation agains ABO blood group is expensive and, due to the increased immunosuppression, increases the infectious and malignancy risk, graft function at five years is slightly similar to transplantation of ABO compatible grafts [68].

2.9. Commercial renal transplantation

World Health Organization condemned the sales of organs since 1989. Sales of organs and tissues has been made illegal in the majority civilized states of the world. The difference between altruistic donation of a kidney and selling off a kidney is viewed as similar to the difference between marriage and prostitution. The first is a sacrament, the second a sin.

Reimbursement for expenses related to the donation process, such as for traveling and lodging is not prohibited, although a formal mechanism to make such reimbursements is not available everywhere, a factor that could act as a decentive to donation for some potential donors.

Iran is currently the only country in which payed donation is officially sanctioned, almost all the donors are pour and uneducated and follow-up studies have shown that their lives are not improved.

Despite the legal constraints on organ sales, commercial kidney transplantation is a common phenomena in many parts of the world, and in some cases has been linked to criminal activity. The donors are typical pour or under great financial stress, the recipients are often wealthy or come from other wealthier countries, and middleman or brokers are often involved.

Arguments against payed donation shows:

- The donor's choice is not voluntary because he is compelled by circumstances of poverty to donate a kidney. Poverty-stricken donors choose what they see as the best of a group of bed options. Compared to some other possibilities such working under unsafe conditions, kidney donation might carry less risk to the donor than other choices and at the same time might accomplish more good for society and for the donor.
- Paid donors are usually pour and uneducated, so making them understand the risks is all but impossible.

- Commercial donation will result in the rich having access to organs for transplantation while the pour do not.
- Donors will be exploited by unscrupulous middleman and sometimes, even by the surgeons. The medical care of both donor and recipient will suffer generally.
- The pour don't know how to handle the money that comes to them and will make no permanent difference in their poverty. This perception may be based on experience with lottery winners and other recipients of a sudden winfall. Donors will have widely differing abilities to plan for the future and would be difficult to predict what they will do with the payment for their donation. The possibility off misuse of money does not justify the overriding the donors wish to give up a kidney.
- During its entire history, transplantation has relayed on the altruism of donors and their families. Commercial donation would change the fundamental character of organ donation and likely would lead to the disappearance of altruistic donor. If any transplants are payed for, all will have to be. Most of payed donors are giving an organ to a specific individual. Payed donors would not have a choice about recipient. Thus, altruistic donation should continue.
- The initial enthusiastic support of organ transplantation has been replaced by suspicion. Although no evidence has proved the charges that are widely accepted urban myths regarding transplantation. This includes stories of people, particularly south-american children being kidnapped and killed for their organs, and people being drugged and kidnaped only to awaken in an alley with a flank incision and no kidney on that side. The myths can only be dispelled by the education, nothing else. Moreover, the possibility exists that skillful paper editors and television producers will exploit current practices for purposes of sensationalism.

Available data on the outcome of organ vending for the donors, indicates that the most of them have a pour outcome. On the other side, recipient of vended organ are subject to an increased risk for complications, particularly infections, likely as a result of a break-down of trust and honesty that is a byproduct of commercialization of organ donation. Evidence from several countries has shown that commercialization of organ donation comes at the expense of program for the related and unpaid living unrelated donation.

3. Cadaveric donation

The modest increase in cadaveric renal transplant in USA has been achieved in principally by extending use of older and younger donors [71]. Fortunately, the death from motor vehicle accidents has decreased over the passed 20 years mainly due to laws meant to increase the safety on the road: the seat belt laws, passive restraints, child safety seats, and stricter drunk driving laws. The greatest number of lives saved by improved highway safety has been specially at the 15 to 40 years old age group. On the other hand, another concern is related to the estimation that 10% of potential donors might be ineligible because of HIV infection [72].

In the same time, the number of older cadaver donors doubled between 1990 and 2000 especially due to a 10 fold increase in donors older than 60 years.

The percentage of donors dying in motor vehicle accidents decreased from 34.4% to 24.00% while the percentage of donors dying from stroke increased from 27% to 42% [71]. Despite the decrease in motor vehicle accidents, enough deaths still occur under circumstances that allow transplantation and could reduce the gap between the need for and the supply of kidneys in all civilized states in the world. The failure to make use of these organs has been attributed to the failure of the intensive care unit staff to recognize potential donors as well as the high refusal rate by families of potential cadaveric donors. Multiple new mechanisms for preventing potential donor from being missed in ICU appear to have been successful. Hospital staff are recognizing over two thirds of potential donors, are asking their families about donation but only half of them agree to donate.

Much attention has been focused on disparity among different ethnic groups as organ donors. A study of 1772 requested donation in come important cities from USA reported a family refusal rate of 17% in whites, 43% in Hispanics, and 45% in blacks [73], but the situation has changed in last period due to intensive efforts done to encourage minority families to donate. As a consequence the rate of cadaver kidney donation became similar for whites, blacks and Hispanics but remained low for Asians. Estimate of the overall refusal rate in the USA is between 38% to 50%. The refusal to donate lead to a 4755 kidneys lost for donation but the true potential in higher since we can't determine the real number of potential donors. This number would have enclosed 81% of the gap between the yearly increase in need and the available kidneys. Even so, the shortage of kidneys can not be closed by eligible donors lost by families refusal to donate and the difference would have to be provided by new cadaveric sources and by living donation.

3.1. Disparity among attitudes regarding cadaver donation

Even it might be only a believing, there is a dichotomy between the public and the medical community regarding cadaveric organ donation. The medical community is preferring cadaver organ donation since there are less concerns on the quality and risks associated with the donor's organs. Physicians don't share the cultural and religious believes of families opposed to organ donation. The doctors are relieved of concerns regarding doing harm to the donor because they often see the main problem as one that may be corrected by education and right information.

Even though over 90% of the public supports allowing living donation [74], many people do have reservations about cadaveric organ donation due to cultural and religious beliefs or beliefs that the dead can still suffer. The concept of brain death remains only a concept when it is about a loved one who has died unexpectedly. Families also express concern that the deceased's own wishes cannot be known or carried out. People might fear that being identified ahead of time as an organ donor would lead the medical team to make less than the maximal effort to save them [75].

3.2. Legislation means

An array of various laws have been passed to maximize the number of cadaveric donor transplants. In USA, the Uniform Anatomical Gift Act, have been passed for over 30 years by american Congress and authorize individuals to give their organs and specified who could give consent if the donor were unable to do so [76]. By now, many states have such a law in place and many of them use the driver license as a donor card.

"Routine inquiry" is active in many hospitals in Europe and USA. Majority of the hospitals who are doing or not transplantation, have routine inquiry policies which qualifies for social reimbursement. Hospitals are required to notify families of potential donors about the possibility of donation and to notify organ procurement agency approved by health care finance administration. In the first years after the passage of required request laws, donation increased slightly but then reached a new plateau.

Another way to approach organ donation, especially in European countries is that of presumed consent. Unless the potential donor has previously expressed a wish not to donate, he is presumed to have agreed to donate. The role of the family is to confirm that the deceased has not expressed an unwillingness to be a donor. The application of the law is variable and approximatively one half of the nations continues to depend on family consent in practice. The effect of donation have been variable; the refusal rate in Austria and Belgium, where the law is strictly applied dropped under 10%. In USA, public opinion shows little support for presumed consent law with only 7% supporting this approach.

An alternative to presumed consent has been proposed in the USA which is mandated choice [77]. When getting or renewing a driving license, a person would have to decide whether to become a potential donor, and the person's choice would take precedence over the family's wishes.

Another law which is active in some states in USA and some countries in Europe, is to provide a compensation for the donor's family. The fund for such thing is obtained by voluntary donations. One thing which is important here that the law makes the distinction between purchasing organs and bestowing a gift to the family in appreciation of its generosity.

3.3. Expanding donation criteria

When efforts that increase the consent rate for cadaver donors, another approach expanding the criteria for an acceptable cadaver donors, also has attempted to increase the number of kidneys available for transplantation. Less than 25% of the increase in cadaveric donors has come from traditional pool age 16 to 50 year age donors. The criteria have been expanded further in some instances by use of donors with encephalitis and core antibody positivity for hepatitis B [78]. Recent data have confirmed that safety of even using kidney from infected donors with blood cultures with pseudomonas and candida, provide appropriate antibiotic treatment is given [79]. There are studies which determined that bacteriemia accounted for 30% of medically unsuitable kidneys in brain death potential donor. There are also transplantation of horse shoe kidney [80] or kidneys from non renal organ transplant recipient which have to be mentioned. From any point you are going to look at this problem, the greatest potential to increase the potential donor pool comprises non-hard beating cadaver kidneys and kidneys from older donor.

Situations requiring edge biopsy
All people with normal renal function regardless of age (graft biopsy in donors over 60 years)
Diabetic donors with normal renal function and without severe proteinuria
All hypertensive donors with normal renal function
All hypotensive donors
Infected donors excluding viral hepatitis, HIV, Jakob-Creutzfeldt disease, viral encephalitis, malaria, disseminated TB
CMV + RPR
Positive urine cultures without pyelonephritis
Bacteremic donors
Donors with abnormal renal function
Donors at high risk for infection (but negative on high sensitive tests)
Donors with a history of malignancy disease-free for two years
Skin tumors without metastases, excluding melanoma
Primary CNS tumors without VP shunt

Adapted from [65]

Table 5. Expanded criteria for cadaveric donors

Non heart beating donors where widely used before the definition of brain death was accepted. They remain the major source of cadaver donors in countries such as Japan and Mexico, where brain death was recognized officially only recently and where social acceptance it is still limited [82]. Non heart beating donors yield about 5% of all cadaveric kidneys transplanted in USA. Use of non-heart beating cadaver donor kidneys has increased in last years. The one year survival of graft from non-heart beating donors was 83% and for brain death donors was 86%. Early function was not as good: 48% of recipient of non-heart beating donor kidneys required dialysis in the first week after transplantation compared to 22% of the recipients of kidneys from brain death donors. Primary non-function was slightly increased also (4% versus 1%). The serum creatinine level at discharge from hospital was higher in the first group. At one year follow-up, the serum creatinine levels for the two groups was, in fact, similar (1.9 mg/dL versus 1.8 mg/dL). When traumatic death were analyzed separately, the one year survival of non heart beating donors kidneys was 89% compared with 70% one year survival for non-traumatic death. Not all programs have found the same results from non-heart beating donors, but the finding of more frequent delayed function and need for dialysis has been universal. The potential for increasing the donor supply from non-heart beating donors has been estimated to be as high as 40% [83].

3.3.1. Older donors

Already, older donors are a major source of cadaveric donation. Some doctors found out an inferior outcome from transplants from cadaveric donors over 55 years of age. Not only did a higher percentage of recipients of such kidneys required dialysis but one year serum creatinine level was higher than that from recipient of transplants from cadaveric donors aged 5 to 55 years and the estimated halve life of the kidney was 5.8 +/- 0.3 years compared to 11+/- 0.3 years. Other analysis have found similar results but suggests that the adverse effects of the donor ages affect only certain subgroups particularly black recipients.

3.3.2. Hypertension

Recipients of kidneys from donors with hypertension were more likely to have anuria and to require dialysis immediately after transplantation. Their serum creatinine level was significant higher at one year than that of recipients of kidneys from donors who were not hypertensive and the predictive graft survival was shorter (halve life of 7.7 +/- 0.5 years versus 10.7 +/- 0.3 years). Graft survival was better with 1 to 5 years of hypertension compared to 6 or more years of hypertension. The difference in serum creatinine and predicted graft survival between kidneys from diabetic and non-diabetic donors was of borderline statistical significance. Serum creatinine at one year was 1.8 +/- 0.8 mg/dL in recipient of kidneys from diabetic donors compared with 1.6 +/- 0.8 mg/dL in recipients of kidney from non-diabetic donors. Predicted halve life in this graft was 8.4 +/- 1.5 years compared with 10.1 +/- 0.3 years.

3.4. Strategies for increasing organ donation

In developing new strategies for increasing kidney available for transplantation we would do well to remember that from its beginning organ transplantation has relied on public good will and support. When public opposition exists, we sometimes avoid using approaches that we find ethically acceptable. Because we really don't know what ideas or practices will strengthen public support for all organ donation the introduction of new practices should be undertaken as pilot projects.

The public already accept living donors who were not considered 50 years ago such unrelated living donors and spouses, which are now widely excepted. Once we accept the donors autonomy and remind ourselves that the risk to the donor is not related to his relationship to the recipient, we will be able to accept the wide arrange and greater number of emotionally related donors. We need to understand that the altruistic donor, although unusual, is not pathologic. The altruistic donor can be considered an emotionally related donor who is emotionally related to all mankind. Thus, this approach to this type of donor is not to keep a registry of willing donors and their HLA types. The altruistic donor is not waiting for the right HLA type but for the right story. The acceptance of donor autonomy would allow for accepting donors with increased risk, but will require careful follow-up thus an increased risk of complications can be recognized.

3.5. Conclusions

During the last period of time, there was a spite of papers from individual countries and registries, which examined the ways in which the number of kidney donors could be increased.

Most studies examined single initiatives, such as changing the transplant law, rather than the development of integrated donor programs. The act of donation is a complex phenomenon depending on many factors and interactions, few of which individually have been proven useful or generally applicable throw the out the european community. Well designed studies are needed urgently. A donation is the result of a chain of events, the final result of which will depend upon its weakest link.

Even when the individual links have been strengthened, each element of the process of donation must be integrated into the operational policies developed in toon with national moral and cultural values. It is easy to set a minimum standard to which countries should aspire. But it is another matter to recommend specific, donor promoting activities for which individual countries and profesional organizational should aim.

Although, living donor rate are no increasing in Europe, rates could be further improved at different stages in the referral process:

- Nephrologist at non transplanting as well as transplanting centers, should be encouraged to discuss openly the subject of living donation with family of patients suffering ESRD, preferably before the patient begins dialysis. This will results in predialysis transplantation, increased transplant rates, and is more efficient in case of reduced dialysis resources.
- Canceling facilities (e.g. by a senior nurse or living donor coordinators) should be available to discuss screening tests, provide information, and arrange eventually reimbursement of donor expenses allowed in law.
- Each transplant center should work to an approved screening protocol, such that the predicted mortality risk of living donation does not exceed 1 in 3000 cases.
- If legally permitted, living unrelated donors should be encouraged. In many countries in Europe, altruistic non related kidney donation is allowed legally, provided that checks are made for altruistic motivation and exclusion as far as possible of the possibility of organ sale.
- Non-directed living donor transplantation between altruistic donor and recipient unknown to the donor is possible and have been developed in few centers. Although controversial, there seem no moral or social reason to exclude such donors. However, there are ethical and legal concerns about this type of donation, which at the moment make it difficult to include in a recommendation list.

Increase supply and use of cadaveric kidneys:

Donor cards. In many countries publicity schemes encourage the population to carry donor cards, or to register their wish to donate (opting-in) on a computerized donor register. Even if in UK 8 mil. of individuals are now registered in the opting-in computer, only 10% of the

http://dx.doi.org/10.5772/55245

population is currently caring donor cards. No more than 50 donor per year results from this initiative. For the success of such schemes, continuous publicity is essential to increase opted-in donors and transplant centers. Intensive care physicians and transplant coordinators should be mandated to access registry routinely, to identify the wishes of potential cadaveric donors.

Improved organization and resources. Services must be more organized and better resourced to increase cadaver donation. In several countries, the number of intensive care beds is probably too low to achieve more than 20 donors per million from intensive care patients. In high donating countries, with better resourced intensive care units, the staff responsible for donation (transplant coordinators), have been expanded and given proper financial support. Transplant coordinators are also to be given the responsibility of public relations, with the aim of avoiding adverse media publicity, and liaising with the coroners.

Opting-out legislation. The introduction of opting-out legislation appears on first site of the data available to be associated with the increased rates of cadaveric donation. In Europe, four countries which exceeded 20 kidneys donor per million population per annum, all have opting-out legislation. In France however, opting-out legislation has not achieved such a successful donation rates. This may be because France choose initially, hard line opting-out, in which donation takes place if the donor has not opted-out irrespective of families wishes. Adverse publicity led to a softening of the practice, which consequently increases the donation rates. Other countries which presumed consent law practices soft presumed consent, in which the families are taking into account in all situations. In general, countries with informed consent do not perform as well, main exception being USA, where kidney donation rates exceed 25 donors per million population.

Criteria for donor suitability. Non-heart beating donors (NHBD) are well known to produce a high rate of primary non-function and their acceptability was low. Recently introduced in situ perfusion of the dead bodies, which has been successfully developed in UK and Holland, are bringing in encouraging results. After harvesting, kidneys may be put into continuous perfusion machine, and their viability assessed using flow measurements and urinary and enzyme excretion. As a matter of fact, presumed consent legislation will allow more NHBD. Rapid intraarterial cold perfusion over recently deceased persons should be allowed before family consent low operate but perfusion without relatives permission is technically unwarranted assault. Agreement by a coroner should allow perfusion without permission and that could expand significantly NHBD.

Elderly donors. Even if long term survival for kidneys from elderly donors (over 60 years old) is 10-15% less than those taken from younger donors, better results may be obtained with carefully selected older donors and shortening of the cold ischemic time.

A good quality organ must be guaranteed to the recipient and every transplant center must established its own guidelines on organ acceptability. If the transplant center uses a less than optimum organs from old subjects to expand the pool of donors, the donors must be evaluated according to age, vascular condition and renal function. The inferior limit for a single kidney transplant is considered creatinine clearance more than 60 mL/min. If the calculated creatinine clearance is between 60 and 50 mL/min. the donor may be considered marginal. If the calculated creatinine clearance is less than 50 mL/min. than the kidney should not be used for a single transplantation, however, as they are organs that nobody wants they can be used for dual transplantation. When this policy is established, it is necessary to inform the patient on the waiting list.

Author details

Lucan Mihai*, Lucan Valerian Ciprian and Iacob Gheorghiță

*Address all correspondence to: mihai.lucan@gmail.com

Clinical Institute of Urology and Renal Transplantation, Cluj-Napoca, Romania

References

[1] Mandal AK, Kalligonis AN, Ratner LE. Expanded criteria donors: attempts to increase the renal transplant donor pool. Adv Ren Replace Ther. 2000;7(2):117-30.

[2] McBride MA, Harper AM, Taranto SE., The OPTN waiting list, 1988-2002. Clin Transpl. 2003:53-64.

[3] Walton-Moss BJ, Taylor L, Nolan MT. Ethical analysis of living organ donation. Prog Transplant. 2005;15(3):303-9.

[4] Lledó-Garcia E, Subirá-Ríos D, Tejedor-Jorge A, del Cañizo-López JF, Hernández-Fernández C. Optimizing outcomes by preconditioning the donor. Transplant Proc. 2011;43(1):349-52.

[5] Brar A, Jindal RM, Abbott KC, Hurst FP, Salifu MO. Practice patterns in evaluation of living kidney donors in United network for organ sharing-approved kidney transplant centers. Am J Nephrol. 2012;35(5):466-73.

[6] Goldfarb DA, Matin SF, Braun WE, Schreiber MJ, Mastroianni B, Papajcik D, Rolin HA, Flechner S, Goormastic M, Novick AC. Renal outcome 25 years after donor nephrectomy. J Urol. 2001;166(6):2043-7.

[7] Hung CJ, Lin YJ, Chang SS, Chou TC, Lee PC. Kidney grafts with multiple renal arteries is no longer a relative contraindication with advance in surgical techniques of laparoscopic donor nephrectomy. Transplant Proc. 2012;44(1):36-8.

[8] Tyson MD, Castle EP, Ko EY, Andrews PE, Heilman RL, Mekeel KL, Moss AA, Mulligan DC, Reddy KS. Living donor kidney transplantation with multiple renal arteries in the laparoscopic era. Urology. 2011;77(5):1116-21.

[9] Modlin CS, Goldfarb DA, Novick AC. The use of expanded criteria cadaver and live donor kidneys for transplantation. Urol Clin North Am. 2001;28(4):687-707.

[10] Lucan M., Tratat de tehnici chirurgicale urologice, ed. Infomedica, Bucuresti, 2001, p513-527.

[11] Nanidis TG, Antcliffe D, Kokkinos C, Borysiewicz CA, Darzi AW, Tekkis PP, Papalois VE. Laparoscopic versus open live donor nephrectomy in renal transplantation: a meta-analysis. Ann Surg. 2008;247(1):58-70.

[12] Dols LF, Kok NF, Ijzermans JN. Live donor nephrectomy: a review of evidence for surgical techniques. Transpl Int. 2010;23(2):121-30.

[13] Giessing M. Laparoscopic living-donor nephrectomy. Nephrol Dial Transplant. 2004;19 Suppl 4:iv36-40.

[14] Tooher RL, Rao MM, Scott DF, Wall DR, Francis DM, Bridgewater FH, Maddern GJ. A systematic review of laparoscopic live-donor nephrectomy. Transplantation. 200415;78(3):404-14.

[15] Moreira P, Sá H, Figueiredo A, Mota A. Delayed renal graft function: risk factors and impact on the outcome of transplantation. Transplant Proc. 2011;43(1):100-5.

[16] Bay WH, Hebert LA. The living donor in kidney transplantation. Ann Intern Med. 1987;106(5):719-27.

[17] Najarian JS, Chavers BM, McHugh LE, Matas AJ. 20 years or more of follow-up of living kidney donors. Lancet. 1992 3;340(8823):807-10.

[18] Fellner CH, Marshall JR. Kidney donors--the myth of informed consent. Am J Psychiatry. 1970;126(9):1245-51.

[19] Frade IC, Fonseca I, Dias L, Henriques AC, Martins LS, Santos J, Sarmento M, Lopes A. Impact assessment in living kidney donation: psychosocial aspects in the donor. Transplant Proc. 2008;40(3):677-81.

[20] Terasaki PI. The HLA-matching effect in different cohorts of kidney transplant recipients. Clin Transpl. 2000:497-514.

[21] 2001 Annual report. Vol. 1. Richmond, Va.: United Network for Organ Sharing, 2002:32.

[22] Abecassis M, Adams M, Adams P, et all; Live Organ Donor Consensus Group. Consensus statement on the live organ donor. JAMA. 2000;284(22):2919-26.

[23] Scheper-Hughes N. Keeping an eye on the global traffic in human organs. Lancet. 2003;361(9369):1645-8.

[24] Cohen L. Where it hurts: Indian material for an ethics of organ transplantation. Daedalus. 1999;128(4):135-65.

[25] Siminoff LA, Chillag K. The fallacy of the "gift of life". Hastings Cent Rep. 1999;29(6): 34-41.

[26] Green RM: What does it mean to use someone as "a means only": rereading Kant. Kennedy Inst Ethics J 2001, 11(3):247-61

[27] Campbell CS: Body, Self, and the property paradigm. Hastings Cent Rep 1992, 22(5): 34-42

[28] Boulware LE, Troll MU, Wang NY, Powe NR. Public attitudes toward incentives for organ donation: a national study of different racial/ethnic and income groups. Am J Transplant. 2006 Nov;6(11):2774-85

[29] Goyal M, Mehta RL, Schneiderman LJ, Sehgal AR. Economic and health consequences of selling a kidney in India. JAMA 2002; 288:1589–1593

[30] National Organ Transplant Act: Public Law 98-507. US Statut Large 1984; 98

[31] Israni AK, Halpern SD, Zink S, Sidhwani SA, Caplan A. Incentive models to increase living kidney donation: Encouraging without coercing. Am J Transplant 2005; 5: 15–20

[32] William Frist, S. 2283 (109th): Gift of Life Congressional Medal Act of 2006, 109th Congress, 2005–2006.

[33] Fortney Stark, H.R. 4753 (109th): Gift of Life Congressional Medal Act of 2006,109th Congress, 2005–2006.

[34] Ross LF, Woodle ES. Ethical issues in increasing living kidney donations by expanding kidney paired exchange programs. Transplantation. 2000;69(8):1539-43.

[35] Smith C. She saves mom, gets fired for it. Seattle Post-Intellinger. November 22, 2001.].

[36] Public law No. 106-56, Organ donor leave act, H.R. 457, USA Congress

[37] Office of the Assistant Secretary for Planning and Evaluation, Depart-ment of Health and Human Services. Standards for Privacy of Individually Identifiable Health Information: Final rule. Fed Regist 2000;65(250): 82475, 82803-5, 82810, 82812-3.

[38] Ellison MD, McBride MA, Taranto SE, Delmonico FL, Kauffman HM. Living kidney donors in need of kidney transplants: a report from the organ procurement and transplantation network. Transplantation. 2002;74(9):1349-51.

[39] Matas AJ, Bartlett ST, Leichtman AB, Delmonico FL. Morbidity and mortality after living kidney donation, 1999-2001: survey of United States transplant centers. Am J Transplant. 2003;3(7):830-4.

[40] Wallis CB, Samy KP, Roth AE, Rees MA. Kidney paired donation. Nephrol Dial Transplant. 2011 Jul;26(7):2091-9

[41] Montgomery RA, Cooper M, Kraus E et al. Renal transplantation at the Johns Hopkins Comprehensive Transplant Center. Clin Transpl 2003: 199–213

[42] Gentry SE, Segev DL, Simmerling M et al. Expanding kidney paired donation through participation by compatible pairs. Am J Transplant 2007; 7: 2361–2370

[43] de Klerk M, Keizer KM, Claas FH et al. The Dutch national living donor kidney exchange program. Am J Transplant 2005; 5: 2302–2305

[44] Montgomery RA. Renal transplantation across HLA and ABO antibody barriers: integrating paired donation into desensitization protocols. Am J Transplant 2010; 10: 449–457

[45] Delmonico FL, Morrissey PE, Lipkowitz GS et al. Donor kidney exchanges. Am J Transplant 2004; 4: 1628–1634

[46] Roth AE, Sonmez T, Unver MU, Delmonico FL, Saidman SL. Util- izing list exchange and nondirected donation through 'chain' paired kidney donations. Am J Transplant 2006; 6: 2694–2705

[47] Gentry SE, Segev DL, Montgomery RA. A comparison of populations served by kidney paired donation and list paired donation. Am J Transplant 2005; 5: 1914–1921

[48] den Hartogh G. Trading with the waiting-list: the justice of living donor list exchange. Bioethics 2010; 24: 190–198

[49] Gilbert JC, Brigham L, Batty DS Jr. et al. The nondirected living donor program: a model for cooperative donation, recovery and allocation of living donor kidneys. Am J Transplant 2005; 5: 167–174

[50] Cecka JM. The UNOS Scientific Renal Transplant Registry--2000. Clin Transpl. 2000:1-18.

[51] Eggers P. Comparison of treatment costs between dialysis and transplantation. Semin Nephrol. 1992;12(3):284-9.

[52] O'Connor KJ, Delmonico FL. Increasing the supply of kidneys for transplantation. Semin Dial. 2005;18(6):460-2.

[53] Fehrman-Ekholm I. Living donor kidney transplantation. Transplant Proc. 2006;38(8):2637-41.

[54] Clayman RV, Kavoussi LR, Soper NJ, Dierks SM, Meretyk S, Darcy MD, Roemer FD, Pingleton ED, Thomson PG, Long SR. Laparoscopic nephrectomy: initial case report. J Urol. 1991;146(2):278-82.

[55] Kerbl K, Clayman RV, McDougall EM, Gill IS, Wilson BS, Chandhoke PS, Albala DM, Kavoussi LR. Transperitoneal nephrectomy for benign disease of the kidney: a comparison of laparoscopic and open surgical techniques. Urology. 1994;43(5): 607-13.

[56] Kavoussi LR, Kerbl K, Capelouto CC, McDougall EM, Clayman RV. Laparoscopic nephrectomy for renal neoplasms. Urology. 1993;42(5):603-9.

[57] Rassweiler J, Fornara P, Weber M, Janetschek G, Fahlenkamp D, Henkel T, Beer M, Stackl W, Boeckmann W, Recker F, Lampel A, Fischer C, Humke U, Miller K. Laparoscopic nephrectomy: the experience of the laparoscopy working group of the German Urologic Association. J Urol. 1998;160(1):18-21.

[58] Benoit G, Blanchet P, Moukarzel M, Hiesse C, Bensadoun H, Bellamy J, Charpentier B, Jardin A. Surgical complications in kidney transplantation. Transplant Proc. 1994;26(1):287-8.

[59] Brown SL, Biehl TR, Rawlins MC, Hefty TR. Laparoscopic live donor nephrectomy: a comparison with the conventional open approach. J Urol. 2001;165(3):766-9.

[60] Levey AS, Danovitch G, Hou S. Living donor kidney transplantation in the United States--looking back, looking forward. Am J Kidney Dis. 2011;58(3):343-8.

[61] Davis CL, Delmonico FL. Living-donor kidney transplantation: a review of the current practices for the live donor. J Am Soc Nephrol. 2005;16(7):2098-110.

[62] Ratner LE, Montgomery RA, Kavoussi LR. Laparoscopic live donor nephrectomy. A review of the first 5 years. Urol Clin North Am. 2001;28(4):709-19.

[63] Montgomery RA, Lonze BE, King KE, Kraus ES, Kucirka LM, Locke JE, Warren DS, Simpkins CE, Dagher NN, Singer AL, Zachary AA, Segev DL. Desensitization in HLA-incompatible kidney recipients and survival. N Engl J Med. 2011;365(4):318-26.

[64] Rapaport FT. The case for living emotionally related international kidney donor exchange registry. Transplant Proc 1986; 18(suppl 2): 5-9.

[65] Gentry S, Segev DL. Living donor kidney exchange. Clin Transpl. 2011:279-86.

[66] Lucan M. Five years of single-center experience with paired kidney exchange transplantation. Transplant Proc. 2007;39(5):1371-5.

[67] Tanabe K, Takahashi K, Sonda K, Tokumoto T, Ishikawa N, Kawai T, et al. Long-term results of ABO-incompatible living kidney transplantation: a single-center experience. Transplantation 1998;65:224-8

[68] Crew RJ, Ratner LE. ABO-incompatible kidney transplantation: current practice and the decade ahead. Curr Opin Organ Transplant. 2010;15(4):526-30.].

[69] Jeon BJ, Kim IG, Seong YK, Han BH. Analysis of the Results of ABO-Incompatible Kidney Transplantation: In Comparison with ABO-Compatible Kidney Transplantation. Korean J Urol. 2010;51(12):863-9.

[70] Genberg H, Kumlien G, Wennberg L, Tyden G. The efficacy of antigen-specific immunoadsorption and rebound of anti-A/B antibodies in ABO-incompatible kidney transplantation. Nephrol Dial Transplant. 2011;26(7):2394-400.

[71] 1998 Annual Report. U.S. Scientific Registry of Transplant Recipients and the Organ Procurement and Transplantation Network. Transplant Data 1988–1997. Richmond, U.S. Department of Health and Human Services, Office of Special Programs, Division of Transplantation, UNOS

[72] Evans RW, Orians CE, Ascher NL. The potential supply of organ donors. JAMA 1992, 267:239–246

[73] Perez LM, Schulman B, Davis F, Olson L, Tellis VA, Matas AJ. Organ donation in three large American cities with large Latino and black populations. Transplantation 1998, 46:553–557

[74] Spital A, Spital M. Living kidney donation: Attitudes outside the transplant center. Arch Intern Med 1988, 148:1077–1080

[75] Callender CO, Hall LE, Yeager CL, Barber JB, Dunston GM, Pinn-Wiggins VW. Organ donation and blacks: A critical frontier. N Engl J Med 1991, 325:442–444

[76] Stuart FP, Veith FJ, Cranford RE. Braindeath laws and patterns of consent to remove organs for transplantation from cadavers in the United States and 28 other countries. Transplantation 1981, 31:238– 244

[77] Spital A. Mandated choice for organ donation: Time to give it a try. Ann Intern Med 1996, 125:66–69

[78] Madayag RM, Johnson LB, Bartlett ST, Schweitzer EJ, Constantine NT, McCarter RJ, Kuo PC, Keay S, Oldach DW. Use of renal allografts from donors positive for hepatitis B core antibody confers minimal risk for subsequent development of clinical hepatitis B virus disease. Transplantation 1967; 64:1781–1786

[79] Freeman RB, Giatras I, Falagas ME, Supran S, O'Conner K, Bradley J, Snydman DR, Delmonico FL. Outcome of transplantation of organs procured from bacteremic donors. Transplantation 1999; 68:1107–1111

[80] Thomson BNJ, Francis DM, Millar RJ. Transplantation of adult and paediatric horseshoe kidneys. Aust NZJ Surg 1997; 67:279–282

[81] Alexander JW. Expanded Donor Criteria: Background and Suggestions for Kidney Donation. Richmond, Report of the UNOS Ad Hoc Donations Committee, 1991

[82] Hiraga S, Kitamura M, Kakuta T, Takebayashi Y, Fukuuchi F, Kitajima N, Hida M: Clinical outcome of cadaveric renaltransplantation with non-heart-beating donors: Special reference to serious complications. Transplant Proc 1997; 29:3561–3564

[83] ChoY W, Terasaki PI, Cecka JM, Gjertson DW. Transplantation of kidneys from donors whose hearts have stopped beating. N Engl J Med 1998; 338:221–225

Chapter 7

Kidney Transplantation Techniques

Farzad Kakaei, Saman Nikeghbalian and
Seyed Ali Malekhosseini

Additional information is available at the end of the chapter

http://dx.doi.org/10.5772/54829

1. Introduction

First successful kidney transplantation was done over 60 years ago and now because of major advances in immunosuppressive medicine, this represents the treatment of choice for patients with end-stage renal disease (ESRD). The kidney was the first organ to be transplanted regularly, and it remains the most common organ transplanted today but the surgical technique has changed very little from the original pelvic operation during this long period.

In most cases kidney is placed retroperitoneally and the iliac arteries and veins are used for perfusion of this organ and the ureter is transplanted directly to the bladder. But the sophisticated intensive care units and advanced perioperative anesthetic techniques lead to the use of more marginal donors for more complicated recipients. Now using a kidney graft from a donor after cardiac death or proceeding to kidney transplantation as a part of multivisceral or other abdominal organ transplantation is a routine procedure in the major transplant centers of the world. In such conditions the kidney grafts are not harvested in an optimized preoperative planning and may be damaged during the surgery. Then we may confront with a graft with 2 or more delicate or very short arteries or veins, ruptured capsule or transected ureter. We may use grafts with congenital anomalies such as horseshoe kidneys or duplicated ureteral system. Also the recipient procedure may be her or his second, third or more transplantation surgery and no more iliac vessels remained for anastomosis and the bladder may be so damaged that makes the anastomosis of the ureter to the bladder impossible. The transplant surgeon should always be ready to conquer such challenges. Using an intraperitoneal space, using the aorta or inferior vena cava or other major arteries and veins such as splenic vessels, and the native ureters for reconstruction of the urine outflow should be an in-hand procedure for every transplant surgeon.

In this chapter we will review basic steps of the standard approach to recipient's procedure from preparing the graft, then the skin incision till the skin closure with special attention to basic vascular and urinary tract re-establishment techniques and also intraoperative care of the patient. Then we proceed to the special and unusual situations including: complex vascular and ureteral reconstruction techniques, using kidneys with congenital and other anatomical anomalies, en bloc double kidney transplantation, using other vasculature for transplanting the kidney in different intraperitoneal spaces, and kidney transplantation conjoint with other abdominal organs.

2. Graft preparation

Preservation of the viability of the graft during the time between explantation and implantation is vital for early and late graft function after transplantation. Most kidney transplant teams consist of at least two separate groups. One group prepares the donor and the other team is doing the recipient operation at the same time or with some delay depending on the duration needs for transferring the graft from the donor operating room to the recipient operation theatre. In many countries such as the United States or in the Euro Zone the kidney grafts from the deceased donors are transferred between hospitals, cities or even countries according to the Human Leukocyte Antigen (HLA) matching or other important criteria for attributing the graft to a preferred recipient. In such conditions it's better to use every effort to improve the graft longevity. Using better preservation solutions or automatic machine perfusion systems are among the routine measurements in such conditions which are discussed in other chapters of this book. The surgeons and coordinators should shorten the ischemic time of the graft as long as possible and during all of this period the temperature of the graft should be maintained between 1-4° centigrade to decrease the injury to the graft.

Simple hypothermia is not enough for preserving the viability of the graft and evacuation of the graft blood and replacing it with a preservation solution is a mandatory step in the graft preparation. Graft cold irrigation in the deceased donors is done during the harvesting operation by irrigation of the clamped aorta and the solution used for this irrigation may be any of the pre-prepared solutions such as Belzer University of Wisconsin's (UW), Histidine-Tryptophan-Ketoglutarate (HTK, Bretschneider or Custodiol), Euro-Collins, Celsior or other newer solutions such as Biolasol® (Dolińska B, et al, 2012)[1]. Table 1 shows the compositions of some of these solutions. All of the blood should be evacuated from the graft during this phase. In the living donor, all of the irrigation is done after removing the graft the donor body in an iced cold basin. In the countries that the living donor still forms over 75% of the donor pool such as China or India, irrigation of the living donor graft is done by more simple solutions such as lactated Ringer's solution and many studies shows that when the total ischemic time is less than 60 minutes (as in most living donor programs) the long-term graft survival is not impacted significantly by using these simple solutions comparing with more complex solutions (Prasad GS, et al, 2007)[2]. In our center we add lidocaine (100 mg/liter), sodium bicarbonate (10 meq/liter) and heparin (5000 IU/liter) to this simple solution. Also, we use intravenous Mannitol and Furosemide in the donor just before the arterial clamping for better diuresis before nephrectomy.

Name	Composition	Claimed advantages
Belzer UW solution (Viaspan®)	Potassium lactobionate: 100 mmol/l KH_2PO_4: 25 mmol/l $MgSO_4$: 5 mmol/l Raffinose: 30 mmol/l Adenosine: 5 mmol/l Glutathione: 3 mmol/l Allopurinol: 1 mmol/l Hydroxyethyl starch: 50 g/l	Allows for kidney preservation time up to 48 hours Allows for liver preservation time up to 24 hours Allows for pancreas preservation time up to 24 hours Provides enough time to admit patients from distant locations Provides enough time to improve recipient matching Provides enough time to operate in a semi-elective situation
Histidine-Tryptophan-Ketoglutarate (Custodiol®)	Sodium chloride: 15 mmol/l Potassium chloride: 9 mmol/l Potassium hydrogen 2-Ketoglutarate: 1mmol/l Magnesium chloride: 4 mmol/l Histidine · HCl:18.0 mmol/l Histidine: 180 mmol/l Tryptophan: 2 mmol/l Mannitol: 30 mmol/l Calcium chloride: 0.015 mmol/l	Rapid homogenous cooling due to low viscosity Superior recovery of function Excellent ischemic tolerance Virtual absence of side effects Simple perfusion technique (ready-to-use, no additives or preparation)
Celsior	Mannitol 60 mmol/l Lactobionic Acid 80 mmol/l Glutamtic Acid 20 mmol/l Histidine 30 mmol/l Calcium Chloride 0.25 mmol/l Potassium Chloride 15 mmol/l Magnesium Chloride 13 mmol/l Sodium Hydroxide 100 mmol/l Reduced Glutathione 3 mmol/l	low potassium comparing with UW prevention of tissue edema prevention of free radical damage prevention of calcium overload with adequate buffer Better for heart and lung transplantation (as depicted by its manufacturer, Genzyme)
Euro-Collins (Renograf®)	Potassium phosphate 42.5 mmol.l Potassium chloride 15 mmol/l Sodium bicarbonate 10 mmol/l Anhydrous glucose 35 g/l Mannitol 31.7 mmol/l Raffinose 3.5 mmol/l	Preserves the kidney up to 48 hours An out of date solution in most US and European centers

Table 1. Composition of the more common organ preservation solutions.

When possible, the donor team should report the detailed graft anatomy (including number of arteries, veins and ureters and any anatomical anomaly or inadvertent injury to the graft during the donor operation) to the recipient team, especially when the graft is transferred from another hospital locally or regionally. It is very important to prevent any more injury to the graft and its capsule, vessels or ureter during the back table procedure, especially in case of deceased donor grafts which usually accompanied with other abdominal organs or at least covered by the peritoneum or peri-renal fats or other non-important tissues. Direct contact of the ice with the graft should be prevented by inserting the graft in a separate basin or organ bag filled with a cold solution and then inserting this bag in another iced filled basin.

First of all, for irrigation of the living donor graft, the surgeon should find the artery and canulate it with an atraumatic olive-headed heparin irrigation needle as shown in figure 1. Using other devices such as Angiocath©, Baranule© or any types of intravenous needles for irrigation should be discouraged because of risk of intimal injury induced by such cannulas. In many cases, it may be difficult to find the artery first because it is hidden by other hilar tissues or retracted to the deeper hilar areas of the graft. In such conditions the irrigation may be started by canulation the more accessible renal vein, till the surgeon finds the artery. All the dissections should better be done after complete irrigation. At this point all of the renal parenchyma will appear in yellow-pink color. All of the dissections should be done delicately by using atraumatic or microvascular instruments, without any more injury to the vessels intima or their major branches and any more unusual traction of the vessel wall.

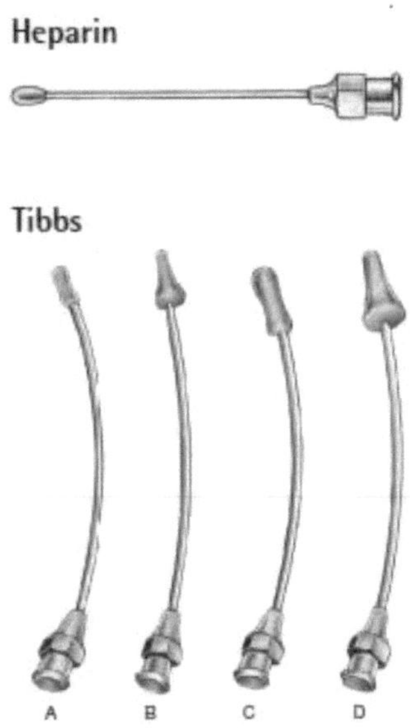

Figure 1. Special olive-headed needles for irrigation (Courtesy of GEISTER Medizintechnik GmbH, Tuttlingen/ Germany)

When using the left kidney of the living donor the adrenal and gonadal vein should be on the graft in order to have a longer vein for future anastomosis. In both right or left kidneys or living donor or deceased donor grafts, the surgeon should make every effort to preserve the connective tissues between the ureter and the gonadal vein to prevent ischemic injury to the delicate collateral vessels of the ureter. Always the ureter should be accompanied by at least one centimeter of the peri-ureteral tissues and also the hilar inferior triangle (e.g. the window between the inferior pole of the graft and the ureteral origin from the renal pelvis) should be maintained intact. Removing peri-renal fat or other tissues should be postponed till complete renal revascularization. These tissues are protective for handling of the graft and might be used for graft covering or anchoring during or after revascularization.

The window between the renal artery and vein in the renal hilum is full of accessory branches and lymphatic vessel. All of the major arterial branches especially of the inferior pole should be maintained intact. Any injury to this branches leads to regional ischemia or necrosis of the kidney or ureter which may lead to future graft dysfunction or ischemia – induced hypertension in the donor or ureteral necrosis, ureteral anastomosis disruption or urine leakage. Some surgeons suggest that all of the major lymphatic vessels should be ligated to prevent future lymphocele, however, the most important measurement for preventing the lymphocele is avoiding excessive dissections around the iliac artery during the preparing the implantation site.

The best approach for prevention of arterial branch injury is to start with dissection of the renal vein and follow its wall through the hilum until sufficient length is achieved by ligating the minor veins. We suture-ligate the accessory minor vein branches and also the major lumbar veins by 6-0 Prolene suture for prevention of postoperative bleeding from hilar vessels.

If the graft has more than one artery, vein or ureter, the surgeon should decide which type of reconstruction is suitable according to the condition of the graft and the recipient. In the deceased donor it's better to use a Carrel patch of aorta and inferior vena cava in line with the graft vessels. But this has two major impacts on future graft implantation. First, this results in a longer than usual artery (especially in the right side) or vein (especially in the left side) which may be results in kinking (and future thrombosis or hypertension) after the anastomosis. And second, it will results in a large Carrel patch in some cases. The surgeon has to remove a large patch from the recipient's vessels for a good anastomosis. If complicated by graft non-function, then future removal of the graft will result in a large defect of the recipient vessels which will be dangerous or even limb life threatening. Also, the Carrel patch of the aorta may be severely atherosclerotic and could not be used for a safe anastomosis. Any reconstruction will elongate the total ischemic time of the graft, and we should do every effort to prevent this by postponing unnecessary dissections and reconstructions to the time after at least partial reperfusion of the graft.

According to these important issues, when possible, we prefer to use no reconstruction prior to implantation to decrease the ischemic time. Every transplant surgeon should be fully trained and familiar with microvascular techniques in such conditions. Every arterial branch should be anastomosed separately. The major artery is anastomosed first usually to the internal iliac artery, which provides a longer arterial conduit and allow more free movements of the graft for venous anastomosis. Smaller arteries are anastomosed after reperfusion of the graft to the external iliac artery or even to the smaller arteries such as inferior epigastric artery (El-Sherbiny M, et al, 2008)[3]. When all arterial branches have the same size, then reperfusion is postponed till the end of anastomosis of all of the arterial branches usually to the external iliac artery but if the kidney has a large artery and some other smaller arteries then reperfusion is started after completion of the large artery anastomosis. Arteries less than 1 mm could be ligated specially in the upper pole. Also ligation of the arteries with resultant ischemic area of less than 15% of the upper or middle pole is acceptable and by reducing the total operation duration will reduce the complications in the recipient comparing with adding a long microvascular anastomosis to the operation. Arteries larger than 1 mm in the lower pole should be reperfused by anastomosis if possible to prevent ischemia of the ureter.

If the surgeon decides to reconstruct the arteries before implantation then multiple varieties of techniques could be used: side to side anastomosis of the same size arteries or end to side anastomosis of a small artery to a larger artery. Using microvascular techniques with a good illumination and at least 4.5X magnification and 7-0 or 8-0 Prolene sutures, all of the ties should be placed out of the intimal surface and the lumen should be protected by a smooth metal probe to prevent inadvertent back-wall suturing. In the deceased donor, the surgeon can use freely every small bifurcated or trifurcated donor artery (such as the celiac artery) for these delicate reconstructions. In such complex situations such as severe atherosclerosis of the renal artery orifice when eversion endarterectomy is not possible (Nghiem DD, Choi SS, 1992) [4] or results in a damaged artery, the best approach for salvage of the graft is transecting the diseased part of the renal artery and using a small branch of the donor artery such as the left gastric or splenic artery as an elongation conduit of the renal artery. In the case of living donors, a short segment of the recipient saphenous vein may be a good choice for this purpose but it has a real risk of future aneurismal transformation in the future (Sharma A, et al, 2010) [5]. Sometimes we could use a combination of these techniques. For example when the graft has 2 large-size and 1 small-size artery, the best option is to perform an anastomosis between the small-size artery and one of the larger size branches and then perform two separate anastomoses in the recipient. This action will reduce the total operative time of the recipient.

Approach to the vein branches is a little different because of intra-parenchymal communications between the vein branches. We could ligate non-major venous branches, but when the vein branches are in the same size we should reconstruct them before venous anastomosis. Some surgeons prefer to mobilize the external iliac vein by ligating the internal iliac vein or superior gluteal vein or other side branches of this vein, but usually these maneuvers are futile in providing better window for venous anastomosis especially when we use the right kidney from a living donor. In such conditions we prefer to perform the venous anastomosis first or placing the graft in an upside down direction (ureter in the upper part) (Webb J et al, 2003) [6]. In the deceased donor, using a part of the donor external iliac, internal jugular or inferior vena cava as an extension graft is more preferable for adding the length of the vein graft. Such reconstructions should be done in the back table prior to implantation.

In our opinion, ureteral reconstruction also should be discouraged in case of multiple graft ureters. When the ureters have insufficient length, or denuded in their entire length, mobilization of the recipient bladder or using of the recipient ureter is preferred.

At the end of graft preparation some authors suggest that the graft should be wrapped in iced or cold saline soaked surgical gauzes or cloth stockinet or surgical glove to remain cold throughout the implantation procedure. In our opinion this is a time consuming and fruitless maneuver when the surgeons could do the anastomoses rapidly. Also using the ice packets in the site of implantation is not necessary.

3. Implantation site

So many factors impact the surgeon's decision on which site he could implant the kidney graft (table 2). These factors include: the graft size comparing with the recipient, the size, length and number of graft arteries, veins and/or ureters, previous surgeries (for example previous failed kidney transplantation, previous pelvic exploration for bladder reconstruction or anti-reflux surgeries), associated abdominal organ (liver, pancreas or small bowel) transplantation, laterality of the donor kidney (left or right), anomalies of the donor graft (horseshoe kidney, double pelvis, double ureter, etc.), and at last the number of kidney grafts (double kidney from a pediatric or old age or marginal donor). Traditionally the right iliac fossa is the standard fossa for a kidney transplantation procedure and the left iliac fossa is the preferred site for simultaneous kidney-pancreas transplantation. In the pediatric recipient when the graft is larger than usual we should use the main abdominal fossa for implantation. The most important limiting factor for each of these procedures is the length of the renal vein and also the length of the donor ureter and mobility of the recipient urinary bladder. In most instances when the recipient internal iliac artery is used as the arterial inflow, it provides a good length for mobilization and would not be a limiting factor. The right iliac fossa is the preferred site because of the more superficial position of the external iliac vein. The deep branches of the iliac vein can be suture ligated and cut if more superficialization is needed. If the recipient ureter is not diseased it can be used for urinary outflow reconstruction if the donor ureter is short.

Factor	Preferred Site	Rationale
Graft size comparing with the recipient	Abdominal fossa if the graft is very large	Prevention of kidney compartment syndrome
The size, length and number of graft arteries and veins	Iliac fossa is preferred	Prevention of entering to the abdominal cavity and postoperative ileus
The size, length and number of ureters	Iliac fossa is preferred if the recipient ureter is not diseased. Retrovesical area if the ureters are short but vessels are long enough	Prevention of urine leakage or ureteral stricture
Previous surgeries	Opposite iliac fossa	Prevention of vessel or visceral injury, prevention of lymphocele, shorter operative time
Associated abdominal organ transplantation	Left iliac fossa and in the retroperitoneal space Abdominal cavity for en bloc or composite grafts	Prevention of adding the complications of each graft on the other graft
Laterality of the donor kidney (left or right)	It's better to use right iliac fossa	More superficial position of iliac vein Some authors use the opposite side because of position of the transplanted graft for future percutaneous interventions on the urinary system
The number of kidney grafts	Retroperitoneal space of right iliac fossa	If the iliac arteries are not large enough it's better to use the abdominal aorta and inferior vena cava
Anomalies of the donor graft	Abdominal cavity if the graft is large, if the graft is small iliac fossa is better.	Enough space for the graft and enough stations for vascular anastomosis

Table 2. Factors influencing the choice of implantation site

4. Skin preparation and incision

Skin preparation and drape is not so different from other clean abdominal operations. The patient should bathe before entering the operation theatre. Hair removal is better done with hair clippers immediately before surgery. We use scrub povidone iodine or any types of alcoholic or polyethylene glycol type solutions (e.g. Decocept®) for initial washing and then normal povidone iodine for 2 times for the final preparation. Also we use a sterile (Opsite®) drape for complete covering of the incision region. The standard skin incision is the traditional hockey-stick Gibson incision or an oblique Rutherford Morison in the right iliac fossa. Gibson incision starts at the tubercule of pubis and continued laterally transverse to inguinal ligament and then upward in a curvilinear manner in the lateral border of the rectus abdominis muscle till 1-2 cm above the level of umbilicus. In larger adults extension till the anterior superior iliac spine may be enough. The epigastric vessels and the round ligament in females usually need to be ligated and transected, but the spermatic cord simply retracted medially by releasing the border of inguinal canal. The surgeon should avoid entering the peritoneal space and any defect in the peritoneum should be repaired before continuing the incision.

All the dissections should be accompanied by strict hemostasis and avoiding extreme injury to the abdominal wall muscles to simplify the future abdominal wall repair at the end of the procedure. All the bleeding sites should be completely hemostatized during this time because at the end of the procedure hemostasis will be very difficult. Also most renal failure patients has bleeding tendency due to platelet dysfunction specially in the first 2 hours after the hemodialysis or in those patient who underwent preemptive renal transplantation. If hemostasis is not complete wound or peri-graft hematoma is inevitable which will lead to the other complications such as infection, dehiscence, hydronephrosis or kidney compartment syndrome due to compression to the graft.

After entering the retroperitoneal space and revealing the anatomy of the iliac vessels and their suitability for transplantation, the iliac vein should be prepared first by ligating all lymphatics around it. It's better to avoid the first major deep iliac lymph node (Cloquet's node). Dissections around the external iliac artery should be limited and if the internal iliac artery has a good contour and length, it's better to use it as the arterial inflow. If this artery has atherosclerotic plaques an endarterectomy could be done. We use the external iliac artery only when the internal iliac artery of the other side is used previously, or when a large size discrepancy is revealed or severe atherosclerosis reduce the arterial flow to a very low and crucial level. Using the internal iliac artery slightly increases the postoperative lymphocele because of more dissections needed for its releasing, but if the surgeon ligate all the lymphatics it would not be a major problem.

Without a good exposure, transplantation is a very difficult procedure and using a, Denis-Browne (Figure 2), Kirschner(Figure 3) or Bookwalter-type (Figure 4) self retaining retractor is a critical step in the implantation procedure. Many manufacturers have invented more powerful retractors. Some of them like Thompson® retractor, although are very useful and unique for liver or kidney-pancreas transplantation, but their use for kidney transplantation alone is time consuming and is best limited to super-obese recipients. Some of them such as Henley or Darling or Gosset abdominal retractor only are useful in pediatric or thin patients with a shallow pelvis. Balfour and Balfour-Baby, Collin and Baby Collin, Ricard and Sullivan- O'Connor have the same problem. Some of them such as Omni-Flex® (Omni-Tract® surgical, Minnesota Scientific, MN, USA) or SynFrame® retractor systems (Synthes® Spine Inc., PA, USA) are modifications to the original Thompson retractor but their use may be more sophisticated.

http://dx.doi.org/10.5772/54829

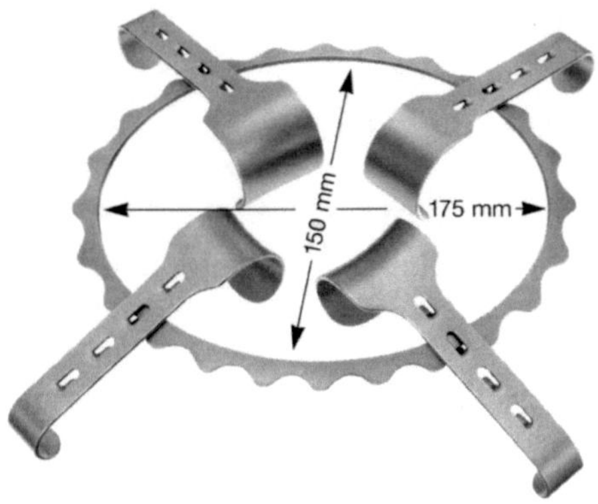

Figure 2. Denis-Browne retractor

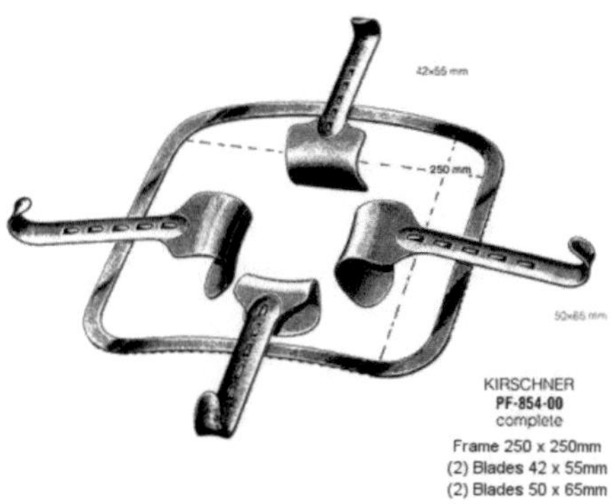

Figure 3. Kirschner retractor

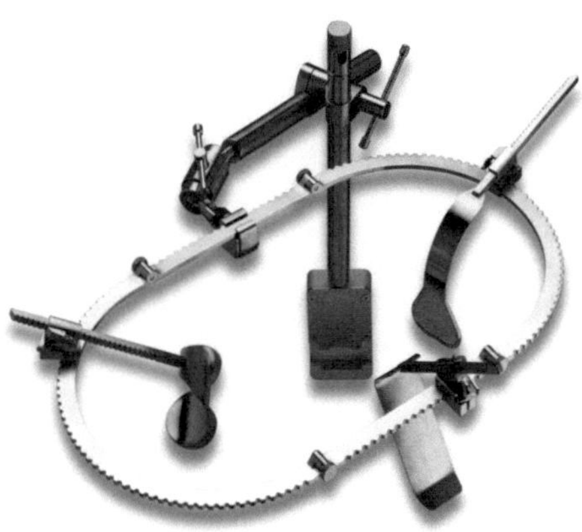

Figure 4. Bookwalter retractor

5. Vascular anastomosis

After preparation of the place of the implantation, the surgeon should transfer the graft to its position transiently for better evaluation of the anastomoses sites. Some authors suggest that slush ice should put in the bed of the graft in the recipient, but we absolutely disagree with this opinion, because the total vascular reconstruction time is usually less than 20 minutes and adding ice only increase the risk of local hypothermic injury. The surgeon should do his best efforts to reduce the total arterial and venous clamping time. First the site of each anastomosis and the position of the graft should be specified accurately according to the size and length of the vessels and also the length of the ureter and position of the recipient bladder or ureter and the final position of the implanted kidney. As described previously, we prefer to use the internal iliac artery and external iliac vein for vascular anastomoses. For reducing the vein clamping time (with subsequent risk of deep vein thrombosis), we perform the arterial anastomosis first. But when the vein is shorter than usual or when the left iliac fossa is used for implantation, or when the abdominal cavity and aorta and inferior vena cava or the external iliac artery are used for implantation, it's better to perform the venous anastomosis first.

The principles of vascular anastomosis are not different from any standard vascular surgery. The best suture size is usually 5-0 and 6-0 Prolene® sutures for venous and arterial anastomosis. The size of the needles depends of the location of the anastomosis but in most cases the needle should be taper-point or taper-cutting-tip round-bodied 3/8 circle with 11 – 13 mm length for better performance. For smaller arteries 7-0 or 8-0, 1/2 circle, 7-9.3 mm needles may be more suitable. For severe atherosclerotic arteries use of special visible Ethicon Visi-Black® Everpoint®, or Tapercut® needles with spatulated heads which is more firm and crash-resistant is needed.

After confirming the exact length and position of the anastomosis site to prevent kinking or rotation, vascular clamps are applied to the first vessel. We prefer to use Bulldog clamps to the internal iliac artery and iliac veins and Satinsky clamps for side-clamping of external iliac and common iliac artery or aorta or inferior vena cava. We discourage systemic heparinization before clamping because of bleeding tendency in chronic renal failure patients, but other authors recommend this. Heparinized saline is enough for irrigation of the vessels during the anastomosis.

For end-to-side anastomoses a patch from the vessel should be removed for preventing future constriction. This patch is removed from the arteries by No. 3, 4 or 5 aortic punches depending on the arterial size and by special Metzenbaum or Potts scissors from the veins. Also we should avoid the venous valve site in the external iliac vein, if possible. The wall of the vein is very thin proximal to the venous valves (sinuses of Valsalva) and may be ruptured during the anastomosis.

For end-to side anastomosis of a renal artery to the external iliac or common iliac or aorta, the graft artery should be spatulated in the direction of its lower corner. For end-to-end anastomosis of the renal artery to the internal iliac artery, the renal artery should be spatulated from the upper corner and the internal iliac artery should be spatulated in the direction of the opposite lower corner (in other words in the direction the deep part of the artery). Renal vein usually needs no spatulation.

An endarterectomy should be done with extreme caution after cutting the internal iliac artery or entering the external iliac artery. No intimal flaps in the opposite direction of the blood flow should be remained at the end of endarterectomy. If such flap is remained, then the surgeon should decide to change the arterial anastomosis site, if possible, or at least the flap must completely secured to the arterial wall with a tagging U-stitch.

Special attention should be paid to the length of the right artery and left renal vein of the deceased donor. They are both too long for anastomosis and if not trimmed or shortened, kinking will be inevitable which will result in postoperative renal dysfunction and hypertension.

Arterial anastomosis is started by two corner stitch in each side of the vessel as described first by Carrel in 1902. Care is taken to include equal bites of all layers of the arterial wall in each passage of the needle and the adventitia remained outside. For this purpose we perform a 1 mm adventitiectomy of both arteries and use microvascular forceps, scissors and needle holders for arterial anastomosis and also recommend using a 4.5-6X loop for magnification and surgical headlights for better illumination. It's so important that the posterior layer suturing of the arterial anastomosis is done first and from outside. The needle should move from inside to outside of the more diseased artery (usually the recipient artery) to tag the intima to the media of the artery and preventing from creating an intimal flap which will be a good trigger point for future thrombosis. The upper suture is tied but the lower is maintained untied till the end of the anastomosis. The posterior layer is sutured first and then anterior layer anastomosis is started from both corners. In the children or for small arteries at least one half of the anastomosis should be done by separate sutures. In all other continuous anastomoses (artery or vein), we tie the last suture loosely and preserve a "Growth factor" or "expansion factor" to prevent purse-string effect of the continuous suture on constricting the anastomosis as first described by Starzl in the portal anastomosis of liver transplantation (Starzl TE, 1984, Zomorrodi, et al, 2012) [7, 8]) [7].

For vein anastomosis we use a somewhat different technique. After inserting the two corner stitches, an anchoring or stay suture is used in the midpoint of the anterior layer of the venotomy site of the external iliac vein to maintain the orifice of the anastomosis site totally exposed and prevent from inadvertent catching of the posterior suture line in the anterior suture line. All the anastomosis is performed circumferentially by a single stitch that used as the proximal corner stitch. Then the surgeon should be cautious when tying this suture that the two remaining part are in the same length. The anastomosis is started from the proximal part by entering tying the corner stitch. Then the needle is entered from the posterior layer of the internal iliac vein into its lumen. Then a four-point technique is used for approximating the two intimal layers of the renal vein and external iliac vein. After completing the posterior layer then the anastomosis is continued from distal and proximal corner to the anterior layer and the anchoring stitch is removed. Again a "Growth factor" is necessary to prevent the purse string effect and also in the pediatric group, the anterior layer stitches should be in separate manner for make future growth possible. If the venotomy site is larger than the orifice of the renal vein, then after completing the posterior layer, the excessive part should be repaired before starting the anterior layer, preferably by another suture line.

6. Unusual situations

In case of thrombosed or fibrotic external iliac vein (due to multiple previous femoral vein canulations or previous DVT) or severe atherosclerotic iliac arteries, the best approach is to use the abdominal major vasculature for renal transplantation. The surgeon may decide to use the common iliac artery or vein if spared from the disease or close the wound and explore the opposite iliac fossa if preoperative Investigations or intraoperative sonographywere negative for the same complication. In extreme cases when the IVC is also thrombosed or fibrotic, or when the infrarenal aorta also is atretic or severely atherosclerotic, using the splenic or native renal vein and artery may be an option, provided that the native ureters has a normal function and anatomy.

Another unusual case is the horseshoe kidney. Anomalous vasculature is the rule in these cases. Crossed fused or non-fused ectopic kidneys have the same problem. One option for approaching this type of anomaly is to incise the ismusth between the two conjoined kidneys and use each kidney for a separate recipient. The major problem is the resultant two grafts with so many arterial and venous branches and also short and multiple ureters. Because of shortage of donor organs most centers prefer this approach. But sometimes dividing the horseshoe kidney is so difficult and may results in damaging both kidneys. In these cases it's better to use the anomalous kidney as an individual graft and use the aorta and IVC as the arterial inflow and venous outflow of the graft. Such large size graft often could not be placed retroperitoneally and should be implanted in an intraperitoneal space. The same principle is applied to double kidney grafts from a pediatric or old age or more marginal donors such as donation after cardiac death (DCD) donors: transplanting each unit separately or using the aorta and IVC as the vascular conduits of the graft. Circumaortic or retroaortic renal veins are other problematic vascular anomalies that make the transplantation procedure more difficult. In experienced hands, these anomalies per se are not contraindication for donation even from the living donors

When a suspicious lesion is found on the kidney graft, it should be incised or excised and sent for frozen section pathologic investigation. Hemostasis could be done by sutures or argon beam coagulators, following the principles of any standard partial nephrectomy. Benign lesions should be removed completely and grafts with any non-benign pathology should be discarded. Solitary cysts are very common and if small, needs no investigation. There are many case reports in the literature about transplanting kidneys from deceased donors with adult polycystic kidney disease, without any short-term complications. These grafts should only be used when the donor kidney function is good and the recipient is fully aware of the donor disease. These cases are best suitable for sedentary recipients with a short life expectancy, provided that no other contraindication such as HLA mismatch is found.

Kidney transplantation may be accompanied by pancreas, liver (Nadim MK, et al, 2012)[9], heart (Florman S, Kim-Schluger L.,2012) [10], lung (Rana RK, et al, 2011) [11] or multiorgan transplantation. In such situations usually the more important transplantation (heart, lung, liver, pancreas or small bowel) is done first. And after stability of the recipient, kidney transplantation is performed. Even when the abdomen is entered during the first procedure, it's better to use the retroperitoneal iliac fossa for the second transplant by the same incision. This will reduce the complications associated with urine leakage. In case of simultaneous kidney –pancreas transplantation the kidney transplant is done first in the left iliac fossa and during the time of this procedure, the other team prepares the pancreas graft by ex vivo surgery for the second transplantation which is usually use the right common or external iliac artery as the inflow. The kidney transplantation combined with multivisceral transplantation is usually is an en-bloc transplantation. This means that the kidney is not separated from the donor aorta and inferior vena cava (IVC). All major vascular anastomoses are done by aorta as the inflow artery and IVC and/or portal vein as the venous outflow. The urinary reconstruction is performed after complete reperfusion of all abdominal organs.

7. Declamping and reperfusion

After completing the vascular anastomoses, the opposite corner stay sutures remained untied until reperfusion. The recipient systolic blood pressure should be at least 120 mmHg and the central venous pressure between 10 to 14 cm H_2O. The use of vasopressors such as dopamine for increasing the blood pressure is controversial. Immunosuppressant is best infused before declamping according to the protocols of each transplant ward. Some authors suggests some over-hydration, infusing Furosemide and Mannitol and correction of acid-base imbalance according to the last arterial blood gas base deficit before declamping to prevent the so called "reperfusion syndrome". Unlike liver or small bowel transplantation, in most cases reperfusion syndrome will not be a problematic issue, because the kidney graft is relatively small, except when using an adult kidney for a pediatric recipient or in cases of a long implantation time with complete aortic or common or external iliac artery clamping time. In such cases the cause of "reperfusion syndrome" is transient ischemia of the lower limbs. The anesthesiologist should prepare sodium bicarbonate, calcium gluconate, and insulin with 50% Glucose before declamping for managing this complication and obtain an arterial blood gas before and after the declamping for estimating the severity of acidosis and monitor the electrocardiogram for diagnosis of hyperkalemia.

Arterial declamping is done first and after complete filling of the graft, veins are also opened. In this phase brisk bleeding is a rule, especially when we applied "growth factors" to the last ties. Most of the bleeding will be stopped spontaneously after complete dilatation of the anastomotic lines. Small bleeding sites may be covered by small parts of any hemostatic agent such as Surgicel®, N-butyl cyanoacrylate glues, Tachosil® or similar agents (Sageshima J, et al, 2011) [13]. All the other larger bleeding sites should be transligated or repaired by fine Prolene® sutures especially near the hilum, but extreme caution should be paid not to include the delicate hilar arterial branches in the sutures.

The kidney should be firm and well-perfused after 1-2 minutes and urine flow usually starts after that. If the graft is flaccid and the patient's blood pressure is good, arterial kinking is the first differential diagnosis. This usually is resolved by repositioning of the graft. Also the surgeon could transiently clamp the renal vein or the distal part of the external iliac artery. If not, thrombosis must be considered and ruled out as soon as possible.

8. Urinary reconstruction

After completing the reperfusion stage usually the urine flow is started. Sometimes, especially in case of deceased donors or when the nephrectomy has been performed with difficulty in the living donors, the urine flow will be delayed. If the color and contour of the graft look good and the arterial and venous flow is good with a well-palpable thrill in the hilum, the surgeon should proceed to urinary reconstruction.

First of all the urinary bladder should be filled with sterile normal saline serum through previously installed urinary catheter. Some surgeons add 10ml/lit povidone iodine and 80 mg/lit Gentamicin or 500 mg/lit Amikacin to the irrigation fluid for better sterility of the bladder (Salehipour M, et al, 2010) [13] but its effect is controversial. The kidney should be positioned in its final expected place to prevent the tension on the remained ureter before cutting the excess length of the ureter. It's better to use the smallest possible length of the ureter to reduce future ischemic complications. If this step is forgotten the final length of ureter may be shorter than expected and this will result in kinking of the vasculature and changing the location of the kidney from its ideal position.

The surgeon has many options for urinary reconstruction: ureteroneocystostomy, ureteroureterostomy, pyeloureterostomy, and pyelocystostomy or even ureteroenterostomy to an ileal conduit or Koch (Manassero F, et al, 2011) [14] or pyelopyelostomy in case of orthotopic kidney transplantation or complicated case (Wagner M, et al, 1994) [15]. The type of reconstruction depends on the position of the graft, the length, condition and number of the donor ureter(s), the condition of the recipient's bladder or bladder substitute (including its capacity and continence), previous operations on the recipient bladder or ureter (and its antireflux condition). The anastomosis should be done by absorbable sutures, usually polydioxanone sutures. Because of the risk of infection, use of any types of stents, such as double J stents or newer antireflux stents are controversial (Parapiboon W, et al, 2012) [16], but we use it in our center and remove it after 3 weeks. At least 4 techniques and their modifications are discussed in the literature for ureteroneocystostomy (Kayler L, et al, 2010) [17]. Prevention of leakage, stricture and reflux is the final goal of all of these techniques. The two most common types are transvesical or Leadbetter-Politano (LP) technique and the extravesical or modified Lich-Gregoir (LG) technique. We use and recommend the second technique because it needs fewer dissections and use only one small cystostomy incision (comparing with 2 large cystostomy incision needs for LP technique) with comparable antireflux characteristics and fewer complications. The LG technique can be performed in a very shorter time. After distending the bladder, the detrusor muscle dissected bluntly in the dome of the bladder approximately for a length of 3 cm till the mucosa bulges out. The ureter shortened to its ideal length and spatulated for a length of 2 cm in its anti-mesoureteral direction and then the bladder mucosa incised. Anastomosis is started near the heel of the spatulated ureter 2-3 mm in the opposite direction of the corner of the ureter. In this manner, the tie is placed outside and with some distance from the corner. The mucosa of the bladder is then sutured to the ureteral end with simple continuous sutures. After completing the anastomosis, an absorbable suture is used for approximating the detrusor muscle to close over the anastomosis and creating a small submucosal tunnel for its antireflux mechanism. The LP techniques and the two other extravesical techniques are better described in the literature (Kayler L, et al, 2010) [17]. In the LP technique, a large anterior cystostomy is done for visualization of the bladder interior and the ureter is transferred through another small posterior cystostomy and then through the mucosa and after anchoring the distal end to the mucosa, the bladder is closed in 2 layers with absorbable sutures. Another extravesical technique is the single or double U-stitch technique. In these techniques after opening the submucosal tunnel by creating by dissection of detrusor muscle and incising the bladder mucosa only 1 U-stitch (Shanfield, 1972) [18] at the toe or 2 U-stitch (MacKinnon et al, 1968) [19] at the toe and heel of the trimmed ureter is used for anchoring the ureter to bladder mucosa and then the detrussor muscle closed as the same manner of the LG technique.

Another extravesical technique uses two parallel incisions in the detrusor muscle, first posterior for transferring the ureter in a submucosal tunnel and the second incision for anastomosis of the ureter to the ureteral mucosa (Barry JM, 1983) [20]. In the last technique, the ureter is anastomosed to the bladder full-thickness wall without any antireflux mechanism (Starzl, et al, 1989) [21]. In our opinion, the surgeon should be familiar with all of these methods and use them as needed, but we have the most experience with the modified LG technique without any major urologic complication (Davari HR, et al, 2006) [22].

When the graft ureter is short, ischemic, or denuded, the surgeon should use the native ureters for ureteroureterostomy or pyeloureterostomy if they are completely in a healthy condition (no stricture, no infection, no dilation or no reflux) or decide to perform a pyeloneocystostomy. This should be done with extreme caution to prevent kinking or pressure on the graft vasculature or repositioning of the graft. A Boari flap or psoas hitch is often necessary in all cases.

In case of previous bladder surgery such as antireflux surgeries or cystoplasty or bladder augmentation, it's very important that the site of final urinary reconstruction is fully depicted before proceeding with vascular anastomosis, or even before proceeding with nephrectomy in the living donor. Also the blood supply of the tissues used for augmentation should be considered. Creating a submucosal flap in the augmented bladder may results in ischemia of the tissues used for augmentation and if possible it's better to use the native bladder area for ureteral anastomosis.

In case of double or multiple ureters (such as horseshoe kidneys or en bloc transplantation of two kidneys), the ureters can be anastomosed separately to the bladder, or one to the bladder and the shorter ones to the native ureter. Another option is anastomosis of the ureters to each other and then anastomosis of the conjoined ureter to the bladder. In our opinion using separate anastomoses (if possible) reduces the future complications.

9. Wound closure

Wound closure is the final step of the procedure. Closing is done by 2-layer repair of the abdominal muscles (first transverse and internal oblique as one layer and then the external oblique muscle), by a No. 0 loop Nylon suture. Using any drain before closure is controversial but if used it should be a closed suction drain such as a Jackson-Pratt drain and every effort should be used that the drain has no compression effect on the renal vasculature and the ureter. The exit site also should be assessed for bleeding. Every bleeding site should be assessed and repaired before closure to prevent postoperative hematoma. Diffuse oozing at the end of operation may be the result of platelet dysfunction or heparin overdose and should be managed accordingly by desmopressin and protamine sulfate, respectively. Excess perirenal fat should be removed, and the graft should be placed in a retroperitoneally created pouch parallel with the psoas muscle, to prevent compression of the kidney between the abdominal wall and the pelvic bones. If the kidney volume is greater than this space, or the renal vasculature or ureter is shorter than usual, then "compartment syndrome" is inevitable is the abdominal muscles repaired in the usual manner. In such situation, the renal artery inflow is good but the outflow will be disturbed because of pressure of the abdominal wall on the renal vein. Renal venous pressure increase and then the graft will be congested and the urine flow will decreased. If remained unmanaged, this will eventually lead to decreasing renal artery flow and finally to renal artery thrombosis and graft loss. If the surgeon could not reposition the graft in to the supravesical area and anchor it to the abdominal wall without vascular kinking, many other options should be tried. One option is to incise the rectus sheath after closing the muscles. Another option is to close the abdominal wall from distal and proximal and let the part which is covering the kidney remains unclosed or closed by an artificial mesh which is used for hernia repair. The last option is to let abdominal musculature remained completely opened and only covered by the skin. The resultant incisional hernia will be repaired in the future, usually 3 months after the transplantation. The best treatment of such conditions is "prevention" by matching the size of the donor and recipient and special attention to the length of the graft vasculature and ureter and also creating the pouch as the first step during the procedure.

Author details

Farzad Kakaei[1], Saman Nikeghbalian[2] and Seyed Ali Malekhosseini[2]

1 Tabriz University of Medical Sciences, Tabriz, Iran

2 Shiraz University of Medical Sciences, Shiraz, Iran

http://dx.doi.org/10.5772/54829

References

[1] Dolińska B, Ostróżka-Cieślik A, Caban A, Cierpka L, Ryszka F. Comparing the effect of Biolasol® and HTK solutions on maintaining proper homeostasis, indicating the kidney storage efficiency prior to transplantation. Ann Transplant. 2012 Jun 29;17(2): 74-8.

[2] Prasad GS, Ninan CN, Devasia A, Gnanaraj L, Kekre NS, Gopalakrishnan G.: Is Euro-Collins better than ringer lactate in live related donor renal transplantation? Indian J Urol. 2007 Jul;23(3):265-9.

[3] El-Sherbiny M, Abou-Elela A, Morsy A, Salah M, Foda A. The use of the inferior epigastric artery for accessory lower polar artery revascularization in live donor renal transplantation. Int Urol Nephrol. 2008;40(2):283-7.

[4] Nghiem DD, Choi SS. Eversion endarterectomy of the cadaver donor renal artery: a method to increase the use of elderly donor kidney allografts. J Urol. 1992 Mar;147(3): 653-5.

[5] Sharma A, King AL, Lee HM, Posner MP. Saphenous vein graft aneurysm after renal transplantation: a case report. Transplantation. 2010 May 15;89(9):1162-3.

[6] Webb J, Soomro N, Jaques B, Manas D, Talbot D. The upside down transplant kidney. Clin Transplant. 2003 Oct;17(5):484.

[7] Starzl TE, Iwatsuki S, Shaw BW Jr. A growth factor in fine vascular anastomoses. Surg Gynecol Obstet. 1984 Aug;159(2):164-5.

[8] Zomorrodi A, Kakei F, Farshi A, Zomorrodi S (2012) Is Placing an Expansion Space at the Anastomosing Site of the Vessel for Prevention of Pursiness, Safe? J Transplant Technol Res 2:113. doi:10.4172/2161-0991.1000113

[9] Nadim MK, Sung RS, Davis CL, Andreoni KA, Biggins SW, Danovitch GM, Feng S, Friedewald JJ, Hong JC, Kellum JA, Kim WR, Lake JR, Melton LB, Pomfret EA, Saab S, Genyk YS Simultaneous Liver-Kidney Transplantation Summit: Current State and Future Directions. Am J Transplant. 2012 Jul 23.

[10] Florman S, Kim-Schluger L. Organ transplantation update, part II: heart and kidney. Mt Sinai J Med. 2012 May-Jun;79(3):303-4.

[11] Rana RK, Ghandehari S, Falk JA, Simsir SA, Ghaly AS, Cheng W, Cohen JL, Peng A, Czer LS, Schwarz ER, Chaux GE. Successful combined heart-bilateral lung-kidney transplantation from a same donor to treat severe hypertrophic cardiomyopathy with secondary pulmonary hypertension and renal failure: case report and review of the literature. Transplant Proc. 2011 Sep;43(7):2820-6. Review.

[12] Sageshima J, Ciancio G, Uchida K, Romano A, Acun Z, Chen L, Burke GW 3rd. Absorbable cyanoacrylate surgical sealant in kidney transplantation. Transplant Proc. 2011 Sep;43(7):2584-6.

[13] Salehipour M, Salahi H, Fathikalajahi A, Mohammadian R, Emadmarvasti V, Bahador A, Nikeghbalian S, Kazemi K, Dehghani M, Malek-Hosseini SA. Is perioperative intravesically applied antibiotic solution effective in the prophylaxis of urinary tract infections after renal transplantation? Urol Int. 2010;85(1):66-9. Epub 2010 Mar 17

[14] Manassero F, Di Paola G, Mogorovich A, Giannarini G, Boggi U, Selli C. Orthotopic bladder substitute in renal transplant recipients: experience with Studer technique and literature review. Transpl Int. 2011 Sep;24(9):943-8. Epub 2011 Jul 1. Review.

[15] Wagner M, Dieckmann KP, Klän R, Fielder U, Offermann G. Rescue of renal transplants with distal ureteral complications bypyelo-pyelostomy. J Urol. 1994 Mar;151(3):578-81.

[16] Parapiboon W, Ingsathit A, Disthabanchong S, Nongnuch A, Jearanaipreprem A, Charoenthanakit C, Jirasiritham S, Sumethkul V. Impact of early ureteric stent removal and cost-benefit analysis in kidney transplant recipients: results of a randomized controlled study. Transplant Proc. 2012 Apr;44(3):737-9.

[17] Kayler L, Kang D, Molmenti E, Howard R: Kidney transplant ureteroneocystostomy techniques and complications: review of the literature. Transplant Proc. 2010 Jun;42(5): 1413-20.

[18] Schanfield I: New experimental methods for implantation of the ureter in bladder and conduit. Transplant Proc 4:637, 1972

[19] MacKinnon KJ, Oliver JA, Morehouse DD, et al: Cadaver renal transplantation: emphasis on urological aspects. J Urol 99:486, 1968

[20] Barry JM: Unstented extravesical ureteroneocystostomy in kidney transplantation. J Urol 129:918, 1983.

[21] Starzl TE, Shapiro R, Tzakis A, et al: A new technique of extravesical ureteroneocystostomy for renal transplantation. Transplant Proc 21:3856, 1989

[22] Davari HR, Yarmohammadi H, Malek-hosseini SA, Salahi H, Bahador A, Salehipour M. Urological complications in 980 consecutive patients with renal transplantation. Int J Urol. 2006 Oct;13(10):1271-5.

Chapter 8

Renal Aging and Kidney Transplantation

Katrien De Vusser and Maarten Naesens

Additional information is available at the end of the chapter

http://dx.doi.org/10.5772/55469

1. Introduction

Kidney transplantation is the preferred therapy for most patients with end-stage renal disease. The demand for kidney grafts however far exceeds the supply of available organs. As a result, transplant teams increasingly use organs from extended criteria donors, of older age or with significant comorbidity. This use of extended criteria organs is not without consequences.

Older donor age is strongly related to impaired kidney graft function and graft failure because older kidneys are limited in their capacity to tolerate injury [1]. Aging is associated with renal structural changes en functional decline. Older kidneys lose renal parenchyma and trough this have a decreased renal plasma flow and tubular dysfunction. The mechanisms required for tissue repair after damage become less reliable, resulting in a decrease in repair capacity. This functional decline in the potential to repair and regenerate is often considered a hallmark of the aging phenotype [2] [3].

Another major component of the aging phenotype is replicative or cellular senescence, which is defined as permanent, irreversible growth arrest. In this chapter we draw the parallel between the aging kidney in the transplantation setting and cellular senescence.

2. Impact of older donor age on transplantation outcome

The success of organ transplantation in patients with end-stage renal damage gave rise to waiting lists and organ shortage. This in itself led to the increasing use of kidneys from older or expanded criteria donors for transplantation. In 2002 the term Expanded criteria donor (ECD) was codified to be deceased donors aged 60 years of older and those aged 50-59 years with at least 2 of the following characteristics: history of hypertension, serum creatinine level greater than 1.5 mg/dL and cerebrovascular cause of death. The risk of graft failure after an ECD kidney transplant is 70% higher than after a non- ECDtransplant [4].

Also Ojo *et al.* have reported on the survival of recipients of marginal kidneys, defined as kidneys with one or more of the following pretransplant factors: donor age >55 years, non-heartbeating donor, cold ischemia time >36 h, and donor hypertension or diabetes mellitus of >10 years duration. Also in this study, marginal kidney transplants had a lower allograft outcomes compared with organs from ideal donors [5].

In another study, Woo *et al.* compared two groups only divided by age. There was a larger increase in graft failure rates of kidneys from donors >55 years of age. Also the mean estimated glomerular filtration rate 6 months post-transplant and the stability of the glomerular filtration rate in the first transplant year were significantly higher in the recipients of donors <55 years [6].

Recent data on 1063 kidney grafts from living donors confirm the association between older donor age and graft outcome even after living donation, where living donors are screened prior to transplantation and comorbidities are avoided. Increasing living donor age was associated with lower kidney function after transplantation, loss of glomerular filtration rate beyond 1 year and reduced graft survival [7].

With the increasing use of older and extended criteria donor kidneys, the intrinsic quality of the kidneys at transplantation is nowadays much more important for the post-transplant histological evolution and long-term graft survival than acute T-cell mediated rejection [1, 8, 9]. The causes by which older kidneys lose function after transplantation remain however incompletely understood. This may involve both early and late-onset processes and is likely to be found mainly in a significant effect of donor age on the subclinical progression of chronic histological damage [10]. In a large study using protocol biopsies, it was not only demonstrated that higher donor age is the major determinant of this non-specific chronic allograft damage, but also that the association between donor age and post-transplant histological damage is independent of the histological quality of the graft at implantation [11]. This suggests that donor age and the aging process in itself are playing an independent role on renal allograft histological progression and long-term outcome. From these studies, it can even be hypothesized that the aging process in itself is accelerated after transplantation, and contributes to transplant outcome [10].

3. Mechanisms of renal aging

It is essential to distinguish aging from age-related disease. Aging itself is not a disease but seems to be the greatest risk factor for age-related pathology [12]. The altered molecules with aging involve many different pathways, including cell integrity, cellular proliferation, cell transport and energy metabolism. Many of these molecules and processes are not unique to aging and are likely general pathways involved in tissue damage and repair. Aging is a programmed biological process that is associated with small transcriptional differences in many genes, rather than large expression changes in a small number of genes [13-16].

The aging phenotype is the consequence of cellular senescence, of increased susceptibility to apoptosis with older age, of impaired regeneration and repair, of decreased functional capacity of stem cells and progenitor cells, of changes in the expression of growth factors with increasing age, of mitochondrial changes, of dysregulation of autoregulatory pathways and of immune system alterations and different immunogenicity of older tissue.

Of the previously mentioned mechanisms of aging, cellular senescence is classically seen as one of the most important drivers of the aging process. Cellular senescence leads to permanent and irreversible growth arrest and was detected in seminal *in vitro* studies by Hayflick and Moorhead [17, 18]. Senescent cells remain viable but show a changed morphology, greater heterogeneity, expression of SA-β-gal, accumulation of lipofuscin granules and lack of response to mitogenic stimuli.

Cellular senescence is a specific response of mitotically active cells to various stressors. It is determined by multiple factors, including the genetic regulation of metabolism, time, the number cell cycles of replication, and most importantly the answer to injury and stress [11, 19]. Examples of these different factors are telomere shortening and telomere dysfunction, non-telomere DNA damage (e.g. due to X-rays, oxidative stress and UV irradiation), mitogenic signals including those produces by oncogens (wich also cause DNA damage) and non-genotoxic stress like chromatin perturbation (epigenetic changes) and other stress factors [20, 21] (. Cellular senescence thus not only comprises exhaustion of a predetermined proliferative capacity (intrinsic senescence or replicative senescence), but can also be induced by extrinsic factors (stress-induced premature senescence).

In this light, the impact of cellular senescence goes beyond the importance for aging. Cellular senescence pathways play essential roles in tumor suppression, tumor promotion and tissue repair.

There is increasing evidence that cellular senescence is a tumor suppressive system (by inducing growth arrest) and a tumor-promoting phenomenon (by secretion of inflammatory cytokines) [22]. To reconcile the apparently conflicting impact of cellular senescence on cancer, Campisi *et al.* suggest that cellular senescence is a biological process that was selected to promote fitness in young organisms (beneficial: tumor suppression, tissue regeneration), but is deleterious in old organisms (harming: aging, tumor promotion) [23]. In the evolution, senescence pathways evolved in an environment where organism lifespan was short. Therefore tumor-suppressor mechanisms needed to be effective for only a relatively short (reproductive) period [21]. Even if this mechanism was harmful later on, this would not affect selective pressure. This concept is the essence of the "antagonistic pleiotropy hypothesis" and makes us understand the senescence concept much better [23].

4. The replicative senescence pathways in renal disease and transplantation

Replicative senescence depends mainly on two pathways: the ARF-p53-p21 signaling pathway that is partially telomere dependent and the p16-pRb pathway, which is independent of telomere dysfunction. These pathways interact but can act independently [21, 24].

1. Replicative senescence pathways ARF-p53-p21 (associated with telomere shortening).

Telomeres comprise tandem TTAGGG repeats of 5000 to 15000 base pairs that normally reside at the ends of chromosome ends as protection and prevent end-to-end fusion of chromosomes. Telomeric DNA is synthesized and its length is regulated by telomerase. Most somatic cells don't express telomerase and mature telomeres tend to progressively shorten with every cell division. The crucial role of telomerase absence in the telomere shortening is proven *in vitro* as telomere shortening can be bypassed by transfection with telomerase [25].

Telomere length reflects several important factors such as heredity, telomerase activity, the efficiency of telomere-binding proteins, the rate of cellular proliferation and oxidative stress in the milieu. Although telomere length is partly heritable, there are major differences in telomere length even among monozygotic twins, which suggests that environmental factors (e.g. hyperglycemie, oxidative stress [26, 27]) play a major role in telomere attrition and aging.

When the telomeres become critically short (reach the "Hayflick limit") a classical DNA-damage response is triggered with participation of several protein kinases (e.g. ATM and CHK2), adaptor proteins (e.g. 53BP1 and MDC1) and chromatin modifiers (e.g. gammaH2AX). Telomere shortening also leads to activation of the p53 pathway (trough p53 phosphorylation) and herewith associated p21 (also termed CDKN1a, p21Cip1, Waf1 or SD11) expression. Also other DNA damage responses (DDRs) and ARF (alternate reading frame, p14) can lead to activation of the p53 pathway. SIRT1 (sirtuin 1) can negatively regulate p53 localization to the nucleus and its function as a transcription factor.

The clinical importance of telomere shortening has been suggested in a very interesting study, where leukocyte telomere length was used as a biomarker of aging. In this study, the association between telomere length and various disease processes was independent of chronological age, which suggests the value of telomere length measurement as a biomarker of biological or cellular age [28].

In contrast to, e.g. blood cells, the association between age and telomere shortening in renal tissue was only studied scarcely. The supposed association with reduced regenerative capacity during aging and chronic diseases, and after acute injury, seems valid but has never been proven in humans. Only Westhoff 's study in telomerase deficient mice suggests that critical telomere shortening in kidneys leads to increased senescence and apoptosis, thereby limiting regenerative capacity [29].

In adult kidneys, telomerase activity is very low, which results in telomere shortening by every cell division, as was demonstrated by Melk *et al* [25]. Also ischemia can induce telomere shortening as has been shown in different animal models [30-32] Finally, glomerular diseases like IgA nephropathy, lupus nephritis and focal glomerulosclerosis are associated with increased p53 expression compared to kidneys without lesions, both in animals [33] and in humans [34, 35] Whether this relates to telomere length has not been studied to date.

After bone marrow transplantation telomere shortening occurs significantly more rapidly than would be expected in graft-derived leukocytes. Probably due to the replicative stress on the blood cell caused the kinetics of haemopoietic engraftment [36]. After solid organ transplantation there are arguments to state that transplantation is associated with accelerated shortening of telomere length in the transplanted cells [12]. In transplanted renal cells, there is

http://dx.doi.org/10.5772/55469

evidence for an increased cell turnover at the time of transplantation and a phase of increased cell regeneration directly after transplantation that correlates with cold ischemia time [37, 38]. Also a small study showed that shorter telomere length in biopsies obtained at implantation was associated with lower graft function at 12 months after transplantation, but no correlation with p21 or p53 was found [39]. These studies need further validation to confirm the role of telomere shortening on transplant outcome.

2. p16-pRB pathways (independent of telomere dysfunction).

DNA damage by environmental stress is the main stressor for activation of the p16-pRB pathway although dysfunctional telomeres can also induce p16 [21]. This telomere-independent senescence pathway is currently often referred to as 'STATIS' (Stress and Aberrant Signaling-Induced Senescence. P16 (encoded by *CDKN2A*) is an important tumor suppressor in the p53 pathway. P16 keeps pRB in an active hypophosphorylated form, which inhibits cell proliferation and induces growth arrest [12]. The p53 and p16-pRB pathways interact witch each other and there is a reciprocal regulation.

In native kidneys increased p16 expression is found in human kidneys with glomerular disease [16], interstitial fibrosis, diabetic nefropathy [40] and animal kidneys with hypertension [41]. Furthermore p16 is induced by cyclosporine, catch up growth in low birth weight and is attenuated by calorie restriction [12]. Finally, p16 expression correlates significantly with kidney age [42].

Like the p53 pathway p16 expression relates to ischemia-reperfusion, at least in mice [43]. Furthermore, a rapid increase in p16 expression after transplantation has been described in murine kidney grafts, which was most pronounced in older animals. Whether these findings are also valid in humans, remains unknown.

5. Summary

In summary, there is extensive data that the outcome of kidney transplantation is heavily influenced by the age of the transplanted kidneys. There is some scant evidence that transplantation in itself increases cell turnover and leads to accelerate replicative senescence. Whether the association between older kidneys and impaired graft outcome relates to this accelerate replicative senescence after transplantation is however not clear, and the few suggestions in the literature need to be validated in large-enough patient cohorts.

Author details

Katrien De Vusser and Maarten Naesens

Department of Nephrology and Renal Transplantation, University Hospitals Leuven, Leuven, Belgium

References

[1] Meier-Kriesche, H.U., et al., Lack of Improvement in Renal Allograft Survival Despite a Marked Decrease in Acute Rejection Rates Over the Most Recent Era. Am J Transplant, 2004. 4(3): p. 378-383.

[2] Epstein, M., Aging and the kidney. J.Am.Soc.Nephrol., 1996. 7(8): p. 1106-1122.

[3] Zhou, W., et al., Predominant role for C5b-9 in renal ischemia/reperfusion injury. Journal of Clinical Investigation, 2000. 105(10): p. 1363-1371.

[4] Port, F.K., et al., Donor characteristics associated with reduced graft survival: an approach to expanding the pool of kidney donors. Transplantation, 2002. 74(9): p. 1281-6.

[5] Ojo, A.O., et al., Survival in recipients of marginal cadaveric donor kidneys compared with other recipients and wait-listed transplant candidates. J.Am.Soc.Nephrol., 2001. 12(3): p. 589-597.

[6] Woo, Y.M., et al., The advanced age deceased kidney donor: current outcomes and future opportunities. Kidney Int, 2005. 67(6): p. 2407-2414.

[7] Noppakun, K., et al., Living donor age and kidney transplant outcomes. Am J Transplant, 2011. 11(6): p. 1279-1286.

[8] Summers, D.M., et al., Analysis of factors that affect outcome after transplantation of kidneys donated after cardiac death in the UK: a cohort study. Lancet, 2010. 376(9749): p. 1303-1311.

[9] Opelz, G. and B. Dohler, Influence of immunosuppressive regimens on graft survival and secondary outcomes after kidney transplantation. Transplantation, 2009. 87(6): p. 795-802.

[10] Naesens, M., et al., Donor age and renal P-glycoprotein expression associate with chronic histological damage in renal allografts. J Am Soc Nephrol, 2009. 20(11): p. 2468-80.

[11] Halloran, P.F., A. Melk, and C. Barth, Rethinking chronic allograft nephropathy: the concept of accelerated senescence. J.Am.Soc.Nephrol., 1999. 10(1): p. 167-181.

[12] Naesens, M., Replicative senescence in kidney aging, renal disease, and renal transplantation. Discov Med, 2011. 11(56): p. 65-75.

[13] Weindruch, R., et al., Microarray profiling of gene expression in aging and its alteration by caloric restriction in mice. J Nutr., 2001. 131(3): p. 918S-923S.

[14] Rodwell, G.E., et al., A transcriptional profile of aging in the human kidney. PLoS.Biol., 2004. 2(12): p. e427.

[15] McCarroll, S.A., et al., Comparing genomic expression patterns across species identifies shared transcriptional profile in aging. Nat.Genet., 2004. 36(2): p. 197-204.

[16] Melk, A., et al., Increased expression of senescence-associated cell cycle inhibitor p16INK4a in deteriorating renal transplants and diseased native kidney. Am J Transplant., 2005. 5(6): p. 1375-1382.

[17] Kawai, T., et al., HLA-mismatched renal transplantation without maintenance immunosuppression. N.Engl.J.Med., 2008. 358(4): p. 353-361.

[18] Hayflick, L. and P.S. Moorhead, The serial cultivation of human diploid cell strains. Exp.Cell Res., 1961. 25: p. 585-621.

[19] Hayflick, L., Biological aging is no longer an unsolved problem. Ann.N.Y.Acad.Sci., 2007. 1100: p. 1-13.

[20] Finkel, T., M. Serrano, and M.A. Blasco, The common biology of cancer and ageing. Nature, 2007. 448(7155): p. 767-774.

[21] Campisi, J. and F.F. dda di, Cellular senescence: when bad things happen to good cells. Nat.Rev.Mol.Cell Biol., 2007. 8(9): p. 729-740.

[22] Coppe, J.P., et al., Senescence-associated secretory phenotypes reveal cell-nonautonomous functions of oncogenic RAS and the p53 tumor suppressor. PLoS.Biol., 2008. 6(12): p. 2853-2868.

[23] Campisi, J., Cellular senescence: putting the paradoxes in perspective. Curr.Opin.Genet.Dev., 2010.

[24] Collado, M. and M. Serrano, Senescence in tumours: evidence from mice and humans. Nat.Rev.Cancer, 2010. 10(1): p. 51-57.

[25] Melk, A., et al., Telomere shortening in kidneys with age. J Am Soc Nephrol, 2000. 11(3): p. 444-453.

[26] Yoshida, T., et al., ATF3 protects against renal ischemia-reperfusion injury. J Am Soc Nephrol, 2008. 19(2): p. 217-224.

[27] Avogaro, A., S.V. de Kreutzenberg, and G.P. Fadini, Insulin signaling and life span. Pflugers Arch., 2010. 459(2): p. 301-314.

[28] Wong, J.M. and K. Collins, Telomere maintenance and disease. Lancet, 2003. 362(9388): p. 983-8.

[29] Westhoff, J.H., et al., Telomere shortening reduces regenerative capacity after acute kidney injury. J Am Soc Nephrol, 2010. 21(2): p. 327-336.

[30] Joosten, S.A., et al., Telomere shortening and cellular senescence in a model of chronic renal allograft rejection. Am J Pathol., 2003. 162(4): p. 1305-1312.

[31] Kelly, K.J., et al., P53 mediates the apoptotic response to GTP depletion after renal ischemia-reperfusion: protective role of a p53 inhibitor. J Am Soc Nephrol, 2003. 14(1): p. 128-138.

[32] Megyesi, J., et al., The p53-independent activation of transcription of p21 WAF1/CIP1/SDI1 after acute renal failure. Am J Physiol, 1996. 271(6 Pt 2): p. F1211-F1216.

[33] Turner, C.M., et al., Increased expression of the pro-apoptotic ATP-sensitive P2X7 receptor in experimental and human glomerulonephritis. Nephrol Dial.Transplant, 2007. 22(2): p. 386-395.

[34] Takemura, T., et al., Proto-oncogene expression in human glomerular diseases. J Pathol., 1996. 178(3): p. 343-351.

[35] Qiu, L.Q., R. Sinniah, and S.I. Hsu, Coupled induction of iNOS and p53 upregulation in renal resident cells may be linked with apoptotic activity in the pathogenesis of progressive IgA nephropathy. J Am Soc Nephrol, 2004. 15(8): p. 2066-2078.

[36] Wynn, R.F., et al., Accelerated telomere shortening in young recipients of allogeneic bone-marrow transplants. Lancet, 1998. 351(9097): p. 178-181.

[37] Oberbauer, R., et al., Apoptosis of tubular epithelial cells in donor kidney biopsies predicts early renal allograft function. J.Am.Soc.Nephrol., 1999. 10(9): p. 2006-2013.

[38] Vinuesa, E., et al., Macrophage involvement in the kidney repair phase after ischaemia/reperfusion injury. J Pathol., 2008. 214(1): p. 104-113.

[39] Koppelstaetter, C., et al., Markers of cellular senescence in zero hour biopsies predict outcome in renal transplantation. Aging Cell, 2008. 7(4): p. 491-497.

[40] Verzola, D., et al., Accelerated senescence in the kidneys of patients with type 2 diabetic nephropathy. AJP - Renal Physiology, 2008. 295(5): p. F1563-F1573.

[41] Westhoff, J.H., et al., Hypertension induces somatic cellular senescence in rats and humans by induction of cell cycle inhibitor p16INK4a. Hypertension, 2008. 52(1): p. 123-129.

[42] Chkhotua, A.B., et al., Increased expression of P21((WAF1/CIP1)) CDKI gene in chronic allograft nephropathy correlating with the number of acute rejection episodes. Transplant Proc., 2003. 35(2): p. 655-658.

[43] Hochegger, K., et al., p21 and mTERT are novel markers for determining different ischemic time periods in renal ischemia-reperfusion injury. AJP - Renal Physiology, 2007. 292(2): p. F762-F768.

Chapter 9

Comparison of Renal Transplantation Outcomes in Patients After Peritoneal Dialysis and Hemodialysis – A Case Control Study and Literature Review

Thomas Rath and Stephan Ziefle

Additional information is available at the end of the chapter

http://dx.doi.org/10.5772/55711

1. Introduction

For patients with end-stage renal disease renal transplantation is the treatment of choice. However, there is still some controversy if mortality rate after renal transplantation is affected by the chosen dialysis modality.

It is widely accepted, that in terms of survival hemodialysis (HD) and peritoneal dialysis (PD) are comparable. Especially in PD-patients with preserved residual renal function, control of hypertension is achieved more easily, whereas patients with diabetes mellitus do better on HD. In general, quality of life for patients is assumed to be better with PD than with HD [1].

In a cost-modeling strategy, incorporating quality of life and social perspective aspects in Scandinavia, it was shown, that the cost per quality-adjusted life year for PD was lower compared to HD in all analyzed age groups, whereas mean survival and frequency of transplantation did not differ [2].

Despite technological advance, only 15 % of the world dialysis population is managed by PD. Therefore, a "integrated approach" suggests starting PD in alarge percentage of patients, especially when renal transplantation is expected in the next 2 or 3 years after initiation of dialysis [3].

A very interesting point became obvious when analyzing data obtained from the Dialysis Morbidity and Mortality Study Wave 2, a national random sample of more than 4000 new dialysis patients in the USA enrolled during 1996 and 1997 and followed up until 2001. There, it was shown, that transplantation rates were significantly higher for patients reporting the greatest contribution to modality selection. These results support the association of patient autonomy with transplantation and survival, probably in favor for patients actively choosing PD as their dialysis modality [4]. Also, a small Japanese single center study in 42 patients analyzed the effect of dialysis modality on rate of kidney transplantation from living donors and transplant outcome. There were no differences between the two modalities prior to transplantation in the graft survival rate, incidence of acute rejection, and complications before and after transplantation.However, The transfer rate from PD to transplantation was significantly ($p = 0.0036$) higher (4.7%) than that of HD (1.9%). Probably reflecting better cooperation between with the patients, their family and the provision of relevant information by nephrologists during PD [5].

2. Mortality on PD and HD

Although in 2005 the European Best Practice Guidelines for Peritoneal Dialysis conclude, on the basis of the available data, that peritoneal dialysis is a good treatment prior to renal transplantation there are contradictory survival rates reported in the literature for patients either on HD or on PD[6].

In 1995, data from the US Renal Data Systems from more than 170,000 patients showed, thatprevalent patients treated with PD had a 19% higher adjusted mortality risk ($p< 0.001$) than those treated with HD [7].

In a comparable analysis obtained from the Canadian Organ Replacement Register, using data from 11,970 ESRD patientswho initiated treatment between 1990 and 1994 and were followed-up for a maximum of 5 years was themortality rate ratio for CAPD/CCPD relative to hemodialysis, as estimated by Poisson regression, was 0.73. There, the increased mortality on hemodialysis compared with CAPD/CCPD was concentrated in the first 2 years of follow-up and was detectable in all subgroups defined by age and diabetes status [8].

In contrast, a study comparing two year mortality rates of patients on the waiting list for renal transplantation to a historical prospective cohort of more than 12000 PD and HD patients disclosed, that especially for patients with a body mass index (BMI) of>= 26 mortality was increased with PD as dialysis modality [9].

Nevertheless, in a cohort of more than 3000 non-diabetic patients starting dialysis there was no difference in survival for patients treated either with PD or HD [10].

Also, in the well-known, prospective Netherlands Cooperative Study on the Adequacy of Dialysis (NECOSAD) adjusted mortality rates between HD and PD patients were similar for the first two years. Thereafter, an increase in mortality especially in patients >= 60 years was detected [11].

Comparable results were seen in a prospective multicenter cohort study in 1041 patients (767 HD, 274 PD). There, the risk of mortality was equal in both groups for the first year with an increase in the second year. In addition, 25% of PD but only 5% of the HD patients switched their type of dialysis modality [12].

3. Renal transplantation in PD–patients – first experience

The first experience about the use of peritoneal dialysis in patients waiting for renal transplantation were published in some very early reports describing the feasibility of PD for patients awaiting renal transplantation[13-15]. Also in a small series of 15 patients the experience with renal transplantation in PD-patients was reported. Despite the fact, that some of the PD patients had peritonitis at the time of transplantation, no differences in graft survival were shown [16].

Similar results were published in an early study with a group of 44 patients, showing comparable results for patients with PD compared to HD patients[17].

Also, a small study in 9 PD patients reported significantly greater and longer wound drainage in PD patients. However, the incidence of acute rejection episodes, delayed graft function, graft arterial thrombosis and graft function recovery was not different [18].

4. PD versus HD and survival after renal transplantation

In a retrospective analysis of 61 PD and 159 HD patients there were no differences in survival of patients or grafts between the two treatment groups. One year after transplantation the percentages of survivors who had received continuous ambulatory peritoneal dialysis and hemodialysis were 88% and 91% respectively, and overall graft survival was 66% and 72%, respectively [19]. Similar results were reported from 42 PD patients, either treated with CAPD for more than 26 weeks or less than 26 weeks in comparison with 55 HD patients, irrespectively if treated with azathioprine + prednisolone or cyclosporine + prednisolone [20]. A retrospective analysis of 389 patients transplanted between Juli,1974, and July 1985, also evaluated the effect of dialysis modality on transplantation and mortality rates. By correcting for the influence of different variables and using time-dependent treatment co-variables, the bias adjusted estimates of the relative risk of death did not differ significantly from one another [21]. A cohort analysis of 500 first renal transplant recipients (241 on CAPD, 259 on HD) showed identical graft and patient survival after five years. However in 37 PD patients post-transplant peritoneal dialysis was necessary, while 10 patients developed peritonitis [22].

In 54 patients with renal transplantation after PD compared to 48 patients after HD with an immunosuppressive regimen consisting of prednisolone, azathioprine and cyclosporine there no significant difference in patient mortality and survival or graft survival between the groups. The incidences of infections were also similar in the two groups [23].

5. PD and complications after renal transplantation

There is some concern with respect for the risk of infections, especially peritonitis caused by the peritoneal catheter in PD patients. In a retrospective single center analysis the experience with 18 renal transplantations in 16 PD patients was reported. In two cases cultures of the peritoneal catheter removed a few days after successful transplantation were positive. Nevertheless, with adequate antibiotic treatment none of the patients ever developed clinical peritonitis [24].

A cohort analysis of 500 first renal transplant recipients (241 on CAPD, 259 on HD) showed identical graft and patient survival after five years. However, 10 PD patients developed peritonitis [21]. Also, in a series of 100 patients undergoing simultaneous pancreas-kidney (SPK) transplantation (25 PD patients, 75 HD patients) frequency of abdominal infections, one year pancreas-graft survival rates, acute rejection episodes, kidney graft survival rates, or length of hospital stay did not differ between the two groups[25].

The question of peritonitis in peritoneal dialysis patients after renal transplantation was also addressed by a retrospective, single center study of 232 PD patients. In total, 30 peritonitis episodes with predominantly Staphylococcus aureus (10/30) or gram-negative bacteria (12/30) were observed. Risk factors associated with post-transplant peritonitis were the total number of peritonitis episodes, previous peritonitis with S. aureus bacteria, male sex, technical surgical problems at the time of transplantation, more than two rejection episodes, permanent graft non-function, and urinary leakage [26].

Comparable results are reported in a two-center study on post-transplant PD-related complications in 137 PD patients. There, only in a minority of the patients (n=19) PD-catheters were removed on the time of transplantation. In the remaining 118 patients the peritonitis rate was 7% [27].

In the European Best Practice Guidelines for Peritoneal Dialysis it is recommended to remove the catheter early after transplantation, nevertheless the catheter could be left in situ for 3–4 months despite a functioning graft. The guidelines also state, that peritonitis and exit site infections in transplanted patients should be treated using the ISPD guidelines 6.

In the last years the problem of post-transplant diabetes mellitus (PTDM) has gained more attention. A single center study reports on the occurrence of PTDM in 72 renal transplant recipients. In univariate analysis, the factors associated with the elevated risk of PTDM appearance were treatment by PD, older recipient age, positive family history of diabetes, hypertensive nephropathy as end-stage renal disease cause, higher body mass index at transplantation, and the graft from an older donor [28].

PD may be associated with an increased risk for graft thrombosis. At least, a single center experience revealed that in 915 consecutive renal transplantations CAPD was associated with a growing frequency of renal allograft thrombosis (7.3% vs. 3.6 %, $p<0.02$). No differences in transplant characteristics, including hemodynamics, hematological parameters, immunosuppressive therapy, graft anatomy and preservation, were observed between the cases with graft thrombosis and a matched control group of 88 patients [29].

After renal allograft failure, patients may chose PD as their primary treatment option again. For this situation, it was shown, that after a failed renal transplantation PD-patients are prone to greater risk of death compared to PD-patients never transplanted. In addition, time to first peritonitis, subsequent episodes of peritonitis, catheter change, or transfer to hemodialysis occurred at a much faster rate in patients with a failed transplant [30].

For patients returning to PD after graft failure, there may be a survival advantage in maintaining them on long-term immunosuppressive therapy. At least, a decision analytic model comparing the use of immunosuppression after transplant failure and return to peritoneal dialysis with immunosuppressive withdrawal, lead the authors to conclude, that there may be a survival advantage in maintaining patients on long-term immunosuppression [31].

6. PD and the occurrence of delayed graft function after renal transplantation

It is well known, that delayed graft function (DGF) and acute renal failure (ARF) after renal transplantation negatively influence short- and long-term graft outcome, therefore it is of interest to know if peritoneal dialysis affects occurrence or severity of DGF after renal transplantation.

A study in 250 patients (70 PD, 180 HD) evaluated the influence of dialysis modality on transplant outcomes. Among HD patients, 16% displayed DGF, versus 12% of PD patients. Multivariate analysis showed that factors affecting DGF were mode of dialysis, serum concentrations of parathyroid hormone and C-Reactive-Protein, and hemoglobin levels. Also after 3 and 5 years follow-up, PD patients showed fewer graft failures than HD patients (14% vs. 20%; and 17% vs. 28%[32].

In an analysis of 92 PD patients and 587 HD patients there was higher immediate graft function, less delayed graft function and less patients with never functioning grafts in the PD group. The groups were comparable except for a higher prevalence of diabetes ($p < 0.05$) and a shorter time on dialysis ($p < 0.01$) in PD patients [33].

A retrospective study in 40 PD and 79 HD patients receiving their first renal transplant analyzed the occurrence and frequency of DGF and acute renal failure. Both, DGF and ARF were observed less in the PD group than in the HD group. In a multivariate model, the authors could show that PD as pre-transplantation modality favorably modified the relative risk of developing DGF and ARF after renal transplantation[34]. A single center analysis in more than 650 patients (92 PD, 587 HD) reports a higher rate of DGF in HD patients (39.5% vs. 22.5%) and a higher rate of never functioning grafts in HD patients compared to PD patients (14% vs. 9%). When potential risk factors for DGF were compared, no relevant differences could be found [33].

Also for PD patients on automated peritoneal dialysis (APD), a retrospective matched-pairs study with 67 APD-patients showed favorable effects for PD on initial graft function (patients with a creatinine clearance below 10 ml/min 6 days after surgery) after post-mortem renal transplantation [35].

A recent retrospective single center analysis in 38 PD and 268 HD patients describes a higher incidence of DGF and primary allograft failure for HD patients, but was no difference in acute rejection episodes, long-term survivals, or renal function [36].

A case control study the incidence of DGF, defined as necessity to perform dialysis after transplantation, was analyzed in 117 PD and HD patients with a follow-up of 6 months. When matching the patients for age, sex, HLA compatibility PD-patients developed less DGF (23.1%) than HD patients (50.4%). In addition the decline of creatinine levels after transplantation was faster in PD patients. However, PD patients developed more acute rejection episodes, than HD patients, but creatinine levels after 6 weeks and 6 months were not different between the groups [37].

Besides a bundle of published single center experiences with renal transplantation in PD patients we do have at least two registry studies reporting on the effect of pre-transplant dialysis modality on renal transplant results.

Data from the United Network of Organ Sharing on all cadaveric graft recipients who were dialysis-dependent at the time of transplantation were analyzed with respect to different outcomes in the immediate post-transplant period for HD or PD patients. In total more than 9000 patients were evaluated, showing that PD patients were on dialysis for a shorter period of time, were more likely to be white, had a better HLA match, and had a lower PRA. After adjusting for comorbidities, the odds of oliguria were 1.60 times higher in black HD patients compared with PD patients and 1.29 times higher in white HD patients. Also, the odds of requiring dialysis in the first week were 1.56 times higher in black HD patients versus PD patients and 1.40 times higher in white HD patients. The rate of acute rejection was similar during the first hospitalization. Therefore, the authors suggest that there may be an association between hemodialysis and delayed graft function assuming that differences in biocompatibility between the two modalities could potentially be responsible [38].

A large retrospective analysis compared transplantation rates in PD and HD and outcomes after transplantation in more than 22000 patients from the years 1995 to 1998 in a US cohort. PD patients were more likely to be transplanted and their death censored graft failure was higher. However, mortality and overall graft failure were not different. Interestingly, the risk for early graft failure was higher for PD patients despite DGF was less common [39].

7. Own experience with PD and renal transplantation

Because of the in part contradictory data published in the literature we analyzed our own population of renal transplant recipients with the means of a retrospective case control study. Therefore, we chose 50 consecutive peritoneal dialysis patients transplanted since 1999. For match-pair-analysis, and as control group we selected the next hemodialysis patient subsequently transplanted after each PD patient. Follow-up data were available with a maximum of ten years after transplantation.

Kruskal-Wallis Test and Chi-Square-Test were calculated, with assuming a $p<0.05$ as significant, for statistical purposes.

The PD-group consisted out of 28 male and 22 female patients with a mean age of 48.7 +/- 11.5 years (HD: 31 m, 19 w, 49,8 +/-13, p=n.s.) quite reflecting the German dialysis population. With respect to time on renal replacement therapy, cytomegalo-virus-status, HLA-mismatch, proportion of living donors, age, sex and initial immunosuppression there were no differences between the groups.

Although, during follow up more less PD-patients (n=3) than HD-patients (n=8) died, this difference did not reach statistical significance. With respect to graft failure, transplant loss (n=18) occurred significantly more in HD patients (n=13) than in PD patients (n=5). Nevertheless, mean serum-creatinine after 1, 2 and 5 years was not significant different between the groups. Also, delayed graft function was reported in only 4 PD patients compared to 10 HD patients ($p<0.05$).

To summarize, in our retrospective match-pair analysis patients on PD before renal transplantation developed less delayed graft function and had less graft loss during follow-up than patients on HD before transplantation.

8. Conclusion

Peritoneal dialysis (PD) is an established method of renal replacement therapy. PD and hemodialysis (HD) seem to be equivalent for long-term survival of the patients. Nevertheless, there is a beneficial effect of PD on patient survival after initiation of dialysis therapy. Probably, better preservation of residual renal function in PD patients compared to HD patients may be responsible for this effect.

Renal transplantation is the best treatment option for patients with endstage renal disease. The potential risk of infectious complications in PD patients after renal transplantation is attributed to the remaining PD catheter. However, this risk seems to be low and without effect on graft survival. For patients on HD a higher percentage of delayed graft function after renal transplantation is constantly reported in the literature. Nevertheless, long time patient and graft survival are not different between both treatment modalities.

Our own long-time clinical experience is congruent with the published literature and proves that peritoneal dialysis is a valuable treatment option for patients with end stage renal disease waiting for renal transplantation.

Author details

Thomas Rath* and Stephan Ziefle

*Address all correspondence to: trath@westpfalz-klinikum.de

Department of Nephrology and Transplantation Medicine, Westpfalz-Klinikum GmbH, Kaiserslautern, Germany

References

[1] Alloatti S, Manes M, Paternoster G, et al. Peritoneal dialysis compared with hemodialysis in the treatment of end-stage renal disease. J Nephrol 2000;13:331-42

[2] Sennfalt K, Magnusson M, Carlsson P. Comparison of hemodialysis and peritoneal dialysis--a cost-utility analysis. Perit Dial Int 2002;22:39-47

[3] Gradaus F, Ivens K, Peters AJ, et al. Angiographic progression of coronary artery disease in patients with end-stage renal disease. Nephrol Dial Transplant 2001;16:1198-202

[4] Stack AG, Martin DR. Association of patient autonomy with increased transplantation and survival among new dialysis patients in the United States. Am J Kidney Dis 2005;45:730-42

[5] Mitome J, Yamamoto H, Kato N, et al. [Dialysis as bridge therapy for renal transplantation: single center experience, a comparison of hemodialysis and continuous ambulatory peritoneal dialysis]. Nippon Jinzo Gakkai Shi 2005;47:813-20

[6] Dombros N, Dratwa M, Feriani M, et al. European best practice guidelines for peritoneal dialysis. 9 PD and transplantation. Nephrol Dial Transplant 2005;20 Suppl 9:ix34-ix35

[7] Bloembergen WE, Port FK, Mauger EA, Wolfe RA. A comparison of mortality between patients treated with hemodialysis and peritoneal dialysis. J Am Soc Nephrol 1995;6:177-83

[8] Fenton SS, Schaubel DE, Desmeules M, et al. Hemodialysis versus peritoneal dialysis: a comparison of adjusted mortality rates. Am J Kidney Dis 1997;30:334-42: published online , doi:S0272638697001686 [pii]

[9] Inrig JK, Sun JL, Yang Q, et al. Mortality by dialysis modality among patients who have end-stage renal disease and are awaiting renal transplantation. Clin J Am Soc Nephrol 2006;1:774-9

[10] Traynor JP, Thomson PC, Simpson K, et al. Comparison of patient survival in non-diabetic transplant-listed patients initially treated with haemodialysis or peritoneal dialysis. Nephrol Dial Transplant 2011;26:245-52: published online , doi:gfq361 [pii]; 10.1093/ndt/gfq361 [doi]

[11] Termorshuizen F, Korevaar JC, Dekker FW, et al. Hemodialysis and peritoneal dialysis: comparison of adjusted mortality rates according to the duration of dialysis: analysis of The Netherlands Cooperative Study on the Adequacy of Dialysis 2. J Am Soc Nephrol 2003;14:2851-60

[12] Jaar BG, Coresh J, Plantinga LC, et al. Comparing the risk for death with peritoneal dialysis and hemodialysis in a national cohort of patients with chronic kidney disease. Ann Intern Med 2005;143:174-83: published online , doi:143/3/174 [pii]

[13] Goldsmith Ei, Whitsell JC, Skelley K, Lubash Gd. Repeated peritoneal dialysis in preparation for renal transplantation. Surg Gynecol Obstet 1965;121:42-6

[14] Brunner FP, Scheitlin W. [Experiences with peritoneal dialysis in the preparation for kidney transplantation]. Z Gesamte Exp Med 1967;143:358-61

[15] Cohen SL, Percival A. Prolonged peritoneal dialysis in patients awaiting renal transplantation. Br Med J 1968;1:409-13

[16] Gokal R, Ramos JM, Veitch P, et al. Renal transplantation in patients on continuous ambulatory peritoneal dialysis. Proc Eur Dial Transplant Assoc 1981;18:222-7

[17] Diaz-Buxo JA, Walker PJ, Burgess WP, et al. The influence of peritoneal dialysis on the outcome of transplantation. Int J Artif Organs 1986;9:359-62

[18] Hrvacevic R, Maksic D, Aleksic S, et al. [Outcome of kidney transplantation in patients on peritoneal dialysis]. Vojnosanit Pregl 2001;58:471-4

[19] Donnelly PK, Lennard TW, Proud G, et al. Continuous ambulatory peritoneal dialysis and renal transplantation: a five year experience. Br Med J (Clin Res Ed) 1985;291:1001-4

[20] Evangelista JB, Jr., Bennett-Jones D, Cameron JS, et al. Renal transplantation in patients treated with haemodialysis and short term and long term continuous ambulatory peritoneal dialysis. Br Med J (Clin Res Ed) 1985;291:1004-7

[21] Burton PR, Walls J. Selection-adjusted comparison of life-expectancy of patients on continuous ambulatory peritoneal dialysis, haemodialysis, and renal transplantation. Lancet 1987;1:1115-9

[22] O'Donoghue D, Manos J, Pearson R, et al. Continuous ambulatory peritoneal dialysis and renal transplantation: a ten-year experience in a single center. Perit Dial Int 1992;12:242, 245-2, 249

[23] Kang Z, Fang G, Chen W. A comparative study of the outcome of renal transplantation in peritoneal dialysis and hemodialysis patients. Chin Med Sci J 1992;7:49-52

[24] Steinmuller D, Novick A, Braun W, et al. Renal transplantation of patients on chronic peritoneal dialysis. Am J Kidney Dis 1984;3:436-9

[25] Padillo-Ruiz J, Arjona-Sanchez A, Munoz-Casares C, et al. Impact of peritoneal dialysis versus hemodialysis on incidence of intra-abdominal infection after simultaneous pancreas-kidney transplant. World J Surg 2010;34:1684-8: published online , doi: 10.1007/s00268-010-0527-z [doi]

[26] Bakir N, Surachno S, Sluiter WJ, Struijk DG. Peritonitis in peritoneal dialysis patients after renal transplantation. Nephrol Dial Transplant 1998;13:3178-83

[27] Warren J, Jones E, Sener A, et al. Should peritoneal dialysis catheters be removed at the time of kidney transplantation? Can Urol Assoc J 2012;6:376-8: published online , doi:cuaj.12112 [pii];10.5489/cuaj.12112 [doi]

[28] Madziarska K, Weyde W, Krajewska M, et al. The increased risk of post-transplant diabetes mellitus in peritoneal dialysis-treated kidney allograft recipients. Nephrol Dial Transplant 2011;26:1396-401: published online , doi:gfq568 [pii];10.1093/ndt/gfq568 [doi]

[29] van der Vliet JA, Barendregt WB, Hoitsma AJ, Buskens FG. Increased incidence of renal allograft thrombosis after continuous ambulatory peritoneal dialysis. Clin Transplant 1996;10:51-4

[30] Sasal J, Naimark D, Klassen J, et al. Late renal transplant failure: an adverse prognostic factor at initiation of peritoneal dialysis. Perit Dial Int 2001;21:405-10

[31] Jassal SV, Lok CE, Walele A, Bargman JM. Continued transplant immunosuppression may prolong survival after return to peritoneal dialysis: results of a decision analysis. Am J Kidney Dis 2002;40:178-83: published online , doi:S0272-6386(02)00022-7 [pii];10.1053/ajkd.2002.33927 [doi]

[32] Sezer S, Karakan S, Ozdemir Acar FN, Haberal M. Dialysis as a bridge therapy to renal transplantation: comparison of graft outcomes according to mode of dialysis treatment. Transplant Proc 2011;43:485-7: published online , doi:S0041-1345(11)00028-5 [pii];10.1016/j.transproceed.2011.01.027 [doi]

[33] Perez FM, Rodriguez-Carmona A, Bouza P, et al. Delayed graft function after renal transplantation in patients undergoing peritoneal dialysis and hemodialysis. Adv Perit Dial 1996;12:101-4

[34] Van Biesen W, Vanholder R, Van Loo A, et al. Peritoneal dialysis favorably influences early graft function after renal transplantation compared to hemodialysis. Transplantation 2000;69:508-14

[35] Lobbedez T, Rognant N, Hurault dL, et al. Impact of automated peritoneal dialysis on initial graft function after renal transplantation. Adv Perit Dial 2005;21:90-3

[36] Freitas C, Fructuoso M, Martins LS, et al. Posttransplant outcomes of peritoneal dialysis versus hemodialysis patients. Transplant Proc 2011;43:113-6: published online , doi:S0041-1345(10)01910-X [pii];10.1016/j.transproceed.2010.12.008 [doi]

[37] Vanholder R, Heering P, Loo AV, et al. Reduced incidence of acute renal graft failure in patients treated with peritoneal dialysis compared with hemodialysis. Am J Kidney Dis 1999;33:934-40

[38] Bleyer AJ, Burkart JM, Russell GB, Adams PL. Dialysis modality and delayed graft function after cadaveric renal transplantation. J Am Soc Nephrol 1999;10:154-9

[39] Snyder JJ, Kasiske BL, Gilbertson DT, Collins AJ. A comparison of transplant outcomes in peritoneal and hemodialysis patients. Kidney Int 2002;62:1423-30

Chapter 10

Overview of Immunosuppression in Renal Transplantation

M. Ghanta, J. Dreier, R. Jacob and I. Lee

Additional information is available at the end of the chapter

http://dx.doi.org/10.5772/54865

1. Introduction

The use of potent induction agents and maintenance immunosuppression has substantially decreased the risk of acute rejection. One year graft survival is greater than 92% in deceased donor and 96% in living donor transplant recipients with current immunosuppressive strategies according to the Scientific Registry of Transplant Recipients, (SRTR, 2009).

Half life appears to be the best way to give the patient a general understanding of how long their transplant may last. The graft half life for deceased donor transplants has increased from 6.6 years in 1989 to 8.8 years by 2005. Significant progress has also been made in high risk transplants where graft half life has improved from 3 years in 1989 to 6.4 years in 2005 for expanded criteria donor recipients. For the standard low risk patient receiving a living donor kidney, current immunosuppression should guarantee a graft half life of at least 11.9 years. [1]

However, the problems of chronic rejection and chronic allograft dysfunction still remain, often leading to graft loss and shortened long-term graft survival.[2] The 5 and 10 year adjusted graft survival for deceased donor transplants were 70% and 43% respectively. The adjusted 5 year and 10 year graft survival for living donor transplant were 82% and 60% respectively. (SRTR, 2009)

Humoral rejection and sensitized patients continue to be a clinical challenge. The management and clinical impact of subclinical rejection also remains unclear. Although there are numerous clinical trials testing different immunosuppressive strategies, a lack of large prospective randomized clinical trials has decreased our ability to generate consensus on the best immunosuppressive strategies for preserving long-term allograft function. This chapter will focus on reviewing multiple aspects of immunosuppressive therapy, such as; 1) mechanism of action, 2) how therapies are being utilized in practice, 3) the advantages and/or disadvantages of different therapies and 4) major clinical trials evaluating the effectiveness of specific regimens. New emerging strategies and therapeutic agents that are being investigated will also be discussed.

2. Induction agents

The goal of induction therapy is to suppress both cellular and humoral responses to prevent episodes of acute rejection. Rabbit anti-thymocyte globulin (rATG), IL-2 receptor blockers, and Alemtuzumab (Campath), are the primary antilymphocyte antibody preparations that are currently used for induction. More than 80% of the transplant centers in the United States use induction agents immediately post transplantation.[3] The specific agent utilized is often based on multiple factors which include recipient risk for rejection, recipient race, presence of chronic infections such as Hepatitis B or C, HIV, and center preference. See Table 1. for common induction agents.

2.1. Thymoglobulin

Thymoglobulin (rATG) is the most commonly used induction agent in United States. (rATG), is an antilymphocyte polyclonal antibody that is derived by injecting rabbits with human thymocytes. rATG contains polyclonal cytotoxic antibodies mainly targeted against various epitopes on human T lymphocytes and works primarily by complement mediated depletion of T lymphocytes. However, the multiple specificities of rATG against a broad range of T-cell antigens can affect multiple pathways involved in T-cell trafficking, adhesion, activation and promotion of certain T-cell subsets that may be more favorable for transplantation such as T-regulatory cells. [4-6] Although primarily a T-cell directed agent, the development of humoral responses which are dependent on T-cell help are likely compromised by rATG as well.

2.1.1. Side effects

Secondary to potential infusion reactions and other toxicities, administration of rATG requires patient monitoring and is administered in an inpatient setting or in an established infusion center. The typical dose is 1.5mg/kg/dose and involves 3-5 doses of rATG, depending on center protocols.

The antibodies in rATG can bind to proteins on the surface of granulocytes as well as platelets and hence leucopenia and thrombocytopenia are commonly encountered after rATG administration. Cytopenias are handled either by dose reduction or holding the dose. Despite premedication, infusion reactions do occur including fevers, chills and arthralgias. Serious reactions such as anaphylaxis, acute respiratory distress syndrome (noncardiogenic pulmonary edema) occur rarely. Typically these reactions are a result of intense cytokine release from lysis of T lymphocytes. Since rATG is obtained from rabbit sera, serum sickness can occur which presents with fever, malaise, diffuse arthralgias and rash. rATG results in prolonged T cell depletion, up to 6 months post administration and recipients are at increased risk for

http://dx.doi.org/10.5772/54865

opportunistic infections and lymphoma. Patients are typically prophylaxed for cytomegalovirus infection and pneumocystis carinii infection post rATG administration.

2.2. Alemtuzumab

Alemtuzumab or Campath is a recombinant humanized monoclonal antibody directed against CD52. It binds to CD52 receptor on the surface of T and B lymphocytes leading to antibody mediated cell lysis. CD52 is present on virtually all B and T cells as well as macrophages, NK cells and some granulocytes. It was initially approved for use in B-cell lymphocytic leukemia and is now used in transplantation. Alemtuzumab induces a rapid and profound depletion of peripheral and central lymphoid cells. It is typically administered as a single 30 mg dose either subcutaneously or intravenously. Just like rATG patients receive premedication to prevent infusion reactions. When used as an induction agent it is given intraoperatively. Single dose administration makes Campath a more convenient option to administer compared to rATG which is typically administered daily for 3-5 days.

2.2.1. Side effects

Potential side effects include thrombocytopenia, vomiting, diarrhea, headache and rarely autoimmune hemolytic anemia. Infection and lymphoma risk is similar to rATG, and patients are similarly prophylaxed for potential infections.

2.3. IL-2 receptor blockers (IL-2RA)

IL-2 receptor blockers, Basiliximab (Simulect) and daclizumab (Zenapax) are humanized anti-CD25 monoclonal antibody preparations. They are targeted against the α-chain (CD25) of the IL-2 receptor. Rather than working by lymphocyte depletion, these agents block IL-2 signaling which is required for T-cell growth, differentiation and expansion. Because both agents are derived from mice and partly humanized, they cause far less infusion reactions compared to rATG. Daclizumab is currently not available for use in United States. Basiliximab is used in the U.S. and is typically administered as 20mg intravenous infusion intraoperatively with subsequent doses given on the third or fourth post operative day. Neither drug has major side effects. Risk of infection and lymphoma is far less than that of lymphocyte depleting agents.

3. Which induction agent?

According to the annual report from SRTR 2009, 83% of transplant recipients received induction agents at the time of kidney transplant. The majority of patients received a T-cell depleting agent, 58%, and 21.2% received an IL-2 receptor blocking agent.

How agents are used in practice is dependent on a number of factors which range from center specific protocols to tailored immunosuppression based on recipient factors. The risks and benefits of each agent must be assessed in every patient individually based on the individuals' immunologic risk and susceptibility to infectious complications. Induction agents clearly possess different mechanisms of action that will have different effects on modulating cellular and humoral immune responses. It may be more advantageous to use more potent induction therapies such as the lymphocyte depleting agents, in those recipients at higher risk for rejection. On the other hand, utilizing such agents may be of concern in recipients with chronic infections such as hepatitis B and/or C or HIV. [7-10]

Induction Agents	Thymoglobulin
	Basiliximab
	Daclizumab
	Alemtuzumab
	Rituximab
Maintenance Agents	Tacrolimus
	Cyclosporine
	Sirolimus
	Mycofenolate Mofetil
	Azathioprine
	Corticosteroids
	Belatacept
	Leflunomide

Table 1. Immunosuppressive agents

Lymphocyte depleting agents such as rATG and Alemtuzumab primarily differ in their ability to deplete specific types of leukocytes. rATG contains polyclonal antibodies directed at thymic antigens and is more T-cell directed, and has little direct effect on B-cell depletion. Alemtuzumab contains a specific monoclonal antibody against CD52 which is expressed by both T and B cells as well as antigen presenting cells (APCs). The effect of Alemtuzumab mechanistically is directed at disabling several arms of the immune response, such as cell mediated (T-cell responses) and humorally mediated (B-cells) responses, as well as affecting antigen presenting cells.

Existing studies however, fail to show greater efficacy of Alemtuzumab compared to rATG in clinical trials. However, case series and other small trials speak of the benefit of utilizing Alemtuzumab in refractory rejection, and in instances of mixed rejection where an agent with activity against both cell mediated and humoral responses are required. Finally, both Alemtuzumab and rATG are agents of choice in patients that are considered higher risk such as African American race, repeat renal transplant, and sensitized patients with high panel reactivity to multiple HLA antigens.

The IL-2 receptor blocker, Basiliximab (Simulect), provides an option for induction therapy in those recipients with history of chronic infections with hepatitis B and or C and HIV, as Simulect is associated with less infectious complications post-transplant compared to lymphocyte depleting agents. Less immunosuppression is also an attractive option for those patients who may not require potent induction therapy, such as recipients that are older,

http://dx.doi.org/10.5772/54865

Caucasian, and those receiving living donor kidneys. When compared to lymphocyte depleting agents, clinical trials suggest more acute rejection episodes with IL-2RA. [11]

Utilizing data from the United Network For Organ Sharing Data Registry, a recent study examining a large cohort of HIV recipients demonstrated higher risk of DGF and death censored graft loss with IL-2 receptor agents.[12] HIV patients also have higher rates of acute rejection with one recent study reporting a 31% incidence at one year.[7] Questions remain as to whether this is driven in part by choosing a less potent induction agent such as Simulect or issues with achieving therapeutic levels and/or avoiding toxic levels of maintenance drugs that interact with many anti-retroviral HIV medications. Thymoglobulin has been used in HIV recipients but can lower the CD4+ cell count dramatically, with recovery occurring as far out as two years. [13] Thymoglobulin use in HIV has also been associated with increased risk of infections requiring hospitalizations. Clearly, more studies are needed to weigh the risks and benefits of IL-2 receptor blockers on long-term graft function and post-transplant infectious complications.

4. Comparison of induction agents; clinical trials

A study by Terasaki et al analyzed the various induction immunosuppression strategies used across centers in the United States [3]. From 2003 onwards, the majority of centers were utilizing Simulect, rATG or Alemtuzumab. According to the OPTN database, recipients who received alemtuzumab had the lowest risk of graft failure, followed by rATG and basiliximab. However, the benefit of one induction agent over the other is not entirely clear because conclusions from small single center studies and retrospective studies utilizing database reviews are often mixed. In addition, studies may be difficult to evaluate secondary to different maintenance regimens that are used after induction.

Larger randomized trials and multicenter trials have been conducted and generally demonstrate that cell-depleting agents are generally more efficacious than IL2RA induction. [3] In a randomized controlled trial, rATG was superior to IL2RA in preventing acute rejection in recipients with high-immunologic risk, and with standard criteria donor kidneys. Two prospective randomized trials demonstrated rATG was superior to basiliximab in preventing biopsy proven acute rejection in standard criteria donor kidney recipients. When comparing Alemtuzumab to rATG, studies are mixed. In a separate single center randomized trial comparing alemtuzumab with rATG induction, Farney et al have shown that alemtuzumab is superior to rATG in preventing biopsy proven acute rejection.[14] However, in a larger randomized multicenter study (INTAC), Hanaway et al compared induction therapy with alemtuzumab to conventional induction (basiliximab or rATG). At one year post transplant, the incidence of biopsy proven acute rejection was lower in the alemtuzumab arm compared to basiliximab induction in low immunologic risk recipients. However in the high immunologic risk recipients, alemtuzumab was as efficacious but not superior to rATG.

5. Induction agents in sensitized patients

Rituximab (Rituxan) is used in the following clinical scenarios; 1) ABO incompatible or positive cross match transplantation, 2) treatment of antibody mediated rejection and 3) desensitization by decreasing titers of preformed alloantibodies prior to transplantation. [15-17] It is an anti-CD20 monoclonal antibody directed against the CD20 antigen present on naive B-cell lymphocytes. It creates a rapid and sustained depletion of circulating naive B cells for approximately 6 months. Because of its specific activity against B-cells, Rituxan is used to target the humoral arm of the immune response by limiting B-cell activity and antibody production. Although widely used in transplantation, the efficacy of this drug when compared with other newer agents in treating humoral responses and decreasing alloantibody production remains to be seen.

Eculizumab, is an anti C5 antibody which leads to terminal complement blockade and prevents formation of the membrane attack complex. Eculizumab protects allografts from complement mediated injury which occurs when pathogenic alloantibodies directed against donor allograft tissue activate complement. Although not widely used yet, the Mayo Clinic published an open label study demonstrating that blockade of terminal complement decreases antibody mediated rejection in sensitized patients and allows for positive crossmatch transplantation to occur. Eculizumab reduced antibody mediated rejection (AMR) to 7.7% compared to historical control groups where the incidence of AMR was 30-40% in the first few months.[18] Compared to long-standing protocols widely used for sensitized patients (e.g, plasmapharesis, IVIG and Rituximab), Eculizumab looks more promising in decreasing AMR rates.

Bortezomib, is a proteasome inhibitor that has specific activity against high affinity antibody producing plasma cells (PC), and induces apoptosis of circulating PC (a small percentage of the PC population) but in addition is able to effect PC that remain in survival niches such as the bone marrow and spleen.[19] Besides affecting the humoral arm, Bortezomib has multiple effects on immune cell function. Proteosome inhibition prevents the function of NFκB, an important transcription factor that transcribes multiple genes important for immune cell function and disrupts the regulation of cell cycle proteins, cell survival signals and expression of adhesion molecules.[20, 21] In transplantation it is used to treat refractory antibody mediated rejection as well as to reduce the burden of preformed alloantibodies to facilitate transplantation of highly sensitized individuals. Studies and case series evaluating the use of Bortezomib for desensitization and treatment of acute rejection have been mixed.[22-25] Although used by some centers, it has not been widely adopted into practice.

6. Maintenance immunosuppression

Maintenance therapy is used to prevent acute rejection and promote long term graft survival. Conventionally, combinations of 2-3 drugs with different mechanisms of action targeting various immune responses are used. Maintenance regimens vary according to the center, immunological risk of the patient, and individual susceptibility to adverse reactions. The

http://dx.doi.org/10.5772/54865

introduction of calcineurin inhibitors (CNI) together with anti-proliferative agents like mycophenolate mofetil has resulted in major improvements in acute rejection rates and short term graft survival over the last three decades in kidney transplant recipients. However, long term graft outcomes have not improved dramatically, partly because of nephrotoxicities associated with the long term use of these drugs. In the year 2009, the initial maintenance regimen for 81% of kidney transplant recipients included tacrolimus and mycophenolate mofetil, per SRTR report, 2009. At one year post transplantation, 72.1% of the kidney transplant recipients remained on tacrolimus and mycophenolate moefetil and only 5.3% were receiving cyclosporine and mycophenolate mofetil. See Table 1 for common maintenance agents.

Although the majority of US centers utilize CNI in combination with mycophenolate moefetil for maintenance, different dosing strategies for CNI, as well as new agents are being explored. A recently FDA approved medication for use in renal transplant, Belatacept, may have a promising role in widescale maintenance immunosuppression in the future. The basic pharmacology, clinical uses, major drug interactions and toxicity profiles of commonly used and new maintenance agents will be discussed in this section.

6.1. Calcineurin inhibitors

Since their introduction in the 1970s, CNI have been the fundamental agents used for maintenance immunosuppression in solid organ transplantation. They played a revolutionary role in transplantation by dramatically reducing the incidence of acute rejection episodes and prolonging allograft survival post-transplant. Cyclosporine and tacrolimus are the available CNI preparations with both having a unique role in maintenance. Currently, tacrolimus is more widely used compared to cyclosporine primarily because there is less nephrotoxicity associated with tacrolimus. Based on recent SRTR reporting, the use of cyclosporine has declined from 66.3% in 1998 to 5.7% in 2009. Notably the use of tacrolimus has increased from 25.9% to 87.8%.

6.2. Mechanism of action of CNI

The target protein of both tacrolimus and cyclosporine is CNI which is a calcium-dependent phosphatase. This enzyme is ubiquitously expressed and associates with calmodulin to form an active enzyme complex that dephosphorylates and activates the transcription factor, nuclear factor of activated T cells (NFAT), after T-cell receptor signaling. Dephosphorylated NFAT can then translocate to the nucleus and initiate transcription of several key cytokine genes (e.g., IL-2, IL-4, TNF- and IFN-γ). Blockade of calcineurin leads to decreased NFAT activity and transcription of critical cytokines affecting T cell function, activation and proliferation. Both these drugs bind to cytoplasmic proteins to mediate their action. Cyclosporin binds to cyclophilin, while tacrolimus binds to FKBP-12.

6.3. Clinical use

Recommended starting dose for tacrolimus is 0.15-0.30 mg/kg, while that of cyclosporine is 6-10 mg/kg. For both drugs, total dose is administered in two divided doses. Intravenous dosing is 1/3rd of the total oral dose, administered as a continuous 24 hour infusion. Patient variability in drug kinetics can be attributed to the heterogeneity of metabolic activity of the enzyme responsible for calcineurin metabolism; the liver enzyme, CYP3A. In general, African Americans may require higher doses of tacrolimus, whereas patients with liver disease and elderly patients may need lower doses. Because of wide patient variability in metabolism, therapeutic drug monitoring is routinely performed with these agents. Most centers check a 12 hr trough level prior to the morning dose. More sophisticated monitoring with area under the curve (AUC) measurements is available but is not routinely performed because of technical and clinical difficulties. During the first 3 months post transplant, our center aims for a 12 hr tacrolimus trough in the range of 8-12 ng/dl, followed by a level of 6-10 ng/dl for months 4 to 12. After the first year, we reduce tacrolimus dosing aiming to achieve maintenance levels of of 4-6 ng/dl. For cyclosporine, a 12 hour trough of 250-350 mg/dl are maintained for the first few months and then target levels are gradually decreased. After the first year post transplantation the usual cyclosporine trough is between 100-200mg/dl. Targeted drug ranges vary across centers and are driven by center protocols that take into account patient risk, type of induction used and the strength of other agents used for maintenance.

6.4. Metabolism of CNIs and major drug interactions

Both tacrolimus and cyclosporine are metabolized by cytochrome P450 (CYP3a) enzymes that are located in the GI tract and liver. Both drugs are excreted in bile so dosage adjustment is not needed in renal insufficiency. Many medications are metabolized by P450 system and therefore many potential and significant drug interactions with CNI can occur. Classes of drugs that induce CYP3a can reduce CNI levels, such that increased dosing may be required to reach therapeutic and adequate ranges. On the other hand, drugs that block the action of CYP3a can lead to increased levels of CNI, which can lead to acute nephrotoxicity among other side effects. Specific blood pressure medications, antibiotics, anti-fungals, anti-convulsants and HIV medications need to be reviewed for p450 interactions, and both CNI and medications need to be adjusted accordingly. Commonly used medications that affect P450, and the subsequent impact on CNI levels are shown in Table 2.

Agents that are not often considered in practice, but having an effect on CNI include, steroids which when withdrawn can lead to increases in drug levels of CNIs, and binders such as cholestyramine and sevelamer which can bind CNIs and prevent absorption leading to sub therapeutic levels. Grape fruit juice increases absorption of tacrolimus and hence it is generally recommended to avoid its use with CNIs. Several herbal medications can also alter the metabolism of these drugs.

Because of the sensitive interactions between CNI and antiretrovirals, mangagement of CNI in HIV recipients can be challenging. CNI toxicity and supra therapeutic levels of CNI are common issues in HIV recipients and most likely contributes to allograft dyfunction. Reduced dosing of Tacrolimus is required with some protease inhibitors, particularly Ritonavir, the most potent blocker of CYP3A, and is dosed once to twice a week as opposed to the normal twice a day dosing.

http://dx.doi.org/10.5772/54865

Increases CNI level by inhibition of P450	Decreases CNI level by induction of P450
* Verapamil	Rifampin
Amlodipine	Rifabutin
* Diltiazem	Barbiturates
Nicardipine	Phenytoin
* Ketoconazole	Carbamazepine
Fluconazole	
Itraconazole	
Voriconazole	
Erythromycin	
Ritonavir	

*Significant increases in CNI level

Table 2. CNI-Drug Interactions

6.5. Adverse effects and toxicities of CNI

CNIs have facilitated the success of transplantation and a greater number of patients are living with functioning transplants for longer periods of time. This has made long term CNI exposure and the associated side effects inevitable. Cyclosporine and tacrolimus possess unique side effect profiles which play an important role in agent selection for individual patients.

One of the most significant side effects of CNIs is nephrotoxicity which contributes to chronic allograft dysfunction and late allograft loss. Acute CNI toxicity is functionally mediated by vasoconstriction of the afferent arteriole leading to reduction in renal blood flow and glomerular filtration rate. Studies demonstrate that CNI increases renin production in the kidney leading to angiotensin II mediated vasoconstriction. [26] Chronic exposure can lead to prolonged vasoconstriction and acute tubular necrosis. Chronic CNI nephrotoxicity can mediate vascular injury, glomerular ischemia, tubular atrophy and chronic interstitial fibrosis. Basic studies do demonstrate that excess production of fibrosing cytokines like transforming growth factor beta (TGF-β) is in part driven by CNI direct role on renin secretion in the kidney. [27] The development of calcineurin minimization and withdrawal protocols as well as the development of new maintenance agents are an attempt to prevent/minimize CNI nephrotoxicity and its impact on long-term allograft survival.

Other adverse renal manifestations of CNIs include thrombotic microangiopathy, which presents with renal dysfunction, microangiopathic hemolytic anemia and thrombocytopenia. CNI can also cause isolated tubular toxicity which manifests in many forms of electrolyte disturbances. The most prominent and clinically significant of these are renal tubular acidosis (RTA) type 4 (typically associated with metabolic acidosis and hyperkalemia) and hypomagnesemia. Proposed mechanisms mediating this effect includes, decreased aldosterone production secondary to cyclosporine, as well as decreased transcription and expression of mineralocorticoid receptor due to prograf.

Since calcineurin is a ubiquitous enzyme, there are other non-renal toxicities associated with CNI use. Tacrolimus is associated with neurotocity, GI side effects and pancreatic islet toxicity. Neurotoxicity can be as benign as tremors, but in some cases can be quite severe and lead to seizures and altered mental status. Finally, Tacrolimus use has been associated with posterior reversible encephalopathy syndrome (PRES) which can present with various neurological manifestations.[28] Another important clinical issue is the development of new onset post-transplant diabetes, or worsening diabetes post-transplant, particularly with tacrolimus. Neuro and pancreatic toxicity of tacrolimus are clinically handled by either dose reduction or conversion to cyclosporine. Cyclosporine use however can cause gingival hyperplasia, hirsutism, hypercholesterolemia, hypertension, salt retention and an increased incidence of gout. Both CNIs have been linked to increased risk of infectious complications as well as post transplant malignancies. Differences in adverse effects among the CNIs as well as other maintenance agents are shown in Table 3.

The current challenge is to mitigate the side effects of CNIs without sacrificing overall graft outcomes. Several novel protocols are recently designed and studied to overcome CNI toxicity. We have summarized these in the section of new evolving protocols.

6.6. Mycophenolate mofetil

Mycophenolate mofetil (MMF) is a maintenance immunosuppressant used often in combination with CNIs and steroids. MMF was introduced in 1995 and has largely replaced azathioprine in transplantation, as clinical trials showed superiority of MMF when compared to azathioprine. [29] Based on a recent SRTR report in 2009, MMF was part of the initial maintenance regimen in 89.9% of kidney transplant recipients.

6.7. Mechanism of action

Mycophenolate mofetil is an inactive prodrug with mycophenolic acid (MPA) being its active component. The mofetil entity significantly increases bioavailability of MPA. There is an enteric coated form of MPA also available for use that may be better tolerated in some patients. MPA is a selective, reversible inhibitor of inosine monophosphate dehydrogenase (IMPDH) which is the rate-limiting enzyme in the denovo synthesis of purines. T- and B-lymphocytes are more dependent on this pathway than other cell types for proliferation since they do not have a salvage pathway for purine synthesis. Moreover, MPA is a more potent inhibitor of the type II isoform of IMPDH, which is predominatly expressed in activated lymphocytes.

6.8. Clinical use

MMF was initially approved for standard dose administration of 1 gram twice daily in adult kidney transplant recipients. Therapeutic drug monitoring for MMF/MPA is not performed routinely since several factors can impact the MPA AUC (detailed in the section below). Recent studies however have shown an association between MPA exposure and clinical outcomes (rejection and toxicity) and therapeutic drug monitoring (TDM) in certain circumstances may be warranted. [30] [31] The APOMYGRE study has shown decreased incidence of acute rejection with individualized MMF dosing based on drug exposure. [32]

When a serious infection develops, MMF or MPA is typically held since the drug's impact on lymphocyte proliferation is reversible and the immunosuppressive effects disappear within a few days. Intravenous formulations are available for MMF and intravenous dosing is the same as oral dosing with 1:1 conversion. Dose adjustment is not necessary in renal insufficiency. These drugs are not dialyzable. Use of MMF in pregnancy is contraindicated since it is associated with congenital malformations in the fetus especially facial abnormalities.[33] Mycophenolate should be discontinued before planned pregnancy in both male and female transplant recipients.

6.9. MMF exposure and metabolism

Mycophenolate moefetil is rapidly absorbed and hydrolysed to yield the active component MPA mainly in the liver, which is detectable in peripheral blood within 1-2 hours. MPA is then converted to 7-0-MPA glucuronide also referred to as MPAG (an inactive metabolite) by UDP-glucuronosyl transferase (UDPGT) in the liver and intestine. MPAG is excreted through the bile and urine. Both MPA and MPAG are protein bound. So factors such as low albumin concentration and high urea levels can decrease protein binding and lead to rapid clearance of the drug. MPAG accumulation in renal failure displaces MPA from protein binding and can lead to an increase in the free fraction of the drug. Once MPAG is excreted in the bile it can be converted back to MPA by bacterial glucuronidases and lead to increased levels of MPA (enterohepatic recirculation). This leads to a second peak in the drug concentration 6 to 12 hours after administration which contributes to more than 30% of the area under the curve. Cyclosporine leads to inhibition of this second peak by blocking the transporters involved in biliary excretion of MPAG. So typically patients on cyclosporine need higher doses of MMF or MPA compared to patients on tacrolimus. Antibiotic therapy is also known to have a similar impact by inhibiting bacterial proliferation in the gut and hence inhibiting enterohepatic recirculation.

There is no significant drug interaction with medications that induce or block the CYP3A pathway. When used in combination with sirolimus both agents can lead to cytopenias. Generally co administration with antacids and cholestyramine should be avoided as they interfere with absorption of MMF.

6.10. Toxicity

The main dose limiting toxicity of MMF or enteric coated MPA is related to gastrointestinal (GI) side effects. More than one third of patients develop diarrhea and in addition some patients have nonspecific GI intolerance in the form of dyspepsia, nausea and vomiting. Indeed, there is evidence demonstrating a correlation between drug exposure and GI toxicity. [31] Most of these side effects are handled with either dose reduction or splitting the dose into 3 to 4 divided doses. Although patients may tolerate enteric coated MPA better, studies curiously do not demonstrate major differences in the GI side effect profile of MMF and enteric coated MPA. [34]

Another major side effect of these preparations is bone marrow suppression mainly manifesting with leucopenia. Typically the dose of MMF is reduced based on the severity of leucopenia. There appears to be a correlation between the incidence of leucopenia and drug exposure. [31] Anemia and thrombocytopenia can occur as well.

6.11. Azathioprine

Azathioprine (Imuran) has been in use in transplantation for more than three decades. With introduction of CNIs and MMF, many centers have moved away from using azathioprine as a first line maintenance agent. SRTR reports from 2009 demonstrate that only 0.6% of the kidney transplant recipients were on Azathioprine. It is commonly used now primarily in patients who are intolerant to MMF. Usual daily dose administered is 2-3 mg/kg once daily.

6.12. Mechanism of action, metabolism and major drug interactions

Azathioprine is an antimetabolite a derivative of 6-mercaptopurine. It gets incorporated into cellular deoxyribonucleic acid (DNA). Once incorporated into DNA it interferes with transcription, purine and ribonucleic acid (RNA) synthesis which are important for T cell activation. Azathioprine is metabolized by xanthine oxidase inhibitor to 6–thiouric acid. Hence allopurinol which is a xanthine oxidase inhibitor should be used with great caution with azathioprine as it can lead to significant toxicity. Typically the dose of azathioprine is reduced when used in combination with allopurinol.

6.13. Adverse drug reactions

The single most severe toxicity of azathioprine is related to suppression of bone marrow. Patients can develop profound leucopenia and thrombocytopenia. It is recommended to monitor white count and platelet count carefully every 2 weeks at initiation. The dose of the drug will need to be decreased if leucopenia occurs and severe leucopenia might necessitate discontinuation of the drug. Cholestasis, hepatic veno occlusive disease, hepatitis and rare cases of pancreatitis have been described with azathioprine use.

6.14. Sirolimus

Sirolimus (Rapamycin) was introduced to transplantation in the late 1990s. It has antitumor, antiproliferative and immunosuppressive actions. Sirolimus plays a key role in immunosuppression especially as an alternative to CNIs to minimize long term CNI induced nephrotoxicity. SRTR database reported that the use of sirolimus as part of initial maintenance regimen peaked in 2001; however it gradually declined to only 3% of kidney transplant recipients receiving it in 2009. In the same report at 1 year post transplantation, 6.5% of recipients were receiving sirolimus. The declining use of sirolimus can be attributed to the side effects encountered with medication usage.

The unique antitumoral properties of sirolimus, however, make it an attractive option for immunosuppression in patients with post transplant malignancies. Recent study reported by Euvrard et al (Tumorapa study) has shown that sirolimus conversion has provided protection against recurrence of skin cancers in patients with squamous cell carcinomas of the skin post transplant. [35]

6.15. Mechanism of action

Similar to CNIs sirolimus binds to cytoplasmic protein FKBP-12 to mediate its action. The sirolimus/FKBP-12 complex then inhibits mTOR (mammalian target of rapamune). This enzyme is a kinase that plays a key role in cell cycle progression (G1-S transition). Blocking mTOR has a profound effect on inhibiting T-cell proliferation and expansion. mTOR is expressed ubiquitously so the antiproliferative effects of sirolimus is not limited to lymphocytes and attributes to several adverse effects of the drug which are detailed below.

The anti-tumor effect of sirolimus is mediated by inhibiting the PI3K-AKT pathway which plays a critical role in cell proliferation, survival, migration and angiogenesis. [36] In addition it inhibits growth of endothelial cells and tumor angiogenesis by interfering with synthesis of vascular endothelial growth factor.

6.16. Clinical use

Sirolimus has a long half life of 60 to 70 hours so consideration is needed when initiating the drug or making dose adjustments. Usually patients receive a loading dose of 3-15mg followed by once daily dosing of 1-5mg per day. The loading and maintenance dose are generally determined by patient weight and immunologic risk. The dose is then adjusted based on drug levels. Therapeutic drug monitoring is routinely used with sirolimus. It is recommended to check 24 hour trough levels several days after initiation or dosage adjustment of sirolimus since it takes longer to achieve a steady state.

The drug is available as oral tablet at 0.5mg, 1mg and 2mgs dose. In addition there is also liquid formulation with strength of 1mg/ml. It is metabolized by CYP3A and hence dose needs to be adjusted in liver disease, but not in renal impairment.

6.17. Metabolism and drug interactions

As both sirolimus and CNIs are metabolized by CYP3A enzyme pathway, concomitant use of both agents can increase exposure to sirolimus 2 to 3 fold. It is generally recommended that sirolimus be administered a few hours after CNI dosing. Similar to CNIs, it interacts with drugs that induce and block the CYP3A pathway. Sirolimus is not renally excreted so dose adjustment is not needed in renal failure. However dose adjustment is recommended in patients with hepatic dysfunction.

6.18. Adverse reactions

Sirolimus is considered to be less nephrotoxic than CNIs, however there are some unique renal side effects related to its use. Sirolimus potentiates CNI nephrotoxicity and can be tubulotoxic leading to hypomagnesemia and hypokalemia. De novo development of proteinuria, or exaggeration of preexisting proteinura is seen with conversion to sirolimus.[37] Use of sirolimus is in fact contraindicated if patient has 24 hour urine protein exceeding 1 gram/day. Sirolimus has been reported to have a direct toxic effect on podocytes. [38] [39] Sirolimus associated cast nephropathy has been reported as well. [40] Thrombotic microangiopathy has also been observed with sirolimus use, likely mediated by its inhibition of VEGF pathway. [41] The discontinuation rate of Sirolimus was as high as 30% in clinical studies due to adverse reactions. [42-44]

Use of sirolimus is not recommended immediately after transplant surgery as sirolimus impairs wound healing (by inhibiting fibroblast proliferation). Sirolimus can increase the risk of lymphocele formation and is also associated with prolonged recovery from delayed graft function. [45]. Due to its effects on tissue repair, sirolimus is generally stopped few weeks prior to any anticipated elective surgery. Metabolic side effects of sirolimus include hyperlipidemia and hyperglycemia. Sirolimus use is also associated with non-infectious atypical pneumonitis. Bactrim is typically prescribed for one year as there are studies observing fatal pneumocystis pneumonia with sirolimus use. Sirolimus also suppresses bone marrow leading to cytopenias. Cell counts should be closely monitored especially when used in combination with MMF. Patients also can develop oral ulcers with this agent.

Adverse Effects	Tac	CsA	mTORi	MMF	Steroids
Nephrotoxicity	↑	↑			
Proteinuria			↑↑		
Hypertension		↑↑			↑↑
Hyperlipidemia		↑	↑↑		↑
New Onset Diabetes	↑↑	↑	↑		↑
Delayed Wound Healing			↑		
Osteopenia	↑	↑			↑↑
Hyperuricemia					
Anemia/Leukopenia			↑	↑	
GI side effects	↑			↑↑	

Tac, Tacrolimus; CsA, Cyclosporine; mTORi, mammalian target of rapamycin inhibitor; MMF, mycophenolate mofetil

↑: mild-moderate adverse effect on the complication

↑↑: moderate-severe adverse effect on the complication

Table 3. Adverse Effects Of Maintenance Immunosuppressive agents

http://dx.doi.org/10.5772/54865

6.19. Everolimus

There are recent studies on use of everolimus in kidney transplant recipients. [46] It is similar to sirolimus in terms of mechanism of action and side effect profile. The only major difference from sirolimus is its shorter half life.

6.20. Corticosteroids

Since the early 1960's, corticosteroids were used in kidney transplantation both as maintenance agents and to treat acute rejections. [47-49]. Corticosteroids down-regulate cytokine gene expression through interference with transcription. Since they are lipophilic they first translocate into cytoplasm and bind to receptors. The steroid –receptor complex then translocates to the nucleus to bind to glucocorticoid responsive elements on DNA to regulate transcription. By dampening cytokine production they blunt the immune response generated by T cells. Long-term steroid use is associated with several adverse effects including hypertension, new onset diabetes after transplantation, osteoporosis, fractures, hyperlipidemia, growth retardation, weight gain, avascular necrosis, cataracts, cosmetic changes, depression, and psychotic behavior. With the advent of potent maintenance and induction agents the transplant community is now moving more and more towards steroid sparing strategies.

6.21. Leflunomide

Leflunomide is used for maintenance immunousppression especially in patients with BK nephropathy. [50, 51] It has both imunosuppressive properties and antiviral activity against BK. It blocks pyramidine synthesis in lymphocytes. The common adverse effects with its use are GI toxicity and neuropathy. There are no major drug interactions with leflunomide.

7. Alternative maintenance regimens

Different immunosuppressive strategies and protocols have evolved over time to address several major concerns with maintenance regimens. Major concerns include the long term side effects of chronic steroid use, as well as long term calcineurin nephrotoxicity which contribute to decreased long-term graft survival. Protocols that have been studied and published include steroid withdrawal and avoidance, as well as studies where calcineurin use is avoided, minimized or replaced with other agents.

7.1. Steroid withdrawal/avoidance (SAW)

Steroid withdrawal typically involves discontinuing steroids several months post transplantation whereas steroid avoidance involves no corticosteroid maintenance at all and only a brief exposure to steroids in the immediate post operative period. Studies demonstrate that early steroid withdrawal is safer than late withdrawal as late withdrawal was associated with increased risk of acute rejections. [52, 53] A recent meta-analysis of 34 randomized controlled studies using SAW regimens published by Knight et al concluded that SAW is associated with increased risk of acute rejection, however this did not impact long term patient or graft survival. [54] There is a more favorable cardiovascular profile with SAW most likely secondary to decreased incidence of hypertension, new onset diabetes and dyslipidemia. As many studies have shown increased risk of acute rejections with SAW it is generally implemented with caution in high immunologic risk recipients (high PRA, repeat transplants, young African American recipients, patients with prior rejections and/or unstable graft function). With use of more potent induction regimens more US centers are currently implementing SAW in immunologically low risk recipients.

7.2. Calcineurin inhibitor avoidance/minimization/withdrawal

Several studies have looked at minimizing exposure to CNIs to over come nephrotoxicity. Complete calcineurin avoidance with de novo use of sirolimus has not been successful and was associated with higher incidence of rejections and graft loss. [43]. Due to this, more centers and studies have favored calcineurin minimization and withdrawal (at 3 to 6 months post transplant) as opposed to complete avoidance. The ELITE-symphony trial was a land mark trial comparing different regimens of calcineurin minimization and withdrawal demonstrating better allograft outcomes at three years of follow up in patients on low dose tacrolimus (in addition to steroids and MMF) than standard dose cyclosporine, reduced dose cyclosporine or low dose sirolimus as primary maintenance agent. [44] A recent meta-analysis evaluating calcineurin minimization strategies concluded that calcineurin minimization decreases rates of graft failure, incidence of delayed graft function, and new onset diabetes post transplant while avoiding an increased risk of acute rejection. [55].

8. Antirejection therapies

Rejection is a common problem with renal allografts, and can be of cellular (lymphocyte) and/ or humoral (circulating antibody) origin. It is well known that if acute rejection is left untreated, eventually graft failure ensues. Rejection can be acute or subclinical. Acute rejection is clinically evident and often presents as a decline in kidney function associated with a rise in creatinine and classic histologic changes seen on renal biopsy. On the other hand, subclinical rejection is subtle; where histologic changes of rejection may be present in grafts that otherwise appear to have stable renal function. Immunosuppressive management for subclinical rejection has not been well delineated. [56-58] Finally, rejection may be mixed and have both cellular and humoral components.

Overall the incidence of acute rejection post-transplant has decreased. However, survival of allografts has not increased to the extent predicted, mostly due to the universal development of chronic allograft dysfunction and late graft loss. Chronic allo-immune injury has been recognized as a major contributor to late graft loss and can present early on in transplantation as demonstrated by several protocol biopsy studies. [59, 60] Compared to cell-mediated rejections, humoral rejection and chronic rejection can be challenging to treat. In addition, the

http://dx.doi.org/10.5772/54865

optimal treatments for humoral rejection, subclinical rejection and chronic rejection have yet to be defined by the transplant community..

8.1. Treatment of cellular rejection

Acute cellular rejection is a T-cell–mediated process, is usually easy to treat, and responds well to therapy. T-cell directed induction therapies, and calcineurin maintenance has substantially decreased the overall incidence of cell-mediated acute rejections. Low grade cellular rejection with out vascular involvement is treated with high dose, intravenous steroids. The dose and duration of treatment with corticosteroids has not been well defined by studies, and is often left to physician discretion. Thymoglobulin in combination with steroids is used to treat severe and high grade acute cellular rejections with a vascular component. Although Thymoglobulin is most widely used for high grade cellular rejections, there are small case series and small studies that favor the use of alemtuzumab for treatment of cellular rejections. [61]

8.2. Treatment of humoral rejection

Humoral rejection mediated by alloreactive B-cells, alloantibodies and complement are more challenging to treat. Humoral rejection is often refractory to treatment and continues to be a significant problem in transplantation due to difficulties in establishing a consensus for safe optimal treatments directed against allosensitization and alloantibody production. Humoral responses also greatly contribute to late acute graft losses and the development of chronic rejection. [62] Humoral rejection has been linked to the presence of donor specific antibody and activation of complement resulting in C4d deposits in renal tissue. Therapeutic strategies have been aimed both at removing alloantibodies as well as decreasing alloantibody production by impairing and/or depleting B-cells. [63, 64]

The best known treatment algorithms to treat antibody mediated rejection include combinations of plasma exchange to remove donor-specific antibody, and/or intravenous immunoglobulins and the anti-CD20 monoclonal antibody (rituximab) to suppress donor-specific antibody production. [65, 66] There are no randomized controlled trials powered to show efficacy or safety of potential different combinations of these different therapeutic strategies. Some side effects of plasmapheresis include hypotension, citrate induced hypocalcemia, complications with access placement, and infections due to removal of immunoglobulins. Adverse reactions of IVIG include anaphylactoid reactions, fevers, chills, flushing, myalgias, malaise, headache, nausea, vomiting, dilutional hyponatremia, pseudohyponatremia, hemolysis and neutropenia. See previous section on Rituximab for side effects.

Bortezomib continues to be a promising agent for acute humoral rejection because of its ability to target multiple pathways involved in B-cell activation and antibody production and its direct activity against CD138+ long lived plasma cells that exist in survival niches such as the bone marrow and spleen. [67] These cells, primarily responsible for producing high affinity alloantibody, are not targeted by Rituximab, the current mainstay treatment for humoral rejection. [68, 69] Initial reports on Bortezomib were in patients with AMR that were refractory to traditional anti-humoral therapies, but recent reports show that Bortezomib can be used as primary therapy for AMR. [70] In terms of its ability to decrease the levels of donor specific antibodies in sensitized patients and patients with AMR, studies have provided mixed results. [71, 72] Part of this may be secondary to differing conditioning regimens that accompany the use of Bortezomib. Another important finding reported by two studies is the differential responses of early versus late AMR after treatment with Bortezomib, with early AMR responding much better than late. [25]

8.3. Treatment of mixed rejection

Rejection may be mixed and have both cellular and humoral components. To date, there are no randomized control studies evaluating different therapies for the treatment of mixed rejection. Case series and small studies suggest that choosing a biologic agent that has activity against both T-cell and B-cell activity would be more favorable. Agents that have broad based activity such as Campath or Bortezomib may be better choices, than T-cell directed agents such as rATG. Plasmapharesis and IVIG may also be added therapies, especially if there is the presence of circulating donor specific antibody. Unfortunately, trials evaluating different combinations of these therapies or head to head comparison of these biologic agents do not exist.

9. Novel immunosuppressive agents

Given substantially decreased rates of acute rejection secondary to potent induction agents and CNI based maintenance regimens, the focus has shifted away from acute rejection to preserving grafts for the long-term. However, many studies are still focused on short term outcomes and there are very few studies looking at which drugs or combinations thereof offer better long term graft function.

Long term graft preservation may be particularly challenging given the nephrotoxic effects of CNIs on allografts. To address this issue, a number of novel agents are undergoing trials currently as a replacement to CNIs. [73] Several biologic agents and fusion proteins have emerged and unfortunately many of these agents have been discarded after preliminary trials due to their toxicity. In addition there are several trials focusing on tolerogenic protocols to avoid use of long term immunosuppression. Table 4 below summarizes the new agents that are currently undergoing clinical trials. Belatacept discussed below, is a newer biologic agent that has been studied the most extensively.

9.1. Belatacept

Belatacept is a recombinant fusion protein with an extracellular domain that consists of human cytotoxic T lymphocyte antigen-4 (CTLA-4) and the Fc fragment of human IgG. The fusion protein Belatacept (CTLA-4Ig) blocks the interaction of CD80/86 present on antigen presenting cells (APC), with the CD28 receptor expressed on T cells. CD80/86 are costimulatory molecules that are necessary for providing costimulation and full activation of T-cells, a requirement for T-cell cytokine production and expansion. The most exciting feature of CTLA4Ig is its known ability to generate immune tolerance particularly in animal models of transplantation and autoimmunity. [74, 75] Whether tolerance can be generated in vivo in humans, however remains to be seen.

Agent	Mechanism of action	Clinical Indication	Studies
TOL101	Target ? T-cell receptor Non-depletional Inactivates Tcell	Induction	Phase 2
Sotrastaurin	ProteinkinaseC inhibitor Blocks T-cell activation	Maintenance	Studies halted secondary to increased rejection rates
Tofacitinib	Inhibitor of the JAKSTAT pathway. Blocks T-cell activation	Maintenance	Phase 2
ASKP1240	Humanized antibody against CD40 on antigen presenting cells	Maintenance	Phase 1

*References [77-79]

Table 4. Novel Immunosuppressive Agents

Belatacept is a relatively new agent used in human transplantation with the first report of its use in human renal transplantation in 2005. The focus of clinical investigative trials utilizing belatacept was to provide a new effective maintenance regimen that would allow for the avoidance of the renal and metabolic side effects of chronic CNI use. Studies such as the BENEFIT and BENEFIT-EXT trials demonstrate its efficacy as a maintenance agent in place of calcineurin inhibitors. [76] The three year follow up data of BENEFIT where belatacept was compared to cyclosporine concluded that patient and graft survival were comparable with better GFR in the belatacept arm. There was however increased incidence of acute rejection and early post transplant lymphoproliferative disease in the belatacept group (especially in EBV sero negative patients). For this reason, belatacept use is approved only for patients who are EBV seropositive. The cost and long term need for intravenous administration of the drug appear to be major obstacles for wide spread use of belatacept. Nevertheless, it still provides a valuable alternative to long term CNI use.

10. Conclusion

Establishing optimal immunosuppressive regimens involves maintaining a delicate balance between over-immunosuppression which increases infection risk and under-immunosuppression which increases risk of allograft rejection. Use of potent induction agents and maintenance therapies that include CNI has led to dramatic decrease in the incidence of acute rejection episodes in the immediate post transplantation period. However, late allograft loss and long-term graft survival are problems that persist despite better immunosuppression. Chronic CNI toxicity, humoral rejection and the development of chronic alloreactivity to donor allograft tissue are major contributing factors to late graft loss.

One challenge with current maintenance regimens is the toxicity related to long term CNI use. Steroid avoidance/withdrawal protocols continue to be evaluated and are being implemented successfully at some centers. Rapamune has been studied in several trials as a CNI sparing agent, but has not gained wide acceptance due to its side effect profile. The predominant trend in recent clinical trials is to find a long term alternative agent to replace CNI. Belatacept was recently approved by the FDA for use as maintenance agent and appears to be a promising alternative to long term CNI use. However, the majority of centers lack experience with belatacept and long term outcome data is lacking.

Other challenges include the rising percentage of sensitized patients on the transplant wait list. Strategies to offer transplantation to these highly sensitized recipients include transplantation against a positive cross match donor, paired kidney exchange and aggressive desensitization to lower alloantibody titers. Immunosuppressive protocols aimed at successfully transplanting sensitized recipients continue to be investigated as these patients present a special immunologic challenge. Sensitized patients are at increased risk of developing antibody mediated rejection and earlier graft loss post-transplant. Several new agents like bortezomib and eculizumab are currently being tested in these patients.

Finally, the optimal immunosuppressive strategy would ideally be one which promotes the development of tolerance to alloantigens such that immunosuppression can be withdrawn successfully. The development of tolerance is certainly possible as the literature supports incidental cases of operational tolerance, where recipients are on minimal or no immunosuppression without evidence of allograft rejection. Currently, the majority of patients will require life long immunosuppressive therapy. Basic mechanisms promoting tolerance are being investigated with the hope that new medications or tolerogenic protocols may be implemented in the near future.

Author details

M. Ghanta, J. Dreier, R. Jacob and I. Lee*

*Address all correspondence to: iris.lee@tuhs.temple.edu

Section of Nephrology, Temple University School of Medicine, Philadelphia, PA, USA

References

[1] Lamb, K. E, & Lodhi, S. Meier-Kriesche HU: Long-term renal allograft survival in the United States: a critical reappraisal. Am J Transplant, , 11, 450-462.

[2] Einecke, G, Sis, B, Reeve, J, Mengel, M, Campbell, P. M, Hidalgo, L. G, & Kaplan, B. Halloran PF: Antibody-mediated microcirculation injury is the major cause of late kidney transplant failure. Am J Transplant (2009).

[3] Cai, J. Terasaki PI: Induction immunosuppression improves long-term graft and patient outcome in organ transplantation: an analysis of United Network for Organ Sharing registry data. Transplantation, , 90, 1511-1515.

[4] Beiras-fernandez, A, & Thein, E. Hammer C: Induction of immunosuppression with polyclonal antithymocyte globulins: an overview. Exp Clin Transplant (2003).

[5] Zand, M. S, Vo, T, Huggins, J, Felgar, R, Liesveld, J, Pellegrin, T, Bozorgzadeh, A, & Sanz, I. Briggs BJ: Polyclonal rabbit antithymocyte globulin triggers B-cell and plasma cell apoptosis by multiple pathways. Transplantation (2005).

[6] Lopez, M, Clarkson, M. R, Albin, M, Sayegh, M. H, & Najafian, N. A novel mechanism of action for anti-thymocyte globulin: induction of CD4+CD25+Foxp3+ regulatory T cells. J Am Soc Nephrol (2006).

[7] Stock, P. G, Barin, B, Murphy, B, Hanto, D, Diego, J. M, Light, J, Davis, C, Blumberg, E, Simon, D, Subramanian, A, et al. Outcomes of kidney transplantation in HIV-infected recipients. N Engl J Med, (2004). , 363, 2004-2014.

[8] Trullas, J. C, Cofan, F, Tuset, M, Ricart, M. J, Brunet, M, Cervera, C, Manzardo, C, Lopez-dieguez, M, Oppenheimer, F, Moreno, A, et al. Renal transplantation in HIV-infected patients: (2010). update. Kidney Int, , 79, 825-842.

[9] Kamar, N, Borde, J. S, Sandres-saune, K, Suc, B, Barange, K, Cointault, O, Lavayssiere, L, Durand, D, & Izopet, J. Rostaing L: Induction therapy with either anti-CD25 monoclonal antibodies or rabbit antithymocyte globulins in liver transplantation for hepatitis C. Clin Transplant (2005).

[10] Roth, D, Gaynor, J. J, Reddy, K. R, Ciancio, G, Sageshima, J, Kupin, W, Guerra, G, Chen, L, & Burke, G. W. rd: Effect of kidney transplantation on outcomes among patients with hepatitis C. J Am Soc Nephrol, , 22, 1152-1160.

[11] Noel, C, Abramowicz, D, Durand, D, Mourad, G, Lang, P, Kessler, M, Charpentier, B, Touchard, G, Berthoux, F, Merville, P, et al. Daclizumab versus antithymocyte globulin in high-immunological-risk renal transplant recipients. J Am Soc Nephrol (2009).

[12] Locke, J. E, Montgomery, R. A, Warren, D. S, & Subramanian, A. Segev DL: Renal transplant in HIV-positive patients: long-term outcomes and risk factors for graft loss. Arch Surg (2009).

[13] Carter, J. T, Melcher, M. L, Carlson, L. L, & Roland, M. E. Stock PG: Thymoglobulin-associated Cd4+ T-cell depletion and infection risk in HIV-infected renal transplant recipients. Am J Transplant (2006).

[14] (Hanaway MJ, Woodle ES, Mulgaonkar S, Peddi VR, Kaufman DB, First MR, Croy R, Holman J: Alemtuzumab induction in renal transplantation. N Engl J Med, 364:1909-1919). 364, 1909-1919.

[15] Vo, A. A, Lukovsky, M, Toyoda, M, Wang, J, Reinsmoen, N. L, Lai, C. H, Peng, A, & Villicana, R. Jordan SC: Rituximab and intravenous immune globulin for desensitization during renal transplantation. N Engl J Med (2008).

[16] Takagi, T, Ishida, H, Shirakawa, H, & Shimizu, T. Tanabe K: Evaluation of low-dose rituximab induction therapy in living related kidney transplantation. Transplantation, , 89, 1466-1470.

[17] Clatworthy, M. R, Watson, C. J, Plotnek, G, Bardsley, V, Chaudhry, A. N, & Bradley, J. A. Smith KG: B-cell-depleting induction therapy and acute cellular rejection. N Engl J Med (2009).

[18] (Stegall MD, Diwan T, Raghavaiah S, Cornell LD, Burns J, Dean PG, Cosio FG, Gandhi MJ, Kremers W, Gloor JM: Terminal complement inhibition decreases antibody-mediated rejection in sensitized renal transplant recipients. Am J Transplant, 11:2405-2413). 11, 2405-2413.

[19] Perry, D. K, Burns, J. M, Pollinger, H. S, Amiot, B. P, Gloor, J. M, & Gores, G. J. Stegall MD: Proteasome inhibition causes apoptosis of normal human plasma cells preventing alloantibody production. Am J Transplant (2009).

[20] Wu J: On the role of proteasomes in cell biology and proteasome inhibition as a novel frontier in the development of immunosuppressants. (2002). *Am J Transplant.*

[21] Wang, X, Luo, H, Chen, H, & Duguid, W. Wu J: Role of proteasomes in T cell activation and proliferation. J Immunol (1998).

[22] Everly, M. J, Everly, J. J, Susskind, B, Brailey, P, Arend, L. J, Alloway, R. R, Roy-chaudhury, P, Govil, A, Mogilishetty, G, Rike, A. H, et al. Bortezomib provides effective therapy for antibody- and cell-mediated acute rejection. Transplantation (2008).

[23] Idica, A, Kaneku, H, Everly, M. J, Trivedi, H. L, Feroz, A, Vanikar, A. V, Shankar, V, Trivedi, V. B, Modi, P. R, Khemchandani, S. I, et al. Elimination of post-transplant donor-specific HLA antibodies with bortezomib. Clin Transpl (2008). , 2008, 229-239.

[24] Lee, I, Constantinescu, S, Gillespie, A, Swami, A, Birkenbach, M, Leech, S, Silva, P, Karachristos, A, & Daller, J. A. Sifontis NM: Bortezomib as therapy for mixed humoral and cellular rejection: should it be first line? Clin Transpl (2009). , 2009, 425-429.

[25] Lee, I, Constantinescu, S, Gillespie, A, Rao, S, Silva, P, Birkenbach, M, Leech, S, Karachristos, A, & Daller, J. A. Sifontis NM: Targeting alloantibody production with bortezomib: does it make more sense? Clin Transpl:, 397-403.

[26] Madsen, K, Friis, U. G, Gooch, J. L, Hansen, P. B, Holmgaard, L, & Skott, O. Jensen BL: Inhibition of calcineurin phosphatase promotes exocytosis of renin from juxtaglomerular cells. Kidney Int, , 77, 110-117.

[27] Khanna, A. K, Cairns, V. R, & Becker, C. G. Hosenpud JD: Transforming growth factor (TGF)-beta mimics and anti-TGF-beta antibody abrogates the in vivo effects of cyclosporine: demonstration of a direct role of TGF-beta in immunosuppression and nephrotoxicity of cyclosporine. Transplantation (1999).

[28] Wu, Q, Marescaux, C, Wolff, V, Jeung, M. Y, Kessler, R, & Lauer, V. Chen Y: Tacrolimus-associated posterior reversible encephalopathy syndrome after solid organ transplantation. Eur Neurol, , 64, 169-177.

[29] Meier-kriesche, H. U, Steffen, B. J, Hochberg, A. M, Gordon, R. D, Liebman, M. N, & Morris, J. A. Kaplan B: Mycophenolate mofetil versus azathioprine therapy is associated with a significant protection against long-term renal allograft function deterioration. Transplantation (2003).

[30] Hale, M. D, Nicholls, A. J, Bullingham, R. E, Hene, R, Hoitsma, A, Squifflet, J. P, Weimar, W, & Vanrenterghem, Y. Van de Woude FJ, Verpooten GA: The pharmacokinetic-pharmacodynamic relationship for mycophenolate mofetil in renal transplantation. Clin Pharmacol Ther (1998).

[31] Van Gelder, T, Hilbrands, L. B, Vanrenterghem, Y, Weimar, W, De Fijter, J. W, Squifflet, J. P, Hene, R. J, Verpooten, G. A, Navarro, M. T, Hale, M. D, & Nicholls, A. J. A randomized double-blind, multicenter plasma concentration controlled study of the safety and efficacy of oral mycophenolate mofetil for the prevention of acute rejection after kidney transplantation. Transplantation (1999).

[32] Le Meur YBuchler M, Thierry A, Caillard S, Villemain F, Lavaud S, Etienne I, Westeel PF, Hurault de Ligny B, Rostaing L, et al: Individualized mycophenolate mofetil dosing based on drug exposure significantly improves patient outcomes after renal transplantation. Am J Transplant (2007).

[33] Coscia, L. A, Constantinescu, S, Moritz, M. J, Frank, A. M, Ramirez, C. B, Maley, W. R, Doria, C, & Mcgrory, C. H. Armenti VT: Report from the National Transplantation Pregnancy Registry (NTPR): outcomes of pregnancy after transplantation. Clin Transpl:, 65-85.

[34] Cooper, M, Deering, K. L, Slakey, D. P, Harshaw, Q, Arcona, S, Mccann, E. L, & Rasetto, F. A. Florman SS: Comparing outcomes associated with dose manipulations of enteric-coated mycophenolate sodium versus mycophenolate mofetil in renal transplant recipients. Transplantation (2009).

[35] Euvrard, S, Morelon, E, Rostaing, L, Goffin, E, Brocard, A, Tromme, I, & Broeders, N. del Marmol V, Chatelet V, Dompmartin A, et al: Sirolimus and secondary skin-cancer prevention in kidney transplantation. N Engl J Med, , 367, 329-339.

[36] Dormond, O, & Madsen, J. C. Briscoe DM: The effects of mTOR-Akt interactions on anti-apoptotic signaling in vascular endothelial cells. J Biol Chem (2007).

[37] Dogan, E, & Ghanta, M. Tanriover B: Collapsing glomerulopathy in a renal transplant recipient: potential molecular mechanisms. Ann Transplant, , 16, 113-116.

[38] (Biancone L, Bussolati B, Mazzucco G, Barreca A, Gallo E, Rossetti M, Messina M, Nuschak B, Fop F, Medica D, et al: Loss of nephrin expression in glomeruli of kidney-transplanted patients under m-TOR inhibitor therapy. Am J Transplant, 10:2270-2278). 10, 2270-2278.

[39] Stallone, G, Infante, B, Pontrelli, P, Gigante, M, Montemurno, E, Loverre, A, Rossini, M, Schena, F. P, & Grandaliano, G. Gesualdo L: Sirolimus and proteinuria in renal transplant patients: evidence for a dose-dependent effect on slit diaphragm-associated proteins. Transplantation, , 91, 997-1004.

[40] Coombes, J. D, Mreich, E, & Liddle, C. Rangan GK: Rapamycin worsens renal function and intratubular cast formation in protein overload nephropathy. Kidney Int (2005).

[41] Reynolds, J. C, Agodoa, L. Y, & Yuan, C. M. Abbott KC: Thrombotic microangiopathy after renal transplantation in the United States. Am J Kidney Dis (2003).

[42] Lebranchu, Y, Thierry, A, Toupance, O, Westeel, P. F, Etienne, I, Thervet, E, Moulin, B, & Frouget, T. Le Meur Y, Glotz D, et al: Efficacy on renal function of early conversion from cyclosporine to sirolimus 3 months after renal transplantation: concept study. Am J Transplant (2009).

[43] Glotz, D, Charpentier, B, Abramovicz, D, Lang, P, Rostaing, L, Rifle, G, Vanrenterghem, Y, Berthoux, F, Bourbigot, B, Delahousse, M, et al. Thymoglobulin induction and sirolimus versus tacrolimus in kidney transplant recipients receiving mycophenolate mofetil and steroids. Transplantation, , 89, 1511-1517.

[44] Ekberg, H, Tedesco-silva, H, Demirbas, A, Vitko, S, Nashan, B, Gurkan, A, Margreiter, R, Hugo, C, Grinyo, J. M, Frei, U, et al. Reduced exposure to calcineurin inhibitors in renal transplantation. N Engl J Med (2007).

[45] Mctaggart, R. A, Tomlanovich, S, Bostrom, A, & Roberts, J. P. Feng S: Comparison of outcomes after delayed graft function: sirolimus-based versus other calcineurin-inhibitor sparing induction immunosuppression regimens. Transplantation (2004).

[46] Mjornstedt, L, & Sorensen, S. S. von Zur Muhlen B, Jespersen B, Hansen JM, Bistrup C, Andersson H, Gustafsson B, Undset LH, Fagertun H, et al: Improved Renal Function After Early Conversion From a Calcineurin Inhibitor to Everolimus: a Randomized Trial in Kidney Transplantation. Am J Transplant.

[47] Goodwin, W. E, & Mims, M. M. Kaufman JJ: Human renal transplantation III. Technical problems encountered in six cases of kidney homotransplantation. Trans Am Assoc Genitourin Surg (1962).

[48] Starzl, T. E, & Marchioro, T. L. Waddell WR: The Reversal of Rejection in Human Renal Homografts with Subsequent Development of Homograft Tolerance. Surg Gynecol Obstet (1963).

[49] Mcgeown, M. G, Douglas, J. F, Brown, W. A, Donaldson, R. A, Kennedy, J. A, Loughridge, W. G, & Mehta, S. Hill CM: Low dose steroid from the day following renal transplantation. Proc Eur Dial Transplant Assoc (1979).

[50] Josephson, M. A, Gillen, D, Javaid, B, Kadambi, P, Meehan, S, Foster, P, Harland, R, Thistlethwaite, R. J, Garfinkel, M, Atwood, W, et al. Treatment of renal allograft polyoma BK virus infection with leflunomide. Transplantation (2006).

[51] Williams, J. W, Javaid, B, Kadambi, P. V, Gillen, D, Harland, R, Thistlewaite, J. R, Garfinkel, M, Foster, P, Atwood, W, Millis, J. M, et al. Leflunomide for polyomavirus type BK nephropathy. N Engl J Med (2005).

[52] Kasiske, B. L, Chakkera, H. A, Louis, T. A, & Ma, J. Z. A meta-analysis of immunosuppression withdrawal trials in renal transplantation. J Am Soc Nephrol (2000).

[53] Pascual, J, Quereda, C, & Zamora, J. Hernandez D: Steroid withdrawal in renal transplant patients on triple therapy with a calcineurin inhibitor and mycophenolate mofetil: a meta-analysis of randomized, controlled trials. Transplantation (2004).

[54] Knight, S. R. Morris PJ: Steroid avoidance or withdrawal in renal transplantation. Transplantation, 91:e25; author reply e, 26-27.

[55] (Sharif A, Shabir S, Chand S, Cockwell P, Ball S, Borrows R: Meta-analysis of calcineurin-inhibitor-sparing regimens in kidney transplantation. J Am Soc Nephrol, 22:2107-2118). 22, 2107-2118.

[56] Rush, D, Nickerson, P, Gough, J, Mckenna, R, Grimm, P, Cheang, M, Trpkov, K, & Solez, K. Jeffery J: Beneficial effects of treatment of early subclinical rejection: a randomized study. J Am Soc Nephrol (1998).

[57] Rush, D. N, Karpinski, M. E, Nickerson, P, Dancea, S, & Birk, P. Jeffery JR: Does subclinical rejection contribute to chronic rejection in renal transplant patients? Clin Transplant (1999).

[58] Kurtkoti, J, Sakhuja, V, Sud, K, Minz, M, Nada, R, Kohli, H. S, Gupta, K. L, & Joshi, K. Jha V: The utility of and 3-month protocol biopsies on renal allograft function: a randomized controlled study. Am J Transplant (2008). , 1.

[59] Joosten, S. A, Sijpkens, Y. W, & Van Kooten, C. Paul LC: Chronic renal allograft rejection: pathophysiologic considerations. Kidney Int (2005).

[60] Mengel, M, Chapman, J. R, Cosio, F. G, Cavaille-coll, M. W, Haller, H, Halloran, P. F, Kirk, A. D, Mihatsch, M. J, Nankivell, B. J, Racusen, L. C, et al. Protocol biopsies in renal transplantation: insights into patient management and pathogenesis. Am J Transplant (2007).

[61] Webster, A. C, Pankhurst, T, Rinaldi, F, & Chapman, J. R. Craig JC: Monoclonal and polyclonal antibody therapy for treating acute rejection in kidney transplant recipients: a systematic review of randomized trial data. Transplantation (2006).

[62] Bartel, G, Regele, H, Wahrmann, M, Huttary, N, Exner, M, & Horl, W. H. Bohmig GA: Posttransplant HLA alloreactivity in stable kidney transplant recipients-incidences and impact on long-term allograft outcomes. Am J Transplant (2008).

[63] Terasaki, P. I. Ozawa M: Predicting kidney graft failure by HLA antibodies: a prospective trial. Am J Transplant (2004).

[64] Everly, M. J, Everly, J. J, Arend, L. J, Brailey, P, Susskind, B, Govil, A, Rike, A, Roy-chaudhury, P, Mogilishetty, G, Alloway, R. R, et al. Reducing de novo donor-specific antibody levels during acute rejection diminishes renal allograft loss. Am J Transplant (2009).

[65] Lehrich, R. W, Rocha, P. N, Reinsmoen, N, Greenberg, A, Butterly, D. W, & Howell, D. N. Smith SR: Intravenous immunoglobulin and plasmapheresis in acute humoral rejection: experience in renal allograft transplantation. Hum Immunol (2005).

[66] Levine, M. H. Abt PL: Treatment options and strategies for antibody mediated rejection after renal transplantation. Semin Immunol, , 24, 136-142.

[67] Ellyard, J. I, Avery, D. T, Phan, T. G, Hare, N. J, & Hodgkin, P. D. Tangye SG: Antigen-selected, immunoglobulin-secreting cells persist in human spleen and bone marrow. Blood (2004).

[68] Ramos, E. J, Pollinger, H. S, Stegall, M. D, Gloor, J. M, & Dogan, A. Grande JP: The effect of desensitization protocols on human splenic B-cell populations in vivo. Am J Transplant (2007).

[69] Faguer, S, Kamar, N, Guilbeaud-frugier, C, Fort, M, Modesto, A, Mari, A, Ribes, D, Cointault, O, Lavayssiere, L, Guitard, J, et al. Rituximab therapy for acute humoral rejection after kidney transplantation. Transplantation (2007).

[70] Everly, M. J. A summary of bortezomib use in transplantation across 29 centers. Clin Transpl (2009). , 2009, 323-337.

[71] Trivedi, H. L, Terasaki, P. I, Feroz, A, Everly, M. J, Vanikar, A. V, Shankar, V, Trivedi, V. B, Kaneku, H, Idica, A. K, Modi, P. R, et al. Abrogation of anti-HLA antibodies via proteasome inhibition. Transplantation (2009).

[72] Sberro-soussan, R, Zuber, J, Suberbielle-boissel, C, Candon, S, Martinez, F, Snanoudj, R, Rabant, M, Pallet, N, Nochy, D, Anglicheau, D, et al. Bortezomib as the sole post-

renal transplantation desensitization agent does not decrease donor-specific anti-HLA antibodies. Am J Transplant, , 10, 681-686.

[73] Webber, A, & Hirose, R. Vincenti F: Novel strategies in immunosuppression: issues in perspective. Transplantation, , 91, 1057-1064.

[74] Martin, S. T, & Tichy, E. M. Gabardi S: Belatacept: a novel biologic for maintenance immunosuppression after renal transplantation. Pharmacotherapy, , 31, 394-407.

[75] Sayegh MH: FinallyCTLA4Ig graduates to the clinic. J Clin Invest (1999).

[76] Vincenti, F, Charpentier, B, Vanrenterghem, Y, Rostaing, L, Bresnahan, B, Darji, P, Massari, P, Mondragon-ramirez, G. A, & Agarwal, M. Di Russo G, et al: A phase III study of belatacept-based immunosuppression regimens versus cyclosporine in renal transplant recipients (BENEFIT study). Am J Transplant, , 10, 535-546.

[77] Vincenti, F. Tedesco Silva H, Busque S, O'Connell P, Friedewald J, Cibrik D, Budde K, Yoshida A, Cohney S, Weimar W, et al: Randomized Phase 2b Trial of Tofacitinib (CP-690,550) in De Novo Kidney Transplant Patients: Efficacy, Renal Function and Safety at 1 Year. Am J Transplant.

[78] Oura, T, Yamashita, K, Suzuki, T, Fukumori, D, Watanabe, M, Hirokata, G, Wakayama, K, Taniguchi, M, Shimamura, T, Miura, T, et al. Long-Term Hepatic Allograft Acceptance Based on CD40 Blockade by ASKP1240 in Nonhuman Primates. Am J Transplant, , 12, 1740-1754.

Chapter 11

Hepatitis C Infection in Kidney Transplantion

A.A. Amir, R.A. Amir and S.S. Sheikh

Additional information is available at the end of the chapter

http://dx.doi.org/10.5772/55648

1. Introduction

Hepatitis C is one of the commonest chronic viral infections world-wide and has major health-care implications. According to World Health Organization (WHO), the estimated prevalence of chronic HCV infection world-wide ranges from 0.1% to more than 12%, equating to approximately 170 million chronic carriers and incidence of 3-4 million new cases per year (Carbone et al., 2011). Chronic kidney disease (CKD) in general is present in approximately 10% of the population with many of these patients requiring renal replacement therapy in the form of dialysis and or kidney transplant. A major cause of morbidity and mortality in dialysis patients and kidney transplant recipients is liver disease secondary to hepatitis C virus (HCV) infection. The prevalence of HCV infection is high among renal transplant donors, recipients, and in end stage renal disease (ESRD) patients on dialysis. When HCV infection is present in this group of patients, it has major implications (Scott et al., 2010; Goodkin et al., 2003; Carbone et al., 2011). The major factors associated with this increased relative risk of HCV infection in dialysis patients as opposed to general population are overall exposure of blood products, age, and duration of dialysis (Periera & Levey, 1997; Finelli et al., 2005; Fissell et al., 2004). On the other hand, some recent reports indicate possible decline in prevalence of HCV infection in dialysis patients (Carbone et al., 2011; Scott et al., 2010; Finelli et al., 2005; Fissell et al., 2004; Jadoul et al., 2004; Fribrizi et al., 2002). This decline could be related to the use of erythropoiesis-stimulating agents that consequently lead to decrease in blood transfusions, and progressive enhancement of dialysis conditions to control infections. In developed countries, the prevalence of HCV infection is higher in renal transplant recipients than in dialysis patients, major contributing factors being longer survival of the former with more exposure to blood products, and most probably dialysis.

2. Natural history of HCV infection, morbidity and mortality in transplant

HCV RNA can be detected in the blood after 1-3 weeks of first exposure. In majority of the HCV acute infection cases the patients are asymptomatic, however the disease can have a fulminant course. The natural history of Hepatitis C infection is quite variable with disease spectrum varying from mild to severe hepatitis, hepatic cirrhosis, and hepatocellular carcinoma. In 60-85% of these cases, HCV RNA can be detected for 6 months or longer. 10-15% of these chronic patients progress to develop liver cirrhosis (National Institute of Health [NIH], 2002). The virus is very slow to progress with almost no signs or symptoms in the first few years or decade. The most reliable tool to examine the progression of HCV liver damage is histologic evaluation of liver biopsy. The activity of liver disease can fluctuate, however, once there is fibrosis the damage is considered to be irreversible and progressive. Poynard, in 2001, reported that the average time of HCV infection to progress to liver cirrhosis is about 30 years, ranging from 13 years (for men who drank and were infected after the age of 40 years) to 42 years (for women who did not drink and were infected before the age of 40) (Poynard et al., 2001).

HCV infection has been associated independently with increased mortality in Hemodialysis patients as shown by several studies including Dialysis Outcomes and Practice Patterns (DOPPS) conducted over three continents (Goodkin et al., 2003; Fibrizi, 2004, 2007).

Transplant recipients from HCV positive donors have a higher rate of fulminant or severe hepatitis and liver disease in general. The literature shows some controversy in results presented by various studies regarding survival. The overall survival and specifically of the allograft survival for HCV infected kidney transplant recipients are much worse than non-infected renal transplant recipients (Figures 1 & 2) (Pedroso et al., 2006). Several studies have shown that although recipients of organs from HCV infected donors have higher rates of liver disease, there is no solid evidence of decreased overall survival rate (Periera, 1991, 1995; Mendez et al., 1995). On the other hand, there are some other studies that show contrary results with recipients of organs from HCV infected donors to have significantly higher morbidity mainly due to liver disease and reduced overall survival with limited life expectancy (Pirsch et al., 1995). The presence of liver damage depending on the severity as determined by biopsy is a strong predictor of liver failure and death post-transplantation. Despite the ongoing controversy, majority of the data shows increased morbidity due to higher rate of liver disease. However, there is no consensus on lack of adverse effect on survival by initial studies that mostly represented comparatively small number of cases and short period of followup. Fabrizi and colleagues pooled these single studies in a meta-analysis and showed that anti HCV positive status is an independent and significant risk factor for death and graft failure after kidney transplantation with estimated relative risk of 1.79 and 1.56 respectively. In a recent study, Scott and colleagues also showed prevalence of HCV infection in renal transplant recipients to be 1.8% and reported the patient survival to be 77% and 90% at 5 years and 50% and 79% at 10 years for HCV antibody positive and HCV antibody negative groups. The most common causes of death in HCV positive kidney transplant recipients were cardiovascular disease, malignancy, and liver failure (Scott et al., 2010). In addition to increased mortality, Zylberberg et al found a significantly increased yearly progression rate of liver inflammation and fibrosis in HCV infected renal transplant recipients than immunocompetent group (Zylberberg et al., 2002). Alric and colleagues, on the contrary, showed the annual progression of liver fibrosis to be significantly lower in renal transplant recipients than patients with HCV and normal renal function (Alric et al., 2002). Reasons for the above mentioned difference is not clear. There is strong evidence that transplantation with kidney from HCV infected donor

http://dx.doi.org/10.5772/55648

is significantly associated with improved survival as opposed to remaining on dialysis on transplant wait list (Abbott et al., 2004; Periera et al., 1998; Knoll et al., 1997; Maluf et al., 2007). Findings suggest that detrimental effect of transplantation in association with HCV infection does not outweigh its long term benefits on survival in end stage renal disease (ESRD) patients on dialysis and therefore anti-HCV positivity should not be considered as an absolute contraindication for renal transplantation (Natov & Periera, 2012; Knoll et al, 1997).

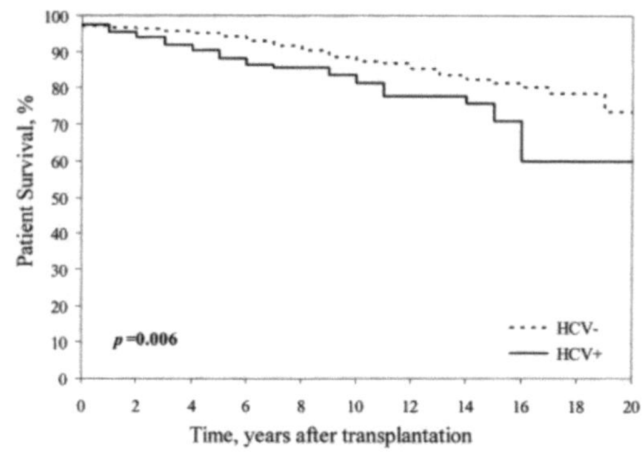

Figure 1. Kaplan-Meier estimate of the cumulative probability of patient survival. Reprinted from Transplantation Proceedings, 38, 1890-1894 (2006), Pedroso S et al., Impact of Hepatitis C Virus on Renal Transplantation: Association with Poor Survival. With permission from Elsevier through Copyright Clearance Center

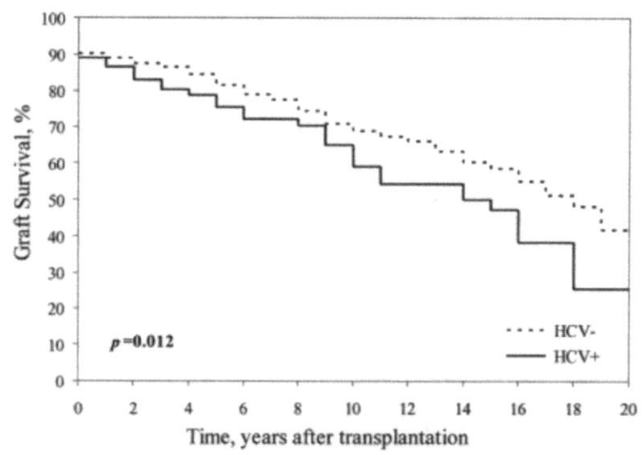

Figure 2. Kaplan-Meier estimate of the cumulative probability of graft survival.Reprinted from Transplantation Proceedings, 38, 1890-1894 (2006), Pedroso S et al., Impact of Hepatitis C Virus on Renal Transplantation: Association with Poor Survival. With permission from Elsevier through Copyright Clearance Center

The increased morbidity and mortality in HCV infection is not only related to liver disease but also extrahepatic complications (Kidney disease: improving global outcome [KDIGO], 2008). HCV infection can predispose to the development of pre and posttransplant diabetes. A 2005 meta-analysis of 2502 patients noted a fourfold increase in the development of New Onset Diabetes mellitus after Transplantation (NODAT) among HCV infected patients when compared to the non-infected group (Gursoy et al., 2000; Abbott et al., 2004). It is suggested that HCV infection might be associated with increased insulin resistance contributing to development of NODAT.

HCV has been associated with renal disease in both native and transplanted kidneys. It is in fact reported to be more associated with glomerular disease in renal transplants than native kidneys. This association is suggested to be secondary to immunosuppressive therapy leading to increased HCV RNA titres (Periera et al., 1995; Burstein & Rodby, 1993). In renal transplant recipients, HCV infection has been implicated in pathogenesis of acute glomerulopathy, de novo immune complex glomerulonephritis in allograft, and chronic allograft nephropathy (CAN) (Cosio et al., 1996; Roth et al., 1995; Ozdemir et al., 2006; Morales et al., 1997; Mahmoud et al., 2005). De novo membranoproliferative glomerulonephritis (MPGN), and de novo membranous glomerulonephritis (MGN), with or without mixed cryoglobulinemia are the most frequent glomerular patterns of injury seen in association with HCV infection in renal allografts. In 2001, one study reported the prevalence of de novo MPGN and MGN to be 45.4% and 18.2% in HCV positive transplant recipients as compared to 5.7% and 7.7% in HCV negative recipients (Cruzado et al., 2001). Subsequently, another study in 2006 reported the prevalence of de novo GN to be 34% in HCV infected recipients and only 6.6% in HCV negative recipients (Ozdemir et al., 2005). In general higher prevalence of autoimmune GN was associated with poor graft outcome, and even worse than de novo GN in HCV negative patients (Carbone et al., 2011).

Proteinuria is a common manifestation of kidney disease in HCV infected patients and renal biopsy is used to establish the diagnosis of glomerular injury, however currently it is impossible to determine HCV as the cause of glomerular damage based solely on morphologic assessment of renal biopsy. (Natov & Periera, 2012).

In 2005, Mahmoud et al reported a higher rate of CAN in HCV infected patients who did not receive interferon (IFN) therapy prior to renal transplant. Recent data also shows increased rate of graft failure due to CAN in HCV positive recipients than HCV negative (Scott et al., 2010). The Spanish Chronic Allograft Nephropathy Group analyzed 4304 renal transplant recipients with 587 of them being HCV positive over a period of 1990 to 2002. The study reported HCV infection to be associated with early proteinuria, lower renal function, de novo GN, chronic rejection, graft loss, and lower survival than HCV negative recipients (Morales et al., 2010). Another implication of HCV infection is its association with development of early graft dysfunction due to acute glomerular lesion. Examples of such lesions include acute transplant glomerulopathy, and de novo renal thrombotic microangiopathy (Cosio et al., 1996, Baid et al., 1995). Acute transplant glomerulopathy is mostly considered to be an atypical variant of acute cellular rejection and is also present more commonly in HCV positive recipients (Cosio et al., 1996a, 1996b).

3. Diagnosis

Detection of HCV infection is based primarily on the type of laboratory test used and its sensitivity and specificity. Any false positive tests will lead to unnecessary waste of precious potential organs for transplant (Natov & Periera, 2012). A large collaborative study was performed in United States that looked at the positive and negative predictive values of antibody screening tests. Eight organ procurement organizations representing different geographical regions studied 3078 cadaver organ donors. Using first generation enzyme linked immunosorbent assay ELISA1 anti-HCV test, the prevalence was found to be 5.1% (1.5-16.7%). Using the second generation ELISA2, the prevalence was 4.2%, with positive predictive value of 55% and negative predictive value of 100%. Some investigators have suggested the use of third generation ELISA3 tests to screen cadavers for HCV that because of its improved specificity showed only 3.7% prevalence. On the other hand, the prevalence of HCV RNA (ribonuclease acid) detection by Polymerase chain reaction (PCR) was only 2.4%. Although discarding all ELISA2 positive organs would eliminate transmission of HCV, there will be waste of 1.8% that will be discarded based on ELISA2 positivity while they are HCV RNA negative. However, it is currently not practical to test cadavers for HCV RNA status prior to organ procurement (Challine et al., 2004). The current practice in major centers is still to screen organ donors for antibodies against HCV. The serum aminotransferase levels are usually normal in uremic patients, and therefore are not considered reliable in determining disease activity and severity of fibrosis in this group. For clinically suspicious patients with elevated serum aminotransferase levels but negative antibody test, an HCV RNA assay with a detection limit of less than 50 IU/mL is recommended to rule out infection (Pawlotsky, 2002).

There is limited data on the impact of different HCV genotypes on survival after transplantation. Data reported by New England Organ Bank had relatively small number of patients and HCV genotype distribution to reach a conclusion (Natov et al., 1999).

Liver biopsy remains the gold standard for assessment of liver damage and fibrosis. Several scoring systems are used for assessment of hepatic fibrosis that use various criteria such as activity index and special stains for collagen deposition. Examples of these scoring systems include hepatic activity index (HAI), Knodell score and the Matavir system. Patients with HCV infection can have evidence of histologic liver disease in the absence of elevated transaminases and abnormal liver function tests. Therefore there may be merit in performing liver biopsy on all anti-HCV positive patients on transplant wait list. In patients with histologic evidence of liver disease, the decision to proceed or not with transplantation should be made with extreme caution as post-transplant immunosuppression may exacerbate liver disease (Zylerberg et al., 2002).

4. Clinical outcome with impact of HCV status before transplantation, and use of allografts from HCV positive donors

HCV has multiple distinct variants that are classified into six major types based on the viral genome sequence analysis. Each type consists of subtypes named in order of discovery such as a,b, c and so on, the subtypes may include individual isolates. Repeated infection or superinfection may occur in the same patient by the same or a different strain as HCV does not provide immunity. Thus transplant recipients that are positive for HCV RNA may have the viral genotype of the donor, same genotype as present pretransplant or both individual genotypes. The impact of superinfection is not clear, however there is some evidence that HCV infection by one or multiple strains does not impact the survival negatively, at least in the short term (Natov et al., 1999; Natov & Periera, 2012; Ali et al., 1998).

The use of renal allografts from HCV positive donors to be transplanted in HCV infected recipients may offer some advantage (Figure 3) (Abbott et al., 2003). This approach is consistent with 2008 Kidney Disease: Improving Global Outcomes (KDIGO) Guideline recommendations (KDIGO, 2008). A survey was performed in United States on 245 transplant centers with response obtained from 147 centers. The data showed that 49% of these centers use HCV seropositive donors (Batiuk et al., 2002). Patients who are HCV positive before transplant have a significantly higher risk of developing posttransplant liver disease, mainly chronic hepatitis and its sequelae. An unusual serious form of liver involvement termed fibrosing cholestatic hepatitis has been reported in such patients. it is characterized by severe cholestasis, extensive fibrosis, and rapidly progressive liver failure, and is most likely related to acute infection under maximum immunosuppression (Toth et al., 1998; Delladetsima et al., 2006). Kidney transplant in HCV positive patients is associated with a 1.8-30.3 fold increase in serum viral titer most likely due to increased viral proliferation secondary to immunosuppressive therapy. However, this increase in viral titer may not be associated with increased risk of posttransplant liver disease, neither does it have any association with transaminase pattern or histologic severity of liver injury (Natov & Periera, 2012; Periera et al., 1995; Rpth et al., 1996).

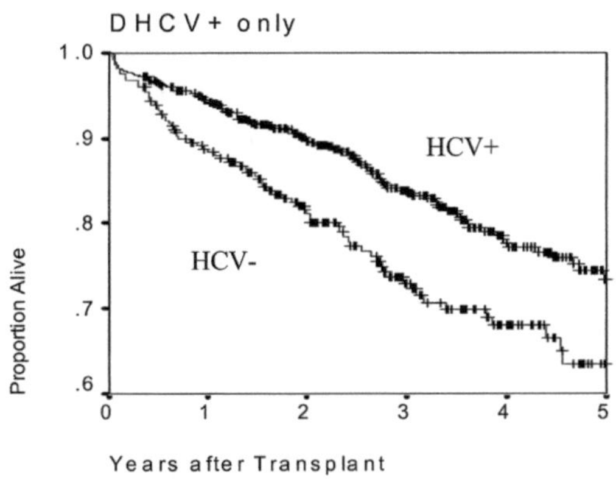

Figure 3. Kaplan-Meier plot of patient survival after renal transplantation, limited to patients who received a kidney positive for hepatitis C (DHCV+; n = 873) stratified by recipients who were HCV+ and HCV–. Reprinted from J Am Soc Nephol, 14, 2908-2918 (2003), Abbott K et al., Hepatitis C and Renal Transplantation in the Era of Modern Immunosuppression. With permission through Copyright Clearance Center

Mycophenolate mofetil and antithymocyte globulin are reported to increase HCV viremia while cyclosporine was found to have a suppressive effect on HCV replicon RNA level and HCV protein expression in cultured human hepatocytes (Figure 4) (Abbott et al., 2003; Rostaing et al., 2000; Geith, 2011; Misiani et al., 1994).

http://dx.doi.org/10.5772/55648

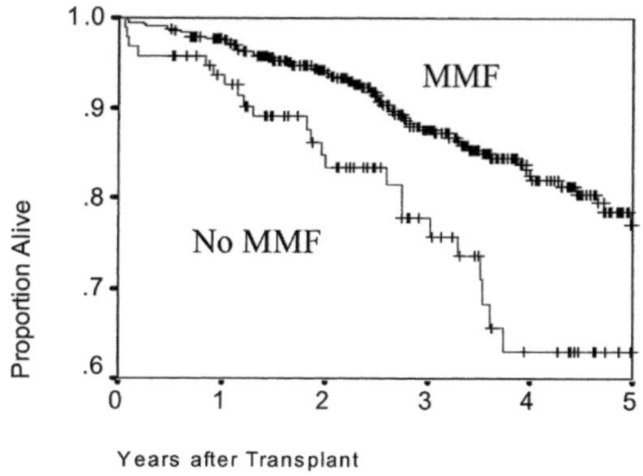

Figure 4. Kaplan-Meier plot of patient survival after renal transplantation, limited to patients who received a kidney positive for hepatitis C (DHCV+; n = 873) stratified by recipients who received mycophenolate mofetil (MMF) or those who did not (no MMF). Reprinted from J Am Soc Nephol, 14, 2908-2918 (2003), Abbott K et al., Hepatitis C and Renal Transplantation in the Era of Modern Immunosuppression. With permission through Copyright Clearance Center

Although there is solid data that shows increased risk of developing liver disease in HCV positive patients, there are conflicting reports and data regarding impact on survival. Some studies failed to show any difference in overall survival in transplant recipients that were HCV positive or negative. Other studies of pretransplant HCV positive recipients reported increased mortality rate mainly due to liver disease and sepsis with a 3.3 fold increased risk of death and 9.9 fold higher risk of mortality due to sepsis (Natov & Periera, 2012; Periera et al., 1995; Legendre et al., 1998). A 2005 meta-analysis on eight clinical trials involving a cohort of 6365 patients showed an increased relative risk of death in HCV positive patients (1.79) mainly due to liver cirrhosis and cancer. In addition the relative risk of allograft failure was 1.56 (Fabrizi et al., 2005).

Studies conducted in the 80s and 90s showed 35% of recipients who received allografts from HCV positive donors developed posttransplant liver disease, 50% became anti HCV positive after transplant, and 73% developed HCV viremia (Natov, 2002; Periera et al., 1994). The wide variation in the rate of transmission could be related to different prevalence among donors, difference in organ preservation and failure to test recipients in some centers. A large registry analysis in 2002 showed increased mortality in recipients of allografts from HCV positive donors regardless of the HCV status of the recipient (Bucci et al., 2002). Using the data from the Organ Procurement and Transplantation Network (OPTN), Maluf reported approximately 300 days shortening of wait time for HCV positive recipients receiving allografts from HCV positive donors compared with HCV negative recipients however there was significantly decreased graft and patient overall survival (Maluf et al., 2010). A larger analysis of the same data from OPTN was performed recently by Northup and colleagues in 2010 that included 19496 HCV positive recipients and 934 HCV positive donors. It showed the adjusted hazard ratio for death to be similar for HCV positive recipients of HCV positive donors and HCV positive recipients of HCV negative donors. The worst survival was seen in HCV negative recipients who received allografts from HCV positive donors (Northup et al., 2010).

In regards to superinfection, HCV genotype 1 is the most common genotype of HCV seen in Western countries and is notorious to be less responsive to antiviral therapy including Pegylated IFN and Ribavirin. Some authorities suggest that genotyping should be done routinely and genotype 1 renal allografts should not be used in recipients with other genotypes. However data is limited regarding this strategy (Carbone et al., 2011).

5. Treatment

In non-transplant setting, the combination therapy with interferon (IFN) and Ribavirin is the standard of care for treatment of initial as well as relapse of HCV infection. Clearance of Ribavirin is impaired in patients with renal dysfunction as the drug itself and its metabolites cannot be removed by Hemodialysis. Therefore, Ribavirin is not recommended in patients with creatinine clearance of less than 50mL/min. IFN therapy is however recommended in dialysis patients. The goal of pretranslant HCV treatment is to attempt to eradicate HCV before transplant subsequently leading to decrease in the risk of progression of HCV-associated liver disease, reduced risk of posttransplant renal dysfunction, and possible reduction in HCV disease progression. The optimal treatment of HCV in dialysis patients is regarded as IFN therapy but it is not known whether there is any added advantage on the use of pegylated IFN over nonpegylated standard IFN. Dialysis patients are not considered candidates of combination therapy owing to concerns regarding development of Ribavirin-induced anemia as the clearance of the drug is impaired in patients with renal dysfunction. A safer but less cost-effective approach is to use IFN therapy to treat HCV positive patients on dialysis who are potential transplant candidates. This strategy seems to have a beneficial effect on the course of liver disease posttransplant, shows higher rates of sustained biochemical and virological response, and seems to have reduced risk of HCV disease progression. At present data on relapse rate on HCV positive patients treated pretransplant is limited and controversial. 2008 KDIGO guidelines suggest HCV positive transplant candidates to be considered for IFN therapy before transplant. Ribavirin is not recommended because of its impaired clearance. Similar concerns apply to pegylated IFN because of its longer half-life and is also not recommended for pretransplant HCV therapy.

Posttransplant HCV treatment is generally not recommended. A major limitation to the use of IFN posttransplant is the potential of developing acute rejection. In addition to antiviral activity, IFN also has pleiotropic effects including antiproliferative and immunomodulatory functions. The National Institute of Health (NIH) Consensus Statement on management of HCV infection lists renal transplant as one of the contraindications to IFN therapy. Most authorities are in line with this approach because of the increased risk of acute rejection, high cost, limited efficacy, and significant side effects that are reported with IFN treatment after transplant. Treatment may be recommended in exceptional and life-threatening cases of HCV complications such as fibrosing cholestatic hepatitis, life-threatening vasculitis, recurrent and progressive HCV-associated glomerulopathy in the transplanted kidney, and advanced histologic stages of liver fibrosis.

2008 KDIGO guidelines recommend monotherapy with standard IFN only to be considered in HCV positive kidney transplant recipients (Terraut & Adey, 2007; Kim et al., 2011; Carbone et al., 2011; Natov & Periera, 2012. Data on efficacy of Ribavirin treatment alone after transplant is limited. Combination therapy is the most likely regimen to achieve a sustained virologic response (SVR), however Ribavirin dosage must be adjusted based on the renal function to minimize the complication of anemia.

Large scale, multicenter clinical trials are needed to determine the optimal treatment approach in these populations. New therapies may offer specific advantages and show decreased incidence of treatment-related side effects than the currently available drugs.

In addition SVR to antiviral therapy in patients with HCV associated renal disease has been associated with improvement in renal histology with reduced inflammation and immune deposits. Recently, five HCV positive renal transplant patients who developed type III cryoglobulinemic MPGN were successfully treated by Rituximab (anti-CD 20) chimeric monoclonal antibody (Basse et al., 2005, 2006).

Transplantation after adequate antiviral therapy followed by minimal immunosuppression can be a good option. Recently, Shah and colleagues evaluated graft function and graft as well as patient survival in retrospective analyses of 132 HCV-positive renal transplant patients who received tolerance induction protocol (TIP) with minimal immunosuppression and compared them with 79 controls transplanted using standard triple immunosuppression drugs. TIP consisted of 1 donor-specific transfusion, peripheral blood stem cell infusion, portal infusion of bone marrow, and target-specific irradiation. In the TIP group patient survival at 1, 5, and 10 years was 92.4%, 70.4%, and 63.7%, respectively, versus 75.6%, 71.7%, and 55.7% in the control group. The graft survival was 92.9%, 81.5%, and 79.1% versus 91.7%, 75.7%, and 67.7%, respectively. Rejection episodes were less frequent in the former group. Abnormal liver enzymes were seen in 22% patients in the TIP group versus 31% of the control group (Shah et al., 2011).

6. Conclusion

HCV infection is relatively common among patients with ESRD on dialysis and kidney transplant recipients. It is a major cause of morbidity and mortality among this group. When indicated, treatment with IFN and antiviral therapy should be commenced prior to kidney transplantation. The optimal treatment of transplant patients with HCV infection is not known. IFN is not recommended posttransplant because of potential risk of rejection. However there are some life threatening HCV related complications that would compel the use of IFN in a renal transplant recipient. In conclusion, Ribavirin is contraindicated in dialysis patients and alternative drugs are needed to enhance antiviral effects of IFN. For renal transplant recipients, Ribavirin can be used in combination with IFN in patients with restored renal function, however the risk of acute rejection with IFN therapy remains a serious concern. Alternative drugs are also needed with better safety and efficacy for treatment of HCV posttransplant. Despite the ongoing dilemma HCV positive renal transplant recipients have a better survival than HCV positive patients awaiting transplantation. Data shows strong evidence that use of allografts from HCV positive donors leads to reduced wait time for HCV positive recipients however there is conflicting data about graft and overall survival that needs to be further studied. In addition transplant of kidneys from HCV positive donors should be restricted to recipients with HCV viremia at the time of transplant.

Author details

A.A. Amir[1], R.A. Amir[2] and S.S. Sheikh[3]

1 Consultant Nephrologist, Dhahran Health Center, Saudi Aramco Medical Services Organization, Dhahran, Saudi Arabia

2 Dammam University, Dhahran, Saudi Arabia

3 Chief, Pathology and Laboratory Services, Dhahran Health Center, Saudi Aramco Medical Services Organization, Dhahran, Saudi Arabia

References

[1] Abbott, K, Bucci, J, Matsumoto, C, et al. Hepatitis C and renal transplantation in the era of modern immunosuppression. Journal of American Society of Nephrology, (2003). doi:ASN.0000090743.43034.72, 14, 2908-2918.

[2] Abbott, K. C, Lentine, K. L, Bucci, J. R, et al. The impact of transplantation with deceased donor hepatitis c-positive kidneys on survival in wait-listed long-term dialysis patients. Am J Transplant (2004).

[3] Abbott, K, Lentine, K, Bucci, J, et al. Impact of diabetes and hepatitis after kidney transplantation on patients who are affected by hepatitis C virus," Journal of the American Society of Nephrology, (2004). , 15(12), 3166-3174.

[4] Ali, M. K, Light, J. A, Barhyte, D. Y, et al. Donor hepatitis C virus status does not adversely affect short-term outcomes in HCV+ recipients in renal transplantation. Transplantation (1998).

[5] Alric, L. DiMartino V, Selves J, et al., "Long-term impact of renal transplantation on liver fibrosis during hepatitis C virus infection," Gastroenterology, (2002). , 123(5), 1494-1499.

[6] Baid, S, Pascual, M, Williams, W, et al. Renal thrombotic microangiopathy associated with anticardiolipin antibodies in hepatitis C virus-infected renal allograft recipients," Transplantation, (1995). , 59, 1676.

[7] Burstein, D. M, & Rodby, R. A. Membranoproliferative glomerulonephritis associated with hepatitis C virus infection. J Am Soc Nephrol (1993).

[8] Basse, G, Ribes, D, Kamar, N, Mehrenberger, M, Esposito, L, Guitard, J, Lavayssière, L, Oksman, F, Durand, D, Dur, D, & Rostaing, L. Rituximab therapy for de novo mixed cryoglobulinemia in renal transplant patients. Transplantation. (2005).

[9] Basse, G, Ribes, D, Kamar, N, Mehrenberger, M, Sallusto, F, Esposito, L, Guitard, J, Lavayssière, L, Oksman, F, Durand, D, & Rostaing, L. Rituximab therapy for mixed cryoglobulinemia in seven renal transplant patients. Transplant Proc. (2006).

[10] Batiuk, T. D, Bodziak, K. A, & Goldman, M. Infectious disease prophylaxis in renal transplant patients: a survey of US transplant centers. Clin Transplant (2002).

[11] Bucci, J, Matsumoto, C, Swanson, S, Agodoa, L, Holtzmuller, K, & Abbott, K. Donor hepatitis C seropositivity: clinical correlates and effect on early graft and patient survival in adult cadaveric kidney transplantation," Journal of the American Society of Nephrology, (2002)., 13(12), 2974-2982.

[12] Carbone, M, Cockwell, P, & Neuberger, J. Hepatitis c and kidney transplantation. *International journal of nephrology, 2011*(593291), 1-17. doi:

[13] "NIH consensus statement on management of hepatitis C: (2002). NIH Consens State Sci Statements, , 19(3), 1-46.

[14] Challine, D, Pellegrin, B, Bouvier-alias, M, et al. HIV and hepatitis C virus RNA in seronegative organ and tissue donors, Lancet (2004).

[15] Cosio, G, Sedmak, D. D, Henry, M. L, et al. The high prevalence of severe early posttransplant renal allograft pathology inhepatitis C positive recipients," Transplantation, (1996)., 62(8), 1054-1059.

[16] Cosio, F. G, Roche, Z, Agarwal, A, et al. Prevalence of hepatitis C in patients with idiopathic glomerulopathies in native and transplant kidneys. Am J Kidney Dis (1996).

[17] Cosio, F. G, Sedmak, D. D, Henry, M. L, et al. The high prevalence of severe early post-transplant renal allograft pathology in hepatitis C positive recipients. Transplantation (1996).

[18] Cruzado, J, Carrera, M, Torras, J, & Griny, J ′ o. Hepatitis C virus infection and de novo glomerular lesions in renal allografts," American Journal of Transplantation, (2001)., 1(2), 171-178.

[19] Delladetsima, I, Psichogiou, M, Sypsa, V, et al. The course of hepatitis C virus infection in pretransplantation antihepatitis C virus-negative renal transplant recipients: a retrospective follow-up study," American Journal of Kidney Diseases, (2006)., 47(2), 309-316.

[20] Fabrizi, F, Poordad, F, & Martin, P. Hepatitis C infection and the patient with end-stage renal disease," Hepatology, (2002)., 36(1), 3-10.

[21] Fabrizi, F, Martin, P, Dixit, V, Bunnapradist, S, & Dulai, G. Meta-analysis: effect of hepatitis C virus infection on mortality in dialysis," Alimentary Pharmacology and Therapeutics,(2004)., 20(11-12), 1271-1277.

[22] Fabrizi, F, Martin, P, Dixit, V, Bunnapradist, S, & Dulai, G. Hepatitis C virus antibody status and survival after renal transplantation: meta-analysis of observational studies," American Journal of Transplantation, (2005)., 5(6), 1452-1461.

[23] Fabrizi, F, Takkouche, B, Lunghi, G, Dixit, V, Messa, P, & Martin, P. The impact of hepatitis C virus infection on survival in dialysis patients: meta-analysis of observational studies," Journal of Viral Hepatitis, (2007)., 14(10), 697-703.

[24] Finelli, L, Miller, J, Tokars, J, & Arduino, M. National surveillance of dialysis-associated diseases in the United States, 2002," Seminars in Dialysis, (2005)., 18(1), 52-61.

[25] Fissell, R, Bragg-gresham, J, Woods, J, et al. Patterns of hepatitis C prevalence and seroconversion in hemodialysis units from three continents: the DOOPS," Kidney International, (2004)., 65(6), 2335-2342.

[26] Gheith, O. Dilemma of HCV infection in renal transplant recipients". International Journal of Nephrology 2011: 471214, (2011). doi:

[27] Goodkin, D, Bragg-gresham, J, Koenig, K, et al. Association of comorbid conditions and mortality in hemodialysis patients in Europe, Japan, and the United States: the dialysis outcomes and practice patterns study (DOPPS)," Journal of the American Society of Nephrology, (2003)., 14(12), 3270-3277.

[28] Gürsoy, M, Köksal, R, Karavelioglu, D, Colak, T, Gür, G, Ozdemir, N, Boyacioglu, S, & Bilgin, N. Pretransplantation alpha-interferon therapy and the effect of hepatitis C virus infection on kidney allograft recipients. Transplant Proc. (2000).

[29] Jadoul, M, Poignet, J, Geddes, C, et al. The changing epidemiology of hepatitis C virus infection in haemodialysis: European multicentre study," Nephrology Dialysis Transplantation, (2004)., 19(4), 904-909.

[30] Kidney disease: improving global outcome (KDIGO)KDIGO clinical practice guidelines for the prevention, diagnosis, evaluation, and treatment of hepatitis C in chronic kidney disease. Kidney Int Suppl (2008). suppl 109):s1

[31] KDIGO clinical practice guidelines for the preventiondiagnosis, evaluation, and treatment of hepatitis C in chronic kidney disease. Kidney Int (2008). Suppl 109):S1.

[32] Kim, E, Ko, H, & Yoshida, E. (2011). Treatment issues surrounding hepatitis c in renal transplantation: A review. Annals of hepatology, 10(1), 5-14.

[33] Knoll, G. A, Tankersley, M. R, Lee, J. Y, et al. The impact of renal transplantation on survival in hepatitis C-positive end-stage renal disease patients. Am J Kidney Dis (1997).

[34] Legendre, C, & Garrigue, V. Le Bihan C, et al. Harmful long-term impact of hepatitis C virus infection in kidney transplant recipients. Transplantation (1998).

[35] Mahmoud, I, Sobh, M, Habashi, A, et al. Interferon therapy in hemodialysis patients with chronic hepatitis C: study of tolerance, efficacy and post-transplantation course," Nephron Clinical Practice, (2005). , 100(4), c133-c139.

[36] Maluf, D. G, Fisher, R. A, King, A. L, et al. Hepatitis C virus infection and kidney transplantation: predictors of patient and graft survival. Transplantation (2007).

[37] Maluf, D, Archer, K, & Mas, V. Kidney grafts from HCV-positive donors: advantages and disadvantages," Transplantation Proceedings, (2010). , 42(7), 2436-2446.

[38] Mendez, R, Shahawy, M, Obispo, E, et al. Four years follow up of hepatitis C positive kidneys into hepatitis C negative recipients- Prospective study. J Am Soc Nephrol (1995).

[39] Misiani, R, Bellavita, P, Fenili, D, Vicari, O, Marchesi, D, Sironi, P. L, Zilio, P, Vernocchi, A, & Massazza, M. Venderamin G: Interferon alfa-2a therapy in cryoglobulinenia associated with hepatitis C virus. N Engl J Med , 330, 751-756.

[40] Morales, J, Pascual-capdevila, J, Campistol, J, et al. Membranous glomerulonephritis associated with hepatitis C virus infection in renal transplant patients," Transplantation, (1997). , 63(11), 1634-1639.

[41] Morales, J. Marc′en R, Andres A, et al., "Renal transplantation in patients with hepatitis C virus antibody. A long national experience," NDT Plus, supplement 2, (2010). , 3, ii41-ii46.

[42] Natov, S. Transmission of viral hepatitis by kidney transplantation:donor evaluation and transplant policies (part 1:hepatitis B virus)," Transplant Infectious Disease, (2002). , 4(3), 124-131.

[43] Natov, S. N, Lau, J. Y, Ruthazer, R, et al. Hepatitis C virus genotype does not affect patient survival among renal transplant candidates. The New England Organ Bank Hepatitis C Study Group. Kidney Int (1999).

[44] Natov, S, & Pereira, B. (2012). Hepatitis c virus infection and renal translpantation. In D. Brennan & A. Sheridan (Eds.), Retrieved from http://www.uptodate.com/contents/hepatitis-c-virus-infection-and-renal-transplantation

[45] Natov, S, & Pereira, B. (2012). Renal disease associated with hepatitis c virus after renal transplantation. In D. Brennan, M. Hirsch & A. Sheridan (Eds.), Retrieved from http://www.uptodate.com/contents/renal-disease-associated-with-hepatitis-c-virus-after-renal-tranplantation

[46] Northup, P, Argo, C, Nguyen, D, et al. Liver allografts from hepatitis c positive donors can offer good outcomes in hepatitis C positive recipients: a us national transplant registry analysis," Transplant International, (2010). , 23(10), 1038-1044.

[47] Ozdemir, B, Ozdemir, F, Sezer, S, Colak, T, & Haberal, M. De novo glomerulonephritis in renal allografts with hepatitis C virus infection," Transplantation Proceedings, (2006). , 38(2), 492-495.

[48] Pawlotsky JM: Molecular diagnosis of viral hepatitis Gstroenterology 122: 1554-1568, (2002).

[49] Pedroso, S, Martins, L, Fonseca, I, et al. Impact of Hepatitis C virus on renal transplantation: Association with poor survival. Transplantation Proceedings, (2006). doi:j.transproceed.2006.06.065, 38, 1890-1894.

[50] Periera, B. J, Milford, E. L, Kirkman, R. L, & Levey, A. S. Transmission of hepatitis C virus by organ transplantation. N Engl J Med (1991).

[51] Periera, B. J, Wright, T. L, Schmid, C. H, et al. Screening and confirmatory testing of cadaver organ donors for hepatitis C virus infection: a U.S. National Collaborative Study, Kidney Int (1994).

[52] Pereira, B, Wright, T, Schmid, C, et al. Screening and confirmatory testing of cadaver organ donors for hepatitis C virus infection: a U.S. national collaborative study," Kidney International, (1994). , 46(3), 886-892.

[53] Periera, B. J, Wright, T. L, Schmid, C. H, & Levey, A. S. The impact of pretransplantation hepatitis C infection on the outcome of renal transplantation. Transplantation (1995).

[54] Periera, B. J, Wright, T. L, Schmid, C. H, & Levey, A. S. Transmission of hepatitis C transmission by organ transplantation. The New England Organ Bank Hepatitis C Study Group. Lancet (1995).

[55] Pereira, B, & Levey, A. Hepatitis C virus infection in dialysis and renal transplantation," Kidney International, (1997). , 51(4), 981-999.

[56] Pereira, B. J, Natov, S. N, Bouthot, B. A, et al. Effects of hepatitis C infection and renal transplantation on survival in end-stage renal disease. The New England Organ Bank Hepatitis C Study Group. Kidney Int (1998).

[57] Pirsch, J, Heisey, D, & Allesandro, D. A, et al. Transplantation of hepatitis C (HCV) kidneys: Defining the risks (abstract). 14th Annual Meeting of the American Society of Transplant Physicians, Chicago, May 14-17, (1995). , 98.

[58] Poynard, T, Ratziu, V, Charlotte, F, Goodman, Z, Mchutchison, J, & Albrecht, J. Rates and risk factors of liver fibrosis progression in patients with chronic hepatitis C," Journal of Hepatology, (2001). , 34(5), 730-739.

[59] Rostaing, L, Izopet, J, Sandres, K, et al. Changes in hepatitis C virus RNA viremia concentrations in long-term renal transplant patients after introduction of Mycophenolate mofetil. Transplantation (2000).

[60] Roth, D, Cirocco, R, Zucker, K, et al. De novo membranoproliferative glomerulonephritis in hepatitis C virus infected renal allograft recipients," Transplantation, (1995)., 59(12), 1676-1682.

[61] Roth, D, Zucker, K, Cirocco, R, et al. A prospective study of hepatitis C virus infection in renal allograft recipients. Transplantation (1996).

[62] Shah, P, Vanikar, A, Gumber, M, Patel, H, Kute, V, Godara, S, & Trivedi, H. (2011). Renal transplantation in hepatitis c positive patients: A single centre experience. Journal of transplantation, doi:, 2011, 1-5.

[63] Scott, D, Wong, J, Spicer, T, et al. Adverse impact of hepatitis C virus infection on renal replacement therapy and renal transplant patients in Australia and New Zealand," Transplantation, (2010)., 90(11), 1165-1171.

[64] Terrault, N, & Adey, D. (2007). The kidney transplant recipient with hepatitis c infection pre- and posttransplantation treatment. American society of nephrology, doi:CJN.02930806, 2, 563-575.

[65] Toth, C. M, Pascual, M, Chung, R. T, et al. Hepatitis C virus-associated fibrosing cholestatic hepatitis after renal transplantation: response to interferon-alpha therapy. Transplantation (1998).

[66] Watashi, K, Hijikata, M, Hosaka, M, et al. Cyclosporin A suppresses replication of hepatitis C virus genome in cultured hepatocytes. Hepatology (2003).

[67] Zylberberg, H, Nalpas, B, Carnot, F, et al. Severe evolution of chronic hepatitis C in renal transplantation: a case control study. Nephrol Dial Transplant (2002).

[68] Zylberberg, H, Nalpas, B, Carnot, F, et al. Severe evolution of chronic hepatitis C in renal transplantation: a case control study," Nephrology Dialysis Transplantation, (2002)., 17(1), 129-133.

Chapter 12

Kidney and Pancreas Transplantation: The History of Surgical Techniques and Immunosuppression

Jean-Paul Squifflet

Additional information is available at the end of the chapter

http://dx.doi.org/10.5772/55347

1. Introduction

Pancreas Transplantation aims at providing Beta cells replacement in diabetic patients, especially for type 1 diabetes recipients in whom Beta cells had been destroyed by an autoimmune process. The final achievement is to restore a normal physiological control of glucose metabolism in order to halt or reverse the secondary complications of diabetes i.e. retinopathy, neuropathy, nephropathy, micro – and macro - angiopathy [1]. That can be achieved by a vascularised pancreas graft (referred as Pancreas Transplantation, PT) or by islet grafting (referred as Islet Transplantation, IT). The former PT includes transplanting 95% of unuseful cells, the exocrine part from one pancreas, while the last one IP, embolizing into the recipient liver, Islets of Langerhans after digestion and purification of several human pancreases. Three types of PT can be performed: the pancreas and a kidney are simultaneously transplanted with a single induction of immunosuppression (IS) therapy in hoping to correct both uremia and diabetes mellitus (SPK = Simultaneous Pancreas and Kidney Transplantation); the pancreas is transplanted after a successful kidney graft allowing two induction therapies along with the basic IS treatment (PAK = Pancreas After Kidney Transplantation) ; and finally the Pancreas can be transplanted alone in pre-uremic recipients with unawareness hypoglycaemic events or with rapidly evolving secondary complications of diabetes such as proliferative retinopathy, or advanced neuropathy (PTA = Pancreas Transplantation Alone) [1].

Moreover, in SPK, both organs the Pancreas and the Kidney are procured from the same deceased donor, either donor after brain death (DBD) or donor after cardiac death (DCD). In some US institutions, a segmental pancreas and the left kidney, are procured in a living donor [2], using a laparoscopic approach in the more recent year [3]. For PAK, in order to avoid an excessive IS load and two induction therapies, other institutions had proposed whenever possible to keep in stand-by the potential live kidney donor until a cadaver whole pancreatic compatible graft is available [1]. By contrast, the number of PTA remains limited in non uremic recipients with life-threatening complications of diabetes, in whom one might hope to avoid the hypoglycaemic events with a successful graft. That can also be achieved with IT. But except for rare cases, insulin independence with IT requires more than a single human pancreas and is limited over time [1]. Moreover, IT needs costly materials, chambers and rooms for preparation. That's why IT will not be included in the present report.

2. The history of surgical techniques in pancreas transplantation

The first pancreas transplantation performed by W. Kelly and R. Lillehei on December 17, 1966 at the University of Minnesota was a duct ligated segmental graft which was implanted in the left iliac fossa along with a kidney coming from the same cadaver donor in a 28 year old female uremic recipient with type 1 diabetic nephropathy [4]. It was the first ever SPK (Fig 1). The recipient was insulin-free for six days; later she needed exogenous insulin, the need being attributed to the high doses of steroids given to prevent rejection. However, she also developed graft pancreatitis, that was most likely related to duct ligation, and for which she received 950 Rads graft irradiation. On February 14, 1967, Kelly and Lillehei removed the pancreas and rejected kidney. The recipient died from pulmonary embolism 13 days after pancreas graft removal [4]. This first case exemplified many of the problems that were associated with TP over the following 2 decades: surgical complications, wound infections, and graft rejection.

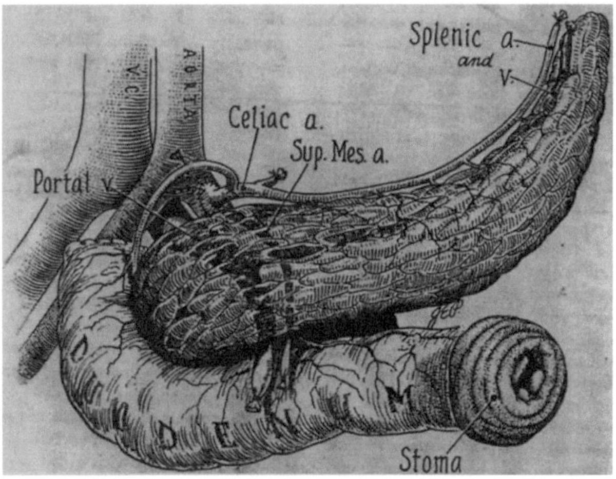

Figure 1. Drawing of the first segmental pancreas transplant (from Kelly et al.) [4].

Lillehei was the lead surgeon in the second pancreas transplant, also done with a kidney (Fig 2). He went on to do a total of 13 cases between the first case of Kelly and 1973, 9 with a kidney and 4 without [5, 6]. Significant changes in surgical techniques were made between the first and the second transplant pertaining to graft size (whole organ versus segmental) and duct management (cutaneous duodenostomy versus duct ligation). Lillehei transplanted the donor's whole pancreas and attached duodenum extraperitoneally to the 32-Year-old recipient's left iliac fossa (Fig 2). This transplant achieved a more prolonged state of graft function, but rejection treatment had to be instituted three and eight weeks post-transplant. Both rejection episodes affected the graft duodenum. The recipient was on insulin when she died four months post transplant from sepsis.

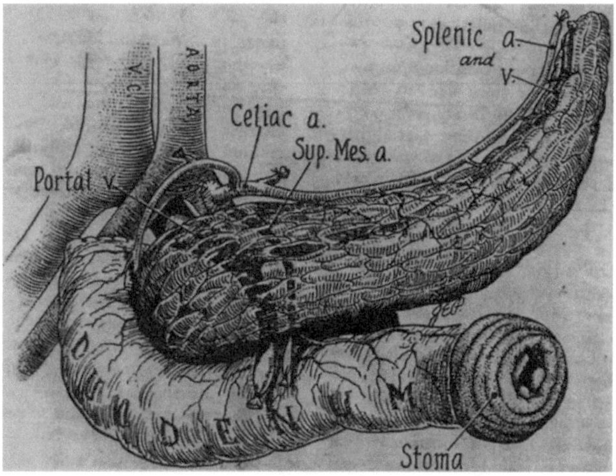

Figure 2. Drawing of the first whole pancreas transplant with cutaneous graft duodenostomy (from Lillelei et al.) [5]

After that series of 13 Pancreas Transplants, R. Lillehei concluded that most complications were associated with kidney graft rejection without pancreas rejection and recipient death [5, 6, 7].

After the first four pancreas transplants at the University of Minnesota, the next four transplants were performed in South America in 1968; [8, 9, 10]; three were performed in Brazil and one in Argentina at the Buenos Aires Hospital. Only one functioned sufficiently to induce insulin-independence and was subsequently lost to rejection at 4 months. [10].

In 1969, two other U.S. institutions performed one SPK transplant each: one at the University of Colorado (Fred Merkel and Thomas Starzl) and one at the University of California, Irvine Medical Center (John Connolly). [8, 11]. The first pancreas transplant in Europe, along with a kidney transplant, was performed in 1972 at Guys Hospital, in London, U.K. (Mick Bewick). [8].

By the 1970s, only 25 pancreas transplants had been performed at six institutions worldwide. Two-thirds of those early pancreas transplants were done along with a simultaneous kidney transplant. Exocrine secretions had been drained by duct ligation, cutaneous duodenostomy, or enteric drainage using a Roux-en-Y loop. Of these 25 grafts, only one, from Lillehei's original series, functioned for almost one year, and none for more than one year.

On November 24, 1971, Marvin Gliedman at Montefiore Hospital and Medical Center in New York performed the first pancreas transplant using urinary drainage via the native ureter [12]. Gliedman and associates performed a total of 11 ureteral pancreas transplants in the early 1970s (Fig 3) with one graft functioning for 22 months and another for 50 months – at that point the longest pancreas graft survival recorded. [13, 14]. However, ureteral drainage did not find widespread application because of tenuous leakage-prone duct-to-ureter anastomosis; leakage from the pancreas cut surface; and the potential need for ipsilateral native nephrectomy. The main conclusion drawn from that original and historical series was the probable evidence of a hierarchy in rejection, the pancreas being less antigenic than the kidney the latter being less antigenic than the duodenum [15]. Therefore, surgical techniques using a segmental pancreatic graft (body and tail) were developed during the next decade.

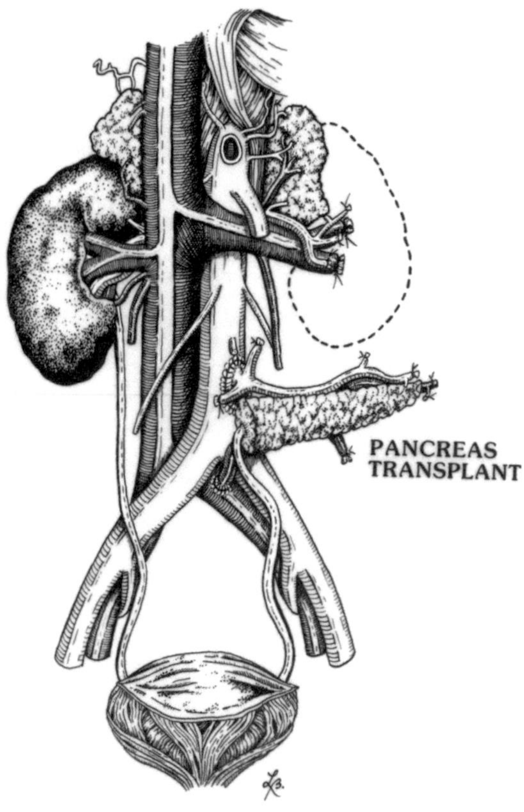

Figure 3. Ureteral pancreas transplant according to Gliedman et al [12] end-to-end distal ureter to pancreatic duct anastomosis.

2.1. The segmental pancreas transplantation reign (from mid 70's to mid's 80's)

In the mid 70's, the segmental pancreas while avoiding the duodenal segment was the most popular technique used for PT [6, 7]. Various procedures were proposed to drain the exocrine secretion: the duct could be left opened with the segmental graft placed intraperitoneally (Fig 4) [16] or blocked by an intraductal injection (Fig 5) of either Neoprene (J.M. Dubernard) [17] or Prolamine (W. Land) [18] or Polyisoprene (P. Mc Master) [19] or Silicone (D.E.R. Sutherland) [20].

http://dx.doi.org/10.5772/55347

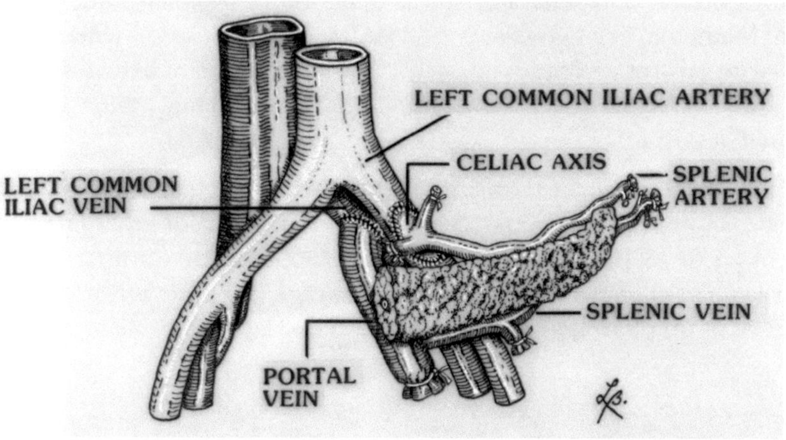

Figure 4. Technique for revascularization in the recipient of a segmental pancreas graft. The celiac axis (on a Carrel patch) and portal vein of the graft are anastomosed to the commun iliac vessels of the recipient through the mesosigmoid [16].

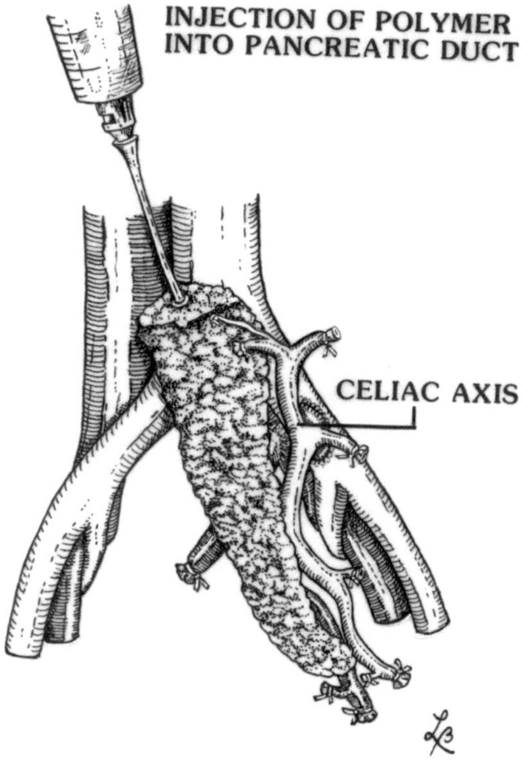

Figure 5. Injection of a synthetic polymer into the duct of a segmental pancreas graft following revascularization. Approximately 4-6 ml of the polymer is injected, followed by ligation of the duct [17-20].

Twelve intraperitoneal open-duct segmental pancreas transplants were performed at the University of Minnesota in a two-year period [16]; four were rejected within 4 months; 3 had to be removed because of peritonitis or ascites. The latter recipient lived insulin-independent for 18 years until in 1996 she died from a trauma, with a functioning graft, the longest duration of function at that time [21].

By contrast the duct occlusion technique became more popular despite numerous leaks, pancreatic fistulae, graft pancreatitis and vascular thrombosis. For managing these complications, Dubernard et al. [17, 7] proposed the omentoplasty in warping the duct-occluted segmental pancreas with the omentum, while Calne et al. [6, 7] was performing an A-V fistula at the distal end of the pancreas tail (Fig 6; panels A and B).

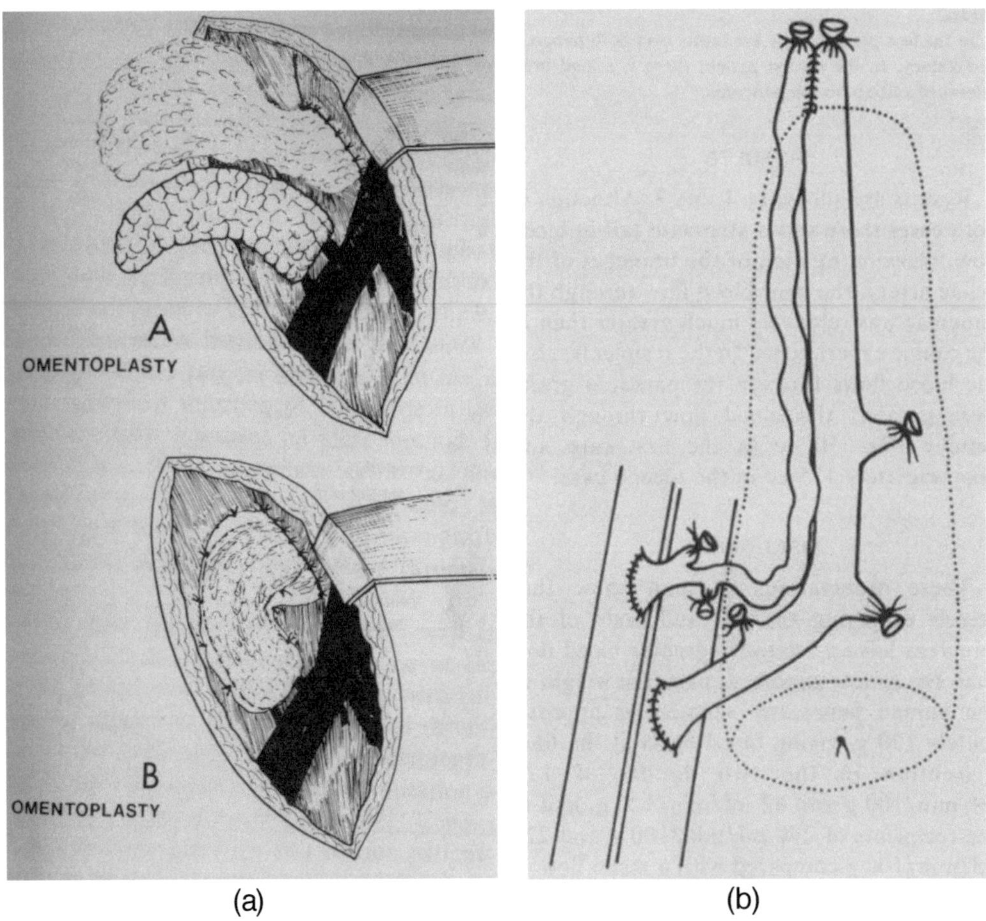

Figure 6. Panel (a): omentoplasty according to Dubernard et al.[7, 17]. Panel (b): AV fistula between the distal splenic artery and vein according to Calne et al. [6, 7].

During the late 70'S, three major events occurred that contributed to the development of PT.

http://dx.doi.org/10.5772/55347

Firstly, in 1979, the clinical use of Cyclosporine A (CsA) by R. Calne et al. [22] as the single immunosuppressant in 36 recipients of cadaveric organs. CsA remained the basic immunosuppressive (IS) drug up to the early 90'S.

Secondly, in 1980, the organization by J.M. Dubernard in Lyon, France, of the first pancreas transplantation meeting, launching the International Pancreas (and Islet) Transplant Registry (IPTR) which was handled by D.E.R. Sutherland at the University of Minnesota [23].

Thirdly and finally, in 1981, the first of a series of 5 workshops – called the Spitzingsee Meeting – organized by W. Land in Kühtai, Austria [24]. The characteristics of these workshops consisted in gathering the world pioneers in PT and allowing them to discuss on not only the successes but also the failures, finding ways to prevent them or improve the results [25]. These meetings were also the basis of creating the International Pancreas and Islet Association (IPITA) and later on, in Europ, the European Study Group in Simultaneous Pancreas and Kidney Transplantation (EuroSPK) [25]. More recently, was created the EPITA, the European Pancreas and Islet Transplantation Association [25].

During one of these workshops, H. Sollinger [26] had the idea to renew an old technique and divert the exocrine secretion of the pancreas into the bladder (Fig 7), while G. Tyden [27] and C. Groth [28] were proposing the enteric drainage (Fig 8). Slowly, both groups moved from the segmental graft [28] to the whole pancreas graft along with a duodenal segment (Fig 9) [26, 27]. This announced the end of the segmental transplantation reign. In the mean time, on November 10, 1982, the first pancreas transplantation was performed in Belgium by J.P. Squifflet and G.P.J. Alexandre [7]. The recipient was a 29 year old female with a 26 year history of type 1 diabetes. She was on peritoneal dialysis since one year and switched to hemodialysis a month before. She received a simultaneous pancreas and kidney transplants from a 22 year old female cadaver donor who died in a car accident from a head trauma. The recipient did not share any HLA antigen with the donor. She received a segmental pancreas graft, anastomosed on a Roux-en-Y loop (Fig 10), according to the technique described by Groth et al. (Fig 8) [23]. The immunosuppressive therapy consisted in a short course of antilymphocytic globulins induction along with cyclosporine A and steroids. She was one of the first few patients who received cyclosporine A in Belgium, at a dose a 14 mgr/kg/day. Following an episode of delayed graft function of the kidney, she fully recovered and was insulin free for a period of 2 years. Than insulin resistance was noticed along with an increase of 15 kg in body weight. Despite Cyclosporin and steroids dose reduction and the introduction of azathioprine, insulin therapy was resumed. She eventually went back on hemodialysis 8 years later and died in June 1992 while waiting for a second kidney transplant. The choice of the surgical technique and IS was based on animal experiments [29–32] but also on the fact that segmental pancreas transplantation was more popular during that period.

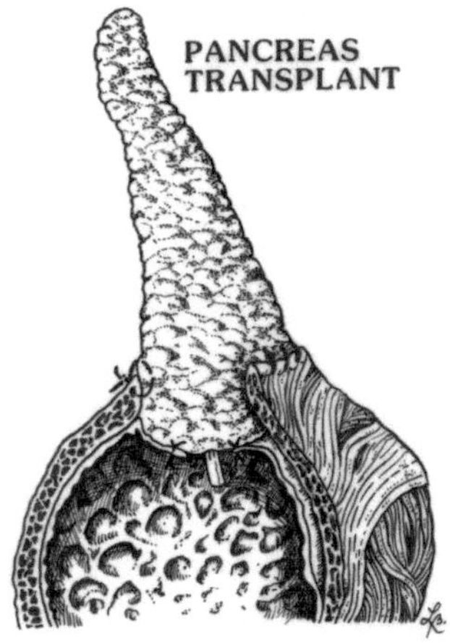

Figure 7. Exocrine secretion of segmental grafts drained directly into the bladder, as first described by Sollinger et al. [26].

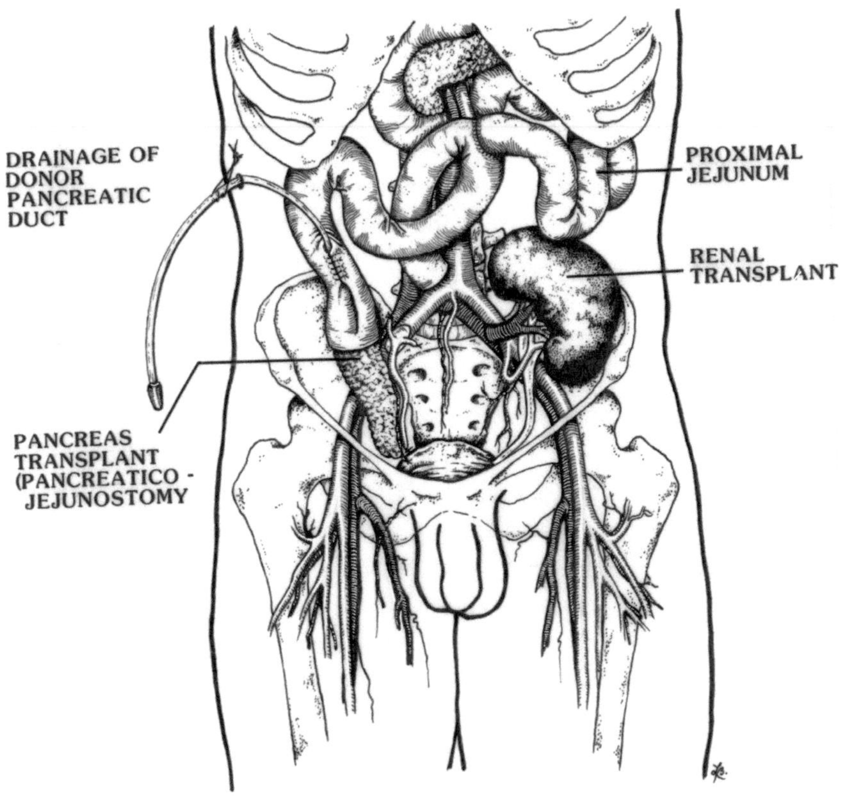

Figure 8. Enteric drainage of a segmental pancreas graft to a Roux-en-Y limb of recipient jejunum. The temporary external drainage of the pancreatic duct secretions to the catheter brought to the Roux-en-Y loop and the abdominal wall is illustrated [28].

2.2. The whole pancreas transplantation reign (from mid 80's)

Thus, in the mid 80's, whole pancreas transplantation with a duodenal segment became the gold standard surgical procedure.

In 1987, Nghiem and Corry at the University of Iowa described the technique of bladder drainage via a graft-to-recipient duodeno-cystostomy for whole pancreaticoduodenal grafts (Fig 9) [33]. Most U.S. and European centers quickly adopted bladder drainage via the graft duodenum. For SPK transplants, the dominant reason to use bladder-drainage was to reduce the risk of anastamotic leaks, since rejection could be monitored by serum creatinine. For solitary pancreas transplants, bladder-drainage had the advantage of urine amylase monitoring for rejection.

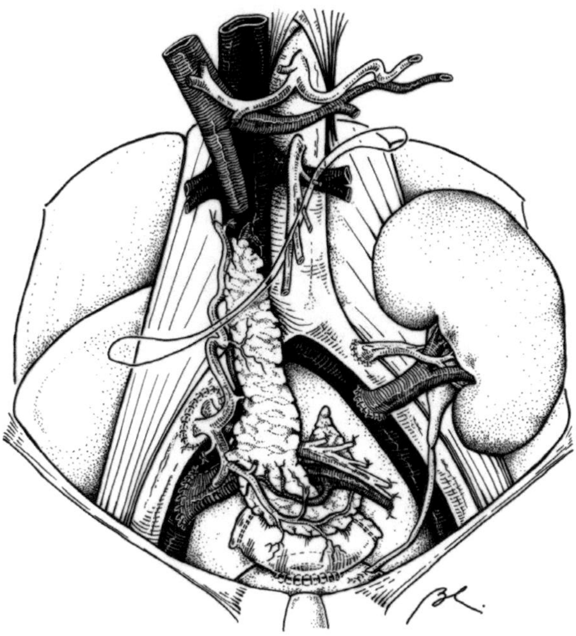

Figure 9. Pancreaticoduodenal transplantation with bladder drainage. A side-to-side anastomosis of the duodenal segment is made to the dome of the bladder [33].

In the mid 80's, Starzl [34] and associates reintroduced in U.S.the technique of enteric-drained whole-organ pancreaticoduodenal transplants, as originally described by Lillehei while the Stockholm group continued to do enteric drainage by direct duodeno-enterostomy [35]. Nearly everyone was convinced that whole pancreaticoduodenal transplants were preferable for PT from cadaver donors, and after en – bloc liver and pancreas procurement (Fig 11), transplant surgeons designed methods for reconstructing the vasculature to both organs (Fig 12) [36 - 39].

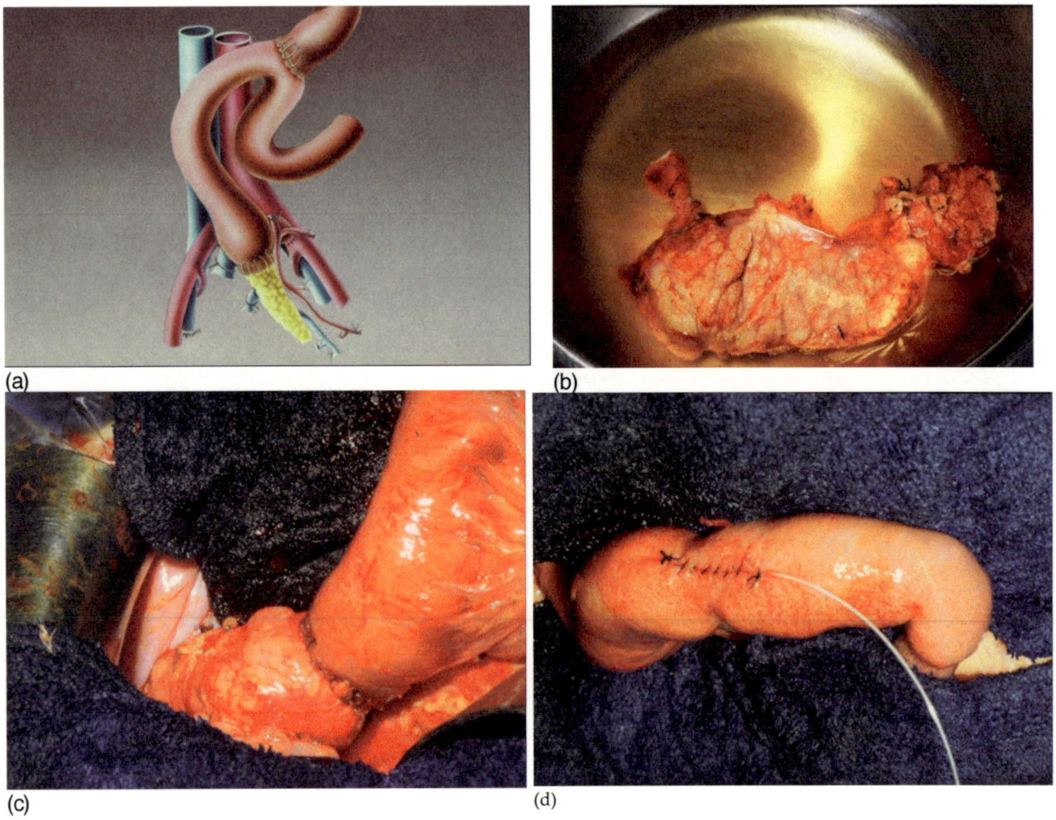

a: drawing of the procedure.
b: the segmental pancreas graft.
c: the end-to-end pancreas graft anastomosis to the Roux-en-Y loop.
d: the anastomosis suture was protected by a catheter inserted into the pancreas duct.

Figure 10. Segmental pancreatic transplant in the first Belgian recipient with enteric diversion of the exocrine secretion, in a Roux-en-Y loop.

From the mid-80s to the mid-90s, bladder drainage became the most common technique worldwide (Fig 9). However, because of chronic complications of bladder drainage (urinary tract infections, cystitis, urethritis (Fig 13), reflux pancreatitis, hematuria, metabolic acidosis and dehydration from fluid and bicarbonate losses), leading to conversion to enteric drainage in approximately a quarter of the recipients, in the mid-1990s, surgeons began to shifted to primary enteric drainage (Fig 14), not only for SPK transplants, but at some institutions also for solitary pancreas transplants [40].

http://dx.doi.org/10.5772/55347

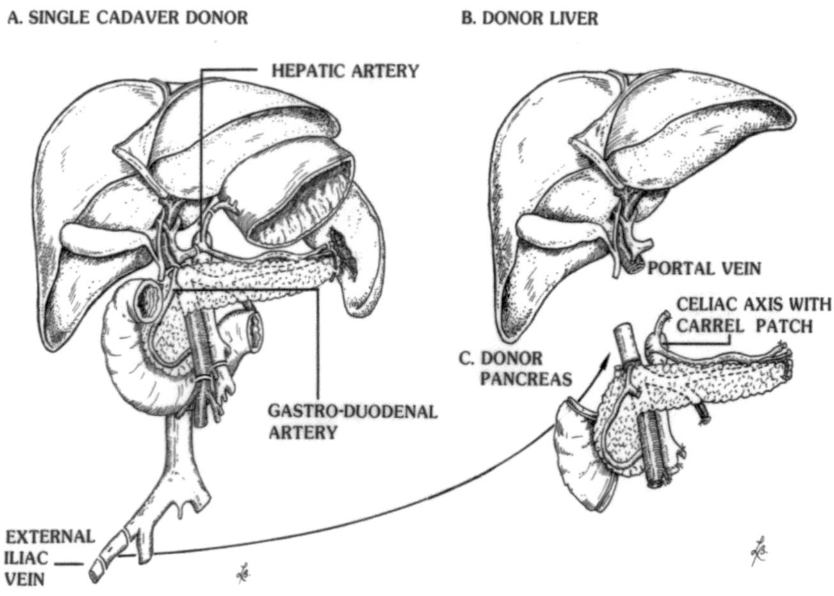

Figure 11. Maneuvers for en-bloc removal of a whole pancreas and a liver from a cadaver donor with normal vascular anatomy.The gastroduodenal artery must be divided so that the common and proper hepatic arteries can remain in continuity and be retained with the liver. The portal vein is divided just superior to the entrance of the splenic vein. Then, the pancreatic portion is lengthened by an iliac vein graft. The celiac and superior mesenteric arteries can remain with the pancreas with a Carrel aortic patch. [38]

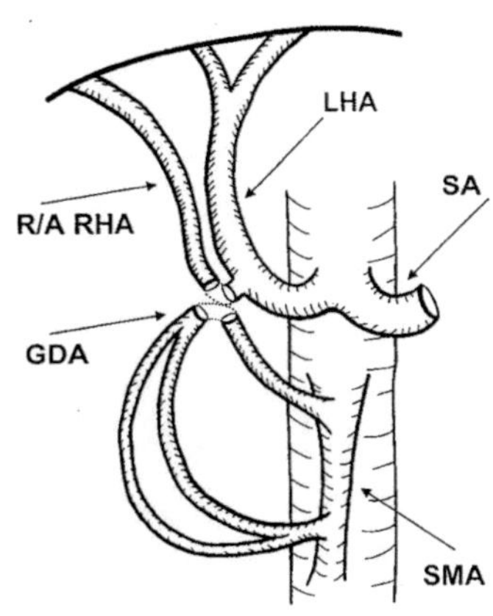

LHA = left hepatic artery.
GDA = gastroduodenal artery
SA = splenic artery
SMA = superior mesenteric artery.[39]

Figure 12. Whole-pancreas procurement and reconstruction of its arterial supply in a donor with a replaced / accessory right hepatic artery (R / A RHA).

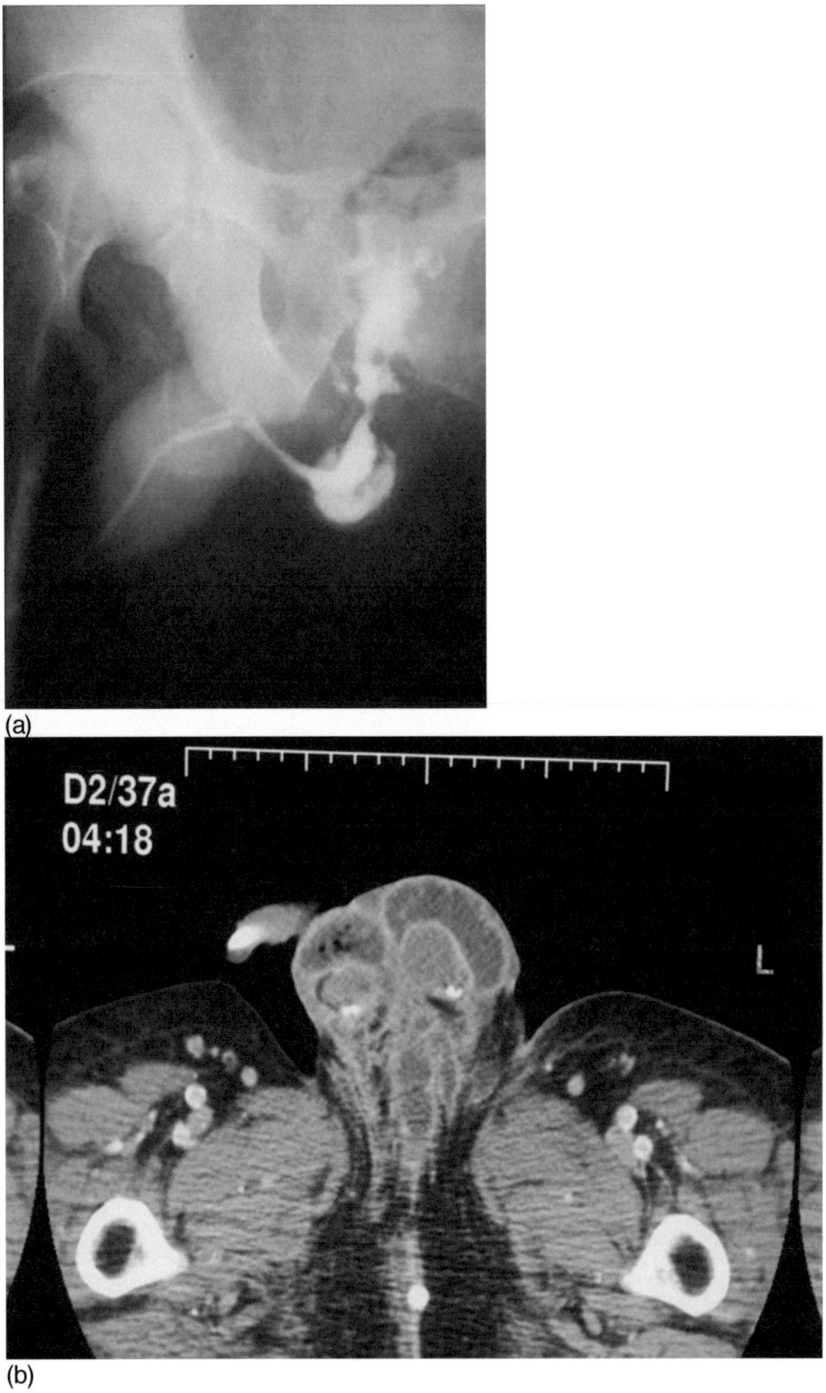

Figure 13. Chemical urethritis in a pancreas recipient with bladder drainage of the exocrine secretion (Panel (a)). CT scan: same recipient (Panel (b)).

http://dx.doi.org/10.5772/55347

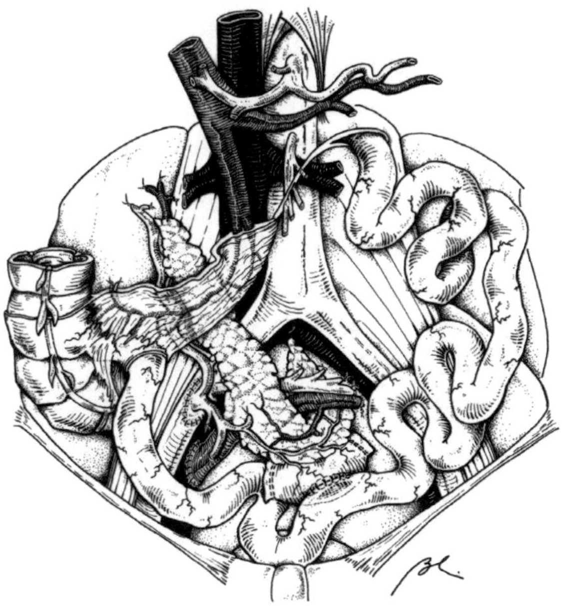

Figure 14. Pancreaticoduodenal transplantation with enteric drainage. A side-to-side anastomosis of the duodenal segment is made to the distal ileon, or the proximal jejeunum. It can also be performed on a Roux-en-Y loop [35].

2.3. The modern era of surgical techniques

Either enteric or bladder drainage is now done for virtually all pancreas transplants using a whole pancreas graft with a duodenal segment. The other techniques are virtually never used unless for salvage of a technical situation (e.g., duct injection might be used to manage a leak). With regard to the venous drainage of pancreas grafts, portal would be the most physiological but the systemic venous system was only accessed during the first two decades. Later on, the use of portal drainage at the junction of the recipient's superior mesenteric and splenic vein was favored in recipients of enteric drained whole-organ pancreaticoduodenal transplants (Fig 15). Surgeons reported on its metabolic and possible immunologic advantage, features also noted at the University of Maryland, where a large program existed of conversion to almost exclusive portal drainage [41]. By the end of the 1990's, almost 20 % of pancreas transplants in U.S. and in Europe were being done with portal drainage but the proportion did not increase nearly as much as the proportion of pancreas grafts that were enteric drained, reaching over 80 % for solitary in U.S. and over 90 % for SPK transplants in Europe (Fig 16). Early diagnosis of pancreas rejection had been difficult from the beginning, in particular for solitary pancreas transplants where serum creatinine could not be used as a surrogate marker like in SPK. That's why there is still room for improvement in surgical techniques. In order to have easy access to the graft for performing biopsies, De Roover et al. [42] proposed recently a technical modification and a side-to-side duodeno-duodenal (D-D) anastomosis while using a whole pancreaticoduodenal transplant with the venous effluent drained into the portal system of the recipient (Fig 17, 18). It offers serial sampling of the duodenal transplant mucosa by simple fibroscopies, a useful tool for monitoring rejection (Fig 18, Panel B). The duodenal anastomosis can be hand-made or performed using a stapler device. But the major drawback of both techniques could be the management of duodenal leaks on graft thrombosis. Our experience in 11 pancreas recipients at the University of Liege, CHU Sart Tilman is summarized in table 1. Peri-pancreatic collections, with or without pancreatitis were managed by surgical exploration and drainage. So far, only one graft thrombosis (PTA) needed prompt removal but was followed by a duodenal leak with cutaneous fistula which required weeks before healing (table 1). Therefore, prospective studies will be useful to specify the place of the D-D and each particular surgical suturing technique.

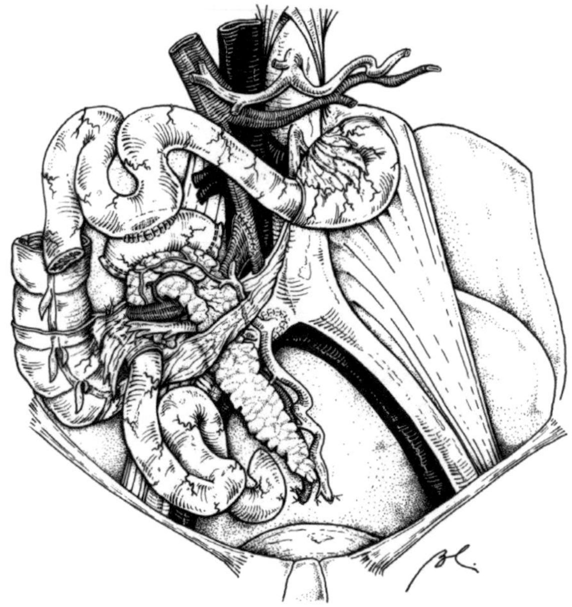

Figure 15. Pancreaticoduodenal transplantation with enteric drainage and portal drainage at the junction of the recipient's superior mesenteric and splenic veins [41].

http://dx.doi.org/10.5772/55347

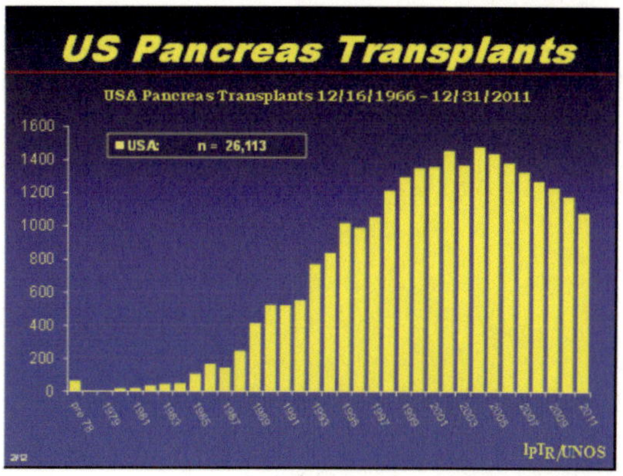

(a)

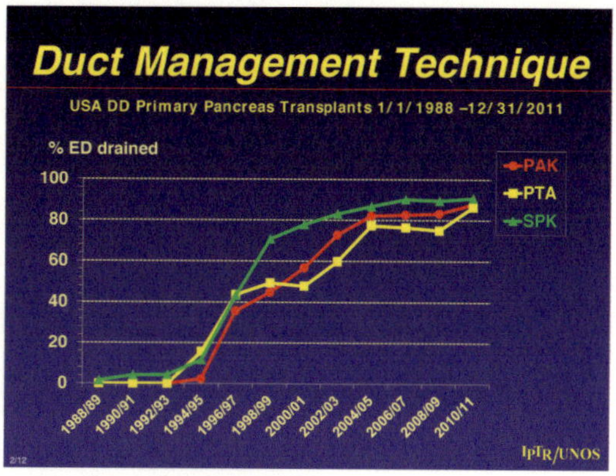

(b)

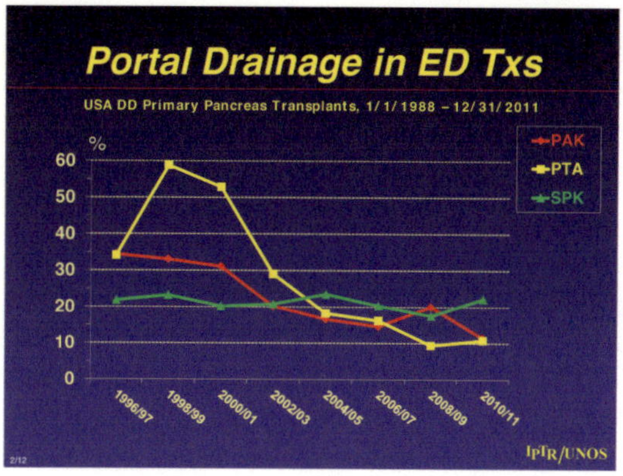

(c)

*By courtesy from A.E. Gruessner
Department of Surgery,
University of Arizona, Tucson, USA.

Figure 16. International Pancreas Transplant Registry * Panel (a): US Pancreas Transplants per year, between 12/16/1966 and 12/31/2011. Panel (b): Duct management techniques (urinary versus enteric drainage) in US primary pancreas transplants, between 1/1/1988 and 12/31/2011. Panel (c): Portal Drainage in enteric drained (ED) transplants. US primary pancreas transplants, between 1/1/1988 and 12/31/2011.

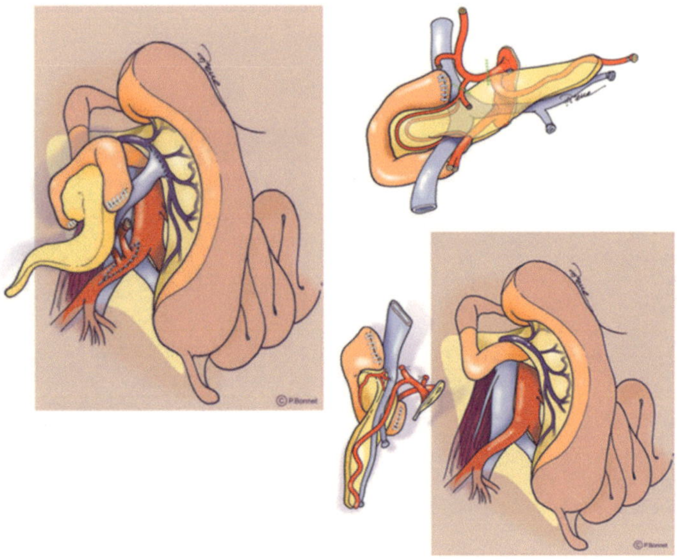

Figure 17. Pancreaticoduodenal transplantation with portal drainage and side-to-side recipient duodenal drainage of the exocrine secretion [23]: schematic representation and positioning.

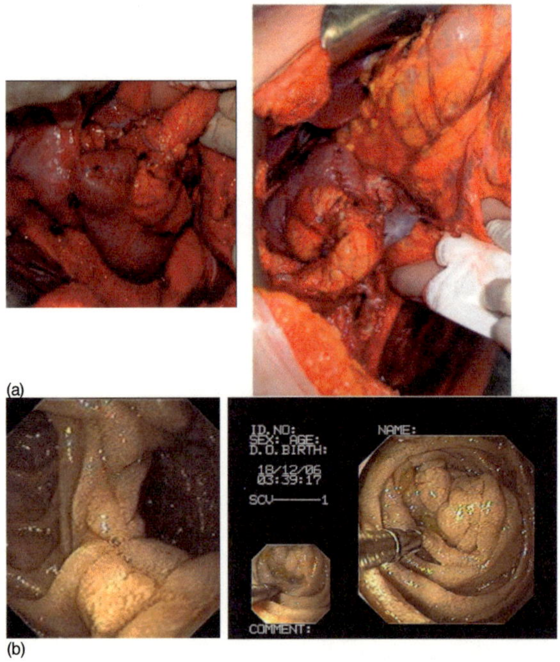

Figure 18. Pancreaticoduodenal transplantation with portal drainage and side-to-side recipient duodenal drainage of the exocrine secretion [23]: Panel (a): per operative view Panel (b): endoscopic view of the duodenum

http://dx.doi.org/10.5772/55347

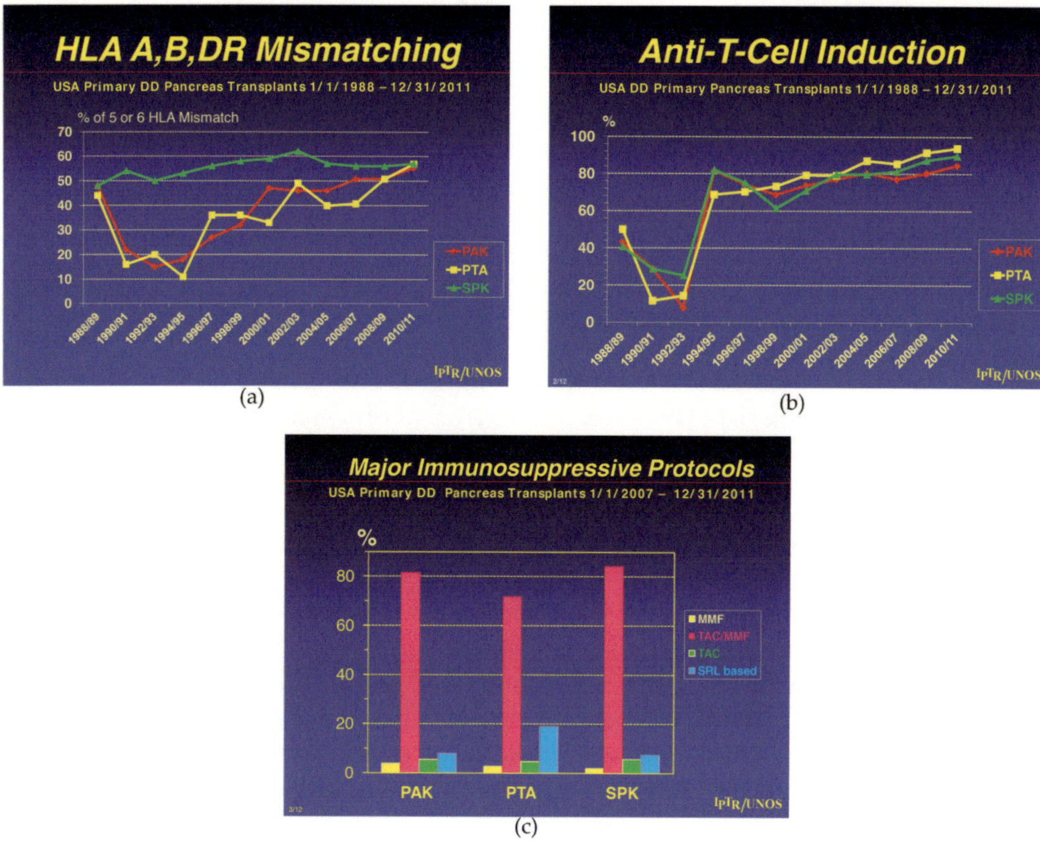

*By courtesy from A.E. Gruessner
Department of Surgery,
University of Arizona, Tucson, USA.

Figure 19. International Pancreas Transplant Registry* Panel (a): Purcentage of 5 or 6 HLA A, B, Dr Mismatching in US primary pancreas transplants between 1/1/1988 and 12/31/2011. Panel (b): Anti-T-Cell induction in US primary pancreas transplants between 1/1/1988 and 12/31/2011. Panel (c): Major immunosuppressive protocols in US primary pancreas transplants between 1/1/2007 and 12/31/2011

PTA hand-made (n=7):	
– Peri-pancreas hematoma + inflammatory syndrome (1)*	Surgical exploration + drainage
– Graft thrombosis (1)*	Transplantectomy
– Pancreatitis + peri-pancreas fluid collection due to partial necrosis of pancreas (1)*	Surgical exploration + drainage
PTA stapler (n=0)	
SPK hand-made (n=1): no.	
SPK stapler (n=3)	
– Peri-pancreas fluid collection + inflammatory syndrome (1)*	Surgical exploration + drainage
– Digestive hemorrhage due to ulcers of the donor duodenal stump (1)	Conservative treatment+transfusion

Table 1. Complications and outcome in 11 recipients of whole pancreas grafts with duodeno-duodenostomy, at the University of Liege, CHU Sart Tilman. The D-D anastomosis was hand-made (n=7) or using a stapler device (n=4)

3. The history of immunosuppression in pancreas transplantation

Advances in immunosuppressive protocols and the introduction of new immunosuppressants have had a major impact on and improved outcome after PT. As already mentioned, in 1979, Calne and associates first reported the successful use of cyclosporine in two pancreas recipients [22]. Due to the large dose of CsA used as a single agent and its nephrotoxicity, Starzl et al. proposed to combined reduced doses of CsA with steroids [43]. Further decreased in CsA dosages by using the synergistic effect of combining CsA to Aza was proposed by Squifflet et al. based on animals experiments [29, 44]. Triple drugs combining CsA, Aza and Steroids and later on quadruple drugs regimen with a short course induction of polyclonal Antibodies was the mainstay IS regimen during the next decade [21]. Starzl and his team first reported the use of Tacrolimus (Tac) in pancreas allograft recipients during the investigative period in 1989. [45] After approval, the first report on the use of Tac for pancreas transplantation was by D. Shaffer and associates, successfully reversing ongoing acute rejection in two SPK recipients. [46].

A major topic of the 4th Spitzingsee Workshop (January 30 – February 02, 1997; Kühtai, Austria) was the IS therapy in PT [25]. At that time, the newly introduced agent mycophenolate mofetil (MMF) was proved to be superior to azathioprine (Aza) for the prevention of acute rejection in kidney transplantation patients [47]. Data comparing Tac with the old (oil-based) formulation of CsA were also available in kidney transplantation, but there were some concerns about Tac having a diabetogenic effect [48], specially for pancreas. A preliminary study investigating the use of Tac in pancreatic transplantation, which was published by Gruessner et al., showed that pancreatic graft survival at 6 months post transplant was higher with Tac (79%) than in a historical group of SPK recipients treated with the oil-based formulation of CsA (65%; p = 0.04)

http://dx.doi.org/10.5772/55347

[49]. During the same era, the new micro-emulsion (Me) formulation of CsA (CsA – Me) had been introduced into clinical practice.

At that period, all European participants to the meeting were performing a limited number of SPK per centre. All realized that local studies would not aim solving the IS problems. Therefore W. Land took the opportunity to propose them the first large international prospective multicentre study in the field of PT, comparing Tac to the new CsA – Me, along with MMF, corticosteroids and a short course of induction therapy with Rabbit – antithymocyte globulines (R-ATG, Fresenius, Germany).

The rationale for induction therapy using anti-T-cell agents was triple: minimizing the risks of early rejection episodes, accelerating recovery of renal and pancreatic allograft function (protection against the ischemic reperfusion injury) and perhaps, inducing a tolerogenic effect to donor alloantigens. Before 1994, choices of maintenance IS agents were limited to a "one size fits all" approach with the combined use of Cyclosporin A (CsA), azathioprine (Aza) and corticosteroids. But, with that regimen, rejection rates were about 75 % to 80 %, with a rate of 25 % to 30 % of recurrence. Therefore, during the early 90's anti-T-cell induction was automatically added in all 3 categories of pancreas transplantation (Fig 19, Panel B). The choice of the anti-T-Cell agent was based more on its accessibility than on any rationale or scientific approach; the anti-T-Cell agents which were used are: MALG®, OKT3®, ATGAM®, R-ATG®, Simulect®, Zenapax®, Thymoglobulin®, Campath®. During the CsA era, single centre studies emphasized the benefit of Quadruple over Triple therapies [50, 51]. Other comparative studies underlined the best efficacy of ATG over OKT3® and MALG® [52 - 54]. During the modern era, during which most centres were using Tacrolimus (Tac), Mycophenolate Mofetil (MMF) and corticosteroids for maintenance therapy, Kaufman et al. designed several multicenter studies [55, 56] in which they confirmed the usefulness of induction therapy in PT. By contrast, the place of Campath®, still remains to be confirmed [57].

The results of the first Euro-SPK study were encouraging [58]. The 1-year incidence of biopsy-proven acute rejection of the kidney or pancreas was lower with Tac (27.2 %) than with CsA-Me (38.2 %; $p = 0.09$). Pancreatic graft survival at 1 year was significantly higher with Tac (91.3 %) than with CsA-Me (74.5 %; $p = 0.0014$). Kidney graft survival was similar in the two groups [58].

At 3 years, fewer patients receiving Tac (36.9 %) than CsA-Me (57.8 %) were discontinued from treatment ($p = 0.003$). The initial episodes of biopsy proven rejection were moderate or severe in just one out of 31 (3 %) Tac-treated patients compared with 11 of 39 (28 %) patients receiving CsA-Me ($p = 0.009$).

While 3-year patient and kidney survival rates were similar in the two treatment groups, pancreas survival was superior with Tac (89.2 vs 72.4 %; $p = 0.002$). Thrombosis resulted in pancreas graft loss in 10 patients receiving CsA-Me and in only 2 treated with Tac ($p = 0.02$). The overall incidence of adverse events was similar in both groups, but MMF intolerance was more frequent with Tac whereas hyperlipidaemia was more frequent with CsA-Me. Acute rejection was more common among CMV-infected patients (66 vs 41 % without infection; $p = 0.001$) and in those not receiving ganciclovir prophylaxis [48, 58].

There were no differences in 3-year kidney pancreas or patient survival between the 0-3 and 4-6 HLA antigen mismatch (MM) groups. Significantly more patients with 0-3 MM (66 %) were rejection-free at 3 years compared to those with 4-6 MM (41 %; $p = 0.003$). The relative risk of acute rejection was 2.6 times higher among patients with 4-6 MM than among those with 0-3 MM [48].

In summary the Euro-SPK study findings provided evidence to support the use of Tac in patients undergoing SPK transplantation.

A second SPK study addressed the issue of the choice of the antiproliferative agent which could be associated to Tac, either MMF or rapamycine (Rapa). Preliminary one and three year results demonstrated more frequent study withdrawal in the Rapa group, due to toxicity [59].

More than 60 % of those patients were rejection free at 1 year. Adequate kidney and pancreas functions were also achieved in both groups while the serum creatinine level was significantly lower in the Rapa group from month 2, the price to pay being hyperlipidemia, delayed wound healing, lymphocoele or hernia.

Corticosteroid withdrawal was possible in both studies in 70 % and 50 % of recipients respectively. Therefore, it can be concluded that steroid withdrawal is feasible in SPK transplantation but not in all patients; further studies must be designed to address that issue completely.

4. Conclusion

The current gold standard IS therapy for all three categories of pancreas transplantation includes induction with polyclonal antibodies and for the maintenance therapy, association of Tac with either MMF or Rapa, the last drug being less popular at least during the first postoperative period due to its possible side-effects (Fig 19).

Based on that potent IS therapy, functional results and patient survival rates of PT are coming closer to those currently achieved in kidney transplantation (Fig 20).

SPK transplantation remains the best therapeutic approach for type 1 diabetic recipients with (pre) end-stage renal failure (creatinine clearance < 50ml/min), up to 55 years of age, without any cardiovascular risk. They have three options: either waiting for the 2 grafts coming from the same -cadaver or live- donor, or one graft –usually the kidney – coming from a live donor who is in stand-by while waiting for the pancreas from a cadaver donor.

PAK can be offered to diabetic recipients who had the opportunity of having a live donor for kidney transplantation.

For other type 1 diabetic recipients, with (pre) end-stage renal failure, more than 55 years of age, with cardiovascular risk factors, they have 2 options: either receiving a kidney transplant alone (and eventually waiting for islet cells) or waiting for a simultaneous islet and kidney transplantation from the same cadaveric donor.

http://dx.doi.org/10.5772/55347

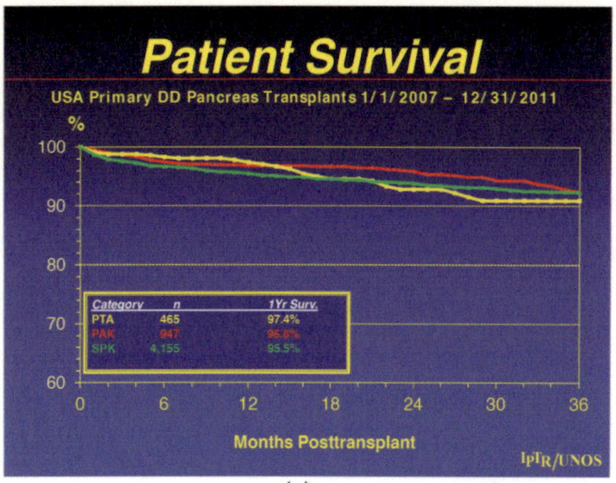

(a)

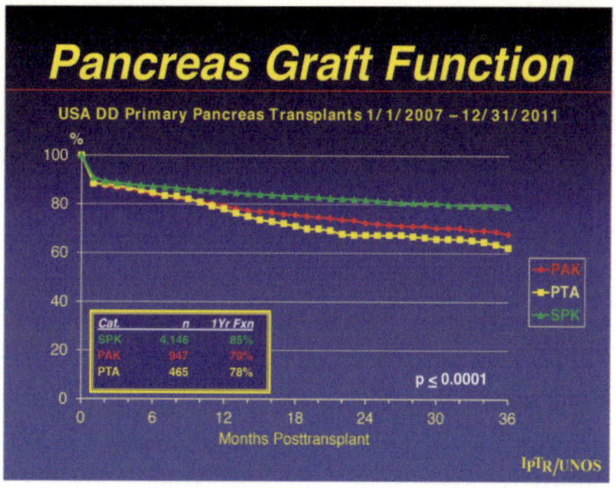

(b)

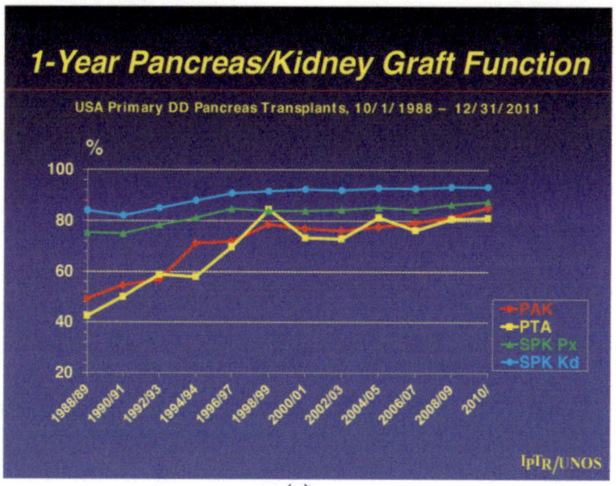

(c)

*By courtesy from A.E. Gruessner
Department of Surgery,
University of Arizona, Tucson, USA.

Figure 20. International Pancreas Transplant Registry* Panel (a): Patient survival in US primary pancreas transplants between 1/1/2007 and 12/31/2011. Panel (b): Pancreas graft function in all 3 categories (SPK, PAK, PTA). Panel (c): One year pancreas and kidney graft function in US primary pancreas transplants, between 10/1/1988 and 12/31/2011.

PTA should be considered for selected type 1 diabetic candidate without nephropathy, with hypoglycemia unawareness syndrom, with proliferative retinopathy. These candidates could be also candidates for islet transplantation, knowing the fact that they will be submitted to the same IS therapy and its long term deleterious side-effects in both options, they might also know that, with islet insulin independence is not always achieved.

Acknowledgements

- Drawings: to Benoit Lengele (BL) and Pierre Bonnet (PB).
- IPTR data : to A.E. Gruessner, and R.W.G. Gruessner, Departement of Surgery, University of Arizona, Tucson, USA.
- EuroSPK data : to all Members of the EuroSPK study group.

Author details

Jean-Paul Squifflet

Department of Abdominal Surgery and Transplantation, University of Liege, Belgium

References

[1] Pancreas transplantation White SA., Shaw J.A. and Sutherland D.E.R. Lancet (2009). , 373, 1808-17.

[2] Gruessner, R. W. G, Kendall, D. M, Drangstveit, M. B, Gruessner, A. C, & Sutherland, D. E. R. Simultaneous pancreas kidney transplantation from live donors Ann Surg (1997). , 226, 471-482.

[3] Gruessner, R. W. G, Kandaswamy, R, & Denny, R. Laparoscopic simultaneous nephrectomy and distal pancreatectomy from a live donor. J Am Cell Surg (2001). , 193, 333-337.

[4] Kelly, W. D, Lillehei, R. C, Merkel, F. K, & Idezuki, Y. And Goetz F.C. Allotransplantation of the pancreas and duodenum along with the kidney in diabetic nephrology. Surgery, (1967).

[5] Lillehei, R. C, Simmons, R. L, Najarian, J. S, Weil, R, Uchida, H, Ruiz, J. O, Kjellstrand, C. M, & Goetz, F. C. Pancreatico-duodenal allotransplantation : experimental and clinical experience. Ann Surg (1970). , 172, 405-436.

[6] Sutherland, D. E. R, & Gruessner, R. W. G. History of Pancreas Transplantation. in:Transplantation of the Pancreas Gruessner R.W.G. and Sutherland D.E.R. (eds), (2004). Springer- Verlag New York, Inc. , 39-68.

[7] Squifflet, J. P, Gruessner, R. W. G, & Sutherland, D. E. R. The history of Pancreas Transplantation: Past, Present and Future. Acta Chir Belg. (2008).

[8] Sutherland DERPancreas and islet transplantation. II. Clinical trials. Diabetologia (1981). , 20, 435-450.

http://dx.doi.org/10.5772/55347

[9] Sutherland DERPancreas and islet transplantation. II. Clinical trials. Diabetologia (1981). , 20, 435-450.

[10] Bortagaray, M. C, Zelasco, J. F, Bava, A, et al. Homotransplante parcial del pancreas en el diabetico. Pren Med Argent (1970).

[11] Connolly, J. E, Martin, R. C, Steinberg, J, et al. Clinical experience with pancreatico-duodenal transplantation. Arch Surg (1973). , 106, 489-493.

[12] Gliedman, M. L, Gold, M, Whittaker, J, Rifkin, H, Soberman, R, Freed, S, Tellis, V, & Veith, F. J. Clinical segmental pancreatic transplantation with ureter-pancreatic duct anastomosis for exocrine drainage. Surgery (1973). , 74, 171-180.

[13] Gliedman, M. L, Tellis, V. A, & Soberman, R. Long-term effects of pancreatic transplant function in patients with advanced juvenile onset diabetes. DiabetesCare (1978). , 1, 1-9.

[14] Tellis, V. A, Veith, F. J, & Gliedman, M. L. Ten-year experience with human pancreatic transplantation. Transplant Proc (1980). suppl 2):78-80.

[15] Lillehei, R. C, Ruiz, J. O, Aquino, C, & Goetz, F. C. Transplantation of the pancreas. Acta Endocrin (1976). suppl 205):303-320.

[16] Sutherland, D. E. R, Goetz, F. C, & Najarian, J. S. Intraperitoneal transplantation of immediately vascularized segmental grafts without duct ligation. A clinical Trial. Transplantation (1979). , 28, 485-491.

[17] Dubernard, J. M, Traeger, J, Neyra, P, Touraine, J. L, Traudiant, D, & Blanc-brunat, N. A new method of preparation of segmental pancreatic grafts for transplantation: Trials in dogs and in man. Surgery (1978). , 84, 633-640.

[18] Land, W, Gebhardt, C, Gall, F. P, Weitz, H, Gokel, M. J, & Stolte, M. Pancreatic duct obstruction with prolamine solution. Transplant Proc (1980). suppl 2): 72-75.

[19] Mcmaster, P, Calne, R. Y, Gibby, O. M, & Evans, D. B. Pancreatic transplantation. Transplant Proc (1980). suppl 2): 58-61.

[20] Sutherland, D. E. R, Goetz, F. C, Rynasiewicz, J. J, Baumgartner, D, White, D. C, Elick, B. A, & Najarian, J. S. Segmental pancreas transplantation from living related and cadaver donors. Surgery (1981). , 90, 159-169.

[21] Sutherland, D. E. Gruessner RWG, Dunn DC, Matas AJ, Humar A, Kandaswamy R, Mauer SM, Kennedy WR, Goetz FC, Robertson RP, Gruessner AC, Najarian JS. Lessons learned from more than 1000 pancreas transplants at a single institution. Ann Surg (2000). , 233, 463-501.

[22] Calne, R. Y, Rolles, K, White, D. J. G, et al. Cyclosporine A initially as the only immunosuppressant in 36 recipients of cadaveric organs : 32 kidneys, 2 pancreas and 2 livers. Lancet (1979). , 2, 1033-1036.

[23] Sutherland, D. E. R. International Human Pancreas and Islet Transplant Registry. Transplant Proc (1980). suppl 2): 229-236.

[24] Land, W, & Landgraf, R. Segmental pancreatic transplantation international workshop Horm Metal Res (1983). , 13, 1-104.

[25] The History of the EuroSPK-Study Group, Squifflet J.P., Malaise J., Van Ophem D., Marcelis V. and Land W.G. Acta Chir Belg, (2008).

[26] Sollinger, H. W, Kamps, D, Cook, K, et al. Segmental pancreatic allotransplantation with pancreatico-cystostomy and high-dose cyclosporine and low-dose prednisone. Transplant Proc (1983). , 15, 2997-99.

[27] Tyden, G, Tibell, A, Sandberg, J, Brattstrom, C, & Groth, C. G. Improved results with a simplified technique for pancreaticoduodenal transplantation with enteric exocrine drainage. Clin Transplant (1996). , 10, 306-309.

[28] Groth, C. G, Collste, H, Lundgren, G, Wilczek, H, Klintmalm, G, Ringden, O, Gunnarsson, R, & Ostman, J. Successful outcome of segmental human pancreatic transplantation with enteric exocrine diversion after modifications in technique.Lancet (1982). , 2, 522-524.

[29] Squifflet, J. P, Sutherland, D. E. R, Rynasiewicz, J. J, Field, M. J, Heil, J. E, & Najarian, J. S. Combined immunosuppressive therapy with cyclosporine A and azathioprine. Transplantation (1982). , 34, 315-318.

[30] Squifflet, J. P, Sutherland, D. E. R, Morrow, C. E, Field, J, & Najarian, J. S. Comparison of rejection of intraportal islet versus immediately vascularized segmental Pancreatic allografts in rats in relation to beta cell mass engrafted. Transplant proc. (1983). , 15, 1344-1346.

[31] Squifflet, J. P, Sutherland, D. E. R, Florack, G, Morrow, C. E, & Najarian, J. S. Physiologic comparison of segmental pancreas and islet transplants in rats. Transplant Proc. (1985). , 17, 378-380.

[32] Squifflet, J. P, Sutherland, D. E. R, Florack, G, & Najarian, J. S. Pancreas Transplantation in the rat: long-term follow-up studies following different methods of management of exocrine drainage. Transplant Proc. (1986). , 18, 1143-1146.

[33] Nghiem, D. D, & Corry, R. J. Technique of simultaneous pancreaticoduodenal transplantation with urinary drainage of pancreatic secretion. Amer J Surg (1987). , 153, 405-406.

[34] Starzl, T. E, Iwatsuki, S, & Shaw, B. W. Jr. , Greene DA, Van Thiel DH, Nalesnik MA, Nusbacher J, Diliz-Pere H, Hakala TR. Pancreaticoduodenal transplantation in humans. Surg Gynecol Obstet (1984). , 159, 265-272.

[35] Tyden, G, Tibell, A, Sandberg, J, Brattstrom, C, & Groth, C. G. Improved results with a simplified technique for pancreaticoduodenal transplantation with enteric exocrine drainage. Clin Transplant (1996). , 10, 306-309.

[36] Sutherland DER, Moudry KC, Najarian JS. Pancreas transplantation. In: Cerilli J, ed. Organ Transplantation and Replacement, Philadelphia: J.B. Lippincott; (1987). , 1987, 535-574.

[37] Delmonico, F. L, Jenkins, R. L, & Auchincloss, H. Jr., Etienne T.J., Russell P.S., Monaco A.B., Cosimi A.B. Procurement of a whole pancreas and liver from the same cadaveric donor. Surgery (1989). , 105, 718-723.

[38] Squifflet, J. P, De Hemptinne, B, Gianello, P, et al. A new technique for en-bloc liver and pancreas harvesting. Transplant Proc (1990). , 22, 2070-71.

[39] Malaise, J, Mourad, M, Van Ophem, D, & Squifflet, J. P. Procurement of Liver and Pancreas Allografts in Donors with Repaced / Accessory right Hepatic Arteries. Transplantation (2005). , 79, 988-991.

[40] Gruessner, A. C, & Sutherland, D. E. R. Pancreas transplant outcomes for United States (US) and non-US cases as reported to the United Network for Organ Sharing (UNOS) and the International Pancreas Transplant Registry (IPTR) as of June 2004. Clin Transplant (2005). , 19, 433-455.

[41] Philosophe, B, Farney, A. C, Schweitzer, E, Colonna, J, Jarrell, B. E, & Bartlett, S. The superiority of portal venous drainage over systemic venous drainage in pancreas transplantation : a retrospective study. Ann Surg (2000). , 234, 689-695.

[42] Deroover, A, Coimbra, C, Detry, O, Van Kemseke, C, Squifflet, J. P, Honore, P, & Meurisse, M. Pancreas graft drainage in recipient duodenum : preliminary experience. Transplantation (2007). , 84, 795-7.

[43] Starzl, T. E, Weil, R, Iwatsuki, S, et al. The use of Cyclosporin A and Prednisone in cadaver transplantation. Surg Gynecol Olstet 180; 151 : 17.

[44] Squifflet, J. P, Sutherland, D. E. R, Field, M. J, Rynasiewicz, J. J, Heil, J. E, & Najarian, J. S. Synergistic immunosuppressive effect of cyclosporine A and azathioprine. Transplant Proc (1983). , 15, 520-522.

[45] Starzl, T. E, Todo, S, Fung, J, Demetris, A. J, Venkatarammn, R, & Jain, A. FK506 for liver, kidney and pancreas transplantation. Lancet (1989). , 2, 1000-1004.

[46] Shaffer, D, Simpson, M. A, Conway, P, et al. Normal pancreas allograft function following simultaneous pancreas kidney transplantation after rescue therapy with tacrolimus (FK506). Transplantation (1995). , 59, 1063-1066.

[47] The Tricontinental Mycophenolate Mofetil Renal Transplantation Study GroupA blinded, randomized clinical trial of mycophenolate mofetil for the prevention of

acute rejection in cadaveric renal transplantation. Transplantation (1996). , 61, 1029-1037.

[48] Malaise, J, Van Ophem, D, & Squifflet, J. P. and the EuroSPK Study Group. Simultaneous Pancreas-Kidney Transplantation in the European Clinical setting : a comprehensive evaluation of long-term outcomes. Nephrol Dial Transplant (2005). Suppl 2) : iiii62., 1.

[49] Gruessner, R. W, Sutherland, D. E. R, Drangstveit, M. B, Troppman, C, & Gruessner, A. C. Use of FK 506 in pancreas transplantation. Transplant Int (1996). Suppl 1): 5251-5257.

[50] Wadstrom, J, Brekke, B, Wramner, L, Ekberg, H, & Tyden, G. Triple versus Quadruple induction immunosuppression in pancreas transplantation. Transplant Proc (1995)., 27, 1317-1318.

[51] Cantarovich, D, Karam, G, Giral- Classe, M, Hourmant, M, Dantal, J, & Blancho, G. Le Normand L. and Soulillou J.P. Randomized comparison of triple therapy and antithymocyte globulin induction treatment after simultaneous pancreas-kidney transplantation. Kidney Int (1998). , 54, 1351-1356.

[52] Lefrancois, N, et al. Prophylactic polyclonal versus monoclonal antibodies in kidney and pancreas transplantation. Transplant Proc (1990). , 22, 632-633.

[53] Fasola, C. G, Hricik, D. E, & Schulak, J. A. Combined pancreas-kidney transplants using quadruple immunosuppressive therapy : a comparison between antilymphoblast and antithymocyte globulins. Transplant Proc (1995). , 27, 3135-3136.

[54] Stratta, R. J, Taylor, R. J, Weide, L. G, Sindhi, R, Sudan, D, Castaldo, P, Cushing, K. A, Frisbie, K, & Radio, S. J. A prospective randomized trial of OKT3 vs ATGAM induction therapy in pancreas transplantation recipients. Transplant Proc (1996). , 28, 917-918.

[55] Kaufman, D. B, Burke, G, Bruce, D, Sutherland, D. E. R, Johnson, C, Gaber, A. O, Merion, R, Schweitzer, E, Marsh, C, Alfrey, E, Leone, J, Concepion, W, Stegall, M, Gores, P, Danovitch, G, Tolzman, D, Scotellaro, P, Salm, K, Keller, A, & Fitzsimmons, W. E. The role of antibody induction in simultaneous pancreas kidney transplant patients receiving tacrolimus + mycophenolate mofetil immunosuppression. Transplantation (2000). S 206.

[56] Kaufman, D. B, & Burke, G. W. III, Bruce D.S., Johnson C.P., Gaber A.O., Sutherland D.E.R., Merion R.M., Gruber S.A., Schweitzer E., Leone J.P., Marsh C.L., Alfrey E., Concepcion W., Stegall M.D., Schulak J.A., Gores P.F., Benedetti E., Smith C., Henning A.K., Kuehnel F., King S., Fitzsimmons W.E. A prospective, randomized, multicenter trial of antibody induction therapy in simultaneous pancreas-kidney transplantation. Am J Transplant. (2003). , 3, 855-864.

[57] Farney, A, Rogers, J, Ashcroft, E, Hartmann, E, Hart, L, Doares, W, Moore, P, Jarett, A, Sundberg, A, Adams, P, & Stratta, R. Alemtuzumab Versus Rabbit Antithymocyte

http://dx.doi.org/10.5772/55347

Globulin Induction in Kidney and Pancreas Transplantation : A prospective Randomized Study. Am J Transplant (2007). Suppl 2) : 233 (330).

[58] Bechstein, W. O, Malaise, J, Saudek, F, et al. Efficacy and safety of tacrolimus compared with cyclosporine microemulsion in primary simultaneous pancreas-kidney transplantation : 1- year results of a large multicentre trial. Transplantation (2004). , 77, 1221-1228.

[59] Pratschke, J, Malaise, J, Saudek, F, Margreiter, R, Arbogast, H, Fernandez-cruz, L, Pisarski, P, Viebahn, R, Peeters, P, Nakache, R, Berney, T, Vanrenterghem, Y, & Bechstein, W. and the EuroSPK Study Group. Sirolimus versus Mycophenolate Mofetil in Tacrolimus based primary simultaneous pancreas-kidney (SPK) Transplantation: 1 year results of a multicentre trial. Transplant Int (2007). Suppl 1): S 270.

Chapter 13

Pregnancy Post Transplant

Rubina Naqvi

Additional information is available at the end of the chapter

http://dx.doi.org/10.5772/54805

1. Introduction

Be a mother is natural desire in female belonging to any community world over. In most cultures, pregnant women have a special status in society and receive particularly gentle care. At the same time, they are subject to expectations that may exert great psychological pressure, such as having to produce a son and heir, and some societies increase female population to fulfill this demand. Rate of ovulation and thus fertility is decreased in female with end stage renal disease, even if pregnancy occurs in dialysis population, only about 23 % were successful till 1980s (European registry). Whereas, after successful renal transplantation not only fertility rate increases with reemergence of better ovulation, but rate of successful childbirth also increases to 70- 80 % (Naqvi 2006,Thopmson 2003).

In this chapter, we aim to review the course of pregnancy and its outcome in renal allograft recipients, in backdrop of different social and cultural values, which we face in this part of world.

2. Status of pregnancy related issues in country

The 2006-07 Pakistan Demographic and Health Survey (PDHS) was undertaken to address the monitoring and evaluation needs of maternal and child health and family planning programs. In 1992-96 marital fertility; reported as 7.6 children per married woman, with a decline of one child over the past decade, PDHS data 2006-2007 reports 6.6 children per married woman. Eight percent of ever-married women report that they had a miscarriage in the past five years; about 2 percent said they had an abortion, and 3 percent reported having a stillbirth. For the most recent five-year period preceding the survey, infant mortality is 78 deaths per 1,000 live births. In interpreting the mortality data, it is useful to keep in mind that sampling errors are quite large. For example, the 95 percent confidence intervals for the under-five mortality estimate of 94 per 1,000 are 86 and 103 per 1,000 indicating that, given the sample size of the 2006-07 PDHS, the true value may fall anywhere between 86 and 103 per 1,000 births. As observed in most studies, the mother's level of education is strongly linked to child survival. Higher levels of educational attainment are generally associated with lower mortality rates because education exposes mothers to information about better nutrition, use of contraceptives to space births, and knowledge about childhood illness and treatment. Similarly, childhood mortality rates decline as the wealth quintile increases. Only 34 percent of births in Pakistan take place in a health facility. Eleven percent is delivered in a public sector health facility and 23 percent in a private facility. Three out of five births (65 percent) take place at home. (Pakistan Demographic and Health Survey 2006-07, National Institute of Population Studies Islamabad, Pakistan. Macro International Inc. Calverton, Maryland USA, published June 2008)

The incidence of low birth weight (defined <2.5 Kg by WHO) in general population reported as high as 31% from South Asia (Badshah, 2008) and 33.9% reported from West Bengal, India. (Pahari 1997)

3. Status of renal transplant in country

The incidence of ESRD in Pakistan and neighboring country India would be expected to be higher since poor socioeconomic status predisposes the population to a number of infection-related glomerulonephritides and the incidence of nephrolithiasis is higher in both countries as they fall in a "stone belt."(Sakhuja, 2003) In addition 6.9 million people in country are affected by diabetes with the International Diabetes Federation estimating that this number will grow to 11.5 million by 2025. With low literacy rate and poor health facilities complications and end organ failure with diabetes and hypertension are more prevalent. If the incidence of ESRD is indeed 100 patients per million population per year, this would mean 18,000 patients for a population of 180 million in Pakistan. There are very few state run dialysis centers and most of them are small units with minimal care facilities, < 5 dialysis stations. The number of patients maintained on dialysis is likely to be < 50 patients per million population since few patients can afford this form of therapy. Sindh Institute of Urology and Transplantation (SIUT) is a semi government organization in country which cater largest population of patients suffering from any kind of kidney ailment. It is running largest hemodialysis and live related renal program not only in country but the region. This organization is unique in terms of providing free health care services to all, be it pre operative preparation, surgical procedure, life long follow up and immunosupression. (www.siut.org) Because of lack of state provided health facilities number of patients seen and treated at this hospital is beyond imagination and for same reason patients do comply during follow up and long term data from this institution is more reliable and representative.

Renal transplant started in country in 1979 from living related donors, initially the activity was as low as < 50 /year, which rose to about 2500 kidney transplants / year in 2007. Most of these were unrelated donor transplants done at private sector. In March 2010 Pakistan was fortunate to have been able to pass a viable and authentic transplant law and activity of unrelated donor transplant decreased. Deceased donor transplant yet has to take off in country, though few have been done from non heart beating donors, organs supplied by Euro-transplant foundation and five local deceased donors.

4. End Stage Renal Disease (ESRD) affecting fertility

Female with ESRD have hypothalamic-pituitary-gonadal dysfunction, associated with high follicle stimulating hormone, luteinizing hormone and prolactin levels. Ovulation is suppressed and mensturation is irregular. Additionally there is sexual dysfunction, suppressed desire and associated psychological factors resulting from chronic ailment. Women on dialysis if conceive present with challenges of worsening of blood pressure controls and anemia, and higher incidences or pre-eclampsia. In 1980, the European Dialysis and Transplant Association reported that only 23% of 115 pregnancies in dialysis ended with surviving infants (European Registry). In 1998, Bagon et al. described a national survey showing a successful outcome in approximately half of the pregnancies in dialysis patients. There are few case series in the new millennium, mainly from single experienced centers, many of which report a successful outcome rate of >70% (Romao 1998, Barua 2008). Our own experience is limited with very poor outcome. (Unpublished)

5. Pregnancy post transplant

Reversal of normal endocrine function has been reported within 4-6 months after renal transplantation. (Ha 1991, Ghafari 2008, McKay 2008) Thus kidney transplant offers best hope for ESRF patients who keen to conceive. First pregnancy in renal transplant recipient was reported by Murray in 1963, since then there are many published reports focusing on impact of pregnancy on renal graft outcome with a conclusion that pregnancy does not have an adverse effect on graft function provided recipient has stable graft function and no adverse event happens during pregnancy. (Table)

6. Optimal timing for pregnancy post transplant

Most transplant centers advise that women can conceive after 2 years of transplant provided graft function is stable i.e. serum creatinine is < 1.5 mg/dl and proteinuria <500 mg/day. At that time, risk of acute rejections generally low, immunosuppression has reduced to minimal, prophylactic anti bacterial and anti viral already completed and women are usually stable. All pregnancies should be considered as high risk and should be managed by multidisciplinary team.

Author	year	Duration	Country	No. of pregnancies reported	outcome
Cararach	1993	25 years	Spain	133	Abortions 10% Preterm 46% Full Term 53%
First	1995	23 years	USA	25	Abortions 3 Live births 22
Saber	1995	25 years	Brazil	25	Abortions 4 Preterm 14 Full term 7
Sturgiss	1996	23 years	UK	18 (compared with 18 non pregnant controls)	Long term graft survival compared in two groups.
Tan	2002	14 years	Singapore	42	Abortions 10 Still birth 1 Ectopic 2
Armenti	2004	14 years	USA NTPR	1125	Abortions 20% Still births 2.5% Ectopic 1% Premature births 53%
Kashanizadeh	2007	6 years	Iran	86	Abortions 24 Full term 62
Sibanda	2007	7 years	UK Transplant Pregnancy Registry	193	Abortions 32 IUDs 3 Ectopic 1 Live Births 149
Draihimh	2008	10 years	5 Middle East Countries	234	Abortions 19.3% Still births 7.3% Live births 74.4%
Naqvi	2010	24 years	Pakistan	68	Abortions 15 Preterm 8 Full term 45 (40 live, 5 IUD or FSB)

Table 1. Published results from world over

7. Risks for mother

Mothers who are renal transplant recipient have certain risks on graft function and survival. Many of renal transplant recipients have hypertension and some degree of renal dysfunction with GFR (Glomerular filtration rate) of not up to the mark, both are affected with pregnancy and blood pressure medications may require alterations and increment in dosages. Some may predispose to pre-eclampsia which is difficult to diagnose especially when few of these women already have some preexisting proteinuria and blood pressure frequently increases after 20th week of gestation. Poorly controlled hypertension can cause preterm delivery.

Women with preexisting graft dysfunction i.e. serum creatinine of > 1.5 mg/dl are at greater risk of developing irreversible worsening of graft function. (Davison 1976) Acute rejection can also occur as blood levels of immunosuppressant may alter with changing volume distribution during pregnancy, this phenomenon is more relevant with calcineurin inhibitors.(Donaldson 1996) However, available reports indicate that rejection rate in pregnant recipient not differ from non pregnant recipients. (Armenti 2004) In our experience of 68 pregnancies in renal transplant recipients, none experienced acute rejection during pregnancy. (Naqvi 2010)

Urinary tract infection rate also increases in pregnant renal transplant recipients, some have reported as high as 42%. (Oliveria 2007)

The transplant recipient is at increased risk for viral infections, therefore, maternal–fetal transmission of infectious agents needs to be considered as a potential risk not only to the mother but also to the fetus. Cytomegalovirus infection is particularly serious because it is associated with hearing/vision loss and mental retardation and can be transmitted from the mother to the fetus through a trans-placental route, as well as during delivery or in breast milk in case mother is feeding to infant. (del Mar Colon 2007, Ross 2006)

Other infections that may pose additional risks in the immunosuppressed mother include toxoplasmosis, primary herpes simplex infection, primary varicella infection, HIV infection, and infection with either hepatitis B or C virus (Gardella 2007, Shiono 2007)

As allograft recipients have increased risk for gestational diabetes, some have recommended that they should be screened every trimester with a 50-g oral glucose load. (del Mar Colon 2007)

8. Risks to fetus

Published reports from UK, USA and European registries persistently highlighted risk of low birth weight of fetus and pre term delivery in renal transplant recipients. (Sibanda 2007, Armenti 2004) Willis et al from Australia reported 44% with low birth weight. (Willis 2000) In our experience we found mean birth weight infants born to transplant recipients was 2.4± 0.57 Kg, with 7 newborns <1.8 Kg. (Naqvi 2010)

Exposure to immunosuppressants: Adrenal insufficiency and thymic hypoplasia have occasionally been described in the infants of transplant recipients, but these problems are unlikely if the dose of prednisone has been decreased to 15 mg (Penn I, 1980). Prednisolone traverses the placenta but 90 % of maternal dose is metabolized within the placenta and not reaching to fetus (Blanford 1977). In addition if pregnancy is occurring after 2 years of transplant, recipient already on very small dose of Prednisolone. Steroids can also aggravate hypertension in mother; mothers are more prone to infections if steroid dose is still high at time of conception. Premature rupture of membrane is another complication reported in relation of steroids. Therefore, it is recommended to get conceive when steroid dose is reduced to minimal. Reports from azathiaprine era through cyclosporine era have not identified specific malformations among infants born to transplant recipients (Armenti 2000). Radioactive labeling studies in humans have shown that 64–93% of Azathioprine administered to mothers appears in fetal blood as inactive metabolites (Sarikoski S, 1973). Cyclosporine metabolism appears to be increased during pregnancy and higher doses may be required to maintain plasma levels in the therapeutic range (Muirhead N, 1992). Data concerning the effect of tacrolimus on pregnancy is scarce. A report of 100 pregnant women (which included all organ transplant recipients), among 84 treated with tacrolimus, 68 progressed to a live birth, with 60% of deliveries being premature (Kainz A, 2000). Teratogenecity of mycophenolate mofetil is not yet confirmed, therefore it is recommended to switch over to azathiaprine in female who are planning to conceive. A study has reported low number of T and B cells at birth in infants born to mothers who were on immunosuppressants, but these were normalized after few months. (Di Paolo 2000) Most published studies related to subject have not described clear cut congenital malformations or autoimmune disorders to children born to transplant recipients, though sporadic case reports which could be related to exposure risk of disease in general population.

9. Breast feeding by transplant recipients

Sparse data is available on recommendations for breast feeding from immunosuppressant mothers. Study published on cyclosporine levels in breast milk reveals cyA levels in milk equivalent to mother's serum. (Moretti 2003) This leads to conclusion that females who are on cyclosporine should not fed their babies, whereas the fact that small amounts of azathiaprine and Prednisolone are excreted in milk (Coulam 1982) can provide an opportunity to consider feeding those babies whose mothers are on these two agents only. French et al. reported the first case of measurement of tacrolimus levels in human milk; suggest that maternal therapy with tacrolimus may be compatible with breast-feeding. (French 2003). Level of Tacrolimus was calculated in breast milk in this case but this was single case report. Data on other drugs is still lacking.

Recommendations

1. preconception counseling is a must
2. good general health for about 2 years after transplant

3. stature compatible with good obstetric outcome
4. no or minimal proteinuria
5. no hypertension or well controlled blood pressure on one agent
6. consider revising anti-hypertensive regimen when pregnant
7. no evidence of recent graft rejection
8. stable graft function with serum creatinine less than 1.5 mg/dl
9. drug therapy at maintenance levels
10. switch immunosuppressants to milder, e.g. MMF should be converted to AZA, Tacrolimus to CyA and Prednisolone in minimal doses
11. once pregnant, transplant recipient should be seen by multidisciplinary team with a frequency of 4 weeks during first trimester and 2 weeks later on.

Author details

Rubina Naqvi*

Nephrology Sindh Institute of Urology and Transplantation (SIUT), Karachi, Pakistan

References

[1] Armenti, V. T, Radomski, J. S, Moritz, M. J, Gaughan, W. J, Hecker, W. P, Lavelanet, A, & Mcgrory, C. H. Coscia LA: Report from the National Transplantation Pregnancy Registry (NTPR): Outcomes of pregnancy after transplantation. Clin.Trans, (2004). , 2004, 103-114.

[2] Bagon, J. A, Vernaeve, H, De Muylder, X, Lafontaine, J. J, Martens, J, & Van Roost, G. Pregnancy and dialysis. Am J Kidney Dis (1998). PubMed: 9590184], 31, 756-765.

[3] Barua, M, Hladunewich, M, Keunen, J, Pierratos, A, Mcfarlane, P, Sood, M, & Chan, C. T. Successful pregnancies on nocturnal home hemodialysis. Clin J Am Soc Nephrol (2008). PMCID: PMC2390936] [PubMed: 18308997], 3, 392-396.

[4] Badshah, S, Mason, L, Mckelvie, K, & Payne, R. Lisboa PJG; Risk factors for low birth weight in public hospitals at Peshawar, NWFP-Pakistan. BMC Public Health. (2008).

[5] Blanford, A. T, & Murphy, B. E. In vitro metabolism of prednisone, dexamethasone, and cortisol by the human placenta. Am J Obstet Gynecol (1977). , 127, 264-7.

[6] Cararach, V, Carmona, F, Monleon, F. J, & Andreu, J. Pregnancy after renal transplantation: 25 years experience in Spain. Br J Obstet Gynaecol. (1993).

[7] Coulam, C. B, Moyer, T. P, Jiang, N. S, & Zincke, H. Breast-feeding after renal transplantation. Transplant Proc (1982)., 14, 605-9.

[8] Donaldson, S, Novotny, D, Paradowski, L, & Aris, R. Acute and chronic lung allograft rejection during pregnancy. Chest (1996)., 110, 293-6.

[9] Di Paolo SSchena A, Morrone LF, Manfredi G, Stallone G, Derosa C, Procino A, Schena FP. Immunologic evaluation during the first year of life of infants born to cyclosporine-treated female kidney transplant recipients: analysis of lymphocyte subpopulations and immunoglobulin serum levels. Transplantation (2000)., 69, 2049-54.

[10] Davison, J. M, & Lind, T. Uldall PR: Planned pregnancy in a renal transplant recipient. Br J Obstet Gynaecol,(1976).

[11] Draihimh, H. A, Ghamdi, G, Moussa, D, Shaheen, F, Mohsen, N, Sharma, U, Stephan, A, Alfie, A, Alamin, M, Haberal, M, Saeed, B, & Kechrid, M. Al-Sayyari A; Outcome of 234 pregnancies in 140 Renal Transplant Recipients from Five Middle Eastern Countries. Transplantation, (2008).

[12] del Mar Colon MHibbard JU: Obstetric considerations in the management of pregnancy in kidney transplant recipients. Adv Chronic Kidney Dis (2007).

[13] European Best Practice Guidelines IVPregnancy in renal transplant recipients. Nephrol Dial Transplant. (2002). suppl.4): 50-5.

[14] French, A. E, Soldin, S. J, Soldin, O. P, et al. Milk transfer and neonatal safety of tacrolimus. Ann. Pharmacotherapy. (2003)., 37(6), 815-8.

[15] First, M. R, Combs, C. A, & Weiskittel, P. Miodovnik M; Lack of Effect of Pregnancy on Renal Allograft Survival or Function. Transplantation. (1995).

[16] Ghafari, A. Sanadgol H; Pregnancy After Renal Transplantation: Ten-Year Single Center Experience. Trans Proc (2008).

[17] Gardella, C. Brown ZA: Managing varicella zoster infection in pregnancy. Cleve Clin J Med 74: 290-296, (2007).

[18] Kainz, A, Harabacz, I, Cowirick, I. S, & Gadgil, S. D. Haqiwara D; Review of the course and outcome of 100 pregnancies in 84 women treated with tacrolimus. Transplantation(2000)., 70, 1718-1721.

[19] Kashanizadeh, N, Nemati, E, Sharifi-bonab, M, Moghani-lankarani, M, Ghazizadeh, S, Einollahi, B, & Lessan-pezeshki, M. Khedmat H; Impact of Pregnancy on the Outcome of Kidney Transplantation. Trans Proceed. (2007).

[20] Moretti, M. E, Sgro, M, Johnson, D. W, Sauve, R. S, Woolgar, M. J, Taddio, A, Verjee, Z, Giesbrecht, E, Koren, G, & Ito, S. Cyclosporine excretion into breast milk. Transplantation (2003)., 75(12), 2144-6.

[21] Muirhead, N, Sabharwal, A. R, Reider, M. J, & Lazarovits, A. I. Hollomby DJ; The outcome of pregnancy following renal transplantation-the experience of a single center.Transplantation(1992). , 54, 429-432.

[22] Naqvi, R. Obstetrics in Renal Transplantation: A Series of Cases of Pregnancy Post Transplant Observed Over 24 Years. WebmedCentral TRANSPLANTATION (2010). WMC00950

[23] Naqvi, R, Noor, H, Ambareen, S, Khan, H, Haider, A, Jafri, N, Alam, A, Aziz, R, Manzoor, K, Aziz, T, Ahmed, E, Akhtar, F, & Naqvi, A. Rizvi A; Outcome of Pregnancy in Renal Allograft Recipients: SIUT Experience. Trans Proceed. (2006).

[24] Oliveira, L. S, Sass, N, Sato, J. L, & Ozaki, K. S. Medina Pestana JO; Pregnancy after renal transplantation: A five year single center experience. Clin Transplant (2007).

[25] Penn, I, Makowski, E. L, & Harris, P. Parenthood following renal transplantation. Kidney Int(1980). , 18, 221-223.

[26] Pahari, K, & Ghosh, A. Study of pregnancy outcome over a period of five years in a postgraduate institute of west Bengal. J Indian Med Assoc. (1997). Jun;, 95(6), 172-4.

[27] Ross, D. S, Dollard, S. C, Victor, M, & Sumartojo, E. Cannon MJ: The epidemiology and prevention of congenital cytomegalovirus infection and disease: Activities of the Centers for Disease Control and Prevention Workgroup. J Womens Health (Larchmt) (2006).

[28] Romão, J. E. Jr, Luders C, Kahhale S, Pascoal IJ, Abensur H, Sabbaga E, Zugaib M, Marcondes M.: Pregnancy in women on chronic dialysis. Nephron (1998). PubMed: 9580542], 78, 416-422.

[29] Successful pregnancies in women treated by dialysis and kidney transplantation: Report from the Registration Committee of the European Dialysis and Transplant AssociationBr J Obstet Gynaecol (1980). PubMed: 7000160], 87, 839-845.

[30] Sibanda, N, Briggs, J. D, Davison, J. M, & Johnson, R. J. Rudge CJ; Pregnancy After Organ Transplantation: A Report From the UK Transplant Pregnancy Registry. Transplantation. (2007).

[31] Sarikoski, S, & Seppala, M. Immunosuppression during pregnancy: transmission of azathioprine and its metabolites from the mother to the fetus. Am J Obstet Gynecol. (1973).

[32] Sakhuja, V, & Sud, K. End stage renal disease in India and Pakistan: burden of disease and management issues. Kidney Int. (2003). Suppl 83):SS118., 115.

[33] Shiono, Y, Mun, H. S, He, N, Nakazaki, Y, Fang, H, Furuya, M, & Aosai, F. Yano A: Maternal-fetal transmission of Toxoplasma gondii in interferon-gamma deficient pregnant mice. Parasitol Int 56: 141-148, (2007).

[34] Sturgiss, S. N. Davison JM; Effect of Pregnancy on the Long-Term Function of Renal Allograft: An Update. Am J Kid Dis. (1996).

[35] Saber LTSDuarte G, Costa JAC, Cologna AJ, Garcia TMP, Ferraz AS; Pregnancy and Kidney Transplantation: Experience in a Developing Country. Am J Kid Dis. (1995).

[36] Thompson, B. C, Kingdon, E. J, Tuck, S. M, & Fernando, O. N. Sweny P; Pregnancy in renal transplant recipients: the Royal Free Hospital experience. Q J Med. (2003).

[37] Tan, P. K, Tan, A. S, Tan, H. K, Vathsala, A, & Tay, S. K. Pregnancy after renal transplantation: experience in Singapore General Hospital. Ann Acad med Singapore, (2002).

[38] Willis, F. R, Findlay, C. A, Gorrie, M. J, Watson, M. A, Wilkinson, A. G, & Beattie, T. J. Children of renal transplant recipient mothers. J Paediatr Child Health. (2000). Jun;, 36(3), 230-5.

Chapter 14

Practical Pharmacogenetics and Single Nucleotide Polymorphisms (SNPs) in Renal Transplantation

María José Herrero, Virginia Bosó, Luis Rojas,
Sergio Bea, Jaime Sánchez Plumed, Julio Hernández,
Jose Luis Poveda and Salvador F. Aliño

Additional information is available at the end of the chapter

http://dx.doi.org/10.5772/54733

1. Introduction

Optimizing balance between therapeutic efficacy and the occurrence of adverse events is the main goal of individualized medicine. This takes even more importance in narrow therapeutic index drugs such as immunosuppressants. These drugs are highly effective in preventing acute graft rejection but tacrolimus, cyclosporine and mycophenolic acid show highly variable pharmacokinetics and pharmacodynamics. Still nowadays the fragile equilibrium between the risks and benefits of immunosuppression makes the management of immunosuppressive pharmacotherapy a challenge.

Therapeutic drug monitoring (TDM) is an essential and indispensable instrument for calcineurin inhibitors dosing, reducing the pharmacokinetic component of variability by controlling drug blood concentrations. But TDM is only possible once the drug is administered and steady state and patient's compliance are achieved, so complementary strategies are needed. Moreover, despite correct TDM, it may take several days or even weeks to reach target blood concentrations. For many patients this time periods are not appropriate in order to achieve sufficiently high concentrations to prevent graft rejection or adverse reactions or, on the other hand, without exposing the patient to excessive toxicity. In this sense, Pharmacogenetics is an interesting approach, helpful to manage immunosuppressant drugs. Changes in expression or function of proteins and enzymes involved in drug transport, metabolism or mechanism of action will cause changes in drug's absorption, metabolism and distribution and, therefore, can lead to changes in the response and toxicity of the treatment. Characterization of these genetic variants, mainly Single Nucleotide Polymorphisms (SNPs), can help to establish effective doses and to minimize adverse effects. Many publications, including our own, have found statistically significant correlations between (SNPs) and tacrolimus and/or cyclosporine dose-corrected blood levels. There are also works correlating certain variants in SNPs with safety and efficacy of the treatment. Even some researchers, working groups and consortia recommend guidelines for initial dosing adjust regarding this SNPs.

Pharmacogenetic tests are becoming cheaper every day, so the cost of performing these assays is getting more assumable, especially when clinically relevant complications are demonstrated. The incorporation of pharmacogenetic studies to the real clinical practice will depend on the creation of well-designed sets of SNPs that, in a cost-effectiveness manner, could correlate clinical complications with genotypes, taking into consideration the whole and complicated treatment in polymedicated patients. Many results contribute to highlight the need of prospective controlled studies, with pharmacogenetic analysis prior to transplantation. This will probably be the critical point for the regulatory agencies to settle the most relevant polymorphisms as validated biomarkers to be widely used in the clinical transplantation setting.

For all this reasons, our aim in this chapter is to provide an easy explanation about what a polymorphism is and an updated view of the most relevant SNPs with evidence of their implication in safety and efficacy of immunosuppressive treatment in renal transplantation. The final goal is to give a summary from basic knowledge to concrete examples that help to improve the medical doctors' knowledge of the clinical impact of Pharmacogenetics in their daily practice.

2. Personalized medicine and pharmacogenetics

The term "Personalized Medicine" was not long ago some "scifi" concept, just expressing the best wishes of the scientific community with an aim of adjusting the pharmacotherapy as best as possible to each single patient. However, in the last years we have seen real advances in this area that have brought to the real clinical practice in most of the "first world" countries, a set of new analysis under the same principle: offering an individualized therapy to each different patient.

In order to understand this new approach in medicine and put it into practice, we necessarily have to take genetics in consideration, and particularly, we have to pay attention to the individual differences that make each patient respond in a different way to a given pharmacological treatment. Here, we arrive to the concepts of Pharmacogenetics and Pharmacogenomics, that can be heard in more and more places each day. They are, and for sure will be, components to be considered in the medical practice. We can define them in many ways, and traditionally they have been employed interchangeably although there are differences between them. They are different but complementary disciplines. The European Medicines Agency, EMA, takes their definitions from The International Conference on Harmonisation of Technical Requirements for Registration of Pharmaceuticals for Human Use (ICH), this is a project with regulatory authorities from Europe, Japan and USA, together with experts from pharmaceuticals that discusses technical and scientific aspects about the products registries. One of its aims is to reach a better harmonization in the interpretation and application of technical guides and requirements for the registries. ICH defines Pharmacogenomics as the study of variations in DNA and RNA characteristics regarding the response to drugs and it defines Pharmacogenetics as a subset inside pharmacogenomics, that studies the variations in the DNA sequence regarding the response to drugs [1-5].

There is another term that is also frequently found: biomarker, genetic or genomic biomarker, whose definition is "a measurable characteristic of DNA and/or RNA which is an indicator of a biological process that can be normal, pathogenic and/or a response to a therapeutic (or other kind) intervention. A genomic biomarker could be, for instance, the measuremente of a gene expression or of its regulation. It can consist in one or more DNA and/or RNA characteristics, as for instance, in DNA, its single nucleotide polymorphisms (SNPs); the variability in the repetition of short sequences; the haplotypes; DNA modifications as methilation; the deletions or insertions of a single nucleotide; the copy number variation; or the cytogenetic rearangements as translocations, duplications, deletions or inversions. Regarding RNA, it could be a particular trait of its sequence; the levels of expression; the processing (as splicing and editing); or the levels of microRNAs. A deeper explanation of some of these terms will be done in the next paragraph.

The aim of pharmacogenomics is to identify the most important genetic elements in the instauration and/or evolution of a pathological process in order to create new strategies for drug evaluation and optimization of the drug development process. These are usually high throughput studies, regarding the simple number and statistical signification but also very exigent with the study subject: the final goal is finding correlation with the disease at a genomic level, not with one single nucleotide but with genes or groups of related genes instead. On the other side, pharmacogenetics studies the influence of genetic factors on the activity of a drug, making attention in concrete changes inside a gene that somehow has already been postulated as a candidate gene, by previous knowledge or by pharmacogenomic studies. Subject of pharmacogenetic studies are especially, the variants in genes related with transport and metabolism of drugs, with the aim that specific drugs can be given to specific groups of genetically defined (or "stratified") patients [6, 7].

To summarize, pharmacogenetics has to be considered as one of the mainstays of personalized medicine, which will let us correlate good or bad response to a drug in a specific population with genetic aspects. It will also let us know which drugs will offer greater therapeutic benefit or lower risk of adverse reactions development for a given population.

3. What are genetic polymorphisms?

We also must review some other basic concepts in genetics and, extensively, pharmacogenetics in order to understand the following information. The most relevant one is Polymorphism, which is defined as a mendelian monogenic character that appears in the population with the presence of more than one allele in the same genetic locus. Applying the term to pharmacogenetics, it makes reference to the different alleles or variants of a gene related to a drug interaction with the body. The frequency of the less common allele in the population must not be higher than 1%. The two main groups of genetic polymorphisms are Single Nucleotide Polymorphisms (SNPs) and Lenght Polymorphisms (repetitions of nucleotide groups). The first group represents 90% of genetic variability in our genome, and each nucleotide change appears approximately in 1 every 1000 nucleotides. Length polymorphisms represent more extensive changes in the DNA sequence and approximately are the remaining 10% of polymorphic variability in our genomes.

The NCBI SNP database (www.ncbi.nlm.nih.gov/snp) contains all the SNPs described, arranged by their Reference number, which names all SNPs starting with the letters "rs", followed by a number code, but also including some classical names that had already been given to some SNPs. By clicking on a SNP code, one can get more information and several links, one of them is called "diversity" and shows the different allele frequencies found depending on the study and especially, depending on the sample's ethnicity. There are polymorphic sites with allelic frequencies quite well conserved amongst different ethnicities, but others have relevant differences and we must always pay attention to this point.

The exact biological difference in meaning between "polymorphism" and "mutation" is not always clearly defined. The term "mutation" is classically associated with pathological significance, while "polymorphism" usually refers to a genetic change without health consequences. The problem is that "polymorphism" has also been employed to describe mostly any newly described genetic variant, without having studied it enough to know if it has a pathological consequence or not. The international research project 1000 genomes (www.1000genomes.org) has been a great effort to sequence the whole genome of a thousand different people, so we are still attending to well quantified frequencies of genetic variants, that in some cases will still be measured in not sufficient people and so, knowing exactly the population frequencies of all our genome variants is still a challenge, moreover due to the fact that the frequencies vary amongst different human ethnicities. In conclusion, we must be cautious when interpreting the term "polymorphism" and not assume that it is just a genetic change without any biological consequences, as it may has not been well characterized yet.

The genetic variants that can influence the behavior of a drug in the body, are mainly related to the interaction of the drug with the receptor/ligand involved in their pharmacological action and/or with the systems involved in its pharmacokinetic process of absorption, distribution, metabolism and excretion. So, transport, metabolism and drug target genes are the three groups of genes whose polymorphisms are of interest in pharmacogenetics. In a very simplistic way, an individual carrying a significant polymorphic variant will suffer from different effects from those suffered by the individuals carrying the "normal" variant at the same polymorphic site, but just in the case of being treated with the particular drug affected by that variant. If that individual is not treated with that drug, he may not manifest any effects related to that polymorphism.

http://dx.doi.org/10.5772/54733

Other relevant concepts to understand pharmacogenetics are Haplotipe and Linkage Disequilibrium (LD). Haplotype refers to those alleles of a chromosome, or part thereof, which are physically close and that tend to be inherited together. In our field, it is especially important that more and more frequently the research is focused not on single SNPs, but on combinations of them, forming haplotypes. Although many research has been simplified, studying SNPs analyzed one by one, the real biological significance of these genetic changes must be seen in the resulting effect of groups of SNPs, since the individual effects of each one can be enhanced, reduced or offset by the effects of others. In addition, the linkage disequilibrium, is the situation in which some alleles are present together in a higher frequency than expected, due to its close location in the chromosomes. This is important in SNPs research, since one can study a SNP that is well know and easy to determine, instead of studying another SNP linked to the first, that is more difficult to assess, and the results can be correlated. For instance, in some cases one SNP, with not known biological significance, is correlated with certain clinical consequence, and after a deeper research it is found that actually that first SNP is in fact in linkage disequilibrium with another SNP, unknown or non studied before, that is directly related to that clinical consequence.

In relation to these concepts, we can now understand that SNPs that have not got a clearly studied functional meaning, for example they do not alter the amino acid sequence or are not regulatory in intronic regions, are usually included in research projects. Maybe these SNPs are linked to others that are not taken into consideration but that do produce a direct effect on the gene product. These studies will be completed when information of LD blocks, provided for instance in public consultation databases as HapMap (www.hapmap.org), would be included. These final integrative approaches require powerful statistical and *in silico* analysis, correlating the large amount of information obtained.

4. Genes and drugs

After understanding the basic concepts, we can now enter the approach to the best known gene-drug relationships. There are currently different reference sources that help us in this welter of information, such as the aforementioned HapMap project, the SNP database of NCBI and, to our knowledge, the best pharmacogenetics website which is the Pharmacogenomics Knowledge Base, PharmGKB (www.pharmgkb.org). This latter website, is a very intuitive way of learning and consulting about gene-drug relationships, by performing searches based on gene, SNP, drug or disease; with research and clinical information, and lots of links to external related sites. There we can find a table of the "well-known drug-gene pharmacogenomics associations" which represents the drugs whose relationship with some polymorphic gene has been clearly defined in the literature and is academically accepted, based on extensive reviews of all available information.

The United States Food and Drug Administration (FDA, www.fda.gov) also publishes a list of drugs where a genetic test is recommended or mandatory for the drug administration, explaining which section of the drug label has the genetic-related information.

DRUG	BIOMARKER	DRUG	BIOMARKER
Abacavir	HLA-B*5701	Irinotecan	UGT1A1
Aripiprazole	CYP2D6	Isosorbide and Hydra-lazine62	NAT1, NAT2
Arsenic Trioxide	PML/RARα	Ivacaftor	CFTR
Atomoxetine	CYP2D6	Lapatinib	Her2/neu
Atorvastatin	LDL receptor	Lenalidomide	Chromosome 5q
Azathioprine	TPMT	Letrozole	ER &/ PgR receptor
Boceprevir	IL28B	Maraviroc	CCR5
Brentuximab Vedotin	CD30	Mercaptopurine	TPMT
Busulfan	Ph Chromosome	Metoprolol	CYP2D6
Capecitabine	DPD	Modafinil	CYP2D6
Carbamazepine	HLA-B*1502	Nilotinib	Ph Chromosome, UGT1A1
Carisoprodol	CYP2C19	Nortriptyline	CYP2D6
Carvedilol	CYP2D6	Omeprazole	CYP2C19
Celecoxib	CYP2C9	Panitumumab	EGFR, KRAS
Cetuximab	EGFR, KRAS	Pantoprazole	CYP2C19
Cevimeline	CYP2D6	Paroxetine	CYP2D6
Chlordiazepoxide and Amitriptyline	CYP2D6	Peginterferon alfa-2b	IL28B
Chloroquine	G6PD	Perphenazine	CYP2D6
Cisplatin	TPMT	Pertuzumab	Her2/neu
Citalopram	CYP2C19, CYP2D6	Phenytoin	HLA-B*1502
Clobazam	CYP2C19	Pimozide	CYP2D6
Clomiphene	Rh genotype	Prasugrel	CYP2C19
Clomipramine	CYP2D6	Pravastatin	ApoE2
Clopidogrel	CYP2C19	Propafenone	CYP2D6
Clozapine	CYP2D6	Propranolol	CYP2D6
Codeine	CYP2D6	Protriptyline	CYP2D6
Crizotinib	ALK	Quinidine	CYP2D6
Dapsone	G6PD	Rabeprazole	CYP2C19
Dasatinib	Ph Chromosome	Rasburicase	G6PD
Denileukin Diftitox	CD25	Rifampin, Isoniazid, and Pyrazinamide	NAT1; NAT2
Desipramine	CYP2D6	Risperidone	CYP2D6
Dexlansoprazole	CYP2C19, CYP1A2	Sodium Phenylacetate and Sodium Benzoate	UCD (NAGS; CPS; ASS; OTC; ASL; ARG)
Dextromethorphan and Quinidine	CYP2D6	Sodium Phenylbutyrate	UCD (NAGS; CPS; ASS; OTC; ASL; ARG)
Diazepam	CYP2C19	Tamoxifen	ER receptor
Doxepin	CYP2D6	Telaprevir	IL28B
Drospirenone and Ethinyl Estradiol	CYP2C19	Terbinafine	CYP2D6
Erlotinib	EGFR	Tetrabenazine	CYP2D6
Esomeprazole	CYP2C19	Thioguanine	TPMT
Everolimus	Her2/neu	Thioridazine	CYP2D6

http://dx.doi.org/10.5772/54733

DRUG	BIOMARKER	DRUG	BIOMARKER
Exemestane	ER &/ PgR receptor	Ticagrelor	CYP2C19
Fluorouracil	DPD	Tolterodine	CYP2D6
Fluoxetine	CYP2D6	Tositumomab	CD20 antigen
Fluoxetine and Olanzapine	CYP2D6	Tramadol and Acetaminophen	CYP2D6
Flurbiprofen	CYP2C9	Trastuzumab	Her2/neu
Fluvoxamine	CYP2D6	Tretinoin	PML/RARα
Fulvestrant	ER receptor	Trimipramine	CYP2D6
Galantamine	CYP2D6	Valproic Acid	UCD (NAGS; CPS; ASS; OTC; ASL; ARG)
Gefitinib	EGFR	Vemurafenib	BRAF
Iloperidone	CYP2D6	Venlafaxine	CYP2D6
Imatinib	C-Kit, Ph Chromosome, PDGFR, FIP1L1-PDGFRα	Voriconazole	CYP2C19
Imipramine	CYP2D6	Warfarin	CYP2C9, VKORC1
Indacaterol	UGT1A1		

Table 1. FDA Pharmacogenomic biomarkers in drug labels (adapted from www.fda.gov)

There is certainly a lot of work done, but there is still much to do. Today, there are many publications and many research articles in the area, and the field is growing exponentially, but most of these studies reflect data from very specific conditions, where sets of patients with convenient features and sometimes far from the clinical reality, where included. It is necessary to validate the actual utility of pharmacogenetics in routine medical practice with serious, well-designed studies [8].

4.1. Genes and drugs in transplantation

In the pharmacogenetics of transplantation, as in other therapeutic areas, three groups of genes specifically involved in the response to immunosuppressive therapy have been identified: the genes encoding drug transporter proteins, inward or outward of the cells; the genes encoding metabolic enzymes involved in drug biotransformation and, finally; those encoding receptors or drug targets. Although the great majority of immunosuppressive drugs are transported and metabolized by a limited set of enzymes which mostly are known genes, the interpretation of the results observed in transplanted patients is complicated in many times. One reason for this is that these patients are highly subjected to polytherapy, and so interactions, both pharmacokinetic and pharmacodynamic, may have great significance and may condition the response to treatment. Another important aspect to consider when interpreting the observed response is the fact that each patient actually contains two different genetic entities: the donor and the recipient. This phenomenon is particularly relevant when the transplanted organs are the liver or the kidney. In these types of transplantation, it must be considered that the drugs administered to the recipient will be metabolized or excreted by the transplanted organ from the donor. In fact, more and more studies in transplantation pharmacogenetics consider both the donor and recipient genotypes to evaluate the response to treatment [9-12].

Moreover, one of the main problems of pharmacogenetic studies is the difficulty to recruit the number of patients needed to achieve sufficient statistical power and demonstrate conclusively the existence of significant clinically relevant differences according the different genotypes, that is, according to the different alleles or variants of a polymorphic site. This is due to the uneven distribution of allele frequencies in the population, which makes it difficult to collect a large enough number of individuals to study minor genotypes. Furthermore, the distribution of allelic frequencies in some genes varies according to ethnicity so, for instance, the expected frequencies of each allele of a polymorphic site in the Caucasian population are not the same as in the Asian. The expected effects of each allelic variant are presumably the same, but the ease for recruiting different genotype patients is not.

Figure 1 shows, in summary, an integrator scheme with the best known genes encoding transporter proteins and enzymes involved in the metabolism of several drugs commonly used in transplantation.

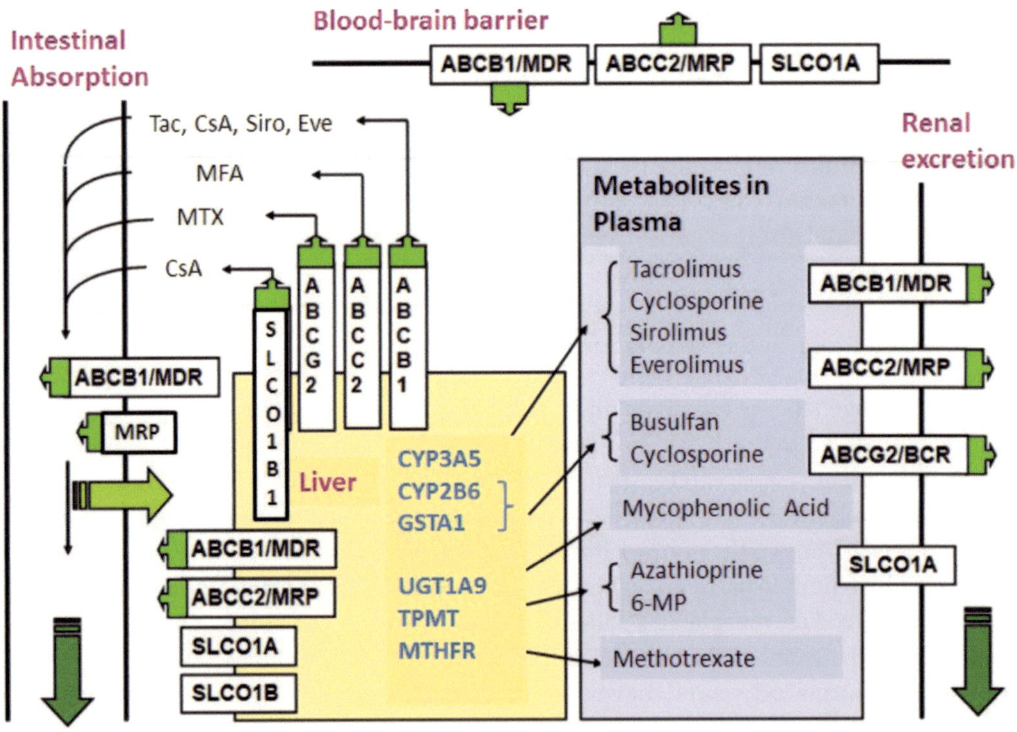

Figure 1. Integrative scheme of pharmacogenetic genes related to transport and metabolism of immunosuppressive drugs for transplantation. (Adapted from ref. 13, ©Astellas Pharma S.A. y Master Line & Prodigio S.L.). The drawing shows a broad view of the location and influence of metabolic enzymes and transporters on the main immunosuppressive drugs used in transplantation. The integrated view of many of the genetic factors that influence the achievement of therapeutic and stationary blood levels, should allow a better interpretation of pharmacogenetic data and also, help improve the safe and effective use of medication.

http://dx.doi.org/10.5772/54733

4.2. Pharmacogenetic examples in renal transplantation

Pharmacogenetic information of immunosuppressants in renal transplantation is mainly related to Tacrolimus, Cyclosporine and Mycophenolic Acid. Sirolimus, Everolimus and Corticoids are also being studied but to a much lesser extent, so we will focus here on the most consolidated conclusion about the first three drugs.

The first two, being both Calcineurin Inhibitors (CNI), share their mechanism of action and so, share transporters, metabolism enzymes and targets and therefore, they also share pharmacogenetic results in most of the cases. The fact that they are both subject of a controlled therapeutic drug monitoring, with "in some way" standardized blood measuring methods, has allowed the publication of many works dealing with correlations between drug levels and polymorphisms [14-23]. To a lesser extent, there are also many works correlating drug adverse effects with SNPs [24-28]. The therapeutic drug monitoring of mycophenolic acid is not as followed as for CNIs, as there is not such a clear consensus about the effects of different blood levels in the possible drug related toxicity. However, many efforts have also been done in the pharmacogenetic studies of this drug [29-36], as it is widely employed in combination with tacrolimus or cyclosporine.

The most consensuated genes regarding polymorphic effects on these three immunosuppressants are shown in table 2.

DRUG	GENE	SNP	Effect
Tacrolimus Cyclosporine	ABCB1 *transport*	rs1045642 C>T; 3435 C>T	C: higher transporter activity, less drug absorption T: lower transporter activity, more drug absorption
	CYP3A5 *metabolism*	rs776746 A>G; *1 (A), *3 (G)	Allele *1 carriers have functional enzyme and require higher drug doses to reach target levels. Allele *3 carriers have nonfunctional allele, the enzyme is not metabolizing the drug, so they need lower doses
	CYP3A4 *metabolism*		Implications not clearly defined
Mycophenolic Acid	UGT1A9 *metabolism*	-275 T>A -2152 C>T	-275A and -2152T: Increased gene expression, lower exposition to MFA and acute rejection in patients with fixed dose MFA+Tac
	ABCC2 *transport*	C-24T C3972T	Implications not clearly defined
	IMPDH1 *target*	rs2278293	Higher risk of leucopenia, lower risk of BPAR
	IMPDH2 *target*	3757 T>C	C: higher IMPDH activity, higher incidence of BPAR (biopsy-confirmed acute rejection)
	SLCO1B1 *transport*	*5	Implications not clearly defined

Table 2. Most studied SNPs related to Tacrolimus, Cyclosporine and Mycophenolic Acid in Renal Transplantation.

As shown in the table, even in these SNPs that are the most extensively studied, the clinical implications are not always well established. Many more other SNPs are currently under research consideration, being what we can call "candidates" to have a clinical meaning. Virtually, every polymorphism of a gene implicated in a drug's route of transport, metabolism or mechanism of action is a potential candidate to be investigated. Especially if the polymorphism is known to have a biological consequence on the gene product as for instance, if it is a polymorphism producing a premature STOP codon or a relevant aminoacid change.

Returning to the SNPs in table 2, we will pay attention now to ABCB1 and CYP3A5 most relevant results. In Figure 2, we can see a schematic example of what happens in the intestine epithelial cells, according to the SNP rs1045642 C>T (also known as 3435 C>T) in ABCB1 gene. This gene codes for glicoprotein P (gp-P)which is an adenosine triphosphate-dependent transporter, that pumps many endogenous substances and also xenobiotics, as drugs, outside of the cell. It is specifically expressed in the intestine, liver and kidney, amongst others, and also in several types of leukocytes so it is postulated to function as a protective barrier by actively extruding different compounds out of the cell, into the gut lumen, bile or urine. The expression of ABCB1 in the kidney plays an important role in the renal elimination of metabolic waste products and toxins. It seems like after renal injury, ABCB1 expression is upregulated, which may represent an adpative response in the renal regeneration process [37]. Parallelly, it has been shown that treatment with CNI induces ABCB1 expression both *in vivo* and *in vitro*, which could serve to protect the kidney from the injurious effects of CNIs by facilitating their extrusion. If we add to this, the polymorphic influence shown in figure 2, we can better understand that a failure to adequately upregulate ABCB1 expression or a constitutively low expression in renal cells (as for instance due to 3435 TT variant), could lead to intrarenal accumulation of CNIs and predispose patients to the occurrence of CNI-related nephrotoxicity [38].

Specifically, in renal transplantation, it has been found a correlation between the genotype of donors TT at this SNP and cyclosporine nephrotoxicity [40], while no consistent relationships were found according to the same SNP in the recipient.

Regarding CYP3A5, there is more statistical evidence, especially regarding its impact on CNIs blood levels and these findings have led to some clinical recommendations, as we will see in the next paragraph. Inside the CYP 450 family, the CYP3A subfamily metabolizes more than 50% of all drugs that are currently in use [41]. CYP3A5 is expressed in the small intestine and the liver but also in the kidney.

One of the most relevant studies regarding CYP3A5 SNP rs776746 A>G (*1 (A), *3 (G)) is the one published by Thervet et al. in 2010 [23]. It is a prospective randomized clinical trial that demonstrates the usefulness of this SNP determination before the first tacrolimus dose in renal transplantation. In this study, the pharmacokinetic parameters were correlated with the recipients' genotype and two arms were constructed, one with the classical management of the patients, adjusting tacrolimus doses according to TDM; and the second arm, where the initial dose was chosen according to a previous genetic analysis to include the patients in "CYP3A5 expresser" or "CYP3A5 non-expresser" cathegories. The expressers were given an initial 0.25mg/kg dose and the non-expressers 0.15mg/kg. As a result, the genetically driven dosage was associated with an earlier obtention of tacrolimus concentrations inside the therapeutic range, also with fewer dose adjustments. Also, it was demonstrated that in the first arm, patients with genotype *1 needed double tacrolimus dose to reach the target levels, as

http://dx.doi.org/10.5772/54733

compared to those patients that were *3. Moreover, there are also consistent data in pediatric renal transplant recipients [42].

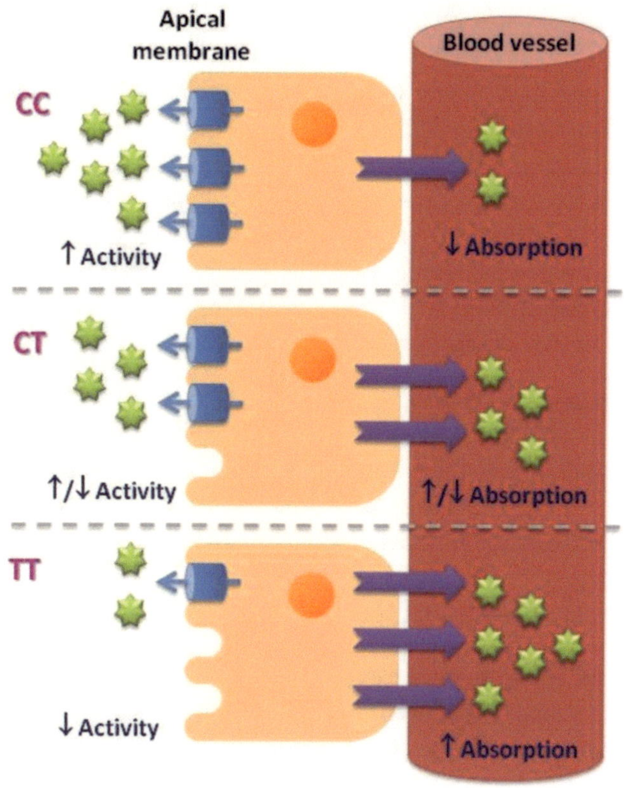

Figure 2. Influence of the functional activity of glycoprotein-P (transporter in apical membrane) in the transport of tacrolimus (green stars) in the intestine epithelium. The diagram shows the different degree of drug absorption due to variations in ABCB1/MDR1 polymorphic site rs1045642. Individuals with TT variant have a decreased transporter activity and hence greater absorption efficiency. CC variant causes more expulsion out of the cell, which decreases absorption. (Figure adapted from ref. 39)

Just as a final remark, we cannot forget to mention the great importance of drug interactions. Although it is not the subject of this chapter, and we are not going to get into it, we just wanted to point here that drug interactions can mask even genetic variations in the clinical practice.

5. Regulatory aspects and final conclusions

5.1. Clinical practice recommendations

We have only seen, with a little bit of detail, two of the SNPs that could actually be influencing the pharmacologic treatment in renal transplantation. And with these two SNPs, only one,

CYP3A5 rs776746, has reached some kind of clinical recommendations. These have not been adopted by any of the regulatory agencies FDA nor EMA, but they already have a strong evidence as to be considered by expert doctors in the area.

The 3rd European Science Foundation- University of Barcelona (ESF-UB) Conference in Biomedicine on Pharmacogenetics and Pharmacogenomics, held in June 2010 in Spain, published a summary of their practical recommendations [43] which include the explained tacrolimus results. They recommend CYP3A5 rs776746 genotyping prior to grafting as it could help to reach steady state plasma tacrolimus concentrations earlier, and therefore prevent overdose (risk of nephrotoxicity) or underdose (risk of acute graft rejection). This recommendation is mainly based on Thervet's publication [23] and suggests the introduction of tacrolimus at 0.15 mg/kg/day when the recpient's genotype is *3/*3, at 0.20 mg/kg/day when it is *3/*1, and at 0.25 mg/kg/day when it is *1/*1; always taking into consideration that the patients will also require the regular TDM.

The Dutch Pharmacogenetics Working Group Guideline from the Royal Dutch Pharmacists Association have also evaluated therapeutic dose recommendations for tacrolimus based on our CYP3A5 SNP [44] and have found evidence to support an interaction between the drug and the gene. However, they do not make dosing recommendations adducing that in dutch transplantation hospitals, the tacrolimus dose is titrated in response to TDM.

5.2. What is a meta-analysis and what is the need of them?

The number of publications is increasing every day in an accelerated manner to limit the ability of researchers and clinicians to assess critically and to assume the results of the studies. This, added to the fact that the knowledge about something is not born due to a single article, but to the integration of many, requires conducting systematic reviews of available evidence, of which there are two types:

- Qualitative systematic reviews, where evidence is presented descriptively
- Quantitative systematic reviews or meta-analyses, which combine the results in a single endpoint and determine the causes of the variations between studies.

Meta-analysis is a summary of different qualitative and quantitative studies (usually randomized controlled trials) that evaluate one aspect whose results are combined using statistic resources to determine the directionality of the effect and the causes of variability between studies. It is the gold standard tool to assess the consistency of an evidence in the effect of a particular intervention, especially when studies are heterogeneous and discordant, when studies evaluating outcomes affect a low number of patients (as it happens when reporting adverse events), when conducting new clinical trials is expensive or when we want to know the existence of patient subgroups responding differently to the intervention analyzed.

- In this way the results allow us to:
- Plan future clinical trials on a related topic.

- Quantify publication bias (as many studies fail to be published because their results are not significant) [45, 46].
- Provide evidence to generate new hypotheses.
- Decide whether further clinical trials are needed on the subject.
- Help to document the approval of the use of interventions by regulatory agents and also expand the knowledge to academics.

Calculate the sample size needed for future clinical trials about a similar topic.

Conducting such studies is cumbersome, it is really time-consuming, requires complex methodological knowledge and its performance is not free of trouble. The main difficulties are the presence of a small number of previously existing studies, the fact that the selected studies to be analysed are usually very heterogeneous and difficult to be combined, and in many of them the necessary information is absent or with low methodological quality. However, meta-analysis studies are low-cost and have high impact.

However, we must be careful as the name "meta-analysis" does not ensure a quality review and readers should critically evaluate it before accepting its results, for which there are currently accessible guides [47, 48]. Its validity largely depends on the quality of the included studies and the absence of bias in its execution [49]. The studies analyzed in the meta-analysis are mostly randomized trials, which are those that offer the best evidence, but there are scenarios where the information comes only from observational studies [50], as studies on etiological hypotheses or adverse events. This represents a challenge as this type of design has a higher risk of bias and lack of essential information for the integration of studies [51]. Furthermore, the inclusion of studies with a large heterogeneity or variability between them, hinders the results interpretation [52], requires the knowledge of statistical tools for proper interpretation [53] and one must know that it is a limitation for the applicability of the results. Meta-analysis is a retrospective process, so it is susceptible to errors of this type of design. It could have biases in any of its stages: in the search and selection of studies, analysis and synthesis of information.

The meta-analysis is the highest level of evidence and summarizes the studies available about a particular matter in a reliable way. Its implementation has its difficulties and limitations, so methodological rigor is required to help reduce the risk of bias and a critical and cautious view of its results.

As far as we know, two meta-analyses have been published regarding clinical implications of CYP3A5 and CNIs in renal transplantation. One is about tacrolimus [54] and its conclusion agrees with the data explained about CYP3A5 expressers/non-expressers dose requirements. The other one deals with cyclosporine [55], and also concludes that there is an association between our SNP and cyclosporine dose-adjusted concentration, where patients carrying *3/*3 genotype will require a lower dose of the drug to reach target levels, compared with *1/*1 or *1/*3 carriers.

5.3. Barriers for the clinical application of Pharmacogenetics

The introduction in the medical practice of new strategies is always difficult, among other reasons due to economic factors and the inertia of much of the professional sector, which is typically conservative. But in the particular case of pharmacogenetics, and genomics in general, there are other social factors that we will now comment, that hinder the implementation of these new techniques.

Contrary to what has usually happened in other fields of biomedicine, in this one we have the paradox that technological progress has gone faster than the advancement of knowledge. Today's technology platforms can just bring in a few days the data that used to take months or even years to achieve. The advances in knowledge of the human genome sequence have been really quick, especially since in February 2001 Nature and Science published simultaneously the results of the Human Genome Project. The enormous progress in data collection through technology could not be accompanied by a corresponding advance in the association of the data with biological effects or implications for medical treatments [56]. A great amount of research investment is still necessary in order to understand and take advantage of this huge avalanche of data.

Clearly, every great discovery is preceded by circumstances that make it possible, and for the deciphering of the human genome, and overall progress of genomics, including Pharmacogenetics-omics, milestones were achieved with the confluence of three fundamental aspects: the opportunity of high performance technologies (high throughput), the multidisciplinary working groups and the development of bioinformatics.

Investment in technology and the big bet of different private companies have been crucial for the rapid performance rate of genetic sequences data collection. In fact, as we have already mentioned, more and more individual human sequences have been obtained, demonstrating the variability of our genome and even small errors in the initial sequencing generations. Anyway, such data cannot give us more information than little white dots on a blackboard, with sometimes very specific information on diseases or even just some predispositions, but little conclusive information for the moment. This is mainly due to two major keys in genetics and biology: the first is that rarely a single gene is responsible for a disease, usually diseases result from the interaction of many genes, with particular variants or defects. The second key is that our phenotype is not an exclusive product of the expression of our genes, instead it is the gene-environment combination. In most cases, the weight of each of the two components in a given disease is difficult to decipher.

Moreover, not only the gene-environment relationship offers serious knowledge gaps, but also the relationships between genes. Everyone knows that life is the result of Systems Biology, waterfalls of activation or repression of components that influence each other. That is the kind of approach that we have to tend to, once we have more experience and results in reductionist studies. Biological systems are complex networks of thousands of routes, many of which are interconnected, biosynthetic pathways, signal transduction pathways, routes of regulating the expression of genes. The integration, representation and modeling of the interconnections of biological information analysis require global, systemic analyses. This is how we enter the era

http://dx.doi.org/10.5772/54733

of "omics" referring to global studies, "whole set", where we pass from the analysis of specific phenomena to the search of the interrelationship of phenomena, where we must integrate not only genomics but also proteomics (the sequences and expression patterns of all proteins), metabolomics (identification and quantification of all metabolites) and even transcriptomics (sequences and expression patterns of all transcripts) and to close the circle, reach the interactome (full set of physical interactions between proteins, DNA sequences and RNA). The review of T. Manolio [57] is very useful for understanding the current situation of genomic studies.

In relation to this need for training and knowledge, we will introduce one of the biggest problems facing the Pharmacogenetics and Pharmacogenomics application in our society: as in any area of knowledge that directly affects Health and Drugs, clinical applications arising from Pharmacogenetics should be well regulated and should be given proper use. Both the patient and the doctor must be well informed of the scope and meaning of the data that can be obtained. It is crucial to know what to expect of a pharmacogenetic analysis, realistically, without creating false hopes.

It is said that in a couple of years, the cost for sequencing a complete human genome will be about 1,000$. It is not difficult to imagine that there will soon be many patients who will consult their physicians with their genome sequence in their hand, asking whether they will have cancer or Alzheimer's or not, according to what is written in their genes. Are we prepared to deal with these situations? The New England Journal of Medicine published a series of articles and editorials addressing these issues on the occasion of the first decade of the publication of the human genome, with very interesting articles written by experts in the field, as the great review of Collins and coworkers [58].

And, if we are not prepared for this new tool yet, how will we discriminate between reliable and fraudulent information? Who should be responsible for setting common guidelines to drive us in making decisions about which tests are acceptable and which are not? We think that the key are not only the regulatory agencies, which do not always agree with each other when defining whether a marker is valid or not. However, other agents, Industry, and especially the scientific societies, should be the ones to influence education on these issues and serve as a reference under the most rigorous scientific method.

At the academic level, many efforts have been demanded to these disciplines because they generated great expectations that were not met as fast as expected. Now, regulatory agencies require a greater statistical significance than that of many other types of studies, to accept the validity of a new marker. That is why well designed clinical studies and meta-analyses are necessary for the agencies to accept new validated markers. We must also be aware of the alarm triggered in relation to commercial proposals that are clearly misleading the consumer. Just a quick search on the Internet to realize that they are on sale genotyping chips that offer scientifically implausible predictions, such as predicting vulnerability to sudden death in athletes, obesity, the ability to succeed at school, etc. The U.S. committee SACGHS (the Secretary's Advisory Committee on Genetics, Health and Society) has already issued several reports concerning with the issue and stressing the need to regulate this area of biomedicine in order to not leave the consumer completely unprotected. There are two excellent publications from Dr. JP Evans, illustrating this problem [59, 60].

5.4. The economical impact

Pharmacogenetics must allow not only the money saving through the prevention of a large number of side effects derived from the use of unsuitable drugs, but also it has to reduce the money spending on unnecessary drugs. In the U.S. there is an incidence of adverse effects of 6.2-6.7% of hospitalized patients, representing two million adverse drug reactions per year [61]. Of these, 0.15 to 0.3% are fatal, leading to about 100,000 deaths annually [62]. In Europe, the data are similar.

Today, there are still few studies on the cost-effectiveness of pharmacogenetic studies, although considerable efforts have been made, including regulatory authorities [63-65]. We cannot forget that everyday genotyping platforms are more compact and economical and, as mentioned, even the whole genome sequencing of a patient will have an assumable cost, so it is not difficult to imagine that the benefits will overcome the costs and that the balance will be tilted towards the realization of these studies [66]. A practical example is found in the studies of mutations in the K-ras gene in colorectal cancer patients to decide about treatment with Cetuximab, which are rendering large amounts of data regarding the savings thanks to the genotyping of patients, avoiding ineffective treatment in 40% of cases.

In conclusion, the economical and clinical benefits of pharmacogenetics are day by day, clearly surpassing its costs. We need to have especialized personnel, to help us know how to interpret the pharmacogenetic information, always in close contact with clinicians and research advances. We cannot obviate this new and real tool for the benefit of our patients' health.

Author details

María José Herrero[1*], Virginia Bosó[1], Luis Rojas[1,2], Sergio Bea[3], Jaime Sánchez Plumed[3], Julio Hernández[3], Jose Luis Poveda[4] and Salvador F. Aliño[5]

*Address all correspondence to: maria.jose.herrero@uv.es

1 Unidad de Farmacogenética, Instituto Investigación Sanitaria La Fe, Servicio de Farmacia, Hospital Universitario y Politécnico La Fe, Valencia, Spain

2 Hospital clínico de la Pontificia Universidad Católica de Chile, Dpto. Medicina Interna, y Centro de Investigaciones Clínicas, Chile

3 Servicio Nefrología, Hospital Universitario y Politécnico La Fe, Valencia, Spain

4 Servicio de Farmacia, Hospital Universitario y Politécnico La Fe, Valencia, Spain

5 Unidad Farmacología Clínica, Hospital Universitario y Politécnico La Fe; Dpto. Farmacología, Fac. Medicina, Universidad de Valencia, Valencia, Spain

References

[1] Herrero, M. J, Marqués, M. R, Sánchez-plumed, J, Prieto, M, Almenar, L, Pastor, A, Galán, J. B, Poveda, J. L, & Aliño, S. F. Farmacogenética/ Farmacogenómica en el trasplante. In: Roche. Bases para la atención farmacéutica al paciente trasplantado. Madrid: (2009). , 331-341.

[2] Aliño, S. F, Herrero, M. J, & Poveda, J. L. De la población al paciente: diferencias individuales en la respuesta a los medicamentos. In: López E., Poveda JL. editors. Evaluación y selección de medicamentos basadas en la evidencia. Madrid: (2008). , 259-282.

[3] Hardy, J, & Singleton, A. Genomewide association studies and human disease. New England Journal of Medicine (2009). , 360, 1759-68.

[4] Herrero, M. J, Aliño, S. F, Poveda, J. L, et al. Farmacogenética: una realidad clínica.., Madrid: Astellas Pharma- Master Line Ed; (2010).

[5] EMEA/CHMP/ICH/437986/(2006). Definitions for genomic biomarkers, pharmacogenomics, pharmacogenetics, genomic data and sample coding categories. www.ema.europa.eu/accessed 20 June 2012)

[6] Aliño, S. F, Dasí, F, & Herrero, M. J. Farmacogenómica y terapia génica en el trasplante.In: Edipharma. Bases para la atención farmacéutica al paciente transplantado, (2006). , 305-316.

[7] Drews, J. Genomic sciences and the medicine of tomorrow. Nat. Biotechnol (1996). , 11, 1516-1518.

[8] Daly, A. K. Pharmacogenetics and human genetic polymorphisms. Biochem. J. (2010). , 429, 435-449.

[9] Provenzani, A, et al. The effect of CYP3A5 and ABCB1 single nucleotide polymorphisms on tacrolimus dose requirements in Caucasian liver transplant patients. Ann Transplant (2009). , 14, 23-31.

[10] Herrero, M. J, Almenar, L, Jordán, C, Sánchez, I, Poveda, J. L, & Aliño, S. F. Clinical interest of pharmacogenetic polymorphisms in the immunosupressive treatment after heart transplantation. Transplantation Proceedings (2010). , 42, 3181-3182.

[11] Herrero, M. J, Sánchez-plumed, J, Galiana, M, Bea, S, Marqués, M. R, & Aliño, S. F. Influence of the pharmacogenetic polymorphisms in the routine immunosuppression therapy after renal transplantation. Transplantation Proceedings (2010). , 42, 3134-3136.

[12] Ran Jun KLee W., Jang M., et al. Tacrolimus concentrations in relations to CYP3A and ABCB1 polymorphisms in solid organ transplant recipients in Korea. Transplantation (2009). , 87, 1225-1231.

[13] Herrero, M. J, Poveda, J. L, García, P, & Aliño, S. F. Metodología, retos y puntos débiles en la aplicación de la Farmacogenética. Madrid: Ergon; (2011).

[14] Anglicheau et alAssociation of MDR1 polymorphism with the tacrolimus dose requirements in renal transplant recipients. J. Am. Soc Nephrol. (2003). , 14(7), 1889-96.

[15] Bouamar, R, Hesselink, D. A, Van Schaik, R. H, Weimar, W, Macphee, I. A, De Fijter, J. W, & Van Gelder, T. Polymorphisms in CYP3A5, CYP3A4, and ABCB1 are not associated with cyclosporine pharmacokinetics nor with cyclosporine clinical end points after renal transplantation. Ther Drug Monit. (2011). , 33(2), 178-184.

[16] Haufroid, V, et al. The effect of CYP3A5 and MDR1 (ABCB1) polymorphism on CYA and Tacrolimus dose requirements and trough blood level in stable renal transplant patients. Pharmacogenetics (2004). , 14, 147-154.

[17] Goto, M, et al. CYP3A5*1-carrying graft liver reduces the concentration/oral dose ratio of tacrolimus in recipients of living-donor liver transplantation. Pharmacogenetics (2004). , 14, 471-478.

[18] Thervet, E, et al. Impact of CYP3A5 genetic polymorphism on TC doses and concentration to dose ratio in renal trasplant recipients. Transplantation (2003).

[19] Zheng, H, et al. Tacrolimus dosing in adult lung transplant patients is related to CYP3A5 gen polymorphisms. Am J. Transplant. (2003). , 3, 477-483.

[20] MacPhee IAet al. Tacrolimus pharmacogenetics polimorphism associated with expression of CYP3A5 and Gly-P correlate with dose requirement. Transplantation (2002). , 74(11), 1486-1489.

[21] MacPhee IAet al. The influence of pharmacogenetics on the time to achieve target tacrolimus concentration after kidney transplantation. Am J. Transplant. (2004). , 4, 914-919.

[22] Haufroid, V, et al. CYP3A5 and MDR1 (ABCB1) polymorphism and tacrolimus pharmacokinetics in renal transplant candidates: guidelines from an experimental study. Am J. Transplant. (2006). , 6, 2706-2713.

[23] Thervet, E, Loriot, M. A, Barbier, S, et al. Optimization of initial tacrolimus dose using pharmacogenetic testing. Clin Pharmacol Ther (2010). , 87(6), 721-726.

[24] Undre, N. A, et al. Low systemic exposure to tacrolimus correlates with acute rejection. Trasplant. Prc. (1999). , 31, 296-298.

[25] Yamauchi, A, et al. Neurotoxicity induced by tacrolimus after liver transplantation: relation to genetic polimorphism of the ABCB1 (MDR1) gene. Trasplantation (2002). , 74, 571-572.

[26] Zheng et alTacrolimus nephrotoxicity is predicted by MDR1 exon 21 polimorphism whereas dosing is predicted by CYP3A5 polimorphism in adult lung transplant patients. American Transplant Congress, Washington DC. Transplantation (2003).

[27] Kuypers et alCYP3A5 and CYP3A4 but not MDR1 polimorphism determine longterm Tacrolimus disposition and drug-related nephrotoxicity in renal recipients. Clin Pharmacol Ther (2007). , 82(6), 711-25.

[28] Glowacki, F, Lionet, A, Buob, D, Labalette, M, Allorge, D, Provo, t F, Hazzan, M, Noe, l C, Broly, F, Cauffiez, C, & Cyp, A. and ABCB1 polymorphisms in donor and recipient: impact on Tacrolimus dose requirements and clinical outcome after renal transplantation. Nephrol Dial Transplant. (2011). , 26, 3046-3050.

[29] Lloberas et alInfluence of MRP2 on MPA pharmacokinetics in renal transplant recipients-results of the Pharmacogenomic Substudy within the Symphony Study. Nephrol Dial Transplant (2011). , 26(11), 3784-3793.

[30] Michellon, H, et al. SLCO1B1 genetic polymorphism influences mycophenolic acid tolerance in renal tranplant recipients. Pharmacogenomics (2010). , 11(12), 1703-1713.

[31] Picard, N. Wah Yee S., Woillard JB., Lebranchu Y., Le Meur Y., Giacomini KM., Marquet P. The role of organic anion-transporting polypeptides and their common genetic variants in mycophenolic acid pharmacokinetics. Clin Pharmacol Ther. (2010). , 87(1), 100-108.

[32] Kagaya, H, Miura, M, Saito, M, Habuchi, T, & Satoh, S. Correlation of IMPDH1 gene polymorphisms with subclinical acute rejection and mycophenolic acid exposure parameters on day 28 after renal transplantation. Basic Clin Pharmacol Toxicol. (2010). , 107(2), 631-636.

[33] Sánchez-fructuoso, A. I, Maestro, M. L, Calvo, N, Viudarreta, M, Pérez-flores, I, Veganzone, S, De La Orden, V, Ortega, D, Arroyo, M, & Barrientos, A. The prevalence of uridine diphosphate-glucuronosyltransferase 1A9 (UGT1A9) gene promoter region single-nucleotide polymorphisms T-275A and C-2152T and its influence on mycophenolic acid pharmacokinetics in stable renal transplant patients. Transplantation Proceedings (2009). , 41, 2313-2316.

[34] Johnson, L'A. A, Oetting, W. S, Basu, S, Prausa, S, Matas, A, & Jacobson, P. A. Pharmacogenetic effect of the UGT polymorphismson mycophenolate is modified by calcineurin inhibitors. Eur J Clin Pharmacol (2008). , 64, 1047-1056.

[35] Miura, M, Satoh, S, Inoue, K, Kagaya, H, Saito, M, Inoue, T, Suzuki, T, & Habuchi, T. Influence of SLCO1B1, 1B3, 2B1 and ABCC2 genetic polymorphisms on mycophenolic acid pharmacokinetics in Japanese renal transplant recipients. Eur J Clin Pharmacol (2007). , 63, 1161-1169.

[36] van Schaik RHN. et alUGT1A9-275T>A/-2152 C>T polymorphisms correlate with low MPA exposure and acute rejection in MMF/Tacrolimus-treated kidney transplant patients. Clinical Phramacology and Therapeutics (2009). , 86(3), 319-27.

[37] Huls, M. van den Heuvel JJMW., Dijkman HBPM., et al. ABC transporter expression profiling after ischemic reperfusion injury in mouse kidney. Kidney Int. (2006). , 69, 2186-2193.

[38] Hesselink, D. A, Bouamar, R, & Van Gelder, T. The pharmacogenetics of calcineurin inhibitor-related nephrotoxicity. Ther Drug Monit. (2010). , 32(4), 387-393.

[39] Galiana, M, Herrero, M. J, Bosó, V, Bea, S, Ros, E, Sánchez-plumed, J, Poveda, J. L, & Aliño, S. F. Pharmacogenetics of immunosuppressive drugs in renal transplantation. In: Long L, editor. Renal Transplantation- Updates and Advances, Rijeka: InTech; (2012)., 143-162.

[40] Hauser, I. A, Schaeffeler, E, Gauer, S, et al. ABCB1 genotype of the donor but not of the recipient is a major risk factor for cyclosporine-related nephrotoxicity after renal transplantation. J Am Soc Nephrol. (2005)., 16, 1501-1511.

[41] Evans, W. E, & Mcleod, H. L. Pharmacogenomics: drug disposition, drug targets, and side effects. N Engl J Med. (2003)., 348, 538-549.

[42] Zhao, W, Elie, V, Roussey, G, et al. Population pharmacokinetics and pharmacogenetics of tacrolimus in de novo pediatric kidney transplant recipients. Clin Pharmacol Ther (2009)., 86(6), 609-618.

[43] Becquemont, L, Alfirevic, A, Amstutz, U, et al. Practical recommendations for pharmacogenomics-based prescription: 2010 ESF-UB conference on pharmacogenetics and pharmacogenomics. Pharmacogenomics (2011).

[44] Swen, J. J, Nijenhuis, M, De Boer, A, et al. Pharmacogenetics: from bench to byte-an update of guidelines. Clinical Pharmacology and Therapeutics (2011)., 89(5), 662-673.

[45] Montori, V. M, Smieja, M, & Guyatt, G. H. Publication bias: a brief review for clinicians. Mayo Clin Proc (2000)., 75(12), 1284-1288.

[46] Egger, M, & Smith, G. D. Bias in location and selection of studies. BMJ (1998)., 316(7124), 61-66.

[47] Liberati, A, Altman, D. G, Tetzlaff, J, Mulrow, C, Gotzsche, P. C, Ioannidis, J. P, et al. The PRISMA statement for reporting systematic reviews and meta-analyses of studies that evaluate healthcare interventions: explanation and elaboration. BMJ (2009). b2700.

[48] Shuster, J. J. Review: Cochrane handbook for systematic reviews for interventions, Version 5.1.0, published 3/2011. Julian P.T. Higgins and Sally Green, Editors. Research Synthesis Methods (2011)., 2(2), 126-130.

[49] Simon, R. Meta-analysis of clinical trials: opportunities and limitations. In: Stangl D, Berry D, editors. Meta-Analysis in Medicine and Health Policy New York; (2000).

[50] Berlin, J. A. Invited Commentary: Benefits of Heterogeneity in Meta-analysis of Data from Epidemiologic Studies. American Journal of Epidemiology (1995). , 142(4), 383-387.

[51] Blettner, M, Sauerbrei, W, Schlehofer, B, Scheuchenpflug, T, & Friedenreich, C. Traditional reviews, meta-analyses and pooled analyses in epidemiology. Int J Epidemiol (1999)., 28(1), 1-9.

[52] Altman, D. G. Matthews JNS. Statistics Notes: Interaction 1: heterogeneity of effects. BMJ (1996).

[53] Higgins, J. P, & Thompson, S. G. Quantifying heterogeneity in a meta-analysis. Stat Med (2002). , 21(11), 1539-1558.

[54] Tang, H. L, Xie, H. G, Yao, Y, & Hu, Y. F. Lower tacrolimus daily dose requirements and acute rejection rates in the CYP3A5 nonexpressers than expressers. Pharmacogenetics and Genomics (2011). , 21, 713-720.

[55] Zhu, H. J, Yuan, S. H, Fang, Y, Sun, X. Z, Kong, H, & Ge, W. H. The effect of CYP3A5 polymorphism on dose-adjusted cyclosporine concentration in renal transplant recipients: a meta-analysis. The Pharmacogenomics Journal (2011). , 11, 237-246.

[56] Varmus, H. Ten years on- the human genome and medicine. N Engl J Med (2010). , 362, 2028-29.

[57] Manolio, T. A. Genomewide association studies and assessment of the risk of disease. N Engl J Med (2010). , 363, 166-176.

[58] Feero, W. G, Guttmacher, A. E, & Collins, F. S. Genomic medicine-an updated primer. N Engl J Med (2010). , 362, 2001-2011.

[59] Evans, J. P, & Green, R. C. Direct to consumer genetic testing: avoiding a culture war. Genet Med (2009). , 11, 568-569.

[60] Evans, J. P, Dale, D. C, & Fomous, C. Preparing for a consumer-driven genomic age. N Engl J Med. (2010). , 363(12), 1099-1103.

[61] Pirmohamed, M, James, S, et al. Adverse drug reactions as cause of admission to hospital: prospective analysis of 18820 patients. Br Med J (2004). , 329, 15-19.

[62] Evans, W. E, & Relling, M. V. Moving towards individualized medicine with pharmacogenomics. Nature (2004). , 429, 646-68.

[63] Ibarreta, D, et al. Cost-effectiveness of pharmacogenomics in clinical practice: a case study of thiopurine methyltransferase genotyping in acute lymphoblastic leukemia in Europe. Pharmacogenomics (2006). , 7, 783-92.

[64] Woelderink, A, Ibarreta, D, Hopkins, M. M, & Rodriguez-cerezo, E. The current clinical practice of pharmacogenetic testing in Europe: TPMT and HER2 as case studies. Pharmacogenomics J (2006). , 6, 3-7.

[65] Hopkins, M. M, Ibarreta, D, Gaisser, S, et al. Putting pharmacogenetics into practice. Nature Biotechnology (2006). , 24, 403-410.

[66] Sheffield, L. J, & Phillimore, H. E. Clinical use of pharmacogenomic tests in (2009). Clin Biochem Rev 2009; , 30, 55.

Chapter 15

Clinical Pharmacology and Therapeutic Drug Monitoring of Immunosuppressive Agents

Ana Luisa Robles Piedras,
Minarda De la O Arciniega and
Josefina Reynoso Vázquez

Additional information is available at the end of the chapter

http://dx.doi.org/10.5772/54910

1. Introduction

Immunosuppressive drugs are used to reduce the immune response in organ transplantation and autoimmune disease. In transplantation, the major classes of immunosuppressive drugs used today are: (1) glucocorticoids, (2) calcineurin inhibitors, (3) antiproliferative/antimetabolic agents, and (4) biologics (antibodies). These drugs have met with a high degree of clinical success in treating conditions such as acute immune rejection of organ transplants and severe autoimmune diseases. However, such therapies require lifelong use and nonspecifically suppress the entire immune system, exposing patients to considerably higher risks of adverse effects [1].

The pharmacokinetics of the immunosuppressive drugs is complex and unpredictable. A narrow therapeutic index unique to each patient, as well as variable absorption, distribution, and elimination, are characteristics of these drugs. Therapeutic drug monitoring plays a key role in helping clinicians maintain blood and plasma levels of immunosuppressive drugs within their respective therapeutic ranges. Variation in concentrations outside the narrow therapeutic ranges can result in adverse clinical outcomes. Therapeutic drug monitoring ensures that concentrations are not too high or too low, thereby reducing the risks of toxicity or rejection, respectively. This chapter briefly reviews some immunosuppressive drugs: cyclosporine, tacrolimus, mycophenolic acid, sirolimus, everolimus, azathioprine, daclizumab and basiliximab, alemtuzumab and glucocorticoids. A general discussion of mechanism of action and side effects of these immunosuppressive agents used more commonly today are described below, followed by an overview of general principles of therapeutic drug monitoring and concluding with brief information about monitoring of individual immunosuppressive agents as well as a brief description of future trends in immunosuppression therapy.

2. Mechanism of action and side effects

2.1. Cyclosporine A (CsA)

CsA is a cyclic polypeptide immunosuppressant consisting of 11 amino acids. It is produced as a metabolite of the fungus species *Tolypocladium inflatum* Gams. CsA generally is recognized as the agent that ushered in the modern era of organ transplantation, increasing the rates of early engraftment, extending kidney graft survival, and making cardiac and liver transplantation possible. Clinical indications for CsA are kidney, liver, heart, and other organ transplantation; rheumatoid arthritis; and psoriasis. The dose of CsA varies, depending on the organ transplanted and the other drugs used in the specific treatment protocols. Dosage is guided by signs of rejection (too low a dose), renal or other toxicity (too high a dose), and close monitoring of blood levels [1].

2.1.1. Mechanism of action

CsA suppresses some humoral immunity, but is more effective against T-cell-dependent immune mechanisms such as those underlying transplant rejection and some forms of autoimmunity. Its actions appear to be dependent upon binding to intracellular sites of action. Because of its high lipophilicity, CsA enters cells easily to gain access to the site of action [1]. The intracellular protein most closely linked to the immunosuppressive activity of CsA is cyclophilin. CsA forms a complex with cyclophilin, a cytoplasmic receptor protein present in target cells. This complex binds to calcineurin to block its phosphatase activity (Table 1). Calcineurin-catalyzed dephosphorylation is required for movement of a component of the nuclear factor of activated T lymphocytes (NFAT) into the nucleus. Calcineurin phosphatase activity is inhibited after physical interaction with the cyclosporine/cyclophilin complex. This prevents Ca^{2+}-stimulated dephosphorylation of the cytosolic component of NFAT such that NFAT does not enter the nucleus, gene transcription is not activated, and the T lymphocyte fails to respond to specific antigenic stimulation. By binding to cyclophilin, the antigenic response of helper T lymphocytes is inhibited; the production of interleukin-2 and interferon-gamma is suppressed [2-3]. In addition, production of the receptor site for interleukin-2 on T lymphocytes is inhibited by CsA and also increases expression of transforming growth factor-β (TGF-β), a potent inhibitor of IL-2–stimulated Tcell proliferation and generation of cytotoxic T lymphocytes (CTL) [4-8].

2.1.2. Side effects

The principal side effects to CsA therapy are hypertension, nephrotoxicity, tremor, hirsutism, hyperlipidemia, nausea and vomiting, gingival hyperplasia, and hepatotoxicity [1,9]. Hypertension is a common adverse effect of CsA, with the incidence decreasing over time. Generally,

http://dx.doi.org/10.5772/54910

mild to moderate hypertension may occur in approximately 50% of renal transplant patients and most cardiac transplant patients. In liver transplant patients (n=75), 27% experienced hypertension. Incidence: 13% to 53% [9]. Discontinuation of CsA therapy may be required for persistent blood pressure elevation despite adjustments in therapy. Antihypertensive agents such as calcium-channel blockers may be used, with isradipine and nifedipine most appropriate since they do not interfere with CsA metabolism. Other calcium-channel blockers (eg, diltiazem and verapamil) may increase cyclosporine levels. Patients with preexisting hypertension controlled by beta-blockers may continue to receive the same therapy. Angiotensin converting enzyme inhibitors and diuretics are not recommended [10]. Probable mechanisms for cyclosporine induced hypertension involve increased prostaglandin synthesis, decreased free water excretion, and decreased sodium and potassium excretion [11]. CsA is nephrotoxic, the mechanism by which CsA causes nephrotoxicity is attributed to changes in vasomotor tone induced by activation of the sympathetic nervous system [12]. Tremor was reported to appear within a few days of initiating CsA therapy and was considered dose dependent. Incidence: 12% to 55% [9].

Immunosuppressive agent	Site of Action
Cyclosporine and tacrolimus	Calcineurin (inhibits phosphatase activity)
Mycophenolic acid	Inosine monophosphate dehydrogenase (inhibits activity)
Sirolimus and everolimus	Protein kinase involved in cellcycle progression (mTOR) (inhibits activity)
Azathioprine	Deoxyribonucleic acid (false nucleotide incorporation)
Daclizumab and basiliximab	IL-2 receptor (block IL-2–mediated T-cell activation)
Alemtuzumab	Cell surface glycoprotein CD52
Glucocorticoids	Glucocorticoid response elements in DNA (regulate gene transcription)

Table 1. Sites of action of immunosuppressive agents on T-cell activation [1]

Administration of CsA adversely affects plasma lipoprotein and cholesterol levels causing hyperlipidemia [9]. In a study CsA increased total cholesterol by 21%, low-density lipoproteins by 31%, and apolipoproteins by 12% over 27 days [13]. Gingival hyperplasia was reported in 4% to 16% of patients treated with CsA [9]. Histologically, CsA-induced gingival overgrowth is characterized by cellular hyperplasia along with myxomatous changes and accumulation of collagen [14]. Reduction of the dose of CsA may result in complete resolution of gingival hyperplasia [15,16].

2.2. Tacrolimus (TRL)

TRL (Prograf®) is a macrolide antibiotic produced by *Streptomyces tsukubaensis*. It is practically insoluble in water. TRL is indicated for the prophylaxis of solid-organ allograft rejection in a manner similar to CsA. The recommended starting dose for TRL injection is 0.03 to 0.05 mg/kg per day as a continuous infusion. Recommended initial oral doses are 0.15 to 0.2 mg/kg per day for adult kidney transplant patients, in two divided doses 12 hours apart. These dosages are intended to achieve typical blood trough levels in the 5 to 15 ng/mL range. Pediatric patients generally require higher doses than do adults [1,17].

2.2.1. Mechanism of action

The compound is chemically distinct from CsA but both agents elicit similar immunosuppressant effects. TRL suppresses both humoral (antibody) and cell-mediated immune responses. Like CsA, TRL inhibits Tcell activation by inhibiting calcineurin [17]. The proposed mechanism for this effect is binding to an intracellular protein FK506-binding protein–12 (FKBP-12), immunophilin structurally related to cyclophilin. A complex of tacrolimus-FKBP-12, Ca2+, calmodulin, and calcineurin then forms, which inhibits the phosphatase activity of calcineurin (Table 1). As described for CsA the inhibition of phosphatase activity prevents dephosphorylation and nuclear translocation of NFAT and inhibits T-cell activation. Thus, although the intracellular receptors differ, CsA and TRL target the same pathway for immunosuppression [1,18]. The immunosuppressive activity of TRL is, however, more marked than that of CsA. Studies on cultured CD4+ (T-helper) lymphocytes have demonstrated that TRL is at least 100 times more potent than CsA (weight basis) in selectively inhibiting secretion of various cytokines (i.e., interleukin-2, interleukin-3, interferon-gamma) [19,20]. The action of TRL on lymphocytes is more difficult to reverse than that of CsA; this may be attributable to the effect of TRL on impairing the expression of interleukin-2 receptors on alloantigen-stimulated T-cells [19]. TRL possesses another important effect in addition to the inhibition of IL-2 gene transcription, to be exact the ability to act as a general inhibitor of the protein secretory pathway, which strongly suggests that the diabetogenic effect of the TRL could be caused by the blockade of insulin secretion. This novel effect also provides an explanation for other side-effects observed in immunosuppressive treatment [1,21,22].

2.2.2. Side effects

TRL is an established immunosuppressant for the prevention and treatment of allograft rejection in organ transplantation. However, TRL therapy also has several adverse effects like nephrotoxicity, hypertension, hyperkalemia, hyperglycemia, hyperlipidemia, neurotoxicity (tremor, headache, dizziness, seizure), gastrointestinal complaints, and diabetes are all associated with TRL use [18].

Nephrotoxicity has been reported with TRL therapy, particularly when used in high doses. Incidence: 36% to 59% [23]. Acute nephrotoxicity is characterized by an increased serum creatinine and/or a decrease in urine output, and is generally reversible. Chronic nephrotoxicity is associated with increased serum creatinine, decreased kidney graft life, and characteristic histologic changes observed on renal biopsy; these changes are usually progressive. Renal function should be monitored closely [23,24]. In systemic formulations hypertension occurred in 13% to 89% of patients receiving TRL in clinical trials. Antihypertensive therapy may be required. Potassium sparing diuretics, ACE inhibitors, and angiotensin receptor blockers should be used with careful consideration since due to the potential to cause hyperkalemia. Calcium channel blockers may be effective in treating TRL associated hypertension, but caution is warranted since interference with TRL metabolism may require a dosage reduction. [23,25]. Hyperlipidemia was reported as one of the more common adverse events in TRL-treated heart transplant recipients. Incidence: 10% to 34% [23]. In clinical trials tremor has occurred in 15% to 56% of patients receiving TRL [23,26]. In systemic formulations headache occurred in 24% to 64% of patients receiving TRL in clinical trials. Headache may respond to a dosage reduction [23]. In clinical trials hyperglycemia occurred in 21% to 70% of patients receiving TRL [23]. New onset diabetes mellitus has been reported in kidney, liver, and heart transplant patients receiving TRL therapy. Incidence: 11% to 22%. Close monitoring of blood glucose concentrations is recommended [23,27].

2.3. Mycophenolic acid (MPA)

MPA is a secondary metabolite produced by *Penicillium brevicompactum*, which has antibiotic and immunosuppressive properties used to prevent rejection of solid organ transplants [28]. It is highly soluble in aqueous media at physiological pH. The drug is marketed as the ester prodrug mycophenolate mofetil (CellCept®) (MMF) for kidney, liver, and heart transplants or enteric-coated mycophenolate sodium (Myfortic®) for kidney transplants [1,29].

2.3.1. Mechanism of action

MPA produces potent selective, noncompetitive, and reversible inhibition of inosine monophosphate dehydrogenase (IMPDH), an important enzyme in the *de novo* pathway of guanine nucleotide synthesis (Table 1). B and T lymphocytes are highly dependent on this pathway for cell proliferation, while other cell types can use salvage pathways; MPA therefore selectively inhibits lymphocyte proliferation and functions, including antibody formation, cellular adhesion, and migration [1,30]. *In vitro* and *in vivo* studies have demonstrated the ability of MPA to block proliferative responses of T and B lymphocytes, and inhibit antibody formation and the generation of cytotoxic T-cells [31]. In a preclinical study in mice, MPA increased survival of heart and pancreatic islet cell allografts. Studies in rats have also demonstrated prolonged heart allograft survival, as well as reversal of acute rejection and prevention of rejection in the sensitized animal. Antirejection effects have been attributed to decreased recruitment of activated lymphocytes to the graft site [32].

2.3.2. Side effects

The principal adverse effects of MPA are gastrointestinal, these include diarrhea, nausea and vomiting; hypertension; hematologic effects (anemia and leukopenia) and neurologic effects (anxiety asthenia dizziness headache insomnia tremor). There also is an increased incidence of some infections, especially sepsis associated with cytomegalovirus [1,33-35]. Diarrhea was reported in 36.1% of renal transplant patients, 45.3% of cardiac transplant patients, and 51.3% of hepatic transplant patients in a clinical study. Vomiting was reported in 33.9% of cardiac transplant patients, and 32.9% of hepatic transplant patients. Nausea was reported in 23.6% of renal transplant patients, 54% of cardiac transplant patients, and 54.5% of hepatic transplant. The incidence of adverse gastrointestinal complications requiring dose reduction. Usually occurs early in therapy and respond to dose reduction or switching from two to three divided daily doses [34].

Hypertension was reported in 28.2% of renal transplant patients, 77.5% of cardiac transplant patients, and 62.1% of hepatic transplant patients [34]. Leukopenia was 23.2% and 34.5% in renal transplant, 30.4% in cardiac transplant, and 45.8% in hepatic transplant in a clinical study. Complete blood counts should be performed weekly during the first month, twice monthly for the second and third months of treatment, then monthly through the first year [34].

2.4. Sirolimus (SRL) and Everolimus (EVL)

SRL(also known as Rapamycin and Rapamune®) is a macrocyclic lactone produced by the actinomycete *Streptomyces hygroscopicus*, with immunosuppressive, antitumor, and antifungal properties. SRL appears to be synergistic with CsA in kidney transplantation, but with a different side-effect profile. It is an immunosuppressive agent of potential benefit in clinical liver transplantation. EVL is an analogue of SRL with immunosuppressive and antiproliferative activity. It is closely related chemically and clinically to SRL but has distinct pharmacokinetics. The main difference is a shorter half-life and thus a shorter time to achieve steady state concentrations of the drug [1,36].

2.4.1. Mechanism of action of SRL

SRL has been demonstrated to block the response of T- and B-cell activation by cytokines, which prevents cell-cycle progression and proliferation. Intracellularly, sirolimus forms a complex with cytosolic FK-binding proteins, primarily FKBP-12, considered essential for functionality; however, the sirolimus–FKBP-12 complex does not affect calcineurin activity. It binds to and inhibits a protein kinase, designated mammalian target of rapamycin (mTOR) (Table 1), which is a key enzyme in cell-cycle progression. Inhibition of mTOR blocks cell-cycle progression at the G1 to S phase transition [37,38]. Specific biochemical steps inhibited by SRL include activation of p70S6 kinase, activation of the cdk2/cyclinE complex, and phosphorylation of retinoblastoma protein [37,38]. SRL appears to be less nephrotoxic than CsA and TRL; this may be related to its lack of effect on calcineurin [1,38]. In preclinical studies (*in vitro* and *in vivo*), additive or synergistic immunosuppressive effects were observed when SRL was combined with TRL, CsA, MMF, and brequinar [37].

2.4.2. Side effects of SRL

The use of SRL in renal transplant patients is associated with a dose-dependent increase in serum cholesterol and triglycerides that may require treatment. Other studies have identified hyperlipidemia and thrombocytopenia as significant SRL side effects [39]. In the other hand, while immunotherapy with SRL *per se* is not nephrotoxic, patients treated with CsA plus SRL have impaired renal function compared to patients treated with CsA and either azathioprine or placebo. Renal function therefore must be monitored closely in such patients. Other adverse effects include anemia, leukopenia, thrombocytopenia, hypokalemia or hyperkalemia, fever, and gastrointestinal effects. Delayed wound healing may occur with SRL use. As with other immunosuppressive agents, there is an increased risk of neoplasms, especially lymphomas, and infections [1,36,37].

2.4.3. Mechanism of action of EVL

Like SRL, EVL binds to the cytosolic immunophyllin FKBP12; both agents inhibit growth factor-driven cell proliferation, including that of T-cells and vascular smooth muscle cells. After binding to and forming a complex with the cytoplasmic protein FKBP-12, this complex binds to and inhibits the mammalian Target Of Rapamycin (mTOR) and phosphorylates P70 S6 ribosomal protein kinase (a substrate of mTOR) (Table 1). The phosphorylation of P70 S6 ribosomal protein kinase by the EVL complex prevents protein synthesis and cell proliferation. The EVL:FKBP-12 complex does not affect calcineurin activity [40,41]. Binding of EVL to FKBP12 is weaker than that of SRL (about 3-fold), related to 40-O-alkylation, and this correlates with a 2- to 3-fold lower in vitro immunosuppressive activity for EVL. However, the oral *in vivo* activity of EVL has been at least equipotent to oral SRL in several animal allotransplantation/autoimmune disease models. This appears related to the chemical modification in EVL (2-hydroxyethyl chain), providing more favorable pharmacokinetic properties (eg, absorption, disposition) which compensate for relatively poor *in vitro* activity [40]. EVL and SRL antagonize TRL based calcineurin inhibition via saturation of FKBP12 [1,42].

2.4.4. Side effects of EVL

Side effects seem to be the same as with SRL [1]. Endocrine abnormalities, including hyperlipidemia and hypertriglyceridemia, have been reported with EVL treatment. Monitoring for hyperlipidemia is recommended in all patients; diet, exercise, and lipid lowering therapy should be initiated if hyperlipidemia occurs. In a clinical study with EVL, the most important causes of discontinuation in 69 patients were severe infections (2.3%), pneumonitis (6.8 %), acute rejection episode (4.1%), proteinuria (4.1%). Although the overall incidence discontinuation due to side effects was higher in the EVL than SRL group, there was no greater frequency of severe side effects [43,44].

2.5. Azathioprine

Azathioprine is a purine antimetabolite. It is an imidazolyl derivative of 6-mercaptopurine. Azathioprine was first introduced as an immunosuppressive agent in 1961, helping to make allogeneic kidney transplantation possible. It is indicated as an adjunct for prevention of organ transplant rejection and in severe rheumatoid arthritis. It has long been used as a steroid sparing agent in a variety of clinical scenarios [1,45]. In the United States azathioprine was usually combined with prednisone and CsA. Azathioprine was regarded as an adjunctive agent to CsA and the combination was often called "triple therapy". The term "adjunctive agent" is used to describe the immunosuppressive drugs that are used, or were developed for use, in combination with a calcineurin inhibitor to enhance the potency of the immunosuppressive protocol, as measured by a decreased incidence of acute rejection episodes [46].

2.5.1. Mechanism of action

Azathioprine inhibits purine metabolism. Following exposure to nucleophiles such as glutathione, azathioprine is cleaved to 6-mercaptopurine, which in turn is converted to additional metabolites that inhibit *de novo* purine synthesis. 6-thio-IMP, a fraudulent nucleotide, is converted to 6-thio-GMP and finally to 6-thio-GTP, which is incorporated into DNA. Cell proliferation is thereby inhibited, impairing a variety of lymphocyte functions. Azathioprine appears to be a more potent immunosuppressive agent than 6-mercaptopurine, which may reflect differences in drug uptake or pharmacokinetic differences in the resulting metabolites [1,45].

2.5.2. Side effects

The major side effect of azathioprine is bone marrow suppression, including leukopenia (common), and thrombocytopenia (less common). Other important adverse effects include increased susceptibility to infections (especially varicella and herpes simplex viruses) and hepatotoxicity [1].

2.6. Anti-IL-2 receptor (Anti-CD25) antibodies

There are two anti–IL-2R preparations for use in clinical transplantation: daclizumab and basiliximab. These are used for prophylaxis of acute organ rejection in adult patients. Basiliximab is considered a chimeric antibody, because it consists of approximately 70% human and 30% murine proteins. This agent has low immunogenicity potential due to the incorporation of human protein sequences. Daclizumab consists of 90% human and 10% murine components. The effectiveness of daclizumab is comparable to that of basiliximab, with an adverse-effect profile comparable to that seen with placebo [1,46].

2.6.1. Mechanism of action

Basiliximab binds with high affinity to the alpha subunit of the IL-2 receptor, also known as CD25, where it acts as a receptor antagonist. The antagonistic effect on the IL-2 receptor prevents T-cell activation and subsequent proliferation without causing lysis or cell destruction. Daclizumab, like basiliximab, is a nondepleting monoclonal antibody that acts as an antagonist at the CD25 subunit of T cells and received marketing approval in 1997 for induction therapy in renal transplant recipients. In Phase III trials, the half-life of daclizumab was 20 days, resulting in saturation of the IL-2Rα on circulating lymphocytes for up to 120 days after transplantation. In these trials, daclizumab was used with maintenance immunosuppression regimens (CsA, azathioprine, and steroids; CsA and steroids). Subsequently, daclizumab was successfully used with a maintenance triple-therapy regimen—either with CsA or TRL, steroids, and MMF substituting for azathioprine. In the Phase III trials, the half-life of basilix-

http://dx.doi.org/10.5772/54910

imab was 7 days. In one randomized trial, basiliximab was safe and effective when used in a maintenance regimen consisting of CsA, MMF, and prednisone [1,47].

2.6.2. *Side effects*

No cytokine-release syndrome has been observed with these antibodies, but anaphylactic reactions can occur. Although lymphoproliferative disorders and opportunistic infections may occur, as with the depleting antilymphocyte agents, the incidence ascribed to anti-CD25 treatment appears remarkably low. No significant drug interactions with anti–IL-2-receptor antibodies have been described [46,47].

2.7. Alemtuzumab

The antibody alemtuzumab is a recombinant DNA-derived humanized monoclonal antibody that is directed against the cell surface glycoprotein CD52, which is expressed on the surface of normal and malignant B and T lymphocytes, NK cells, monocytes, macrophages, and tissues of the male reproductive system; thus, the drug causes extensive lympholysis by inducing apoptosis of targeted cells. It has achieved some use in renal transplantation because it produces prolonged T- and B-cell depletion and allows drug minimization [1,47].

2.7.1. *Mechanism of action*

Alemtuzumab antibody binds to CD52, it triggers an antibody-dependent lysis of these cells. The depletion of lymphocytes is so marked that it takes several months or up to one year postadministration for a patient's immune system to be fully reconstituted ([1,47].

2.7.2. *Side effects*

Alemtuzumab's mechanism of depletion is so profound that its adverse-effect profile occurs frequently and with a high level of severity. Adverse effects associated with alemtuzumab use include neutropenia (70%), thrombocytopenia (52%), anemia (47%), nausea (54%), vomiting (41%), diarrhea (22%), headache (24%), dysesthesias (15%), dizziness (12%), and autoimmune hemolytic anemia (<5%) [47].

2.8. Glucocorticoids

The introduction of glucocorticoids as immunosuppressive drugs in the 1960s played a key role in making organ transplantation possible. Steroids are a cornerstone of immunosuppressive therapy in kidney transplantation despite their side effects and morbidity. More than 95% of transplant recipients are treated with steroids as a usual component of clinical immunosuppressive regimens. Prednisone, prednisolone, and other glucocorticoids are used alone and in combination with other immunosuppressive agents for treatment of transplant rejection and autoimmune disorders [1,48]. Transplantation specialists are now moving toward protocols that reduce the incidence of infections and minimize adverse events. Most immunosuppressive regimens are currently based on the combination of calcineurin inhibitors (CsA, TRL) with antiproliferative agents (azathioprine, MMF) and steroids (prednisone) [49].

2.8.1. Mechanism of action

Glucocorticoids lyse (in some species) and induce the redistribution of lymphocytes, causing a rapid, transient decrease in peripheral blood lymphocyte counts. To effect longer-term responses, steroids bind to receptors inside cells; either these receptors, glucocorticoid-induced proteins, or interacting proteins regulate the transcription of numerous other genes. Additionally, glucocorticoid-receptor complexes increase IκB expression, thereby curtailing activation of NF-κB, which increases apoptosis of activated cells. Of central importance, key proinflammatory cytokines such as IL-1 and IL-6 are down regulated. T cells are inhibited from making IL-2 and proliferating. The activation of cytotoxic T lymphocytes is inhibited. Neutrophils and monocytes display poor chemotaxis and decreased lysosomal enzyme release. Therefore, glucocorticoids have broad anti-inflammatory effects on multiple components of cellular immunity [1].

2.8.2. Side effects

Steroids are effective in reducing the incidence of acute rejection but are an important cause of morbidity and probably mortality. Moreover, they have adverse effects on cardiovascular risk factors such as hypertension, hyperglycemia, or hyperlipidemia, deleterious effects on bone metabolism, and may contribute to an increased risk of infection [1,48].

3. General principles of Therapeutic Drug Monitoring (TDM)

A basic tenet of clinical pharmacology is that the pharmacologic activity of an exogenously administered agent is related to the free drug concentration available at its receptor or ligand-binding site. A mayor underlying hypothesis in clinical pharmacokinetics is that the concentration of the agent in blood, serum or some other measurable compartment is related to the concentration of free (or non-bound) drug at its effector site [50]. Drugs are administered to achieve a therapeutic objective. Once this objective is defined, a drug and its dosage regimen are chosen for the patient. Drug therapy is subsequently managed together with steps required to initiate therapy, this management is usually accomplished by monitoring incidence and intensity of both therapeutic and toxic effects.

3.1. Therapeutic range

The therapeutic range (therapeutic index) is the ratio between the toxic dose and the therapeutic dose of a drug. The closer this ratio is to 1, the more difficult the drug is to use in clinical practice. The therapeutic index for immunosuppressant drugs is very low, whereas that for amoxicillin is extremely high. Clinical use of drugs with a narrow therapeutic index has led to the monitoring of drug concentrations in patients – therapeutic drug monitoring – in which the plasma concentration of a drug is measured and the dose adjusted to achieve a desired therapeutic drug concentration. Generally defined as the range of drug concentrations associated with maximal efficacy and minimal toxicity, there is currently no standard defining

http://dx.doi.org/10.5772/54910

an acceptable level of toxicity or efficacy, nor are there consistent procedures used to establish a therapeutic range [51].

In general, a therapeutic range should never be considered in absolute terms, as it represents no more than a combination of probability charts. In other words, a therapeutic range is a range of drug concentrations within which the probability of the desired clinical response is relatively high and the probability of unacceptable toxicity is relatively low [52].

Since the development of the range is probabilistic in nature, a concentration that is within the "therapeutic range" for a given drug does not exclude the possibility that signs and symptoms of toxicity experienced by an individual patient are related to the monitored drug. A concentration outside of the range also does not indicate that a patient will experience toxicity or reduced efficacy; however, the likelihood of either is certainly lower [51]. It is important to recognize that the therapeutic range is not necessarily valid outside of the population used to establish it. This is particularly critical for immunosuppressive drugs, as most patients that are treated with these drugs receive additional immunosuppressive agents. A change in dosing of one drug may have a profound impact on the pharmacodynamic relationship of another. The nature of the transplanted organ (e.g., cadaveric versus living-related donor kidneys), age, and co-morbid illness can all have important influences on the pharmacodynamic response. The importance of these factors should not be ignored [51].

3.2. Interpretation of plasma drug concentration

The process of selecting the most appropriate dosage regimen to achieve concentrations in a relatively narrow range may be complicated by unpredictable intrapatient and interpatient variability in the drug's pharmacokinetics. A sophisticated application of pharmacokinetic principles, incorporating prior and subsequent measures of drug concentration and effects, can improve the quality of one's predictions. Although a single "best" approach to using drug concentrations does not exist for every drug, it is imperative to realize that without a systematic approach to therapeutic drug concentration monitoring, drug concentrations may be uninterpretable, unhelpful and potentially harmful. It thus becomes essential to recognize the key elements of clinical pharmacokinetics and pharmacodynamics, and to develop strategies to perform and use them most effectively [52].

There are a number of advantages to therapeutic drug monitoring that provide the clinician with clinically useful information. Plasma drug concentrations in conjunction with a thorough assessment of the patient's clinical status and the therapeutic goals to be achieved provide a means of successfully and rapidly individualizing a patient's therapeutic regimen to assure optimal benefits con minimal risk. Therapeutic drug measuring is only one part of therapeutic drug monitoring that provides expert clinical interpretation of drug concentration as well as evaluation based on pharmacokinetic principles. Expert interpretation of a drug concentration measurement is essential to ensure full clinical benefit. Clinicians routinely monitor drug pharmacodynamics by directly measuring the physiological indices of therapeutic responses, such as lipid concentrations, blood glucose, blood pressure, and clotting [53].

Anyone involved in the utilization of information derived from TDM must always bear in mind that the interpretation of plasma drug concentration must always be carried out in conjunction with an assessment of the clinical status of the patient. Therapeutic ranges should more correctly be described as optimal concentrations. According to the definition mentioned above, the therapeutic range (optimal concentration) of a drug is that concentration of drug present in plasma or some other biologic fluid or tissue that provides the desired therapeutic response in most patients. The severity of the disease process determines the amount of drug necessary to achieve a given therapeutic effect. Thus, it is quite possible that a patient may achieve the desired therapeutic effect at a plasma concentration well below the optimal range. Conversely, some patients will not achieve the desired therapeutic effect even when plasma concentrations are elevated into the toxic range. If the desired therapeutic effect is achieved at suboptimal plasma concentrations, every attempt should be made to avoid the prescription of additional drugs simply to increase the plasma concentration into what is commonly referred to as the therapeutic range. Obviously, the interpretation of plasma drug concentration must take into account the various factors that can alter the steady state plasma concentrations achieved on a given dosage form [54].

3.3. Therapeutic Drug Monitoring (TDM)

Individualizing a patient's drug therapy to obtain the optimum balance between therapeutic efficacy and the occurrence of adverse events is the physician's goal. However, achieving this goal is not always straight forward, being complicated by within and between patient variability in both pharmacokinetics and pharmacodynamics. In the early 1960's new analytical techniques became available allowing the measurement of the low drug concentrations seen in biological fluids during drug treatment. This offered the opportunity to reduce the pharmacokinetic component of variability by controlling drug therapy using concentrations in the body rather than by dose alone. This process became known as therapeutic drug monitoring [55].

The aim of TDM is to optimize pharmacotherapy by maximizing therapeutic efficacy, while minimizing adverse events, in those instances where the blood concentration of the drug is a better predictor of the desired effect(s) than the dose. The reasons why these principles have gained wide acceptance include the following: (1) although imperfect, a better relationship often exists between the effect of a given drug and its concentration in the blood than between the dose of the drug and the effect; (2) a thorough understanding of pharmacokinetics, i.e., the processes of drug absorption, distribution, metabolism, and drug excretion in individual patients and in patient populations is available; and (3) the development of reliable and relatively easy to use drug-monitoring assays. In addition, TDM can also be useful in cases in which compliance is in question, where it is not clear if the right drug is being taken, where dosage adjustment is required as a result of drug–drug or drug–food interactions, and where intoxication is suspected.

TDM is more than simply the analysis of a single drug concentration in the blood of a patient and a report of this number. It also comprises interpretation of the value measured using the mathematical (pharmacokinetic) principles mentioned above, drawing the appropriate conclusions about the result, and advising the physician who ordered the test how to optimize treatment. It is important to apply a uniform definition of TDM here, because different definitions have previously been used in cost-effectiveness studies and reviews of TDM. Consequently, comparisons have been made based on different approaches, which may influence the results. The International Association for Therapeutic Drug Monitoring and Clinical Toxicology has adopted the following definition:

Therapeutic drug monitoring is defined as the measurement made in the laboratory of a parameter that, with appropriate interpretation, will directly influence prescribing procedures. Commonly the measurement is in a biologic matrix of a prescribed xenobiotic, but it may also be of an endogenous compound prescribed as replacement therapy in an individual who is physiologically or pathologically deficient in that compound. This definition places TDM within the total therapeutic approach and should give not only more emphasis to the medication and patient-safety aspects of pharmacotherapy, but also more insight into why there are differences in efficacy among different patients. This definition implies that clinical pharmacologists have an active involvement in drug therapy, something that is not yet realized in many countries [56].

3.3.1. Why TDM for immunosuppressants?

For a drug to be a suitable candidate for therapeutic drug monitoring it must satisfy the following criteria [55]:

1. There should be a clear relationship between drug concentration and effect.
2. The drug should have a narrow therapeutic index; that is, the difference in the concentrations exerting therapeutic benefit and dose causing adverse events should be small.
3. There should be considerable between-subject pharmacokinetic variability and, therefore, a poor relationship between dose and drug concentration/response.
4. The pharmacological response of the drug should be difficult to assess or to distinguish form adverse events.

The most commonly used immunosuppressants require TDM because of their narrow therapeutic index and significant variability in blood concentrations between individuals. In transplant recipients, both supratherapeutics and subtherapeutics drug concentrations can have devastating results. At subtherapeutics drug concentrations, the transplant recipient is at risk for allograft rejection. At supratherapeutics drug concentrations, the patient is at risk for over-immunosuppression which can potentially lead to infection or drug specific side effects. It is it known that neurological and gastrointestinal side effects occur more frequently at higher concentrations of TRL [53]. Immunosuppressants display significant interindividual variability in plasma drug concentrations, which creates the demand for TDM when such drugs are used.

3.3.2. Factors contributing to the variability

Immunosuppressants display significant interindividual variability in plasma drug concentrations, which creates the demand for TDM when such drugs are used. It is appropriate to look into the multitude of factors that contribute to the interindividual variability. Some of the factors include drug-nutrients interactions, drug-disease interactions, renal insufficiency, inflammation and infection, gender, age, polymorphism and liver mass. Drug nutrient interactions are becoming very widely appreciated. The metabolism of drugs sometimes also depends on the type of diet taken by the patients. Renal transplant patients may have reduced oral bioavailability for TRL. When given with meals, especially with high fat content food, oral bioavailability of TRL decreases [57].

To avoid the possible effect of food on TRL bioavailability, the drug should be given at a constant time in relation to meals. Several studies have demonstrated that grapefruit juice can increase plasma concentrations of CsA by inhibiting CYP3A-mediated metabolism and by increasing drug absorption via inhibition of P-glycoprotein (P-gp) efflux transporters. Also, oral TRL should not be taken with grapefruit juice since this vehicle inhibits CYP3A4 and/or P-gp contained in the gastrointestinal tract and markedly increases bioavailability. Similarly, drug disease interactions can also contribute to interindividual variability in plasma concentration of immunosuppressants. Renal insufficiency can result in an altered free fraction of MPA due to the reduction in protein binding. MMF is rapidly converted to its active form, MPA, upon reaching the systemic circulation. MPA is metabolized to its glucuronide metabolite, MPA glucuronide (MPAG), by glucoronyl transferases in the liver and possibly elsewhere. MPAG is then excreted by the kidney. MPA is extensively and avidly bound to serum albumin. Previous studies have demonstrated that it is only the free (non-protein-bound) fraction of MPA that is available to exert its action. *In vivo* and *in vitro* studies demonstrate that renal insufficiency decreases the protein binding of MPA and increases free drug concentrations. This decrease in protein binding seems to be caused both by the uremic state itself and by competition with the retained metabolite MPAG. The disposition of MPA in patients with severe renal impairment may be significantly affected by this change in protein binding [58]. The concomitant administration of TRL and nonsteroidal anti-inflammatory drugs has been described as a possible cause of increased TRL nephrotoxicity because of the reduction of vasodilator prostaglandin synthesis through a blockade of the enzyme cyclo-oxygenase. Coadministration of ibuprofen and TRL has resulted in acute renal failure. Drugs such as aminoglycosides, cotrimoxazole (trimethoprim/sulfamethoxazole), amphotericin B and aciclovir, which cause significant renal dysfunction on their own, may also enhance TRL nephrotoxicity in the absence of careful monitoring of both renal function and drug concentrations [59].

It has been demonstrated that the *in vitro* metabolism of CsA in human liver microsomes was significantly reduced by TRL [60]. Interaction between MMF and TRL or CsA is probably related to a possible inhibitory effect of TRL on MPA metabolism and an inhibition of the enterohepatic recirculation of MPA by CsA, resulting in a substantial reduction in the MMF dosage when associated with TRL as compared with CsA. This has been reported in pediatric renal allograft patients and animal models [61,62].

Gender also influences drug concentration. Biologic differences exist between men and women that can result in differences in responses to drugs. Both pharmacokinetic and pharmacodynamic differences between the sexes exist, with more data on pharmacokinetic differences. Bioavailability after oral drug dosing, for CYP3A substrates in particular, may be somewhat higher in women compared to men [63]. It is known that MPA is primarily metabolized in the liver to its MPAG derivative. Morissette et al., found that men treated with MMF and TRL showed a lower ratio than patients treated with this couple of drugs, confirming that TRL inhibits glucuronidation of MPA. Because MPAG can favor the elimination of MPA, they concluded that gender differences and cotreatment with TRL must be taken into consideration when MMF is being administered [64]. Velickovic et al., investigated the gender differences in pharmacokinetics of TRL, their result show remarkable gender-related differences between women and men after the first oral dose among kidney transplant recipients on quaternary immunosuppressive therapy, including TRL, MMF, methylprednisolone and basiliximab [65].

Likewise, age can also contribute to interindividual difference in immunosuppressant plasma concentration. Pharmacokinetic parameters observed in adults may not be applicable to children, especially to the younger age groups. In general, patients younger than 5 years of age show higher clearance rates regardless of the organ transplanted or the immunosuppressive drug used [66]. Young children (1–6 years of age) appear to need higher doses per kilogram body weight of TRL than older children and adults to maintain similar trough concentrations. The reason for this age-related faster clearance rate is unknown [67]. Pediatric transplant recipients require higher doses of CsA to maintain blood concentrations equal to those found in adults [68]. Studies using intravenous CsA demonstrate that this is not because of any metabolic differences, as CsA clearance is not related to age [69].

Polymorphism has demonstrated functional consequences of many drug metabolizing enzymes. For example, CsA is known substrate for CYP3A4/5 and P-gp. CYP3A5 is one of the main CYP3A enzymes and its expression is clearly polymorphic and shows ethnic dependence. TRL is primarily metabolized by cytochrome P450(CYP)3A enzymes in the gut wall and liver. It is also a substrate for P-gp, which counter-transports diffused TRL out of intestinal cells and back into the gut lumen. Age-associated alterations in CYP3A and P-gp expression and/or activity, along with liver mass and body composition changes would be expected to affect the pharmacokinetics of TRL in the elderly [70]. The importance of interethnic differences in the pharmacokinetics of immunosuppressants has been recognized as having a significant impact on the outcome of transplantation. In a retrospective analysis Fitzimmons et al., found that the oral bioavailability of TRL in African American healthy volunteers and kidney transplant patients was significantly lower than in non-African Americans, but there was no statistically significant difference in clearance [71]. These results were confirmed in a healthy volunteer study. The absolute oral bioavailability of TRL in African American and Latin American subjects was significantly lower than in Caucasians. The results suggested that the observed ethnic differences in TRL pharmacokinetics were, instead, related to differences in intestinal P-glycoprotein-mediated efflux and CYP3A-mediated metabolism rather than differences in hepatic elimination [72].

Other ethnic groups such as the Japanese populations are not different from the Caucasian population because their transplant outcomes were comparable under usual TRL dosages [73]. All this factors contribute to the variability of immunosuppressant concentrations which has to be maintained within therapeutic range in order to achieve the optimal benefit of drug therapy, rendering TDM necessary for these drugs.

4. Monitoring of individual immunosuppressive agents

4.1. Cyclosporine (CsA)

The introduction of CsA in the early 1980s was immediately associated with an enhanced one year renal allograft survival; however, the argument for the therapeutic monitoring to optimize efficacy and safety, has been discussed in the last 25 years and it is still debated [74].

4.1.1. Therapeutic monitoring

4.1.1.1. Trough concentration (C_0) monitoring

Over the past two decades, there have been changes to recommended CsA dosing, changes in concomitant medications, and one major change to the oral drug formulation. Lately, there has also been the introduction of generic formulations of CsA [75]. In 1988, in a prospective study showed that although C_0 (trough concentration) levels of CsA correlated poorly with dose, Cmax was significantly correlated with dose, Area Under the Curve (AUC) and elimination half-life ($t_{1/2}$). Those who suffered acute rejection had a significantly lower Cmax by 15–31% [76]. The problem with this method for adjusting the dosage of CsA is that it relies on only one aspect of CsA pharmacokinetics, the predose or trough concentration. With the original formulation of CsA, Sandimmune®, this was the best practice, but during the conversion of patients from that formulation to the improved formulation, Neoral® the 2 h post-dose concentration has been advocated as a single concentration monitoring alternative to C0 [77]. The microemulsion formulation of CsA, Neoral®, makes CsA pharmacokinetics more predictable and reduces the effects of bile and food on absorption [78]. Nevertheless the predose concentration is still widely used in clinical practice. Currently, most transplant centers measure a single steady-state CsA concentration as either a C_0 predose trough or 2 hours postdose, while some conduct multiple measurements to determine CsA AUC estimates [79]. The target predose concentrations varied not only with transplanted organ and time after transplant but also with the analytical method used. The therapeutic range of CsA used by clinicians varies greatly according to the type of assay used to measure CsA and whether blood or serum concentrations are determined by the clinical laboratory.

Thus, it has reported by high pressure liquid chromatography, monoclonal fluorescence polarization immunoassay (monoclonal TDx assay, Abbott Diagnostics®), or monoclonal radioimmunoassay (various manufacturers), the level of therapeutic concentrations in blood are 10-400 ng/mL. By high pressure liquid chromatography, monoclonal fluorescence polarization immunoassay (monoclonal TDx assay, Abbott Diagnostics®), or monoclonal radioimmunoassay (various manufacturers), the level of therapeutic concentrations in serum are 50-150 ng/mL. By polyclonal fluorescence polarization immunoassay (monoclonal TDx assay, Abbott Diagnostics®), or polyclonal radioimmunoassay (various manufacturers) the level of

http://dx.doi.org/10.5772/54910

therapeutic concentrations in blood are 200-800 ng/mL, and by polyclonal fluorescence polarization immunoassay (monoclonal TDx assay, Abbott Diagnostics®), or polyclonal radioimmunoassay (various manufacturers), the level of therapeutic concentrations in plasma are 100-400 ng/mL [79].

4.1.1.2. Area under the blood concentration-time curve (AUC)

The first steps towards the development of a more precise monitoring strategy for CsA resulted from the landmark studies by Lindholm and Kahan and Kahan et al., which identified a link between the pharmacokinetics of CsA and clinical outcomes in the individual transplant recipient [80,81]. The area under the concentration-time curve for CsA over a 12-hour drug administration interval (AUC_{0-12h}) was a more precise predictor of graft loss and incidence of acute rejection than other parameters, including the C_0. Since then, subsequent studies on the pharmacokinetics of CsA in renal transplant patients have identified that intrapatient variability in AUC values over time was directly correlated with the risk of chronic rejection [77,82].

Proper calculation of AUC requires administration of a dose, followed by blood collection according to an intensive sampling strategy. Concentration values obtained are used to calculate AUC, usually by the trapezoidal method [78]. Some advantages of AUC monitoring are that it is the most precise indicator of drug exposure, can characterize abnormal absorption patterns, appears to be a predictor of clinical outcomes, generates a concentration-time profile, allows calculation of oral pharmacokinetic parameters, and reduces the problems associated with laboratory errors and single concentrations [74,83,84].

Despite its appealing potential advantages, the major disadvantage of AUC monitoring is its inherent need for multiple blood samples. The increased number of samples required, makes AUC monitoring impractical for routine clinical use, more expensive in the short term because of increased sample collection, analysis and interpretation of results, and inconvenient for patients, especially those in an outpatient setting [77,85]. AUC has been advocated as a better parameter to monitor than trough concentrations, because trough concentrations give no indication of exposure to CsA. For example, 2 patients could have the same trough concentration, but one could have a much lower AUC and, therefore, exposure to CsA. Unfortunately, AUC monitoring is not clinically feasible because of the added time, expense and inconvenience required to collect a sufficient number of samples to properly calculate AUC. Although the full AUC for CsA has been demonstrated as being a sensitive monitoring tool, there may be an alternative approach to the determination of the degree and variability of CsA exposure in the individual patient [77,83].

4.1.1.3. Two hours post dose concentration monitoring (C_2)

This approach, which is termed 'absorption profiling', has the underlying rationale that the 4-hour absorption phase following administration provides measurements that are more informative than C_0 monitoring in the assessment of likely CsA exposure and subsequent clinical response [86,87]. AUC_{0-4h} monitoring is a sensitive tool used to optimize CsA immunosuppression in renal transplant recipients. However, the tool is not practical in the clinical setting because of 3 drawbacks: (1) it requires multiple sampling of blood for determination of the AUC_{0-4h}, (2) the actual value requires a mathematical calculation step, and (3) the test may be too expensive for many clinical hospitals or institutions because of the use of added costly laboratory tests for CsA concentrations and the subsequent increase in workload. Therefore, the search for a single blood-sampling point that best reflects the sensitivity of AUC_{0-4h} was the focus of several research initiatives that resulted in a broad approval for C_2 monitoring [82,85]. This method is done by measuring either the area under the blood CsA concentration-time curve in the first hours after dose, AUC_{0-4} or, more simply, by measuring the blood CsA concentration at 2 hours after dose, C_2 [82].

In *the novo* patients this monitoring method has led to result in the following clinical benefits compared with trough concentration monitoring [88]: (1) reduced incidence of acute rejection, (2) reduced severity of rejection episodes and (3) reduced incidence of nephrotoxicity.

4.1.1.4. Bayesian forecasting

The initial pharmacokinetic models for CsA were complicated by the nonlinear, segmented, zero order absorption of the drug from the gut [77,89]. Bayesian forecasting is a TDM tool that has been successfully used clinically in the monitoring of drugs that have a narrow therapeutic index, including antiepileptic drugs, theophylline and aminoglycosides; however, although Bayesian forecasting has proven useful clinically with other drugs, this is not the case with CsA [78]. Bayesian forecasting, in its modern form, was first proposed in 1979 by Sheiner et al. [90]. Since that time, user-friendly computer programs that perform this technique have become widely available. These programs are capable of calculating dosage regimens and pharmacokinetic parameters, as well as predicting drug concentrations by blending population values with patient-specific values [78]. However, these methods were technically complex and were not practical or successful for individualizing CsA therapy in a routine clinical setting and therefore did not gain widespread use. The introduction of Neoral, with its less variable and more predictable blood concentration profile, has rekindled interest in the pharmacokinetic modeling of CsA and in the use of Bayesian forecasting to predict CsA blood concentrations [77].

4.2. Tacrolimus (TRL)

The therapeutic range for TRL used by most transplantation centers is 5–20 ng/mL in blood. Although, plasma TRL concentrations have been measured and an equivalent therapeutic range in this matrix suggested (0.5–2 ng/mL), the two most widely used assays for the drug use blood samples. Because this drug is extensively bound to erythrocytes, blood concentrations average about 15 times greater than concurrently measured serum or plasma concentrations [57,79,91]. As a result, whole blood has become the principal sample used for TRL concentration monitoring, with extraction accomplished through cell lysis and protein denaturation steps that are similar or identical to those used for CsA analysis [51]. The pharmacokinetics of TRL is highly variable. Since TRL shares many of the pharmacokinetic and pharmacodynamic problems associated with CsA the rationale for TDM is similar. Although the feasibility of a limited sampling scheme to predict AUC has been demonstrated, as yet, through or predose whole blood concentration monitoring is still the method of choice [55].

4.2.1. *Therapeutic monitoring*

TRL whole-blood through concentrations have been found to correlate well with the area under the concentration-time curve measurements in liver, kidney and bone marrow transplant recipients (r= 0.91-0.99). Thus, through concentrations are good index of overall drug exposure, and are currently used for routine monitoring as part of patient care posttransplantation [91,92]. This approach offers the opportunity to reduce the pharmacokinetic variability by implementing drug dose adjustments based on plasma/blood concentrations. Drug levels are obtained as predose (12 hours after previous dose) trough concentrations in whole blood [88]. These trough levels correlate reasonably well with area under the curve, with total area under the curve being an accurate measure of drug exposure [94].

Therapeutic ranges of TRL after kidney transplantation are reported as a range for various times after transplant: 0-1 month, 15-20 μg/L; 1-3 months, 10-15 μg/L; and more than 3 months, 5-12 μg/L [95]. TRL blood concentrations are monitored 3 to 7 days a week for the first 2 weeks, at least three times for the following 2 weeks, and whenever the patient comes for an outpatient visit thereafter [96]. On the basis of the terminal half-life of TRL, it was suggested to start monitoring blood concentrations 2 to 3 days after initiation of TRL treatment after the drug has reached steady state. However it is important to reach effective drug concentrations early after transplantation to decrease the risk of acute rejection and to avoid excessive early calcineurin inhibitors concentrations that may be severely damaging after reperfusion of the transplanted organ [97].

The frequency of TDM of TRL should be increased in the case of suspected adverse events or rejection, when liver function is deteriorating, after dose adjustments of the immunosuppressants, change of route of administration, or change of drug formulations, when drugs that are known to interact with CYP3A or P-gP are added or discontinued, or when their doses are changed, in case of severe illness that may affect drug absorption or elimination such as severe immune reactions and sepsis, or if noncompliance is suspected [98].

4.3. Mycophenolic acid (MPA)

In 1995, for preventing rejection in renal transplant patients, MMF, the morpholinoethyl ester prodrug from MPA was approved for clinical use. This drug has since become the predominant anti-metabolite immunosuppressive used in the transplant setting. Although the current labeling information for MMF does not indicate any need for therapeutic monitoring of plasma MPA concentrations, there were a number of studies showing a relationship between MPA pharmacokinetics and clinical outcome [99]. Definitive determination of the pharmacokinetics of the drug in renal allograft recipients after transplantation is not without difficulty. In principle, substantial changes in pharmacokinetics could be produced by changes following transplantation, both in the immediate post-transplant period (reflecting rapid alterations in drug therapy, renal function, hemodynamics and gastrointestinal motility) as well as more gradual changes (reflecting change in bodyweight, plasma proteins and organ function) [100]. The greatest variability in MPA pharmacokinetic is noted in the initial 2 months following transplantation, when adequate immunosuppression is critical to graft function and survival. It has also become apparent from longer term pharmacokinetic studies that exposure to MPA increases over time due to reduced clearance of the drug. A possible additional factor that could contribute to the higher oral clearance of MPA early after transplantation is corticosteroid therapy, which is significantly higher in that period but then is tapered to low dose levels or completely withdrawn. Based upon the marked pharmacokinetic variability observed with MPA and the pharmacodynamic relationship of pharmacokinetic parameters to rejection outcome, several scientific societies and consensus conferences have advocated the use of concentration monitoring for patients undergoing treatment with MMF or enteric-coated MPA [101].

4.3.1. Therapeutic monitoring

The incorporation of MMF into immunosuppressive regimens has been associated with decrease rates of acute rejection and decreased chronic allograft loss. Indications for TDM of mycophenolates were reviewed in a consensus meeting [101]. They included high-risk patients, patients with delayed graft function, or patients with immunosuppressive protocols excluding induction therapy or steroids or calcineurin inhibitor or patients with calcineurin minimization. Most of these patients (especially high-risk patients) are often excluded from the clinical trials. In fact, MPA TDM is currently only used in a few transplant centers on a routine basis, whereas a few others only checked MPA exposure in case of unexpected acute rejection or adverse event or drug interaction. Most of the centers never measure MPA. It is clear that the use of MPA TDM is conditioned by the faith of the physicians in its use, local availability of MPA measurements, and organization of the nursing staff [102].

4.3.1.1. Trough concentration (C_0) monitoring

Although a relationship between AUC and outcome exists, the clinical utility of concentration monitoring, particularly C_0 monitoring for MMF, has been questioned. Over the past decade, several studies were conducted to evaluate the clinical utility of prospective concentration controlled MMF therapy. While these studies were anticipated to fully clarify the utility of monitored MMF therapy, the outcomes from these studies are conflicting and have done little to settle the controversies surrounding this area of therapeutic drug monitoring [100]. With trough concentration, plasma concentration of MPA is measured immediately before a dose, it is easy to measure because only -ask patient to return to give sample, it is immediately before a dose, and only requires single simple possible association between C_0 and decreased rejection noted in transplant recipients. However this method represents some disadvantages. Timing may not be accurate (depends on remembering time of last dose). Timing may vary from the "ideal" (12 h after last dose) by several hours. There is no high-level evidence of a strong association between C_0 and outcome, or between C_0 and AUC_{0-12}, C_0 is not a very informative time point for estimation of individual pharmacokinetic parameters. Single time-point samples such as the trough concentration or others do not correlate well with the MPA AUC, especially in the early posttransplantation period [103].

4.3.1.2. Limited sampling strategies for estimation of MPA AUC

The dose interval MPA $AUC_{0\text{–}12}$ h is generally regarded as the most reliable pharmacokinetic parameter index of risk for acute rejection but is impractical to measure in routine clinical practice. Single time-point samples such as the trough concentration or others, do not correlate well with the MPA AUC, especially in the early posttransplantation period renal transplant patients and for regimens that include MMF plus CsA, TRL, or SRL [104]. Therefore, assessment of whether C_0 concentrations or other single time points correlate well with the AUC is important for establishing routine monitoring of the drug. Apart of the C_0 level other single time points after MMF dosing are examined for their ability to predict full AUC values. A full MPA AUC typically requires at least eight blood samples during 12 hour dose interval. In clinical practice this is impractical; therefore, abbreviated sampling schemes involving the collection of there to five plasma samples have been investigated. The abbreviated sampling approach has provided estimations of MPA AUC with high correlations (r^2>0.8). Several models have been developed all of them in renal transplant patients [105-108].

4.4. Sirolimus (SRL)

SRL (formerly known as rapamycin) is a macrolide antibiotic with immunosuppressive properties that was introduced relatively recently (September 1999) into clinical practice for maintenance therapy in organ transplantation [109]. Pharmacokinetics studies of SRL in renal transplant patients have been shown great variability between patients. Several features contribute to the interpatient pharmacokinetic variability observed with SRL and can include any combination of the following: absorption, distribution, metabolism and/or excretion [110].

This drug presents a rapid gastrointestinal absorption (t_{max} from 0.33 to 5 hours) as well as a low (mean value 14%) and variable bioavailability. It has been reported that SRL is a substrate for the multidrug P-glycoprotein transporter and that the biotransformation of SRL is mediated by CYP3A enzymes. Accordingly, considerable variability in its pharmacokinetic parameters may be expected (apparent blood clearance rates after oral administration from 87 to 416 mL/h/kg). In addition, the disposition of SRL in humans includes a large volume of distribution, a long half-life (35 to 95 hours) and dose proportionality for Cmax and AUC. Also, some interracial variability and an influence of hepatic dysfunction have been noted with SRL [111]. Although structurally similar to TRL, SRL has a novel mechanism of action, which leads to synergy with CsA. The long half-life of the drug necessitates a loading dose to achieve therapeutic concentrations quickly, and also allows for once daily administration. Highly variable absorption and metabolism of the drug result in large differences in blood concentrations among patients receiving the same dose. Efficacy for the prevention of acute rejection episodes, and the rate of common adverse effects (thrombocytopenia, leucopenia and hypertriglyceridemia), are concentration-dependent [112].

4.4.1. Therapeutic monitoring

Clinical data suggest that the immunosuppressive efficacy and the occurrence and severity of adverse effects of SRL correlate with blood concentrations [112]. Drug interactions with concomitant immunosuppressant medications will alter SRL whole blood concentrations. The appropriate SRL through concentration at steady state (Cmin,ss) for acute rejection episode prophylaxis is a function of the concomitant immunosuppressive regimen. When it is used as base therapy with azathioprine and prednisone, a regimen stipulating initial Cmin,ss values equal to 30 μg/L during the first 2 months, and 15 μg/L(LC/UV assay) thereafter, led to a 41% rate of acute rejection episodes among 41 cadaveric kidney transplant recipients [113].

When combined with MMF and prednisone, this SRL regimen was associated with a 27.5% rate of acute rejection episodes among 40 cadaveric renal transplant recipients. Indeed, the combination of SRL (Cmin,ss of 10 to 20 μg/L; LC/UV assay) and basiliximab with late introduction of low dosage CsA has provided excellent prophylaxis of acute rejection episodes and renal function for primary, non-African-American recipients of cadaveric kidney transplants that displayed delayed graft function [112,114,115].

In purely Caucasian low-risk liver and kidney-pancreas transplant recipients, Cmin,ss of 6 to 12 μg/L (IMx® assay) in combination with low dosage TRL has been reported to yield low rates of acute rejection episodes and toxicity [116]. Because of the long half-life and extensive tissue distribution of the drug, steady-state concentrations are not reached before day 6 after initiation of therapy or after a dosage change. Thus, daily concentration monitoring is not necessary; the first SRL measurements should not be obtained before day 4 after inception of, or change in therapy. Thereafter, recommend monitoring Cmin,ss weekly for the first month and bi-weekly for the next month, targeting a 5 to 15 μg/L range if CsA is being used concomitantly at Cmin,ss concentrations of 75 to 150 μg/L. If the patient fails to attain these values despite a dosage of 20mg/day, a full pharmacokinetic study should be performed to assess whether the defect is due to limited absorption or rapid clearance rates [112]. Modest correlation ($r = 0.59$) exists between SRL dose and peak plasma concentration (Cmax) or AUC, but a good correlation ($r = 0.85$) exists between trough concentration prior to the dose (minimum Cmin,ss and AUC. For this reason, Cmin,ss is a simple and useful index for therapeutic monitoring of SRL [112,117,118].

4.5. Everolimus (EVL)

In April 2010, EVL, a more water-soluble analog of SRL was approved for use in CsA-sparing regimens, including the requirement for adjusting EVL doses using target trough blood concentrations in renal transplant patients [51]. EVL, which has greater polarity than SRL, was developed in an attempt to improve the pharmacokinetic characteristics of SRL, particularly to increase its oral bioavailability. After a single oral dose of EVL 4mg in 12 healthy volunteers, it was absorbed rapidly (within 30 minutes after drug intake). The Cmax of EVL amounted to 44.2 ± 13.3 μg/L and was reached (t_{max}) after 30 minutes (range 0.5–1 hour). The AUC was 219 ± 69 μg* h/L. The overall absorption of EVL, like that of SRL, is probably affected by the activity of P-gp. It is recommended that patients should take the drug consistently with or without food to reduce fluctuations in drug exposure [119]. In an international study, the pharmacokinetics of EVL, were characterized over the first 6 months post-transplant in 731 patients receiving either 0.75 or 1.5mg bid EVL in addition to CsA and corticosteroids. The within- and between-patient variability of dose interval AUC was 27% and 31% respectively. There was no detectable influence of sex, age (16–66 years), or weight (42-132 kg) on AUC, but EVL exposure was significantly lower by an average of 20 % in blacks. In a study of 659 AUC profiles the correlation between trough concentration and overall exposure (AUC) there was a significant linear correlation with a regression coefficient of 0.89 and corresponding coefficient of determination of 0.79 [120].

For example, see [121] reported that multiple daily dosing of EVL, in doses up to 5 mg/day, is adequately well tolerated as add-on therapy in stable renal transplant patients receiving maintenance Neoral® immunosuppression. Similar degrees of correlation between EVL trough concentration and thrombocytopenia, leukopenia, hypertriglyceridemia, or hypercholesterolemia in 54 stable renal transplant patients (18-68 years) were found.

4.5.1. Therapeutic drug monitoring

EVL is a drug with a narrow therapeutic index. The limited and variable bioavailability, intrinsic interindividual pharmacokinetic variability, the number of factors affecting the pharmacokinetics, and the number of drug interactions limits the use of fixed doses of this drug. The EVL Cmin is a good surrogate marker of EVL exposure (AUC), and correlates with pharmacological response and clinical outcomes. Therefore, prospective dose adjustments to obtain and maintain a therapeutic EVL Cmin have the potential to improve efficacy and reduce toxicity [122].

A role for EVL drug monitoring has been suggested because of the potential for improving efficacy and reducing adverse effects, the EVL Cmin is a good surrogate marker of EVL exposure (AUC), and correlates with pharmacological response and clinical outcomes. Therefore, prospective dose adjustments to obtain and maintain a therapeutic EVL Cmin have the potential to improve efficacy and reduce toxicity [123]. Mere clinical monitoring of efficacy is insufficient because clinical presentations of graft rejection vary for each patient and are nonspecific. Thus, some authors have used a previously published 9-step decision-making algorithm to evaluate the utility of TDM for EVL. The recommended therapeutic range for EVL is a trough concentration of 3 to 8 ng/mL, as concentrations over 3 ng/mL have been associated with a decreased incidence of rejection, and concentrations >8 ng/mL with increased toxicity. Patients on EVL who have problems with absorption, who take concurrent cytochrome P450 inhibitors or inducers, or are noncompliant will attain the greatest benefit from therapeutic drug monitoring [124].

5. Advances in immunosuppression – Future trends

Maintenance immunosuppressive therapy over the past decade has become more diversified. Until the mid-1990s, CsA and azathioprine were the cornerstones in maintenance immunosuppressive therapy. Today, these agents have been largely replaced by the newer agents TRL and MMF. Triple immunosuppression continues to be the standard, and corticosteroids are still part of most widely used immunosuppressive protocols. More effective immunosuppression has reduced the incidence of acute rejection without a reduction in patient survival [125]. Calcineurin inhibitors are still the cornerstone of current immunosuppressive therapy, but have important cardiovascular and oncogenic side effects and nephrotoxicity effects that contributes to the multifactorial process called "chronic allograft dysfunction", the leading cause of chronic allograft failure among kidney transplant recipients. New drugs, with a different mechanism of action, are being developed focusing on a better balance between drug efficacy and toxicity. These novel compounds interfere with either T-cell mediated or antibody-mediated rejection [126].

A number of novel drugs are currently under investigation in Phase I, II, or III clinical trials primarily to replace the nephrotoxic but highly effective calcineurin inhibitors. ISA247 (voclosporine) is a CsA analog with reduced nephrotoxicity in Phase III study. AEB071 (sotrastaurin), a protein kinase C inhibitor, and CP-690550, a JAK3 inhibitor, are small molecules in Phase II studies EVL is derived from the mTOR inhibitor SRL and is in Phase III study. Belatacept is a humanized antibody that inhibits T-cell costimulation and has shown encouraging results in multiple Phase II and III trials. Alefacept and Efaluzimab are humanized antibodies that inhibit T-cell adhesion and are in Phase I and II clinical trials [127]. Finally, the exciting field of tissue engineering and stem cell biology with the repopulation of decellularized organs is ushering in a new paradigm for transplantation. The era of simplified immunosuppression regimens devoid of toxicities is upon us with the promise of dramatic improvement in long term survival [128].

6. Conclusions

Monitored drug therapy has undergone a tremendous change over the past quarter of a century with the increasing availability of advanced techniques like liquid chromatography with tandem mass spectrometry detection and immunoassays. Currently, the possibility of accurately and specifically measuring almost any drug in any biological fluid is a reality, and while TDM has become a standard of care for most immunosuppressive drugs, TDM practices will continue to evolve with the field of transplantation. New immunosuppressives, such as sotrastaurin, exhibit pharmacokinetic variability comparable to that seen with currently used immunosuppressive drugs and may benefit from monitoring therapy [129]. Although TDM of biologic drugs such as belatacept have not been reported in clinical trials to date, potentially useful pharmacodynamic assays that can be performed on blood specimens have been described [51,130]. The information gained through further study in these complex regimens should provide innovative strategies and new immunosuppressive agents that will serve to extend the functional life of allografts without toxicity or infection.

http://dx.doi.org/10.5772/54910

Author details

Ana Luisa Robles Piedras*, Minarda De la O Arciniega and Josefina Reynoso Vázquez

*Address all correspondence to: roblesa@uaeh.edu.mx

Academic Area of Pharmacy, Institute of Health Sciences, Autonomous University of Hidalgo State, Mexico

References

[1] Krensky AM, Vincenti F, Bennett WM. Immunosuppressants, Tolerogens, and Immunostimulants. In: Brunton L. (ed) Goodman and Gilman's The Pharmacological Basis of Therapeutics 11th ed. McGraw-Hill Co. New York, NY. 2006. p1405-1431.

[2] Kahan BD. Cyclosporine. New England Journal of Medicine 1989;32:1725-1738.

[3] Khanna A, Li B, Stenzel KH, Suthanthiran M. Regulation of new DNA synthesis in mammalian cells by cyclosporine. Demonstration of a transforming growth factor beta-dependent mechanism of inhibition of cell growth. Transplantation 1994;57:577-582.

[4] Freeman DJ. Pharmacology and pharmacokinetics of cyclosporine. Clinical Biochemistry 1991;24:9-14.

[5] Fairley JA. Intracellular targets of cyclosporine. Journal of the American Academy of Dermatology 1990;23:1329-1334.

[6] Halloran PF, Madrenas J. The mechanism of action of cyclosporine: a perspective for the 90's. Clinical Biochemistry 1991;24:3-7.

[7] Schreiber SL, Crabtree GR. The mechanism of action of cyclosporin A and FK506. Immunology Today 1992;13:136-142.

[8] Aszalos A. Cyclosporin: some aspects of its mode of action. A review. Journal of Medicine 1988;19:297-316.

[9] Product Information. Sandimmune® oral capsules, oral solution, intravenous injection, cyclosporine oral capsules, oral solution, intravenous injection. Novartis Pharmaceuticals Corporation, East Hanover, NJ. 2010.

[10] Cush JJ, Tugwell P, Weinblatt M, Yocum D. US consensus guidelines for the use of cyclosporin A in rheumatoid arthritis. Journal of Rheumatology 1999;26(5):1176-1186.

[11] Charnick SB, Nedelman JR, Chang CT, Hwang DS, Jin J, Moore MA, Wong R. Description of blood pressure changes in patients beginning cyclosporin A therapy. Therapeutic Drug Monitoring 1997;19:17-24.

[12] de Mattos AM, Olyaei AJ, Bennett WM. Nephrotoxicity of immunosuppressive drugs: long-term consequences and challenges for the future. American Journal of Kidney Diseases 2000;35(2):333-346.

[13] Ballantyne CM, Podet EJ, Patsch WP, Harati Y, Appel V, Gotto AM Jr, Young JB. Effects of cyclosporine therapy on plasma lipoprotein levels. The Journal of the American Medical Association 1989;262:53-56.

[14] McGaw WT, Porter H. Cyclosporine-induced gingival overgrowth: an ultrastructural stereologic study. Oral Surgery, Oral Medicine, Oral Pathology 1988;65(2):186-190.

[15] Daly CG. Resolution of cyclosporin A (CsA)-induced gingival enlargement following reduction in CsA dosage. Journal of Clinical Periodontology 1992;19:143-145.

[16] Wong W, Hodge MG, Lewis A, Sharpstone P, Kingswood JC. Resolution of cyclosporin-induced gingival hypertrophy with metronidazole. Lancet 1994;343:986.

[17] Shapiro R. Tacrolimus in pediatric renal transplantation: A review. Pediatric Transplantation 1998;2:270-276.

[18] Plosker GL. Foster RH. Tacrolimus: a further update of its pharmacology and therapeutic use in the management of organ transplantation. Drugs 2000;59:323-389.

[19] Tocci MJ, Matkovich DA, Collier KA, Kwok P, Dumont F, Lin S, Degudicibus S, Siekierka JJ, Chin J, Hutchinson NI. FK-506 selectively inhibits expression of early T cell activation genes. The Journal of Immunology 1989;143:718-726.

[20] Kay JE, Moore AL, Doe SE, Benzie CR, Schönbrunner R, Schmid FX, Halestrap AP. The mechanism of action of FK 506. Transplantation Proceedings 1990;22(1):96-99.

[21] Peters DH, Fitton A, Plosker GL, Faulds D. Tacrolimus: a review of its pharmacology, and therapeutic potential in hepatic and renal transplantation. Drugs 1993;46:746-794.

[22] Rauch MC, San Martín A, Ojeda D, Quezada C, Salas M, Cárcamo JG, Yañez AJ, Slebe JC, Claude A. Tacrolimus causes a blockage of protein secretion which reinforces its immunosuppressive activity and also explains some of its toxic side-effects. Tacrolimus causes a blockage of protein secretion which reinforces its immunosuppressive activity and also explains some of its toxic side-effects. Transplant Immunology 2009;22(1-2): 72-81.

[23] Product Information: PROGRAF® oral capsules, IV injection, tacrolimus oral capsules, IV injection. Astellas Pharma US, Inc. (per manufacturer), Deerfield, IL. 2011.

[24] Henry ML. Cyclosporine and tacrolimus (FK506): a comparison of efficacy and safety profiles. Clinical Transplantation 1999;13:209-220.

[25] Pham SM, Kormos RL, Hattler BG, Kawai A, Tsamandas AC, Demetris AJ, Murali S, Fricker FJ, Chang HC, Jain AB, Starzl TE, Hardesty RL, Griffith BP. A prospective trial of (FK 506) in clinical heart transplantation: intermediate-term results. The Journal of Thoracic and Cardiovascular Surgery 1996;111:764-772.

[26] AM, Furth SL, Case BW, Wise B, Colombani PM, Fivush BA. Evaluation of neurotoxicity in pediatric renal transplant recipients treated with tacrolimus (FK506). Clinical Transplantation 1997;11:412-414.

[27] Krentz AJ, Dousset B, Mayer D, McMaster P, Buckels J, Cramb R, Smith JM, Nattrass M. Metabolic effects of cyclosporin A and FK 506 in liver transplant recipients. Diabetes 1993;42:1753-1759.

[28] Ardestani F, Fatemi SS, Yakhchali B. Evaluation of mycophenolic acid production by Penicillium brevicompactum MUCL 19011 in batch and continuous submerged cultures. Biochemical Engineering Journal 2010;50(3):99-103.

[29] Oremus M, Zeidler J, Ensom MHH. Utility of monitoring mycophenolic acid in solid organ transplant patients. Evidence Report/Technology Assessment No. 164. AHRQ Publication No.08-E006. Rockville, MD: Agency for Healthcare Research and Quality. 2008. http://www.ahrq.gov/downloads/pub/evidence/pdf/mpa/mpaorgan.pdf (accessed 3 August 2012).

[30] Groth CG, Ohlman S, Gannedahl G, Ericzon BG. New immunosuppressive drugs in transplantation. Transplantation Proceedings 1993;25:2681-2683.

[31] Eugui EM, Mirkovich A, Allison AC. Lymphocyte-selective antiproliferative and immunosuppressive effects of mycophenolic acid in mice. Scandinavian Journal of Immunology 1991;33:175.

[32] Bumgardner GL, Roberts JP. New immunosuppressive agents. Gastroenterology Clinics of North America 1993;22:421-449.

[33] Butani L, Palmer J, Baluarte HJ, Polinsky MS. Adverse effects of mycophenolate mofetil in pediatric renal transplant recipients with presumed chronic rejection. Transplantation 1999;68:83-86.

[34] Product Information. CellCept® oral tablets, capsules, suspension and intravenous injection, mycophenolate mofetil oral tablets, capsules, suspension, mycophenolate mofetil hydrochloride intravenous injection. Roche Laboratories Inc., Nutley, NJ. 2009.

[35] Kuypers DR, Le Meur Y, Cantarovich M, Tredger MJ, Tett SE, Cattaneo D, Tönshoff B, Holt DW, Chapman J, Gelder T; Transplantation Society (TTS) Consensus Group on TDM of MPA. Consensus report on therapeutic drug monitoring of mycophenolic acid in solid organ transplantation. Clinical Journal of the American Society of Nephrology 2010;5:341-358. http://ebookbrowse.com/transplante-consensus-report-therapeutic-drug-monitoring-mycophenolic-acid-pdf-d322644574 (accessed 3 August 2012).

[36] Watson CJ, Friend PJ, Jamieson NV, Frick TW, Alexander G, Gimson AE, Calne R. Sirolimus: a potent new immunosuppressant for liver transplantation. Transplantation 1999;67(4):505-509. http://www.centerspan.org/pubs/transplantation/1999/0227/tr0499005050.pdf (accessed 3 August 2012).

[37] Kelly PA, Gruber SA, Behbod F, Kahan BD. Sirolimus, a new potent immunosuppressive agent. Pharmacotherapy 1997;17:1148-1156.

[38] Morris RE. Mechanisms of action of new immunosuppressive drugs. Kidney International 1996;49(53):S26-S38.

[39] Brattström C, Wilczek H, Tydén G, Böttiger Y, Säwe J, Groth CG. Hyperlipidemia in renal transplant recipients treated with sirolimus (Rapamycin). Transplantation 1998;65(9):1272-1274.

[40] Schuler W, Sedrani R, Cottens S, Häberlin B, Schulz M, Schuurman HJ, Zenke G, Zerwes HG, Schreier MH. SDZ RAD, a new rapamycin derivative. Transplantation 1997;64(1): 36-42.

[41] Eisen HJ, Tuzcu EM, Dorent R, Kobashigawa J, Mancini D, Valantine-von Kaeppler HA, Starling RC, Sørensen K, Hummel M, Lind JM, Abeywickrama KH, Bernhardt P; RAD B253 Study Group. RAD B253 Study Group. Everolimus for the prevention of allograft rejection and vasculopathy in cardiac-transplant recipients. The New England Journal of Medicine 2003;349:847-858.

[42] van Rossum HH, Romijn FP, Smit NP, de Fijter JW, van Pelt J. Everolimus and sirolimus antagonize tacrolimus based calcineurin inhibition via competition for FK-binding protein 12. Biochemical Pharmacology 2009;77(7):1206-1212.

[43] Sánchez-Fructuoso AI, Ruiz JC, Pérez-Flores I, Gómez Alamillo C, Calvo Romero N, Arias M. Comparative analysis of adverse events requiring suspension of mtor inhibitors: everolimus versus sirolimus. Transplantation Proceedings 2010;42(8): 3050-3052.

[44] Moldawer NP, Wood LS. Management of key adverse events associated with everolimus therapy. Kidney Cancer Journal 2010;8(2):51-59. http://www.kidney-cancer-journal.com/emag/v8n2/pageflip.htm (accessed 3 August 2012).

[45] Afzali B, Taylor AL, Goldsmith DJ. What we CAN do about chronic allograft nephropathy: Role of immunosuppressive modulations. Kidney International, 2005;68:2429-2443.

[46] Danovitch GM. Immunosuppressive medications for renal transplantation: A multiple choice question. Kidney International 2001; 59:388-402.

[47] Gabardi S, Martin ST, Roberts KL, Grafals M. Induction immunosuppressive therapies in renal transplantation. American Journal of Health-System Pharmacy 2011;68(1): 211-218.

[48] Helal I, Chan L. Steroid and calcineurin inhibitor-sparing protocols in kidney transplantation. Transplantation Proceedings 2011;43:472-477.

[49] Ponticelli C. Present and future of immunosuppressive therapy in kidney transplantation. Transplantation Proceedings 2011;43: 2439-2440.

[50] Budde K, Glander P. Pharmacokinetic principles of immunosuppressive drugs. Annals of Transplantation 2008;13(3):5-10.

[51] Milone MC., Shaw LMJ. Therapeutic Drug Monitoring for Immunosuppressive Agents. In: Kaplan B., Burkhart JG., Lakkis FG. (ed.) Immunotherapy in Transplantation: Principles and Practice. USA: Wiley-Blackwell; 2012. p95-113.

[52] Evans W. General Principles of Clinical Pharmacokinetics. In: Burton ME., Shaw LM., Schentag JJ., Evans WE. (ed) Applied Pharmacokinetics and Pharmacodynamics. Principles of Therapeutic Drug Monitoring. USA: Williams and Wilkins; 2006. p3-7.

[53] Kang JS, Lee MH. Overview of Therapeutic Drug Monitoring. The Korean Journal of Internal Medicine 2009;24(1):1-10. http://www.ncbi.nlm.nih.gov/pmc/articles/PMC2687654/pdf/kjim-24-1.pdf (accessed 6 July 2012).

[54] Peppinger C., Massoud N. Therapeutic Drug Monitoring. In: Benet L., Massoud N., Gambertoglio J. (ed.) Pharmacokinetic Basis for Drug Treatment. New York: Raven Press; 1985. p367-393.

[55] Johnston A, Holt DW. Therapeutic drug monitoring of immunosuppressant drugs. British Journal of Clinical Pharmacology 1999; 47(4): 339–350.

[56] Neef C, Touw DJ, Stolk LM. Therapeutic Drug Monitoring in Clinical Research. Pharmaceutical Medicine.2008;22(4):235-44. http://adisonline.com/pharmaceuticalmedicine/Abstract/2008/22040/Therapeutic_Drug_Monitoring_in_Clinical_Research.4.aspx (accessed 6 July 2012).

[57] Venkataramanan R, Swaminathan A, Prasad T, Jain A, Zuckerman S, Warty V, McMichael J, Lever J, Burckart G, Starzl T. Clinical pharmacokinetics of tacrolimus. Clinical Pharmacokinetics 1995;29(6):404-30.

[58] Meier-Kriesche HU, Shaw LM, Korecka M, Kaplan B. Pharmacokinetics of mycophenolic acid in renal insufficiency. Therapeutic Drug Monitoring 2000;22(1):27-30.

[59] Mignat C. Clinically significant drug interactions with new immunosuppressive agents. Drug Safety 1997;16:267-78

[60] Omar G, Shah IA, Thomson AW, Whiting PH, Burke MD. FK 506 inhibition of cyclosporine metabolism by human liver microsomes. Transplantation Proceedings 1991;23(1 Pt 2):934-5.

[61] Filler G, Lampe D, Mai I, Strehlau J, Ehrich JH. Dosing of MMF in combination with tacrolimus for steroid-resistant vascular rejection in pediatric renal allografts. Transplant International 1998;11 Suppl 1:S82-5.

[62] van Gelder T, Klupp J, Barten MJ, Christians U, Morris RE. Comparison of the effects of tacrolimus and cyclosporine on the pharmacokinetics of mycophenolic acid. Therapeutic Drug Monitoring 2001;23(2):119-28.

[63] Schwartz JB. The influence of sex on pharmacokinetics. Clinical Pharmacokinetics 2003;42(2):107-21.

[64] Morissette P, Albert C, Busque S, St-Louis G, Vinet B. In vivo higher glucuronidation of mycophenolic acid in male than in female recipients of a cadaveric kidney allograft

and under immunosuppressive therapy with mycophenolate mofetil. Therapeutic Drug Monitoring 2001;23(5):520-5.

[65] Velicković-Radovanović R, Mikov M, Paunović G, Djordjević V, Stojanović M, Cvetković T, Djordjević AC. Gender differences in pharmacokinetics of tacrolimus and their clinical significance in kidney transplant recipients. Gender Medicine 2011;8(1):23-31.

[66] del Mar Fernández De Gatta M, Santos-Buelga D, Domínguez-Gil A, García MJ. Immunosuppressive therapy for paediatric transplant patients: pharmacokinetic considerations. Clinical Pharmacokinetics 2002;41(2):115-35.

[67] de Wildt SN, van Schaik RH, Soldin OP, Soldin SJ, Brojeni PY, van der Heiden IP, Parshuram C, Nulman I, Koren G. The interactions of age, genetics, and disease severity on tacrolimus dosing requirements after pediatric kidney and liver transplantation. European Journal of Clinical Pharmacology 2011;67(12):1231-41.

[68] Cooney GF, Habucky K, Hoppu K. Cyclosporin pharmacokinetics in paediatric transplant recipients. Clinical Pharmacokinetics 1997;32(6):481-95.

[69] Jacqz-Aigrain E, Montes C, Brun P, Loirat C. Cyclosporine pharmacokinetics in nephrotic and kidney-transplanted children. European Journal of Clinical Pharmacology 1994;47(1):61-5.

[70] Staatz CE, Tett SE. Clinical pharmacokinetics and pharmacodynamics of tacrolimus in solid organ transplantation. Clinical Pharmacokinetics 2004;43(10):623-53.

[71] Fitzsimmons WE, Bekersky I, Dressler D, Raye K, Hodosh E, Mekki Q. Demographic considerations in tacrolimus pharmacokinetics. Transplantation Proceedings 1998;30(4): 1359-64.

[72] Mancinelli LM, Frassetto L, Floren LC, Dressler D, Carrier S, Bekersky I, Benet LZ, Christians U. The pharmacokinetics and metabolic disposition of tacrolimus: a comparison across ethnic groups. Clinical Pharmacology and Therapeutics 2001;69(1): 24-31.

[73] Ochiai T, Fukao K, Takahashi K, Endo T, Oshima S, Uchida K, Yokoyama I, Ishibashi M, Takahara S, Iwasaki Y. Phase III study of FK 506 in kidney transplantation. Japanese FK 506 Study Group. Transplantation Proceedings 1995;27(1):829-33.

[74] Citterio F. Evolution of the therapeutic drug monitoring of cyclosporine. Transplantation Proceedings 2004;36(2 Suppl):420S-425S.

[75] Trevillian P. Therapeutic drug monitoring. Nephrology 2007; 12, S57–S65.

[76] Kasiske BL, Heim-Duthoy K, Rao KV, Awni WM. The relationship between cyclosporin pharmacokinetic parameters and subsequent acute rejection in renal transplant recipients. Transplantation 1988;46: 716–22.

[77] Johnston A., Holt DW. Cyclosporine. In: Burton ME., Shaw LM., Schentag JJ., Evans WE. (ed) Applied Pharmacokinetics and Pharmacodynamics. Principles of Therapeutic Drug Monitoring. USA: Williams and Wilkins; 2006. p512-528.

http://dx.doi.org/10.5772/54910

[78] Dumont RJ, Ensom MH. Methods for clinical monitoring of cyclosporin in transplant patients. Clinical Pharmacokinetics 2000;38(5):427-47.

[79] Bauer LA. Applied Clinical Pharmacokinetics. USA: McGraw-Hill; 2001.

[80] Lindholm A, Kahan BD. Influence of cyclosporine pharmacokinetics, trough concentrations, and AUC monitoring on outcome after kidney transplantation. Clinical Pharmacology and Therapeutics 1993;54:205-18.

[81] Kahan BD, Welsh M, Schoenberg L, Rutzky LP, Katz SM, Urbauer DL, Van Buren CT. Variable oral absorption of cyclosporine. A biopharmaceutical risk factor for chronic renal allograft rejection. Transplantation 1996; 62:599-606.

[82] Levy GA. C2 monitoring strategy for optimizing cyclosporin immunosuppression from the Neoral formulation. BioDrugs 2001;15(5):279-90.

[83] David-Neto E, Araujo LP, Feres Alves C, Sumita N, Romano P, Yagyu EM, Nahas WC, Ianhez LE. A strategy to calculate cyclosporin A area under the time-concentration curve in pediatric renal transplantation. Pediatric Transplantation 2002;6(4):313-18.

[84] Weber LT, Armstrong VW, Shipkova M, Feneberg R, Wiesel M, Mehls O, Zimmerhackl LB, Oellerich M, Tönshoff B; Members of the German Study Group on Pediatric Renal Transplantion. Cyclosporin A absorption profiles in pediatric renal transplant recipients predict the risk of acute rejection. Therapeutic Drug Monitoring 2004;26(4):415-24.

[85] Mahalati K, Belitsky P, West K, Kiberd B, Fraser A, Sketris I, Macdonald AS, McAlister V, Lawen J. Approaching the therapeutic window for cyclosporine in kidney transplantation: a prospective study. Journal of the American Society of Nephrology 2001;12(4):828-33.

[86] Dunn CJ, Wagstaff AJ, Perry CM, Plosker GL, Goa KL. Cyclosporin: an updated review of the pharmacokinetic properties, clinical efficacy and tolerability of a microemulsion based formulation (neoral)1 in organ transplantation. Drugs 2001;61(13): 1957-2016.

[87] Keown PA. New concepts in cyclosporine monitoring. Current Opinion in Nephrology and Hypertension. 2002;11(6):619-26.

[88] Belitsky P, Dunn S, Johnston A, Levy G. Impact of absorption profiling on efficacy and safety of cyclosporin therapy in transplant recipients. Clinical Pharmacokinetics 2000;39(2):117-25.

[89] Grevel J, Post BK, Kahan BD. Michaelis-Menten kinetics determine cyclosporine steady-state concentrations: a population analysis in kidney transplant patients. Clinical Pharmacology and Therapeutics 1993;53(6):651-60. ABSTRACT

[90] Sheiner LB, Beal S, Rosenberg B, et al. Forecasting individual pharmacokinetics. Clinical Pharmacology & Therapeutics 1979;26:294-305.

[91] Jusko WJ, Thomson AW, Fung J, McMaster P, Wong SH, Zylber-Katz E, Christians U, Winkler M, Fitzsimmons WE, Lieberman R. Consensus document: therapeutic monitoring of tacrolimus (FK-506). Therapeutic Drug Monitoring 1995;17(6):606–614.

[92] Staatz C, Taylor P, Tett S. Low tacrolimus concentrations and increased risk of early acute rejection in adult renal transplantation. Nephrology Dialysis and Transplantation 2001;16(9):1905-9.

[93] Cattaneo D, Perico N, Remuzzi G. From pharmacokinetics to pharmacogenomics: a new approach to tailor immunosuppressive therapy. American Journal of Transplantation 2004;4(3):299-310.

[94] Kapturczak MH, Meier-Kriesche HU, Kaplan B. Pharmacology of calcineurin antagonists. Transplantation Proceedings 2004;36(2 Suppl):25S-32S.

[95] Scott LJ, McKeage K, Keam SJ, Plosker GL. Tacrolimus: a further update of its use in the management of organ transplantation. Drugs 2003;63(12):1247-97.

[96] Jusko WJ, Kobayashi M. Therapeutic monitoring of tacrolimus (FK 506). Therapeutic Drug Monitoring 1993;15(4):349.

[97] Shaw LM, Holt DW, Keown P, Venkataramanan R, Yatscoff RW. Current opinions on therapeutic drug monitoring of immunosuppressive drugs. Clinical Therapeutics 1999;21(10):1632-52.

[98] Christians U., Pokaiyavanichkul T., Chan l. Tacrolimus. In: Applied Pharmacokinetics and Pharmacodynamics: Principles of Therapeutic Drug Monitoring, 4th Ed., edited by Burton ME, Shaw LM, Schentag JJ, Evans WE, Philadelphia, Lippincott Williams & Wilkins, 2006, pp 563–594.

[99] Bullingham RES, Nicholls A, Hale M. Pharmacokinetics of mycophenolate mofetil (RS-61443): a short review. Transplantation Proceedings 1996;28:925-29.

[100] Bullingham RE, Nicholls AJ, Kamm BR. Clinical Pharmacokinetics of Mycophenolate Mofetil. Clinical Pharmacokinetics 1998;34(6):429-455.

[101] van Gelder T, Le Meur Y, Shaw LM, Oellerich M, DeNofrio D, Holt C, Holt DW, Kaplan B, Kuypers D, Meiser B, Toenshoff B, Mamelok RD. Therapeutic drug monitoring of mycophenolate mofetil in transplantation. Therapeutic Drug Monitoring 2006;28(2): 145-54.

[102] Le Meur Y, Borrows R, Pescovitz MD, Budde K, Grinyo J, Bloom R, Gaston R, Walker RG, Kuypers D, van Gelder T, Kiberd B. Therapeutic drug monitoring of mycophenolates in kidney transplantation: report of The Transplantation Society consensus meeting. Transplantation Reviews 2011;25(2):58-64.

[103] Nawrocki A., Korecka M., Solari S., Kang J., Shaw LM.: Mycophenolic acid. In: Applied Pharmacokinetics and Pharmacodynamics: Principles of Therapeutic Drug Monitoring, 4th Ed., edited by Burton ME, Shaw LM, Schentag JJ, Evans WE, Philadelphia, Lippincott Williams & Wilkins, 2006, pp 563–594.

[104] Shaw LM, Figurski M, Milone MC, Trofe J, Bloom RD. Therapeutic drug monitoring of mycophenolic acid. Clinical Journal of the American Society of Nephrology 2007;2(5): 1062-72.

[105] Filler G, Mai I. Limited sampling strategy for mycophenolic acid area under the curve. Therapeutic Drug Monitoring 2000;22(2):169-73.

[106] Yeung S, Tong KL, Tsang WK, Tang HL, Fung KS, Chan HW, Chan AY, Chan L. Determination of mycophenolate area under the curve by limited sampling strategy. Transplantation Proceedings 2001;33(1-2):1052-3.

[107] Musuamba FT, Rousseau A, Bosmans JL, Senessael JJ, Cumps J, Marquet P, Wallemacq P, Verbeeck RK. Limited sampling models and Bayesian estimation for mycophenolic acid area under the curve prediction in stable renal transplant patients co-medicated with ciclosporin or sirolimus. Clinical Pharmacokinetics 2009;48(11):745-58.

[108] Pawinski T, Hale M, Korecka M, Fitzsimmons WE, Shaw LM. Limited sampling strategy for the estimation of mycophenolic acid area under the curve in adult renal transplant patients treated with concomitant tacrolimus. Clinical Chemistry 2002;48(9): 1497-504.

[109] Vasquez EM. Sirolimus: a new agent for prevention of renal allograft rejection. American Journal of Health System Pharmacy 2000; 57(7):437-48.

[110] Stenton SB, Partovi N, Ensom MH. Sirolimus: the evidence for clinical pharmacokinetic monitoring. Clinical Pharmacokinetics 2005;44(8):769-86.

[111] Ingle GR, Sievers TM, Holt CD. Sirolimus: continuing the evolution of transplant immunosuppression. Annals of Pharmacotherapy 2000;34:1044-55.

[112] Mahalati K, Kahan BD. Clinical Pharmacokinetics of Sirolimus. Clinical Pharmacokinetics 2001;40(8):573-585.

[113] Groth CG, Bäckman L, Morales JM, Calne R, Kreis H, Lang P, Touraine JL, Claesson K, Campistol JM, Durand D, Wramner L, Brattström C, Charpentier B. Sirolimus (rapamycin)-based therapy in human renal transplantation: similar efficacy and different toxicity compared with cyclosporine. Sirolimus European Renal Transplant Study Group. Transplantation 1999;67(7):1036-42.

[114] Hong JC, Kahan BD. Use of anti-CD25 monoclonal antibody in combination with rapamycin to eliminate cyclosporine treatment during the induction phase of immunosuppression. Transplantation 1999;68:701-4.

[115] Hong JC, Kahan BD. A calcineurin-free strategy for induction immunosuppression for delayed graft function in cadaveric kidney transplantation. Transplantation Proceedings 2001;33:1271-2.

[116] McAlister VC, Gao Z, Peltekian K, Domingues J, Mahalati K, MacDonald AS. Sirolimus-tacrolimus combination immunosuppression. Lancet 2000;355(9201):376-7.

[117] Zimmerman JJ, Kahan BD. Pharmacokinetics of sirolimus in stable renal transplant patients after multiple oral dose administration. Journal of Clinical Pharmacology 1997;37(5):405-15.

[118] Yatscoff RW, LeGatt DF, Kneteman NM. Therapeutic monitoring of rapamycin: a new immunosuppressive drug. Therapeutic Drug Monitoring 1993;15(6):478-82.

[119] Kirchner GI, Meier-Wiedenbach I, Manns MP. Clinical pharmacokinetics of everolimus. Clinical Pharmacokinetics. 2004;43(2):83-95.

[120] Kovarik JM, Kaplan B, Silva HT, Kahan BD, Dantal J, McMahon L, Berthier S, Hsu CH, Rordorf C. Pharmacokinetics of an everolimus-cyclosporine immunosuppressive regimen over the first 6 months after kidney transplantation. American Journal of Transplantation 2003;3(5):606-13.

[121] Budde K, Neumayer HH, Lehne G, Winkler M, Hauser IA, Lison A, Fritsche L, Soulillou JP, Fauchald P, Dantal J; RADW 102 Renal Transplant Study Group Tolerability and steady-state pharmacokinetics of everolimus in maintenance renal transplant patients. Nephrology Dialysis Transplantation 2004;19(10):2606-14.

[122] Helio Tedesco-Silva Jr, Claudia Rosso Felipe, Tainá Veras de Sandes, Freitas, Marina Pontello Cristeli, Carolina Araújo Rodrigues, José Osmar Medina Pestana. Impact of everolimus: update on immunosuppressive therapy strategies and patient outcomes after renal transplantation. Transplant Research and Risk Management 2011;3:9-29.

[123] Kovarik JM, Tedesco H, Pascual J, Civati G, Bizot MN, Geissler J, Schmidli H. Everolimus therapeutic concentration range defined from a prospective trial with reduced-exposure cyclosporine in de novo kidney transplantation. Therapeutic Drug Monitoring 2004;26(5):499-505.

[124] Mabasa VH, Ensom MH. The role of therapeutic monitoring of everolimus in solid organ transplantation. Therapeutic Drug Monitoring 2005;27(5):666-76.

[125] Shapiro R, Young JB, Milford EL, Trotter JF, Bustami RT, Leichtman AB. Immunosuppression: evolution in practice and trends, 1993-2003. American Journal of Transplantation 2005;5(4 Pt 2):874-86.

[126] Metalidis C, Kuypers DR. Emerging immunosuppressive drugs in kidney transplantation. Current Clinical Pharmacology 2011;6(2):130-6.

[127] Cooper JE, Wiseman AC. Novel immunosuppressive agents in kidney transplantation. Clinical Nephrology. 2010;73(5):333-43.

[128] Webber A, Hirose R, Vincenti F. Novel strategies in immunosuppression: issues in perspective. Transplantation 2011;91(10):1057-64.

[129] Kovarik JM, Steiger JU, Grinyo JM, Rostaing L, Arns W, Dantal J, Proot P, Budde K; Sotrastaurin Renal Transplant Study Group. Pharmacokinetics of sotrastaurin combined with tacrolimus or mycophenolic acid in de novo kidney transplant recipients. Transplantation 2011;91(3):317-22.

[130] Vincenti F, Charpentier B, Vanrenterghem Y, Rostaing L, Bresnahan B, Darji P, Massari P, Mondragon-Ramirez GA, Agarwal M, Di Russo G, Lin CS, Garg P, Larsen CP. A phase III study of belatacept-based immunosuppression regimens versus cyclosporine in renal transplant recipients (BENEFIT study). American Journal of Transplantation 2010;10(3):535-46.

Section 3

Advances in Transplantation Immunology

Chapter 16

The Evolution of HLA-Matching in Kidney Transplantation

Hung Do Nguyen, Rebecca Lucy Williams,
Germaine Wong and Wai Hon Lim

Additional information is available at the end of the chapter

http://dx.doi.org/10.5772/54747

1. Introduction

In this chapter, we will explore the effect of human leukocyte antigen (HLA) matching on renal transplant outcomes. The importance of HLA matching has been clearly established in renal transplantation and the extent of HLA mismatches at the A, B and DR loci form an important part in the assessment of the immunological risk of potential transplant candidates. Increasing number of HLA mismatches has been shown to be associated with poorer graft and patient survival following kidney transplantation but the ongoing importance of this association in the era of more potent immunosuppression and improved donor selection remains unclear. Nevertheless, HLA mismatches remain a crucial component of deceased donor kidney allocation in most countries including the United States and Australia. As a result of major advances in technology, HLA-typing has evolved from serological-based typing to molecular HLA-typing and solid-phase anti-HLA-antibody-detection assays, which have had a major influence in both allocation and outcome of transplanted kidneys. The identification of donor-specific anti-HLA-antibody (DSA) has become standard practice and cross-matching assays to establish the presence of DSA has evolved from complement-dependent cytotoxicity (CDC) assay to the exquisitely sensitive flow-cytometric and solid-phase assays. The availability of these sensitive assays has enable clinicians to perform calculated panel reactive antibody and virtual cross-match, which has led to a more accurate assessment of immunological risk of potential transplant candidates and improvement in the allocation of deceased donor kidneys. Defining the appropriate threshold values for clinically relevant DSA assignment, the ongoing significance of HLA-matching in the presence of DSA and the importance of anti-HLA-Cw, HLA-DQ and HLA-DP antibodies remain poorly defined. Finally, we will discuss the process of identifying acceptable HLA-mismatches using HLAMatchmaker, which determines HLA-compatibility at the level of polymorphic amino acid triplets or eplets in antibody-accessible regions, and the benefit of acceptable HLA-mismatch programs in improving the transplant potential of highly sensitized transplant candidates.

2. Basic transplant immunology

Immune protection against foreign antigens in humans relies on a coordinated response of both innate and adaptive immune system [1]. The innate system, comprising of anatomical barriers (e.g. skin), phagocytic cells (e.g. macrophages), and soluble compounds (e.g. complements and interferons [IFN]) provide an efficient initial defence against foreign antigens such as donor antigens in solid organ transplantation but this response lacks specificity. In contrast, subsequent adaptive immune response has the ability to create a large diversity of antigen-specific responses upon antigenic challenge to the host, with the development of immunological memory consequent on subsequent exposure to the same antigen. This response involves predominantly lymphocytes and antibodies, and is characteristically more intense, leading to a more rapid elimination of the foreign antigen (Figure 1).

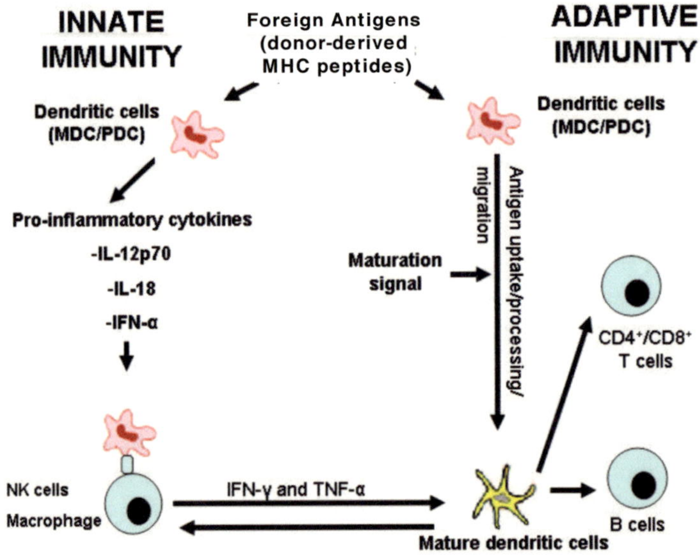

The ability of dendritic cells to coordinate innate and adaptive immune system. Upon exposure to foreign antigens, dendritic cells secrete pro-inflammatory cytokines ± cell-cell contact, activate effector cells including natural killer cells and macrophages (innate immunity). Immature dendritic cells capture and process antigens for presentation to T cells via major histocompatibility complexes. DC undergo maturation and migrate to secondary lymphoid tissues (enhanced by inflammatory cytokines produced by natural killer cells and CD40 ligand expressed by activated T cells). Mature dendritic cells drive the expansion of antigen-specific, major histocompatibility complex-restricted T and B cell responses and the development of immunologic memory (adaptive immunity).

Figure 1. Innate and adaptive immune response to foreign antigens.

2.1. Dendritic cells (Figure 2)

Dendritic cells (DC) are a group of rare, heterogenous population of professional antigen-presenting cells (APC) that can initiate primary immune responses, and hence have the ability to regulate both innate and adaptive immune responses [2-4]. Precursor DC (pre-DC), arising from bone marrow progenitors, enter tissues as immature DC with superior phagocytic capabilities. DC encounter foreign antigens such as donor antigens (in solid organ transplantation), bacteria and tumour antigens resulting in the secretion of cytokines (e.g. IFN) and activation of natural killer (NK) cells, macrophages and eosinophils. Following antigen capture and processing, DC undergo maturation and migrate to secondary lymphoid tissues where they present processed antigen/peptide coupled to major histocompatibility complexes (MHC) to T cells, allowing for selection and expansion of antigen-specific cluster designation $(CD)4^+$ T-helper cells. These $CD4^+$ T-helper cells subsequently amplify the immune responses by regulating antigen-specific (e.g. $CD8^+$ cytotoxic T cells, B cells), and antigen non-specific (e.g. macrophages, NK cells, and eosinophils) effector cells.

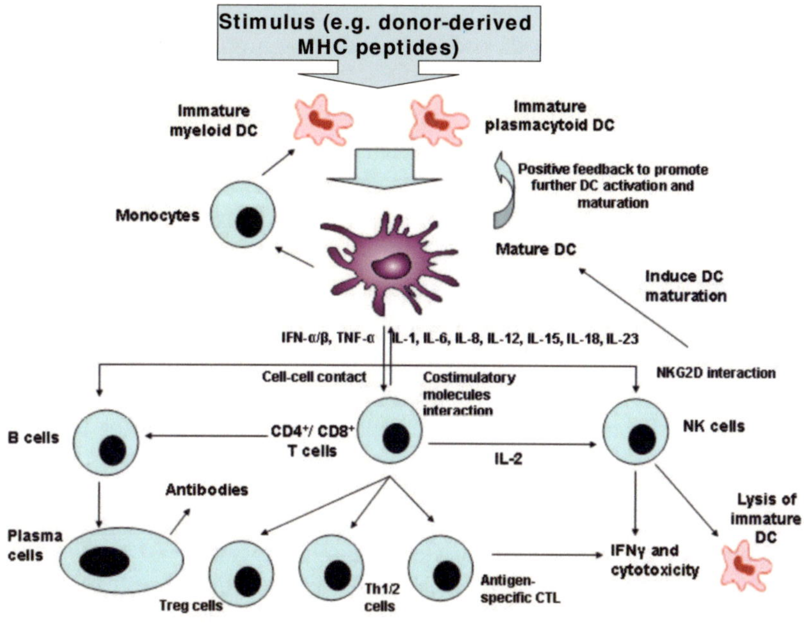

Overview of the complex relationship between dendritic cells and effector T and B cells. Immature DC (MDC and PDC) maturate in response to appropriate stimuli (e.g. microbial products, TLR ligands). Mature DC secretes immunoregulatory cytokines (including IFN-α and IL-12] and with cell-cell contact, modulates effector cell response including NK cells, B and T cells as well as providing a positive feedback to DC to initiate ongoing activation and maturation. Activated effector cells could in turn modulate DC activation, maturation, and survival as well as enhancing other effector cell functions through the production of cytokines (IFN-γ) and/or via cell-cell contact.

Figure 2. Interaction between dendritic cells and effector T and B cells.

DC play a critical role in the initiation and regulation of adaptive T cell responses, the maintenance of central and peripheral tolerance in normal steady-state and hence are essential in regulating immune responses in solid organ and cellular transplantation. DC have dual roles in organ transplantation. They are responsible for allorecognition and presentation of foreign antigens to T cells, which may initiate allograft rejection; but are also involved in the promotion of transplant tolerance.

2.2. Role of T and B cells in allograft rejection

2.2.1. T cells

The most common form of acute rejection of allogeneic tissues and allografts involve the activation of recipient's T cells (i.e. adaptive immune response) directed against donor MHC antigens or MHC-derived peptides presented by either the donor's or recipient's APC [5]. DC are considered the most potent form of APC in humans through their capacity for antigen uptake and processing of foreign antigens into peptides which can then be presented to antigen-specific T cells via MHC complexes, leading to activation and clonal expansion of naïve and memory T cells (i.e. primary and secondary immune responses) [2]. During steady state, DC reside as functionally immature cells in most tissues. Following organ transplantation, the systemic effects of donor brain death and/or ischaemia-reperfusion injury are sufficient to generate an inflammatory response to mature these DC during their migration carrying donor antigens from the transplanted organ to the recipient's secondary lymphoid organs including the draining lymph nodes and spleen [6, 7]. DC may also be activated via CD40-CD40L interaction, with activated cells (e.g. platelets, T cells, mast cells) within transplanted allografts the potential source of CD40L. This interaction may regulate DC migration possibly via tumour necrosis factor (TNF)-α production by DC [8]. DC maturation and immunostimulatory capacity are dependent on nuclear factor kappa B (NF-κB)-dependent gene transcription including genes involved in the expression of adhesion molecules, chemotactic factors and the production of various cytokines [9]. Although DC are very efficient in presenting donor antigens to T cells, other cell types including tubular epithelial cells, endothelial cells, macrophages and also B cells can participate in T cell interaction, the latter by capturing and presenting foreign antigens via their surface immunoglobulins and MHC class II molecules [10-12].

Direct and indirect allorecognition of allogeneic antigens are mediated by donor-derived and recipient's DC respectively. Donor DC present donor peptide mounted on donor MHC molecules to recipient's T cells following migration of donor DC to T cell areas of lymphoid tissues ('passenger leukocytes') in response to surgery [13]. This mode of presentation is termed *direct allorecognition* and is particularly important in the initiation of acute rejection resulting from a powerful alloantigen-specific T cell response directed against allogeneic antigens [14]. The finding of >90% of infiltrating recipient's T cells involved in recognising donor-derived MHC molecule directly presented by donor DC during acute rejection of allogeneic skin graft in mice support the existence of this direct pathway [15]. Furthermore, the frequency of direct donor-specific hyporeactivity is similar between long-term renal transplant recipients with good graft function compared to those recipients with established chronic rejection suggesting that direct allorecognition is not the predominant response in

http://dx.doi.org/10.5772/54747

chronic rejection [16]. In contrast, recipient's DC may acquire allogeneic donor antigens following migration into the allograft in response to proinflammatory cytokines and chemokines. Recipient's DC present donor MHC-derived peptides (e.g. regions of MHC class II molecules) loaded to self-MHC molecule to recipient's T cells. This mode of presentation is termed *indirect allorecognition* and may be more important in establishing chronic rejection. Unlike direct allorecognition, indirect allorecognition involves a less potent T cell response with a reduced proportion of recipient's T cells involve in the immune response directed against the donor-derived antigens [17, 18]. The finding of a higher frequency of T cells with indirect anti-donor reactivity in transplant recipients with established chronic rejection support this finding [16]. Similarly, studies in non-human primates demonstrated that inhibition of direct anti-donor reactivity can prolong graft survival, but does not prevent late graft loss to chronic rejection [19]. In both direct and indirect allorecognition pathways, DC can internalise extracellular donor antigens, process them and present them to either $CD4^+$ or $CD8^+$ T cells through MHC class I or II molecules respectively. However, the contribution of direct and indirect pathway in acute and chronic allograft rejection remains controversial with studies demonstrating that indirect pathway may also be important in the initiation of acute rejection [20].

Following activation of naïve T cells, activated $CD4^+$ T cells proliferate and differentiate into different cell types with distinct cytokine profiles. Subtypes of helper T cells include type I helper T (Th1], Th2 cells, Th17 cells and regulatory T (Treg) cells. Although Th1 cells may be more important in allograft rejection by producing inflammatory cytokines capable of driving a cellular immune response such as IFN-γ and interleukin (IL)-2, Th2 cells may also be involved in rejection through the activation of eosinophils and promoting a humoral immune response (via cytokines IL4, 5 and 13) [21, 22]. There is increasing evidence that Th17 cells contribute to allograft rejection although the susceptibility of these cells to immune regulation remains unclear [23]. Although Treg cells are capable of inducing immune tolerance in animal models of transplantation, the role of these cells in humans remains unclear [24, 25]. Both $CD4^+$ and $CD8^+$ T cells can mediate allograft injury either directly or indirectly through the production of cytokines or by activating vascular endothelial cells. $CD8^+$ T cells can directly cause cell death by promoting caspase-induced cell apoptosis by releasing perforin and granzymes A and B intracellularly or via Fas-ligand/Fas-receptor interaction between $CD8^+$T cells and allograft [26]. Similarly, $CD4^+$ T cells can directly induce cell apoptosis via Fas-ligand/Fas-receptor interaction but they can also cause indirect cell damage by secreting TNF-α and TNF-β, which subsequently bind to TNF-receptors on endothelial or tubular cells resulting in cell apoptosis [27, 28].

2.2.2. B cells

There is increasing evidence that in solid organ transplantation, B cells play an important role in the immune response to an allograft through the production of antibodies (resulting in the development of acute and chronic antibody mediated rejection [AMR]), but these cells may also have an important role in the support of T cells (resulting in the development of acute cellular rejection) [29]. Most peripheral B cells are produced in the bone marrow and continuously circulate as immature cells through secondary lymphoid organs until they encounter antigen. Once activated, B cells become efficient APC by capturing antigen via B-cell receptor, then interacts with naïve T cells through the presentation of antigen by MHC class II molecules to T-cell receptor respectively. Through this interaction coupled with the ability to produce cytokines such as IL-2, B cells are critical for optimal T cell activation and development of T cell memory [30, 31]. Activated B cells may also differentiate into memory B cells or plasma cells, a small proportion of the latter cell type may persist as long-lived plasma cells that reside in the bone marrow ± allografts indefinitely, continuously producing IgG antibodies [32]. APCs such as DC, monocytes and macrophages produce BAFF (B-cell-activating factor belonging to the tumour necrosis factor family), a cytokine which enhances B cell survival [33]. Antibodies produced by terminally differentiated B cells, especially directed against donor antigens, are critical mediators of AMR and associated graft damage through complement activation and Fc-receptor cross-linking, the latter resulting in proinflammatory cytokine release, DC maturation, macrophage phagocytosis and NK cell-mediated antibody-dependent cellular cytotoxicity [34]. Like Treg cells, there is a recently described subset of B cells in humans and mouse known as regulatory B cells, which are capable inhibiting T cell responses, possibly through the production of IL-10 [35]. The clinical significance of these regulatory B cells in organ transplantation remains unclear.

3. Human Leukocyte Antigen (HLA)

The HLA system is the name given to the human MHC, which was first described by Jean Dausset in 1952 after observing the development of alloantibodies to leukocytes following blood transfusions [36]. The HLA system comprises a group of cell-surface antigen-presenting proteins encoded by a region on the short arm of chromosome 6 and is divided into class I and class II molecules. Humans have three class I HLA (A, B, C) that are present on all nucleated cells and six class II HLA (DPA1, DPB1, DQA1, DQB1, DRA, DRB1) that are present only on antigen-presenting cells and lymphocytes. Class I HLA presents intracellular antigens while class II HLA present extracellular antigens. HLA are highly polymorphic with almost 6000 HLA Class I and over 1500 HLA Class II alleles having been identified [37]. Three of the seven heterodimers (HLA-A, -B, and -DRB1) contribute to the majority of the immunogenicity of mismatched antigens and therefore traditional HLA-typing methods have primarily focussed on these alleles.

HLA play an important role in the immune system by controlling immune responses through antigen presentation and distinguish "self" from "non-self". Since its introduction after the first International Histocompatibility Workshop (IHWS) in 1964, HLA matching has formed the cornerstone of deceased-donor kidney allocation policies worldwide [38]. By the first World Health Organization nomenclature meeting in 1970, 27 HLA antigens were identified. The discovery of new antigens on occasion splits previously known 'broad' antigens into two or more antigens, termed 'split' antigens. For example, the A9 broad antigen was split to A23 and A24 split antigens, whereas the DR2 broad antigen was split to DR15 and DR16 split antigens [39]. HLA matching criteria may vary with regards to consideration of broad or split antigens. Split antigen matching appears to be more common and clinically important for HLA-A and-B antigens than for HLA-DR antigens [40]. Not surprisingly, utilization of matching for broad antigens increases the probability of identifying HLA-matched recipients for any given donor [41].

Although 0 HLA-mismatched grafts have been shown to have superior graft outcomes compared with grafts with ≥1 HLA-mismatch, a proportion of 0 HLA-mismatched grafts may be complicated by acute rejection, possibly reflecting potential allorecognition of incompatibilities at other minor HLA loci. On the contrary, many HLA-mismatched grafts have excellent graft outcomes without acute rejection, suggesting that under specific circumstances, certain HLA mismatches may be permissible, such as the lack of immunologic response against non-inherited maternal HLA antigens (NIMA) as a result of prenatal tolerance development. However, verification of this association between NIMA and graft outcomes remains inconclusive [42-44].

HLA compatibility has also been defined by mismatch acceptability known as acceptable HLA-mismatch. These are mismatched HLA antigens that do not result in a positive complement dependent cytotoxicity (CDC) crossmatch [42]. Identification of acceptable HLA-mismatches has been utilised to improve the transplant potential of highly sensitized patients, and this concept and application will be discussed in greater details later in this chapter.

In most countries worldwide including Australia, the number of HLA-mismatches is calculated by the sum of the total number of HLA-mismatches between donor-recipient at HLA-A, B, and DR loci. Large single centre and registry studies have consistently demonstrated an inverse association between increasing number of mismatches and graft and/or patient survival [43-45]. However, with the evolution from serological to molecular-based HLA-typing over time resulting in improved immunological risk stratification of transplant candidates, coupled with the availability of more potent immunosuppression and donor selection has created uncertainty regarding the ongoing clinical importance of HLA-mismatches in the modern era.

4. Effect of HLA-mismatches and renal transplant outcomes

Large registry reports including analysis from the Collaborative Transplant Study (CTS) and more recently from the Australia and New Zealand Dialysis and Transplant (ANZDATA) registry have consistently demonstrated a strong association between HLA-matching at the HLA-A, B and DR loci and graft and patient outcomes, independent of donor type, initial immunosuppression, transplant era and even the presence of DSA [46-48].

The advantage of improved HLA-matching in reducing acute rejection risk has been demonstrated predominantly in renal transplant recipients receiving cyclosporine-based immunosuppressive regimen [49, 50]. Recent retrospective single centre study of live and deceased donor renal transplants has demonstrated that HLA-mismatches remained an important determinant of acute rejection risk in renal transplant recipients receiving quadruple immunosuppression involving the use of interleukin-2 receptor antibody induction, tacrolimus, mycophenolate mofetil and corticosteroids [51]. In this study, increasing number of HLA mismatches was an independent predictor of acute rejection (OR 1.65 for every single HLA-mismatch; 95% CI: 1.15 to 2.38; P=0.007), with HLA-mismatches at the HLA-DR locus associated with the highest risk of acute rejection compared to mismatches at the HLA-A and HLA-B loci in the adjusted model. Analysis of the CTS data of 135,970 deceased donor renal transplant recipients demonstrated that the effect of HLA-mismatches on acute rejection risk remained highly significant over two consecutive decades (1985-1994 vs 1995-2004), independent of 'intention to treat' immunosuppressive regimen [47]. Similarly, recent analysis of ANZDATA registry of live and deceased donor renal transplants between 1998 and 2009 demonstrated that the association between HLA-mismatches and acute rejection risk appeared to be independent of transplant era and initial immunosuppression, but this association appeared to be much stronger for live-donor transplants compared to deceased donor transplants (Figure 3A). The reduced benefit of 0-HLA-mismatched kidneys in recipients of deceased compared with live donor kidneys may be explained by the presence in unrelated deceased donors of apparently matched but actually mismatched splits of antigens, which is less frequently observed in biologically related living donors [46]. However, the association between HLA mismatches and rejection was not linear, with the greatest benefit of HLA matching appeared to be confined to those with <4 HLA mismatches [46, 47].

Large retrospective studies have consistently demonstrated the importance of HLA-matching in determining deceased donor renal allograft survival [52-54]. Analysis of the United Network for Organ Sharing (UNOS) registry between 1991 to 1997 demonstrated an 11% reduction in 3-year graft survival rate (p<0.001) between transplants involving 6 compared to 0 HLA-mismatches, with the most discernible difference in survival was observed between recipients with 0 to 1 HLA-mismatch [55]. In the UNOS study, the association between HLA-mismatches and reduced graft survival appeared to be related to mismatches at the HLA-DR locus within the first year post-transplant, whereas mismatches at the HLA-AB loci were more important beyond the first year post-transplant. However, the association between HLA-mismatches and graft survival in the era of modern immunosuppression remains contradictory [56]. Analysis of the CTS data demonstrated that the importance of HLA-matching on graft outcomes remained strong during the two decades of 1985-1994 and 1995-2004, suggesting that association between HLA-mismatches and graft survival remains robust in the era of modern immunosuppression [47]. Unlike the other large registry studies that had focused on deceased donor renal transplants, the study by *Lim WH et al* using ANZDATA registry data evaluated both live and deceased donor renal transplants. Similarly, the authors demonstrated a strong association between HLA-mismatches and overall graft survival for both live and deceased donor renal transplants (Figure 3B), especially between those receiving 0-HLA-mismatched kidneys compared to those receiving ≥1 HLA-mismatched kidneys [46]. In contrast, analysis of the UNOS data suggested that the relative importance of HLA-mismatches and reduced graft survival may have diminished in recent years, whereas other factors such as donor age retained their statistical significance over time prompting the suggestion that kidney allocation algorithms based predominantly on HLA-matching should be modified [57]. However, this study focused on era between 1994 and 1998 whereby the use of induction therapy and/or tacrolimus was limited.

http://dx.doi.org/10.5772/54747

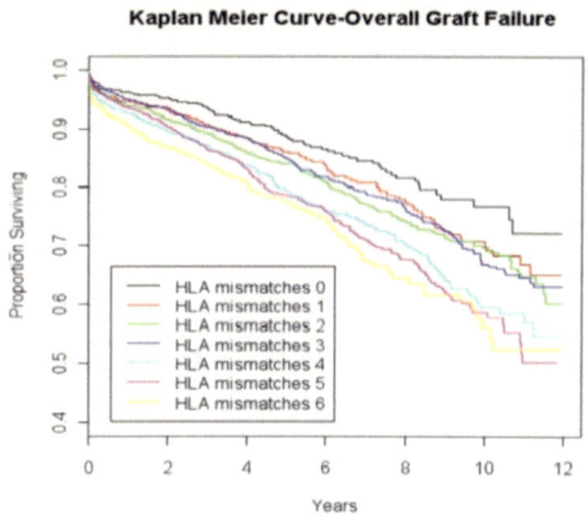

Years	0 HLA-MM	1 HLA-MM	2 HLA-MM	3 HLA-MM	4 HLA-MM	5 HLA-MM	6 HLA-MM
0	550	734	1795	1792	1181	1330	654
4	337	432	900	1042	601	611	285
8	140	194	360	439	225	189	82

(a)

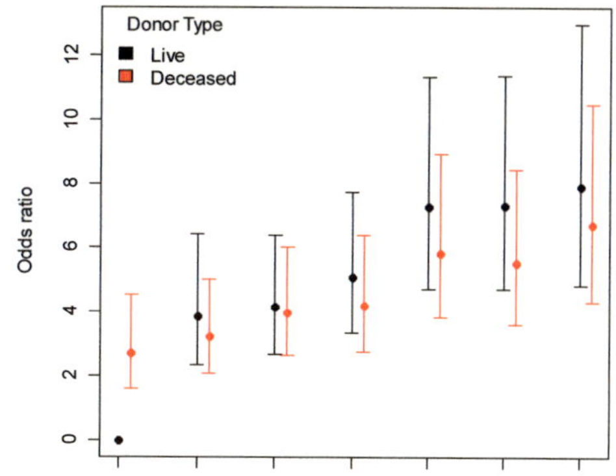

HLA-mismatches	Live donor	Deceased donor
0	1.00	1.00
1	4.00 (2.38, 6.67)*	1.19 (0.79, 1.79)
2	4.17 (2.71, 6.67)*	1.47 (1.01, 2.13)*
3	5.26 (3.33, 7.69)*	1.54 (1.04, 2.27)*
4	7.14 (4.76, 11.11)*	2.13 (1.43, 3.12)*
5	7.69 (4.76, 11.11)*	1.96 (1.33, 2.86)*
6	8.33 (5.00, 12.50)*	2.38 (1.56, 3.57)*

(b)

Figure 3. (a) Odds ratio plot of HLA mismatches and acute rejection according to donor type (reference live donor 0 HLA mismatch) and corresponding table of the adjusted odds ratio between HLA mismatches and acute rejection according to donor type (reference live or deceased donor 0 HLA mismatch; adapted from *Lim WH et al* Clin Transplant 2012) [46]. (b) Kaplan–Meier survival curve of overall graft failure according to the number of HLA mismatches with corresponding numerical table of the number at risk at 0, 4 and 8 years post-transplant (adapted from *Lim WH et al* Clin Transplant 2012) [46].

The association between acute rejection and graft survival appears well established. In the study by *Wissing et al*, the authors had shown rejection within the first year post-transplant was independently associated with a significant reduction in overall (57% vs 83%; p=0.0004) and death-censored graft survival (63.5% vs 91.2%; p<0.0001) [51], a finding corroborated by ANZDATA registry analysis [46].

Although HLA-DR mismatches appear to be of greater importance in predicting graft outcomes compared to HLA-AB mismatches, the current kidney allocation algorithm in Australia specifically favours fully HLA-DR matched recipients but still takes into account HLA-AB matching, therefore confers an appropriate concession to allow satisfactory HLA-matching but avoiding discrimination to potential recipients with rare HLA combinations as HLA-DR locus has fewer polymorphisms compared to HLA-AB loci [58]. Previous studies have demonstrated that allocation based predominantly on HLA-DR matching, as implemented in the United States, may eliminate any advantage of HLA-AB matching but this remains controversial [59, 60]. Analysis of Scientific Registry of Transplant Recipients (SRTR) of 108,701 deceased donor renal transplant recipients demonstrated that the elimination of allocation priority for HLA-B mismatches improved the transplant potential of ethnic minorities and this policy had achieved comparable renal allograft survival compared to historical graft outcomes prior to the change in allocation policy [61]. Although the presence of HLA-

Cw, DP and DQ DSA have been shown to be associated with poorer graft outcomes [62, 63], matching at the HLA-Cw, DP and DQ loci are not routinely performed and therefore is not explicitly included in the allocation of deceased donor kidneys in any countries.

5. Serological and molecular HLA typing and the detection of donor-specific anti-HLA antibodies (Figure 4)

The evolution in our understanding of the HLA system is closely linked to advancements in technology. Traditional serological-based low resolution HLA typing methods can be completed relatively quickly but are dependent on the availability of specific cell types, viability and appropriate anti-sera that are capable of recognising HLA antigens. The emergence of molecular HLA typing techniques over the past two decades has allowed for a more specific, flexible and robust means of high resolution HLA typing. In 1982, *Wake et al* described restriction fragment length polymorphism (RFLPs), which eventually highlighted the shortcomings of serology-based methods ensuing the establishment of molecular-based HLA-typing for routine clinical practice [64]. Data generated via the genome project and the initiation of polymerase chain reaction (PCR) techniques through the 1980s further refined DNA-based techniques for HLA-typing, which has led to the development of a number of PCR-based techniques still in use to the present day.

Alongside advances in the typing of HLA alleles, the techniques used to detect anti-HLA antibodies has also evolved from CDC assays to more sensitive techniques including flow-cytometry and solid-phase assays (e.g. enzyme-linked immunosorbent assay [ELISA] or Luminex), which has allowed a more accurate assessment of transplant candidate's immunological risk pre-transplantation (e.g. calculated panel reactive antibodies to determine level of sensitization and application of virtual cross-match to determine transplant suitability) (Figure 4).

Since the recognition of the clinical importance of CDC assay in kidney transplantation in the 1960s, CDC cross-match has become the cornerstone of determining transplant suitability in both live and deceased donor renal transplantation [65]. The underlying principle of CDC cross-match is to detect clinically relevant donor-specific anti-HLA antibodies that could result in hyperacute rejection following transplantation. Donor T and B cells are incubated in the presence of recipients' sera and complements. If donor-specific anti-HLA antibodies are present, these will bind to donor cells and initiate the complement cascade resulting in lysis of donor lymphocytes. The percentage of lysis will be quantified and forms the basis of determining transplant candidate's suitability for transplantation. Many laboratories perform CDC assays in the presence of anti-human globulin (enhances the sensitivity of assay by enhancing the number of Fc receptors available to bind with complements) and/or dithiothreitol (breaks down the disulfide bonds in IgM antibodies of no clinical significance) to improve the accuracy and reduce the false negative rates associated with these assays [66, 67]. Initial data using the CDC assay revealed that 80% of CDC cross-match–positive transplants and 4% of CDC cross-match–negative transplants were associated with early graft loss (within 48 hours post-transplant), thereby establishing the clinical significance of anti-HLA antibodies

http://dx.doi.org/10.5772/54747

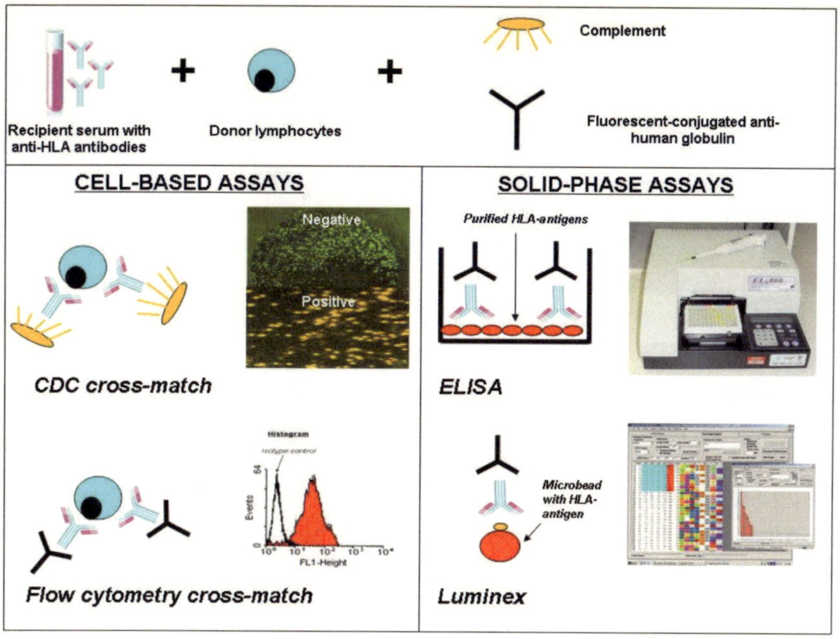

Cell-based assays	Solid-phase assays
• CDC-XM reduced the incidence of hyperacute rejection • Inability to identify the antigen causing positive	• Sensitive with high degree of specificity to donor antigens, luminex more sensitive than ELISA • Capable of quantifying anti-HLA antibodies level

HLA – human leukocyte antigen, CDC-XM – complement-dependent cytotoxicity cross-match, ELISA – enzyme-linked immunosorbent assay.

Figure 4. Detection of anti-HLA antibodies – differences between cell-based and solid-phase assays.

in renal transplantation. The inability to correlate all graft losses with anti-HLA antibodies has led to the development of more sensitive cross-match assays, including flow cytometric cross-match assays. It is noteworthy that 20% of patients transplanted across a positive cross-match did not lose their grafts [68]. Because T cells express class I antigens and B cells express both class I and II antigens, the interpretation of T cell together with B cell cross-match will help to establish whether class I and/or II anti-HLA antibodies are present. A positive B cell CDC cross-match invariably accompanies a positive T cell CDC cross-match but this may reflect either anti-HLA antibodies to class I antigens and/or multiple antibodies to class I and/or II antigens. However, a positive B cell CDC cross-match may occur in the absence of a positive T cell CDC cross-match and suggest the presence of class II antigens or low levels class I antigens. The presence of a positive T cell CDC cross-match is an absolute contraindication for transplantation whereas a positive B cell cross-match is a relative contraindication because of the uncertainty regarding the clinical significance and the possibility of false-positive results [69, 70]. In the allocation of deceased donor kidneys in Australia, the presence of a positive T cell CDC cross-match is an absolute contraindication for transplantation whereas B cell cross-match is not routinely performed and therefore not utilized in the decision-making process for transplantation. With the increasing recognition of the potential importance of a positive CDC B cell cross-match, these results are now often interpreted in the context of solid phase assays.

The basic principle of flow cross-match technique is similar to CDC assay. Since the description of this assay in the early 1980s, this technique has been widely adopted to determine transplant suitability [71]. Similar to CDC assay, flow assay requires the addition of donor cells to recipients' sera, followed by the addition of a secondary fluorescein-labelled antibody allowing for the detection by flow cytometry and quantification of antibodies expressed as channel shifts. Unlike CDC cross-match, flow cytometric cross-match identifies both complement-fixing and non-complement-fixing anti-HLA donor-specific antibodies. However, the availability of different subtypes of detection antibodies has allowed for the differentiation between complement-fixing versus non-complement-fixing antibodies [72]. Although an universal cut-off value for a positive flow cross-match has not been determined, it is agreed that the use of a low cut-off point will result in increased sensitivity but reduced specificity for predicting graft outcomes (especially in the presence of negative CDC cross-match) as this may identify anti-HLA donor specific antibodies of no clinical significance. Nevertheless, renal transplant recipients with positive flow cross-match but negative CDC cross-match have a significantly greater risk of antibody-mediated rejection (AMR) and early graft loss with a positive predictive value for predicting AMR of 83% [72, 73].

To avoid problems associated with the viability of the donor cells, which could affect the accuracy of cell-based assays, the introduction of solid-phase assays have largely circumvented these problems and improved the sensitivity of detection of anti-HLA antibodies [74]. The identification of anti-HLA antibodies using ELISA was first described in 1993 where purified HLA antigens were directly immobilized on the surface of microtitre plates but the basic principle of antibody detection was similar to cell-based assays [75]. The Luminex platform is a solid-phase assay that utilizes polystyrene microspheres (beads), each embedded with fluorochromes of differing intensity attached to one (single-antigen beads) or several HLA molecules (screening beads) to determine anti-HLA antibody specificity. Similar to other assays, the addition of recipients' sera containing anti-HLA antibodies are added to the bead mix, these antibodies will bind to the appropriate beads expressing specific antigen(s). A second phycoerytherin-labelled anti-human IgG is then added to this mixture and these antibodies will bind to the primary anti-HLA antibody already attached to the beads. The sample is then passed through lasers, which would independently excite the beads and the phycoerytherin therefore allowing the laser detector to define antibody specificity [76, 77]. Unlike the CDC assays, Luminex assay detect both complement-fixing and non-complement-fixing anti-HLA antibodies but does not detect IgM autoantibodies or non-HLA antibodies. With the continued reliance on using cell-based cross-match assays, especially CDC cross-match assays to determine transplant suitability, a potential disadvantage of virtual cross-match is that transplants may be excluded based on antibody results with unknown clinical relevance [78]. It is generally accepted that solid phase virtual cross-match to identify anti-

http://dx.doi.org/10.5772/54747

HLA donor specific antibodies complements the results of cell-based assays to help inform decision-making process with regards to transplant suitability.

6. Clinical significance of anti-HLA donor-specific antibodies

It is well known that the presence of high levels of pre-transplant class I (HLA-A and B) ± II (HLA-DR) donor-specific antibodies (DSA; i.e. anti-HLA antibodies with reactivity against the potential donor leading to positive cross-match often as a result of prior sensitization events including previous HLA-mismatched transplants, blood transfusions or pregnancy) is associated with poorer graft outcomes, including the development of acute AMR, chronic AMR, transplant glomerulopathy and late graft loss (Table 1) [79-81]. However, few studies have suggested that the association between pre-transplant DSA and graft survival was restricted to recipients who had developed early AMR, within the first 30-days post-transplantation [82]. In addition, the authors queried the cost-effectiveness of pre-transplant screening for preformed DSA by demonstrating that the additional cost associated with quarterly screening for anti-HLA antibodies would be between 3200 to 6700 Euros, which would equate to an additional 83,000 to 130,000 Euros per avoided AMR because of preformed non-lymphocytotoxic DSA in transplant candidates on the transplant wait-list for >5 years [82]. There is also increasing evidence demonstrating that the development of *de novo* DSA (occurring post-transplantation), especially development of DSA directed against HLA-DQ graft molecules in HLA-class II incompatible graft transplantations, are both associated with acute and subclinical AMR and graft loss in kidney transplant only and/or simultaneous pancreas-kidney transplant recipients [80, 83-85]. Although there is no current consensus on the level of clinically significant DSA identified by flow cytometric or Luminex assays, most studies have demonstrated that increasing single, peak or total DSA levels were associated with an incremental risk of rejection and/or graft loss [86, 87]. Recent studies have suggested that the detection of C1q-fixing DSA (i.e. the potential to identify DSA that can activate complements by binding C1q) may be more specific in predicting acute rejection, biopsy C4d-deposition, transplant glomerulopathy and late graft failure following kidney transplantation but this remains controversial and not routinely performed in many transplanting centres [88, 89]. The clinical benefit of routine regular surveillance for *de novo* DSA in improving graft survival following kidney transplantation remains unclear although a recent study of 72 live-donor renal transplant recipients suggested that the appearance of *de novo* DSA was inversely proportional to the amount of maintenance immunosuppressive drugs (especially in the weaning phase of immunosuppression minimization particularly prednisolone) such that DSA monitoring may be highly effective for detecting escape from tolerance and reappearance of the immune response in weaned patients [90]. With the greater understanding of HLA antigens and anti-HLA antibodies, innovative techniques have been established to allow transplantation across positive CDC and/or flow cross-match barriers but this is beyond the scope of this chapter.

Study	Cohort	Rejection	Graft survival
Eng H et al (n=471 DD renal transplant recipients) [*79*]	83 T-B+ XM vs 386 T-B- XM; IgG HLA DSA in 33% of T-B+ XM patients	Vascular: 19% T-B- vs 32% T-B+ (p=0.01); DSA was a significant predictor for vascular or glomerular rejection	Graft loss: T-B+ - 44%; T-B- 27% (especially class I DSA)
Lefaucheur C et al (n=402 DD renal transplant recipients) [*80*]	83 (21%) positive DSA by Luminex by peak sera vs 76 (19%) by current sera	The presence of SAB HLA-DSA on the peak and current serum has a PPV for AMR of 35% and 32% respectively. Prevalence of AMR 1% in patients with MFI <465, 19% MFI between 466 and 3000, 36% MFI between 3001 and 6000, and 51% MFI "/>6000. Peak HLA-DSA Luminex MFI predicted AMR better than current HLA-DSA MFI.	5 and 8-year DCGS were 89% and 84% in non-sensitized patients, 92% and 92% in sensitized patients with no peak HLA-DSA, and 71% and 61% in patients with peak HLA-DSA. Relative risk (RR) for graft loss for patients who had an episode of AMR was 4.1 (95% CI 2.2 to 7.7) as compared with patients without AMR.
Lefaucheur C et al (n=237 LD and DD renal transplant recipients) [*81*]	All negative T and B-cell CDC-XM. 27% class I or II anti-HLA antibody with 52% DSA.	The incidence of AMR among patients with preformed DSA was 35%, 9-fold higher than in patients without DSA (3%) (p < 0.001).	Overall graft survival at 8 years was 68% in patients with DSA and 77% in those with no DSA. Graft survival of patients with DSA and AMR was significantly worse than in DSA patients without AMR and in non-DSA patients.
Amico P et al (n=334 LD and DD renal transplant recipients) [105]	332 negative T and B cell CDC-XM, 67 DSA vs 267 no DSA by Luminex	Overall incidence of clinical/ subclinical rejection (i.e., AMR and acute T-cell mediated rejection) at day 200 post-transplant was significantly higher in patients with HLADSA (48/67; 71%) than in patients without HLA-DSA (94/267; 35%).	DCGS at 5 years was 89% in those without DSA, 87% with DSA but no AMR and 68% with DSA and AMR.

HLA – human leukocyte antigen, DD – deceased donor, LD – live-donor, CDC-XM – complement dependent cytotoxicity cross-match, DSA – donor-specific antibodies, SAB – single antigen bead, AMR – antibody mediated rejection, DCGS – death-censored graft survival, MFI – mean fluorescent intensity, PPV – positive predictive value.

Table 1. Association between donor-specific antibodies and graft outcomes.

7. HLA-matching in kidney allocation from deceased donors

Most renal transplant programs preferentially allocate kidneys from deceased donors to transplant candidates with favourable HLA compatibility. The current allocation of deceased-

http://dx.doi.org/10.5772/54747

donor kidneys in most countries, including Australia and the Eurotransplant group (Germany, The Netherlands, Belgium, Luxembourg, Slovenia, and Austria), is weighted largely on the degree of mismatched antigens at the HLA-A, -B and -DR loci, with less emphasis on other factors such as time on dialysis, prior sensitization and even ischaemic time. When a potential deceased-donor kidney is available in Australia, transplant candidates on the wait-list are ranked according to an allocation score calculated from a combination of factors including the number of HLA-mismatches, age of recipient, degree of sensitization and time on wait-list [91]. Approximately 20% of deceased donor kidneys are allocated on a national level to highly sensitized transplant candidates (around 20% of kidneys allocated) but the remaining 80% of deceased donor kidneys are allocated through individual state allocation algorithms.

Despite efforts to achieve equity of access to transplantation in many countries, the inclusion of HLA matching in the allocation of deceased donor kidneys is believed to disadvantage transplant candidates with uncommon HLA phenotypes [92]. Consequently, indigenous populations and ethnic minorities often have a much longer transplant wait-list time and are less likely to receive well-matched kidneys [97-100]. The elimination of the allocation priority for HLA-B mismatches has been shown to improve the transplant potential of ethnic minorities but this approach has not been widely adopted by other countries [61].

In Australia, unacceptable class I HLA-mismatches are defined using the Luminex platform and the presence of class I DSA against HLA-A and -B antigens with >2000 mean fluorescent intensity (MFI) excludes transplant candidates from receiving these donor kidneys, independent of the CDC-cross match results. At present, class II DSA is not explicitly considered in the allocation of kidneys from deceased donors in Australia but many centres have already adopted the policy of avoiding transplantation of kidneys into transplant candidates with high levels of class II DSA.

8. Acceptable HLA-mismatch and highly sensitized transplant candidates

Highly sensitised transplant candidates (defined as those having a panel reactive antibody [PRA] level of >80%) on the deceased donor transplant wait-list are less likely to receive donor kidneys (greater likelihood of obtaining a positive complement-dependent cytotoxicity [CDC]-cross-match result with any given donor) and have a much longer wait-list time compared to unsensitized transplant candidates, resulting in a greater risk of mortality whilst remaining on the transplant wait-list [93]. In Australia, highly sensitized transplant candidates represent approximately 5% of the wait-listed candidates and are more likely to wait on average twice as long as unsensitized transplant candidates despite an increase in the number of deceased donors over time (202 donors in 2006 compared to 309 donors in 2010) [6].

Although HLA matching has traditionally been performed at the broad antigen level, a model considering cross-reacting groups (CREGs) may increase the probability of identifying more compatible kidneys for ethnic minorities and highly sensitized transplant candidates. HLA antigens comprise of multiple serologic epitopes made of polymorphic amino acid residues, and it is these structures and their conformation and position that determine antibody

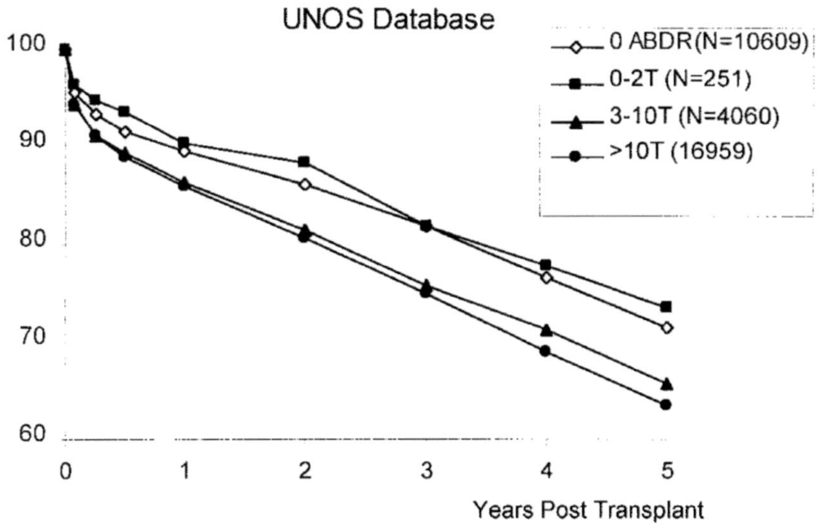

HLA – human leukocyte antigen, UNOS – United Nation Organ Sharing, T - triplets.

Figure 5. Impact of HLA-A, -B triplet (T) matching on 5-year graft survival rates in zero-HLA-DR-mismatched kidney transplants in a cohort of United Nation of Organ Sharing (UNOS) renal transplant recipients between 1987 and 1999 (adapted from *Duquesnoy et al* Transplantation 2003) [101].

accessibility, recognition, and subsequent reactivity [94]. Almost 200 class I and II epitopes have been defined by Luminex technology [95]. Some epitopes are shared across different HLA alleles while some are unique to single or more restricted numbers of HLA alleles. While there are considerable differences in HLA antigen frequencies between different ethnic groups, CREGs are more evenly distributed [96].

The concept of acceptable HLA-mismatch identifies mismatched HLA-antigens that could be considered as compatible at a structural or functional level. It is based on the principle that each HLA antigen is structurally unique and that an individual cannot mount an immunological response against an epitope expressed by their own HLA, i.e. one cannot react against shared 'self' epitopes [105, 106]. It has been demonstrated that such acceptable HLA-mismatches would result in a negative CDC cross-match and therefore allow transplantation to safely proceed [97, 98].

Acceptable HLA-mismatches can be identified using HLAMatchmaker or the Luminex platform. HLAMatchmaker is a computer algorithm that regards each HLA antigen as a string of polymorphic amino acid configurations in antibody-accessible positions (epitopes) formed by triplets or eplets [99, 100]. For any given set of HLA antigens, HLAMatchmaker can define the number of triplet or eplet mismatches present against any foreign HLA antigen and hence define the HLA antigens that are mismatched at the broad antigen level but matched at the eplet level, i.e. acceptable HLA-mismatches. Graft outcomes of HLAMatchmaker-identified 0-2 triplet-mismatched kidney transplant recipients are similar compared to recipients with 0 HLA-mismatch at the HLA-A, -B and –DR loci (Figure 5) [101]

http://dx.doi.org/10.5772/54747

The Luminex platform determines specificity and quantifies anti-HLA antibodies present in potential transplant candidates and is used in Australia to define unacceptable class I HLA-mismatches. Although it may be logical to consider Luminex-define DSA with MFI of <500 as acceptable mismatch, the utlilization of this technique or the appropriate thresholds of Luminex-determined acceptable mismatch remain unknown [102].

In highly sensitized transplant candidates, the identification of acceptable HLA-mismatch has been shown to improve their transplant potential by reducing the number of HLA-mismatches therefore identifying additional donors likely to produce a negative CDC cross-match.

9. Acceptable HLA-mismatch programs

Successful acceptable HLA-mismatch programs have been implemented in many countries, including Europe, United Kingdom and United States [45, 114-116]. Eurotransplant Acceptable Mismatch Program was established in mid 1970 to improve the transplant potential of highly sensitized transplant candidates. Over the ensuing decade, eleven other similar programs were introduced throughout Europe [103]. Although there is considerable variation in PRA cut-off to define highly sensitized transplant candidates, it is generally accepted that PRA >80% may be the most appropriate cut-off. Table 2 highlights the results of the established acceptable mismatch programs.

Scheme	Initiation	Reference	Eligibility	Outcomes/Activity
UK Transplant SOS Scheme (UKT:SOS)	Feb 1984	[*106*]	PRA"/>85% (historic or current sera)	• 65% graft survival at 1year • 42% transplanted within 1year
Collaborative Transplant Study Highly Immunized Trial (CTS:HIT)	1985	[*107*]	PRA"/>80% (current sera)	• 5-year graft survival comparable to unsensitized recipients (59% vs 60%)
Eurotransplant Acceptable Mismatch Program (ET:ACMM)	1985	[*100*]	PRA≥85% (historic or current sera)	• 2-year graft survival comparable to unsensitized recipients (87%) • 45% transplanted in 1year, mean 8.9 months reduction in mean wait time
South Eastern Organ Procurement Foundation High Grade HLA Match algorithm (SEOPF:HGM)	Jan 1994	[*108*]	PRA≥40% (current sera)	• 2-year graft survival comparable to unsensitized recipients (86% vs 88%)

PRA – panel reactive antibody, HLA – human leukocyte antigen

Table 2. Description of allocation schemes based on acceptable HLA-mismatch.

The Eurotransplant Acceptable Mismatch Program is the largest and most successful program and runs in parallel with the Eurotransplant Kidney Allocation System (ETKAS) to identify acceptable HLA-mismatches in potential highly sensitized transplant candidates through comprehensive serum screening for acceptable mismatches. The introduction of the acceptable mismatch program has significantly reduced waiting time for highly sensitized transplant candidates whilst achieving comparable short and long-term graft outcomes to unsensitized transplant recipients [100].

The deceased donor kidney allocation algorithm in Australia does not consider acceptable HLA-mismatches for highly sensitized transplant candidates. We are currently investigating the impact of identifying and incorporating acceptable mismatches into the deceased-donor kidney allocation model and our preliminary data suggest that an acceptable mismatch program could result in an improvement in transplant potential of 1 in 10 highly sensitized renal transplant recipients (PRA >80%) with a potential reduction in average transplant wait-list time of 33 months [104].

10. Conclusion

Despite the evolution of more sensitive molecular-based HLA-typing and the ability to detect DSA, there continues to be an important association between HLA-matching and graft and patient outcomes in kidney transplantation. Nevertheless, the application of molecular-based typing in kidney transplantation is already being mandated by most of the transplant community and may provide greater accuracy in the assessment of individual's immunological risk as well as improving transplant outcomes.

Author details

Hung Do Nguyen[1,2], Rebecca Lucy Williams[1], Germaine Wong[3] and Wai Hon Lim[1,2]

*Address all correspondence to: wai.lim@health.wa.gov.au

1 Department of Renal Medicine, Sir Charles Gairdner Hospital, Australia

2 School of Medicine and Pharmacology, University of Western Australia, Perth, Australia

3 Sydney School of Public Health, University of Sydney; Centre for Kidney Research, The Children's Hospital at Westmead; Centre for Transplant and Renal Research, Westmead Hospital, Sydney, Australia

http://dx.doi.org/10.5772/54747

References

[1] Fearon D, Locksley R. The instructive role of innate immunity in the acquired immune response. Science 1996; 272 (5258): 50.

[2] Banchereau J, Briere F, Caux C, et al. Immunobiology of dendritic cells. Ann Rev Immunol 2000; 18: 767.

[3] Banchereau J, Steinman RM. Dendritic cells and the control of immunity. Nature 1998; 392: 245.

[4] Coates PTH, Thomson AW. Dendritic cells, tolerance induction and transplant outcome. Am J Transplant 2002; 2 (3): 299.

[5] Morelli A, Thomson A. Dendritic cells: regulators of alloimmunity and opportunities for tolerance induction. Immunol Rev 2003; 196: 125.

[6] Gallucci S, Lolkema M, Matzinger P. Natural adjuvants: endogenous activators of dendritic cells. Nat Med 1999; 5: 1249.

[7] Gallucci S, Matzinger P. Danger signals: SOS to the immune system. Curr Opin Immunol 2001; 13: 114.

[8] Morelli A, Zahorchak A, Larregina A, et al. Regulation of cytokine production by mouse myeloid dendritic cells in relation to differentiation and terminal maturation induced by LPS or CD40 ligation. Blood 2001; 98 (5): 1512.

[9] Rescigno M, Martino M, Sutherland C, Gold M, Ricciardi-Castagnoli P. Dendritic cell survival and maturation are regulated by different signaling pathways. J Exp Med 1998; 188: 2175.

[10] Nankivell B, Alexander S. Rejection of the kidney allograft. N Engl J Med 2010; 363 (15): 1451.

[11] Hagerty D, Allen P. Processing and presentation of self and foreign antigens by the renal proximal tubule. J Immunol 1992; 148: 2324.

[12] Kreisel D, Krupnick A, Balsara K, et al. Mouse vascular endothelium activates CD8+ T lymphocytes in a B7-dependent fashion. J Immunol 2002; 169 (11): 6154.

[13] Larsen C, Morris P, Austyn J. Migration of dendritic leukocytes from cardiac allografts into host spleens. A novel pathway for initiation of rejection. J Exp Med 1990; 171: 307.

[14] Suciu-Foca N, Colovai A, Ciubotariu R, Cortesini R. Mapping of HLA-DR determinants recognized via the indirect pathway. Graft 1999; 2: 28.

[15] Benichou G, Valujskikh A, Heeger PS. Contributions of direct and indirect T cell alloreactivity during allograft rejection in mice. J Immunol 1999; 162: 352.

[16] Baker R, Hernandez-Fuentes M, Brookes P, Chaudhry A, Cook H, Lechler R. Loss of direct and maintenance of indirect alloresponses in renal allograft recipients: implications for the pathogenesis of chronic allograft nephropathy. J Immunol 2001; 167 (12): 7199.

[17] Gould D, Auchincloss HJ. Direct and indirect recognition: the role of MHC antigens in graft rejection. Immunol Today 1999; 20: 77.

[18] Lechler R, Ng W, Steinman R. Dendritic cells in transplantation - friend or foe. Immunity 2001; 14 (4): 357.

[19] Montgomery S, Xu H, Tadaki D, et al. Combination induction therapy with monoclonal antibodies specific for CD80, CD86, and CD154 in nonhuman primate renal transplantation. Transplantation 2002; 74 (10): 1365.

[20] Auchincloss H, Lee R, Shea S, Markowitz J, Grusby M, Glimcher L. The role of "indirect" recognition in initiating rejection of skin grafts from major histocompatibility complex class II-deficient mice. Proc Natl Acad Sci U S A 1993; 90: 3373.

[21] Zhai Y, Ghobrial R, Busuttil R, Kupiec-Weglinski J. Th1 and Th2 cytokines in organ transplantation: paradigm lost? Crit Rev Immunol 1999; 19: 155.

[22] Goldman M, Le Moine A, Braun M, Flamand V, Abramowicz D. A role for eosinophils in transplant rejection. Trends Immunol 2001; 22 (5): 247.

[23] Chadha R, Heidt S, Jones N, Wood K. Th17: contributors to allograft rejection and a barrier to the induction of transplantation tolerance? Transplantation; 91 (9): 939.

[24] Wood K, Sakaguchi S. Regulatory T cells in transplantation tolerance. Nat Rev Immunol 2003; 3: 199.

[25] Wood K, Bushell A, Hester J. Regulatory immune cells in transplantation. Nat Rev Immunol 2012; 12 (6): 417.

[26] Barry M, Bleackley R. Cytotoxic T lymphocytes: all roads lead to death. Nat Rev Immunol 2002; 2: 401.

[27] Al-Lamki R, Wang J, Skepper J, Thiru S, Pober J, Bradley J. Expression of tumor necrosis factor receptors in normal kidney and rejecting renal transplants. Lab Invest 2001; 81: 1503.

[28] Jagger A, Evans H, Walter G, et al. FAS/FAS-L dependent killing of activated human monocytes and macrophages by CD4+CD25- responder T cells, but not CD4+CD25+ regulatory T cells. J Autoimmun 2012; 38 (1): 29.

[29] Caltworthy M. Targeting B cells and antibody in transplantation. Am J Transplant 2011; 11: 1359.

[30] Ng Y, Oberbarnscheidt M, Chandramoorthy H, Hoffman R, Chalasani G. B cells help alloreactive T cells differentiate into memory T cells. Am J Transplant 2010; 10: 1970.

[31] Lund F, Randall T. Effector and regulatory B cells: modulators of CD4+ T cell immunity. Nat Rev Immunol 2010; 10 (4): 236.

[32] Vinuesa C, Linterman M, Goodnow C, Randall K. T cells and follicular dendritic cells in germinal center B-cell formation and selection. Immunol Rev 2010; 237: 72.

[33] Parsons R, Vivek K, Redfield Rr, et al. B-lymphocyte homeostasis and BLyS-directed immunotherapy in transplantation. Transplant Rev 2010; 24 (4): 207.

[34] Smith K, Clatworthy M. FcgammaRIIB in autoimmunity and infection: Evolutionary and therapeutic implications. Nat Rev Immunol 2010; 10: 328.

[35] DiLillo D, Matsushita T, Tedder T. B10 cells and regulatory B cells balance immune responses during inflammation, autoimmunity, and cancer. Ann N Y Acad Sci 2010; 1183: 38.

[36] Dausset J. Les thrombo-anticorps: Acta Haematologica, 1958.

[37] EMBL-EBI. IMGT HLA sequence data.

[38] Bontadini A. HLA techniques: Typing and antibody detection in the laboratory of immunogenetics. METHODS 2012: 1.

[39] Terasaki PI. Histocompatibility testing, 1980, 1980.

[40] Hata Y, Cecka JM, Takemoto S, Ozawa M, Cho YW, Terasaki PI. Effects of changes in the criteria for nationally shared kidney transplants for HLA-matched patients. Transplantation 1998; 65 (2): 208.

[41] Takemoto S, Terasaki P. Equitable allocation of HLA-compatible kidneys for local pools and for minorities. New England Journal … 1994.

[42] Claas FHJ, Claas FH, Witvliet MD, Duquesnoy RJ, Persijn GG, Doxiadis IIN. The acceptable mismatch program as a fast tool for highly sensitized patients awaiting a cadaveric kidney transplantation: short waiting time and excellent graft outcome. Transplantation 2004; 78 (2): 190.

[43] Lim W, Chadban S, Clayton P, et al. Human Leukocyte Antigen Mismatches Associated with Increased Risk of Rejection, Graft Failure and Death Independent of Initial Immunosuppression in Renal Transplant Recipients. Unpublished: 1.

[44] Opelz G. Impact of HLA compatibility on survival of kidney transplants from unrelated live donors. Transplantation 1997; 64 (10): 1473.

[45] Paramesh AS, Zhang R, Baber J, et al. The effect of HLA mismatch on highly sensitized renal allograft recipients. Clinical transplantation 2010; 24 (6): E247.

[46] Lim W, Chadban S, Clayton P, et al. Human leukocyte antigen mismatches associated with increased risk of rejection, graft failure, and death independent of initial immunosuppression in renal transplant recipients. Clin Transplant 2012; e-pub.

[47] Opelz G, Dohler B. Effect of human leukocyte antigen compatibility on kidney graft survival: comparative analysis of two decades. Transplantation 2007; 84 (2): 137.

[48] Dunn T, Noreen H, Gillingham K, et al. Revisiting Traditional Risk Factors for Rejection and Graft Loss After Kidney Transplantation. Am J Transplant 2011; 11 (10): 2132.

[49] Beckingham I, Dennis M, Bishop M, Blamey R, Smith S, Nicholson M. Effect of human leucocyte antigen matching on the incidence of acute rejection in renal transplantation. Br J Surg 1994; 81 (4): 574.

[50] McKenna R, Lee K, Gough J, et al. Matching for private or public HLA epitopes reduces acute rejection episodes and improves two-year renal allograft function. Transplantation 1998; 66 (1): 38.

[51] Wissing K, Fomegné G, Broeders N, et al. HLA mismatches remain risk factors for acute kidney allograft rejection in patients receiving quadruple immunosuppression with anti-interleukin-2 receptor antibodies. Transplantation 2008; 85 (3): 411.

[52] Held P, Kahan B, Hunsicker L, et al. The impact of HLA mismatches on the survival of first cadaveric kidney transplants. N Engl J Med 1994; 331 (12): 765.

[53] Gjertson D, Terasaki P, Takemoto S, Mickey M. National allocation of cadaveric kidneys by HLA matching. Projected effect on outcome and costs. N Engl J Med 1991; 324 (15): 1032.

[54] Takemoto S, Terasaki P, Gjertson D, Cecka J. Twelve years' experience with national sharing of HLA-matched cadaveric kidneys for transplantation. N Engl J Med 2000; 343 (15): 1078.

[55] Schnitzler M, Hollenbeak C, Cohen D, et al. The economic implications of HLA matching in cadaveric renal transplantation. N Engl J Med 1999; 341 (19): 1440.

[56] Gillich M, Heimbach D, Schoeneich G, Müller S, Klehr H. Comparison of blood group versus HLA-dependent transplantation and its influence on donor kidney survival. Nephrol Dial Transplant 2002; 17 (5): 884.

[57] Su X, Zenios S, Chakkera H, Milford E, Chertow G. Diminishing significance of HLA matching in kidney transplantation. Am J Transplant 2004; 4 (9): 1501.

[58] Corte G, Damiani G, Calabi F, Fabbi M, Bargellesi A. Analysis of HLA-DR polymorphism by two-dimensional peptide mapping. Proc Natl Acad Sci 1981; 78 (1): 534.

[59] Doxiadis I, de Fijter J, Mallat M, et al. Simpler and equitable allocation of kidneys from postmortem donors primarily based on full HLA-DR compatibility. Transplantation 2007; 83 (9): 1207.

[60] Vereerstraeten P, Abramowicz D, Andrien M, Dupont E, De Pauw L, Kinnaert P. Allocation of cadaver kidneys according to HLA-DR matching alone would result in optimal graft outcome in most recipients. Transplant Proc 1999; 31 (1-2): 739.

http://dx.doi.org/10.5772/54747

[61] Ashby V, Port F, Wolfe R, et al. Transplanting Kidneys Without Points for HLA-B Matching: Consequences of the Policy Change. Am J Transplant 2011; 11: 1712.

[62] Frohn C, Fricke L, Puchta J-C, Kirchner H. The effect of HLA-C matching on acute renal transplant rejection. Nephrol Dial Transplant 2001; 16: 355.

[63] Takemoto S, Port F, Claas F, Duquesnoy R. HLA Matching for kidney transplantation. Hum Immunol 2004; 65: 1489.

[64] Wake C, Long E. Allelic polymorphism and complexity of the genes for HLA-DR β-chains—direct analysis by DNA–DNA hybridization. 1982.

[65] Patel R, Terasaki P. Significance of the positive crossmatch test in kidney transplantation. N Engl J Med 1969; 280 (14): 735.

[66] Bryan C, Martinez J, Muruve N, et al. IgM antibodies identified by a DTT-ameliorated positive crossmatch do not influence renal graft outcome but the strength of the IgM lymphocytotoxicity is associated with DR phenotype. Clin Transplant 2001; 15 (Suppl 6): 28.

[67] Mulley W, Kanellis J. Understanding crossmatch testing in organ transplantation: A case-based guide for the general nephrologist. Nephrology 2011; 16: 125.

[68] Gebel H, Bray R. Laboratory assessment of HLA antibodies circa 2006: making sense of sensitivity. Transplant Revs 2006; 20 (4): 189.

[69] Eng H, Bennett G, Chang S, et al. Donor HLA Specific Antibodies Predict Development and Define Prognosis in Transplant Glomerulopathy. Hum Immunol 2011.

[70] Le Bas-Bernardet S, Hourmant M, Valentin N, et al. Identification of the antibodies involved in B-cell crossmatch positivity in renal transplantation. Transplantation 2003; 75 (4): 477.

[71] Garovoy M, Bigos M, Perkins H, Colombe B, Salvatierra O. A high technology crossmatch technique facilitating transplantation. Transplant Proc 1983; XV: 1939.

[72] Limaye S, O'Kelly P, Harmon G, et al. Improved graft survival in highly sensitized patients undergoing renal transplantation after the introduction of a clinically validated flow cytometry crossmatch. Transplantation 2009; 87 (7): 1052.

[73] Karpinski M, Rush D, Jeffery J, et al. Flow cytometric crossmatching in primary renal transplant recipients with a negative anti-human globulin enhanced cytotoxicity crossmatch. J Am Soc Nephrol 2001; 12 (12): 2807.

[74] Schlaf G, Pollok-Kopp B, Manzke T, Schurat O, Altermann W. Novel solid phase-based ELISA assays contribute to an improved detection of anti-HLA antibodies and to an increased reliability of pre- and post-transplant crossmatching. NDT Plus 2010; 3: 527.

[75] Kao K, Scornik J, Small S. Enzyme-linked immunoassay for anti-HLA antibodies-an alternative to panel studies by lymphocytotoxicity. Transplantation 1993; 55: 192.

[76] Gibney E, Cagle L, Freed B, Warnell S, Chan L, Wiseman A. Detection of donor-specific antibodies using HLA-coated microspheres: another tool for kidney transplant risk stratification. Nephrol Dial Transplant 2006; 21 (9): 2625.

[77] Muro M, Llorente S, Gónzalez-Soriano M, Minguela A, Gimeno L, Alvarez-López M. Pre-formed donor-specific alloantibodies (DSA) detected only by luminex technology using HLA-coated microspheres and causing acute humoral rejection and kidney graft dysfunction. Clin Transpl 2006: 379.

[78] Lee P, Ozawa M. Reappraisal of HLA antibody analysis and crossmatching in kidney transplantation. Clin Transplant 2007: 219.

[79] Eng H, Bennett G, Tsiopelas E, et al. Anti-HLA donor-specific antibodies detected in positive B-cell crossmatches by Luminex predict late graft loss. Am J Transplant 2008; 8 (11): 2335.

[80] Lefaucheur C, Loupy A, Hill G, et al. Preexisting donor-specific HLA-antibodies predict outcome in kidney transplantation. J Am Soc Nephrol 2010; 21: 1398.

[81] Lefaucheur C, Suberbielle-Boissel C, Hill G, et al. Clinical relevance of preformed HLA donor-specific antibodies in kidney transplantation. Am J Transplant 2008; 8 (2): 324.

[82] Ziemann M, Schonemann C, Bern C, et al. Prognostic value and cost-effectiveness of different screening strategies for HLA antibodies prior to kidney transplantation. Clin Transplant 2012; e-pub.

[83] Cantarovich D, De Amicis S, Aki A, et al. Posttransplant donor-specific anti-HLA antibodies negatively impact pancreas transplantation outcome. Am J Transplant 2011; 11: 2737.

[84] Ntokou I-SA, Iniotaki A, Kontou E, et al. Long-term follow up for anti-HLA donor specific antibodies postrenal transplantation: high immunogenicity of HLA class II graft molecules. Transplant Int 2011; 24: 1084.

[85] Wiebe C, Gibson I, Blydt-Hansen T, et al. Evolution and clinical pathologic correlations of de novo donor-specific HLA antibody post kidney transplant. Am J Transplant 2012; 12: 1157.

[86] Lefaucheur C, Loupy A, Hill G, et al. Preexisting donor-specific HLA antibodies predict outcome in kidney transplantation. J Am Soc Nephrol 2010; 21 (8): 1398.

[87] Mujtaba M, Goggins W, Lobashevsky A, et al. The strength of donor-specific antibody is a more reliable predictor of antibody-mediated rejection than flow cytometry crossmatch analysis in desensitized kidney recipients. Clin Transplant 2011; 25 (1): E96.

[88] Yabu J, Higgins J, Chen G, Sequeira F, Busque S, Tyan D. C1q-fixing human leukocyte antigen antibodies are specific for predicting transplant glomerulopathy and late graft failure after kidney transplantation. Transplantation 2011; 91 (3): 342.

[89] Sutherland S, Chen G, Sequeira F, Lou C, Alexander S, Tyan D. Complement-fixing donor-specific antibodies identified by a novel C1q assay are associated with allograft loss. Pediatr Transplantation 2012; 16: 12.

[90] Hoshino J, Kaneku H, Everly M, Greenland S, Terasaki P. Using donor-specific antibodies to monitor the need for immunosuppression. Transplantation 2012; 93: 1173.

[91] Organ Transplantation from Deceased Donors: Consensus Statement on Eligibility Criteria and Allocation Protocols, 2011.

[92] Gaston R, Ayres I, Dooley L. Racial equity in renal transplantation. JAMA: the journal of the … 1993.

[93] Smits JM, van Houwelingen HC, De Meester J, Persijn GG, Claas FH. Analysis of the renal transplant waiting list: application of a parametric competing risk method. Transplantation 1998; 66 (9): 1146.

[94] Duquesnoy RJ. Clinical usefulness of HLAMatchmaker in HLA epitope matching for organ transplantation. Current Opinion in Immunology 2008; 20 (5): 594.

[95] Duquesnoy RJ, Marrari M. Correlations between Terasaki's HLA class I epitopes and HLAMatchmaker-defined eplets on HLA-A, -B and -C antigens. Tissue Antigens 2009; 74 (2): 117.

[96] Rodey GE, Neylan JF, Whelchel JD, Revels KW, Bray RA. Epitope specificity of HLA class I alloantibodies. I. Frequency analysis of antibodies to private versus public specificities in potential transplant recipients. Human Immunology 1994; 39 (4): 272.

[97] Gebel HM, Bray RA, Nickerson P. Pre-transplant assessment of donor-reactive, HLA-specific antibodies in renal transplantation: contraindication vs. risk. American journal of transplantation : official journal of the American Society of Transplantation and the American Society of Transplant Surgeons 2003; 3 (12): 1488.

[98] Lobashevsky AL, Senkbeil RW, Shoaf JL, et al. The number of amino acid residues mismatches correlates with flow cytometry crossmatching results in high PRA renal patients. Human Immunology 2002; 63 (5): 364.

[99] Duquesnoy RJ. HLAMATCHMAKER: a molecularly based donor selection algorithm for highly alloimmunized patients. Transplantation proceedings 2001; 33 (1-2): 493.

[100] Claas F, Witvliet M, Duquesnoy R, Persijn G, Doxiadis I. The acceptable mismatch program as a fast tool for highly sensitized patients awaiting a cadaveric kidney transplantation: short waiting time and excellent graft outcome. Transplantation 2004; 78 (2): 190.

[101] Duquesnoy RJ, Takemoto S, de Lange P, et al. HLAmatchmaker: a molecularly based algorithm for histocompatibility determination. III. Effect of matching at the HLA-

A,B amino acid triplet level on kidney transplant survival. Transplantation 2003; 75 (6): 884.

[102] Claas FHJ, Doxiadis IIIN. Human leukocyte antigen antibody detection and kidney allocation within Eurotransplant. Human Immunology 2009; 70 (8): 636.

[103] Gore SM, Bradley, Benjamin A. Renal transplantation : sense and sensitization. Strasbourg Dordrecht; Boston: Council of Europe; Kluwer Academic Publishers, 1988.

[104] Do Nguyen H, Fidler, S, Irish, A, D'Orsogna, L, Christiansen, FT, Martinez, P, Lim, W. The Idenfication of Acceptable HLA-Mismatches Improves Transplant Potential of Highly-Sensitised Renal Transplant Recipients: Sir Charles Gairdner Hospital, Royal Perth Hospital, University of Western Australia, 2012.

[105] Amico P, Hönger G, Mayr M, Steiger J, Hopfer H, Schaub S. Clinical relevance of pretransplant donor-specific HLA antibodies detected by single-antigen flow-beads. Transplantation 2009; 87 (11): 1681.

[106] Klouda P, Corbin S, Ray T, Rogers C, Bradley B. Renal transplantation in highly sensitized pati... [Clin Transpl. 1990] - PubMed - NCBI. Clinical transplantation 1990: 69.

[107] Opelz G. Five-year results of renal transplantation in highly sensitized recipients. Collaborative Transplant Study. Transplant international : official journal of the European Society for Organ Transplantation 2007; 9 (Suppl 1): S16.

[108] Tardif GN, McCalmon RT. SEOPF high-grade HLA match algorithm: effective kidney sharing using ROP trays with HLA matching for highly sensitized patients. Transplantation proceedings 1997; 29 (1-2): 1406.

Chapter 17

Transplantation Antigens and Histocompatibility Matching

Bhadran Bose, David W. Johnson and
Scott B. Campbell

Additional information is available at the end of the chapter

http://dx.doi.org/10.5772/54738

1. Introduction

Since the discovery of the major histocompatibility complex (MHC) in 1967, there has been significant development in the field of organ and tissue transplantation. In humans, the MHC is called the human leukocyte antigen system and is located on the short arm of chromosome 6, near the complement genes. These cell surface proteins are the principal antigenic determinants of graft rejection.

The presence of donor-specific HLA antibodies in kidney transplant recipients can be identified by crossmatch. Since 1969, pre-transplant crossmatch has become a mandatory component of the transplant work-up process. It has largely eliminated hyperacute rejection. Crossmatch techniques have expanded from basic complement-dependent microcytotoxicity (CDC) assays to additionally include flow crossmatches and virtual crossmatches derived using the luminex assay. The improved sensitivity and specificity of virtual crossmatch when compared to CDC and flow crossmatches has revolutionised the pre-transplant crossmatch process, but also greatly increased its complexity.

2. HLA antigens

HLA molecules are membrane bound glycoproteins that bind processed antigenic peptides and present them to T cells. The essential role of the HLA antigens lies in the control of self-recognition and thus defence against microorganisms. Based on the structure of the antigens produced and their function, there are two classes of HLA antigens, HLA Class I and Class II.

The overall size of the MHC is approximately 3.5 million base pairs. Within this is the HLA Class I genes and the Class II genes each spread over approximately one third of this length. The remaining section, sometimes known as Class III, contains loci responsible for complement, hormones, intracellular peptide processing and other development characteristics [1]. Thus the Class III region is not actually a part of the HLA complex, but is located within the HLA region, because its components are either related to the functions of HLA antigens or are under similar control mechanisms to the HLA antigens.

2.1. HLA Class I antigens

The cell surface glycopeptide antigens of the HLA A, B and C series are called HLA Class I antigens [2]. HLA Class I antigens are expressed on all nucleated cells of the body. Additionally, they are found in soluble form in plasma and adsorbed onto the surface of platelets. Erythrocytes also adsorb HLA Class I antigens to varying degrees depending on the specificity (e.g. HLA-B7, A28 and B57 are recognizable on erythrocytes as so called "Bg" antigens). Immunological studies indicate that HLA-B (which is also the most polymorphic) is the most significant HLA Class I locus, followed by HLA-A and then HLA-C. There are other HLA Class I loci (e.g. HLA E, F, G, H, J, K and L), but most of these may not be important as loci for "peptide presenters".

The HLA Class I antigens comprise a 45 Kilodalton (Kd) glycopeptide heavy chain with three domains, which is non-covalently associated with β_2-microglobulin, which plays an important role in the structural support of the heavy chain [3]. The HLA Class I molecule is assembled inside the cell and ultimately sits on the cell surface with a section inserted into the lipid bilayer of the cell membrane and has a short cytoplasmic tail.

The general structure of HLA Class I, HLA Class II and IgM molecules show such similarity of subunits, that a common link between HLA and immunoglobulins, back to some primordial cell surface receptor is likely. The full 3-dimensional structure of HLA-A Class I molecules has been determined from X-ray crystallography [4]. This has demonstrated that the molecule has a cleft on its outermost surface, which holds a peptide. Consequently, if a cell becomes infected with a virus, the virally induced proteins within the cell are broken down into small peptides which are then inserted into this cleft during the synthesis of HLA Class I molecules. The HLA Class I molecules then translocate these virally (or self) induced peptides to the cell surface leading to activation of cytotoxic (CD8) T cells [5]. This role of HLA Class I, in identifying cells, which are changed (e.g. virally infected), is the basis for their expression on all cells [4]. Epitopes on certain expressed HLA Class I molecules also act as ligands for killer inhibitory receptors expressed on natural killer [6] cells, thereby influencing NK cell function [7].

2.2. HLA class II antigens

The cell surface glycopeptide antigens of the HLA DR, DP and DQ loci are termed HLA Class II [1]. The tissue distribution of HLA Class II antigens is confined to the "immune competent" cells, including B-lymphocytes, macrophages, and endothelial cells and activated T-lymphocytes. The expression of HLA Class II, on cells, which would not normally express them, is stimulated by cytokines like interferon-γ and is associated with acute graft rejection in the

http://dx.doi.org/10.5772/54738

setting of transplantation. HLA Class II molecules consist of two chains each encoded by genes in the "HLA Complex" on Chromosome 6 [3]. The T Cells, which link to the HLA Class II molecules, are Helper (CD4) T cells. This role of HLA Class II, in initiating a general immune response, is the rationale for their limited expression on "immunologically active" cells (B lymphocytes, macrophages, etc.) and not on all tissues [4].

2.3. Recent changes to HLA nomenclature

A new HLA nomenclature was introduced in April 2010, replacing a system which had been in use since the 1990's. The main drive for the change was that the old system could no longer accommodate the increasing number of HLA alleles that were being described. There are currently over 5,700 alleles described across all the classical and non classical HLA loci.

The old system was based on assigning significance to pairs of digits in the allele nomenclature (Fig 1). For example in the allele HLA-A*02010102L, the designation 'HLA' identifies the allele as a HLA allele. The dash (-) separates the HLA designation from the gene, in this case the 'A' gene. The '*' is a separator. Of the actual allele name, the first two digits (02010102L) represents the allele group and in most instances, was synonymous with the Serological type (A2 in this case). The third and fourth digits (02010102L) identified the specific allele. All alleles whose nomenclature differed in these first four positions (02010102L) must code for proteins with different sequences. Alleles whose nomenclature differed in the fifth and sixth position (02010102L) code for proteins with silent mutations within the coding sequences. A sequence which differed by mutations in the introns or in the untranslated regions flanking the 3' and 5' ends of the exons were identified by different digits in the seventh and eighth positions (02010102L). In addition, a number of suffixes were used to identify sequences that were null, i.e. not expressed (N), those that had low expression (L), those that were secreted (S), those found only in the cytoplasm (C), those with questionable expression and those with aberrant expression (A).

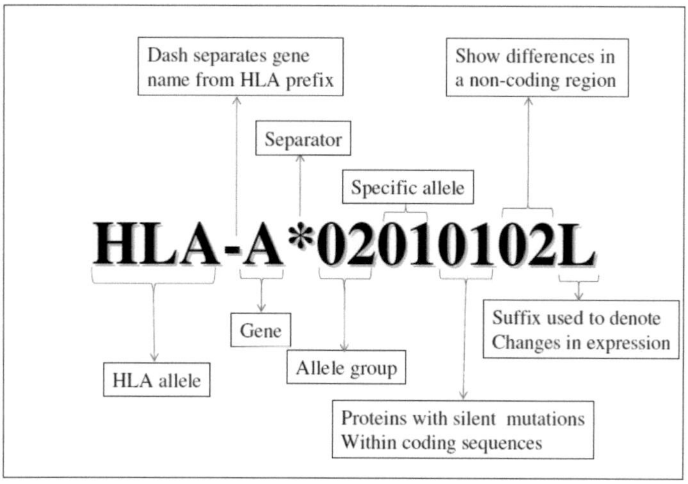

Figure 1. Old HLA nomenclature

A key limitation of this old system was that it only allowed for up to 99 alleles which differ in any of the pairs of positions. The HLA-A*02 and B*15 allele groups were the first to run into this problem when more than 99 alleles were detected. At that time, the WHO Nomenclature Committee for the HLA system decided to adopt the rollover sequences A*92 and B*95 respectively for A*02 and B*15. When A*0299 was identified, the next A*02 allele described was named A*9201. Similarly when B*1599 was identified the next B*15 allele described was named B*9501. Recently however, a number of other HLA types started to fast approach 99 alleles. These include A*03, B*40, B*44 and DRB1*11. Adopting rollover sequences for all of these was impractical. A rollover system of sorts had already been adopted for HLA-DPB1. When HLA-DPB1*9901 was identified, the next HLA-DPB1 allele was named 'within the existing sequences' as HLA-DPB1*0102.

In 2010, a new nomenclature system was adopted (Fig 2) [8, 9]. This introduced colons ':' as separators between pairs of digits. HLA-A*02010102L therefore became HLA-A*02:01:01:02L. The pairs of digits separated by colons are known as Fields. The first and second digits of the old nomenclature form the 1st Field of the new nomenclature. The third and fourth digits of the old nomenclature form the 2nd Field of the new nomenclature. To help reduce confusion in adopting the new nomenclature, the leading '0' in alleles 1-9 of each allele group was kept.

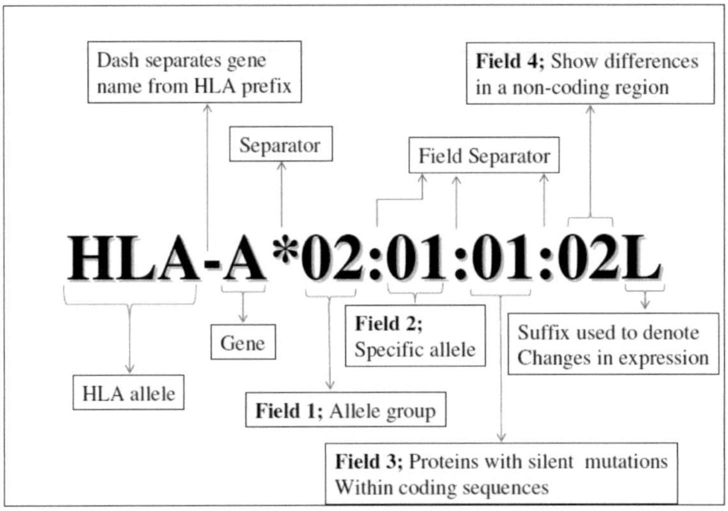

Figure 2. New HLA nomenclature

The introduction of the colons means that each Field is no longer restricted to 99 digits but can be expanded limitlessly. Once HLA-A*03:99 was identified, the next A3 allele could be named HLA-A*03:100.

With the introduction of colons and therefore the removal of the artificial restriction of 99 digits, there is no more need for rollover sequences. HLA-A*92 and B*95 were renamed A*02 and B*15 respectively and their associated alleles remapped. A*9201 became A*02:101. A*9202 became A*02:102 etc. HLA-B*9501 became B*15:101. HLA-B*9502 became B*15:102 etc. HLA-

A*02:100 and B*15:100 were not used to help make the remapping easier. However other HLA types which exceed 99 alleles will use allele 100. HLA-DPB1 alleles were also remapped. HLADPB1*0102 became HLA-DPB1*100:01.

A number of other changes were made to the nomenclature. The 'w' was dropped from HLA-Cw alleles but not from Cw antigens. HLA-Cw*0102 became HLA-C*01:02. The 'w' was kept in antigen names to avoid confusion with complement factors as well as with KIR ligand groups. For ambiguous allele strings, the codes 'P' and 'G' were introduced. A group of alleles that share the same nucleotide sequences within exons 2 and 3 for HLA class I and exon 2 for HLA class II were named after the first allele in the sequence and given a code of 'G' as a suffix. E.g. HLA-A*02:01:01 and HLA-A*02:01:02 could be named HLA-A*02:01G. A group of alleles that share the same protein sequences in the $\alpha 2$ and $\alpha 3$ domains, irrespective of the nucleotide sequence differences could be named after the first allele in the sequence and given a code of 'P' as a suffix e.g. HLA-A*02:01:01P.

2.4. Clinical relevance of the HLA system

The most important function of MHC molecule is in the induction and regulation of immune responses. T-lymphocytes recognize foreign antigen in combination with HLA molecules.

In an immune response, foreign antigen is processed by and presented on the surface of a cell (e.g. macrophage). The presentation is made by way of a HLA molecule. The HLA molecule has a section, called its antigen (or peptide) binding cleft, in which it has these antigens inserted. T-lymphocytes interact with the foreign antigen/HLA complex and are activated. Upon activation, the T cells multiply and by the release of cytokines, are able to set up an immune response that will recognize and destroy cells with this same foreign antigen/HLA complex, when next encountered. The exact mode of action of HLA Class I and HLA Class II antigens is different in this process. HLA Class I molecules, by virtue of their presence on all nucleated cells, present antigens that are peptides produced by invading viruses. These are specifically presented to cytotoxic T cells (CD8) which will then act directly to kill the virally infected cell. HLA Class II molecules have an intracellular chaperone network which prevents endogenous peptide from being inserted into its antigen binding cleft. They instead bind antigens (peptides) which are derived from outside of the cell (and have been engulfed). Such peptides would be from a bacterial infection. The HLA Class II molecule presents this "exogenous" peptide to helper T cells (CD4) which then set up a generalized immune response to this bacterial invasion. Thus it is apparent that MHC products are an integral part of immunological health and therefore it is no surprise to see a wide variety of areas of clinical and genetic implications.

2.5. HLA and renal transplants

HLA typing was applied to kidney transplantation very soon after the first HLA determinants were characterized [10-12]. The importance of reducing mismatched antigens in donor kidneys was immediately apparent with superior survival of grafts from HLA identical siblings compared to one haplotype matches or unrelated donors. It is apparent that the effect of HLA matching is significant, even with the highly efficient immunosuppression used today. The important things include need for ABO compatibility and the need for a negative T-lymphocyte crossmatch (using cytotoxicity). Complement binding anti-HLA Class I antibodies present at the time of transplant will cause "hyperacute rejection" of the graft (i.e. when the T cell crossmatch is positive).

3. HLA antibody detection and identification

3.1. Lymphocytotoxicity (serological testing)

In this serological test, lymphocytes are added to sera, which may or may not have antibodies directed to HLA or other cell surface antigens [13]. If the serum contains an antibody specific to an HLA (Class I or Class II) antigen on the lymphocytes, the antibody will bind to this HLA antigen. Complement is then added. If there is a cell bound antibody that is able to fix complement, the complement pathwayis activated causing membrane damage. The damaged cells are not completely lysed but suffer sufficient membrane damage to allow uptake of vital stains such as eosin or fluorescent stains such as Ethidium Bromide. Microscopic identification of the stained cells, indicates the presence of a specific HLA antibody. The cells used for the test are lymphocytes because of their excellent expression of HLA antigens and ease of isolation compared to most other tissue. The most important use of this test is to detect specific donor-reactive antibodies present in a potential recipient prior to transplantation.

This test has long been used to type for HLA Class I and Class II antigens, using antisera of known specificity. However, the problems of cross-reactivity and non-availability of certain antibodies have led to the introduction of DNA-based methods.

3.2. Mixed Lymphocyte Culture (MLC)

When lymphocytes from two individuals are cultured together, each cell population is able to recognize the "foreign" HLA class II antigens of the other. As a response to these differences, the lymphocytes transform into blast cells, with associated DNA synthesis. Radio-labelled thymidine, added to the culture, will be used in this DNA synthesis. Therefore, radioactive uptake is a measure of DNA synthesis and the difference between the HLA Class II types of the two people. This technique can be refined by treating the lymphocytes from one of the individuals to prevent cell division, for example by irradiation. It is thus possible to measure the response of T lymphocytes from one individual to a range of foreign lymphocytes. It has thus proved possible by using the mixed lymphocyte culture (MLC) test to use T lymphocytes to define what were previously called HLA-D antigens. The "HLA-D" defined in this way is actually a combination of HLA-DR, DQ and DP.

An important use of the MLC is in its use as a "cellular crossmatch" prior to transplantation especially bone marrow. By testing the prospective donor and recipient, an in-vitro transplant model is established which is an extremely significant indicator of possible rejection or Graft-Versus-Host reaction.

http://dx.doi.org/10.5772/54738

3.3. Molecular genetic techniques

3.3.1. RFLP (Restriction Fragment Length Polymorphism)

Restriction Fragment Length Polymorphism (RFLP) methods rely on the ability of certain enzymes to recognize exact DNA nucleotide sequences and to cut the DNA at each of these points [14]. Thus, the frequency of a particular sequence will determine the lengths of DNA produced by cutting with a particular enzyme.

The DNA for one HLA (Class II) antigen, e.g. DR15, will have these particular enzyme cutting sites (or "restriction sites") at different positions compared to another antigen, e.g. DR17. Consequently, the lengths of DNA observed when DR15 is cut by a particular enzyme, are characteristic of DR15 and different to the sizes of the fragments seen when DR17 is cut by the same enzyme [15].

3.3.2. Polymerase chain reaction

The Polymerase Chain Reaction (PCR) is a revolutionary system for investigating the DNA nucleotide sequence of a particular region of interest in any individual [16]. Very small amounts of DNA can be used as a starting point, such that it is theoretically possible to tissue type using a single hair root. Sequencing DNA has been transformed from a long and laborious exercise to a technique that is essentially automatable.

The first step in this technique is to obtain DNA from the nuclei of an individual. The double stranded DNA is then denatured by heat into single stranded DNA. Oligonucleotide primer sequences are then chosen to flank a region of interest. The oligo- nucleotide primer is a short segment of complementary DNA, which will associate with the single stranded DNA to act as a starting point for reconstruction of double stranded DNA at that site.

If the oligonucleotide is chosen to be close to a region of special interest like a hypervariable region of HLA-DRB then the part of the DNA, and only that part, will become double stranded DNA, when DNA polymerase and deoxyribonucleotide triphosphates are added. From one copy of DNA it is thus possible to make two. Those two copies can then, in turn, be denatured, reassociate with primers and produce four copies. This cycle can then be repeated until there is a sufficient copy of the selected portion of DNA to isolate on a gel and then sequence or type.

There are a number of PCR based methods in use. For example:

- *Sequence Specific Priming (SSP)* - In this test, the oligonucleotide primers used to start the PCR have sequences complimentary to known sequences which are characteristic to certain HLA specificities. The primers, which are specific to HLA-DR15, for example, will not be able to instigate the PCR for HLA-DR17. Typing is done by using a set of different PCR's, each with primers specific for different HLA antigens.

3.4. Sequence Specific Oligonucleotide (SSO) Typing

By this method, the DNA for a whole region (e.g. the HLA DR gene region) is amplified in the PCR. The amplified DNA is then tested by adding labeled (e.g. Radioactive) oligonucleotide probes, which are complementary for DNA sequences, characteristic for certain HLA antigens. These probes will then "type" for the presence of specific DNA sequences of HLA genes.

3.5. Panel Reactive Antibodies (PRA)

PRA has been used to measure patient HLA sensitisation ever since pre-formed donor specific HLA antibodies were associated with hyperacute rejection in renal transplantation in the 1960's [17]. As traditionally defined, PRA refers to the percentage of an antibody screening panel with which the patient's serum reacts. A kidney patient with a PRA > 85% is considered highly sensitised. This measure of PRA however relies on the composition of the panel which may not necessarily reflect the antigen frequencies in the donor population. This measure of PRA is not therefore a good reflection of the chances of the patient finding a compatible donor. Variations in cell panels, both commercial and in house, result in wide variations in recorded PRA for patients on the waiting list.

The calculated PRA (cPRA) was introduced to overcome this problem [18]. The cPRA can be calculated in a number of different ways, but relies on the identification of a potential recipient's anti-HLA antibody profile. This has been made much easier by the wide adoption of solid phase assays such as Luminex. Luminex assays, especially those involving the use of single antigen beads (SABs) allow fine specificity definition and allow the strength of the reactions (MFI) to be used to assess immunological risk and help decide whether or not specificity should be listed. The cPRA is then calculated by defining a set of unacceptable mismatches for that recipient, and weighting those mismatches according to the frequency of the antigen in the donor population. This could be based on the frequency of different HLA antigens in the most recent 10,000 deceased donors.The cPRA therefore gives a measure of the chances of a patient finding a compatible donor in the donor pool.

cPRA removes some of the variability between laboratories using different panels and allows a PRA value to be assigned which reflects the patients' transplantability.

4. Non-HLA antibodies

Acute and chronic allograft rejection can occur in HLA-identical sibling transplants implicating the importance of immune response against non-HLA targets. Non-HLA anti-bodies may occur as alloantiboides, yet they seem to be predominantly autoantibodies. Antigenic targets of non-HLA antibodies described thus far include various minor histocom-patibility antigens, vascular receptors, adhesion molecules, and intermediate filaments. Non-HLA antibodies may function as complement and non-complement-fixing antibodies and they may induce a wide variety of allograft injuries, reflecting the complexity of their acute and chronic actions.

4.1. The KIR receptor complex

The adaptive immune response recognises infection through presentation of pathogen-derived peptides in association with MHC to the host T cells. One of the mechanisms

http://dx.doi.org/10.5772/54738

which pathogens use to evade this immune response is to down regulate their MHC cell surface expression. Natural Killer cells are able to detect altered expression of MHC through a number of cell surface receptors leading to target cell lysis [19]. These receptors include the killer immunoglobulin like receptors (KIR), which are also expressed on some effector T cells. In humans, the KIR gene cluster is located on chromosome 19. KIR genes are both polygenic and polymorphic [20]. The KIR gene cluster codes for 15 expressed KIR genes and 2 pseudo genes.

The ligands for KIR receptors are HLA class I molecules [21]. These include HLA-C locus antigens with either Asn (Group 1 HLA-C antigens) or Lys (Group 2 HLA-C antigens) at position 80, the HLA-Bw4 epitope and some HLA-A antigens. KIR receptors binding to HLA class I are either inhibitory or are stimulatory with the overall effect of NK cell interaction with the target cell dependent on the balance between these inhibitory and stimulatory signals. It is thought that the inhibitory KIR's bind class I with greater affinity than the corresponding activating KIR with the effect that under normal circumstances the inhibitory signal prevails. The 'missing self' hypothesis holds that NK cell alloreactivity occurs when the ligand for inhibitory KIR receptors is down regulated or 'missing', leading to activation. This however requires that KIR receptors engage their cogent HLA class I molecules during maturation to acquire effector function. NK cells that express only inhibitory KIRs for absent HLA class I molecules are hypo responsive in the non transplant setting.

Inhibitory KIR receptors possess long cytoplasmic tails with immunoreceptor tyrosine based inhibitory motifs (ITIMs). Activating KIR receptors have short cytoplasmic tails that pair with adaptor molecules with immunoreceptor tyrosine based activating motif (ITAMs). The nomenclature for KIR receptors therefore includes an 'L' (long tail) for inhibitory KIR's and an 'S' (short tail) for activating KIR's. The nomenclature also includes 'P' for pseudo genes. The inhibitory and activating KIR receptors share sequence and structural similarities in their extracellular domains. KIR's have either 2 or 3 extracellular immunoglobulin domains and this is reflected in their nomenclature as either '2D' or '3D', giving KIR receptors nomenclature such as KIR2DL1, KIR2DS2 and KIR3DL1, where the final digit indicates the order in which the genes were described.

The KIR genes assemble into haplotypes with two haplotypes described, 'A' and 'B'. The 'A' haplotype has only one activating KIR (2DS4), while the 'B' haplotype has a higher number of activating KIRs and generally possess more KIRs than the 'A' haplotype.

4.2. MICA/B

The major histocompatibility complex class I related chain was first described in the 1990's [22]. The genes are located centromeric to the HLA class I B gene. The only two MIC genes which are expressed are MICA and MICB. MICA and MICB share a significant amount of sequence homology with HLA class I and have some similarity in their conformation. MICA and MICB antigens have α1, 2 and 3 domains like classical HLA antigens but do not associate with β2 microglobulin and do not bind peptide for presentation to T cells. Instead, MIC antigens serve as ligands for the NKG2D receptor on NK cells and on some T cells.

MICA and MICB genes are polymorphic but not as much as the classical HLA class I genes. Over 70 MICA alleles and over 30 MICB alleles have been described [23]. Unlike HLA class I where the polymorphic residues are located mainly in the region that forms the peptide binding groove, polymorphism in MIC is more dispersed throughout the $\alpha2$ and $\alpha3$ domains. There is also polymorphism in the trans-membrane region. Many MIC antigens have the same extracellular domains with the only differences lying in the trans-membrane regions.

MICA and MICB antigens are constitutively expressed on epithelial cells, especially those of the gastrointestinal tract and on fibroblasts, monocytes, dendritic cells and on endothelial cells. They are not constitutively expressed on lymphocytes. They are however up regulated in stressed cells.

The structure of MICA is similar to that of HLA class I but has some striking differences. Like HLA class I, MICA has three extracellular domains ($\alpha1$, 2 and 3), a transmembrane region and a cytoplasmic domain. Unlike HLA class I, the MICA protein does not associate with $\beta2$ microglobulin. The MICA $\alpha1$ and 2 domains form a platform that is analogous to the platform formed by HLA class I $\alpha1$ and 2 domains. In HLA class I, this platform forms the peptide binding groove. The MICA molecule however has extensive disordering of sections of the alpha helix in the $\alpha2$ domain resulting in a very shallow groove, incapable of binding peptide. The MICA $\alpha1$ and 2 platform domains do not interact with the $\alpha3$ domain except for being linked together through a short linker chain. This allows for some flexibility in the structure.

The NKG2D receptor forms a complex with MICA by binding orthogonal to the alpha helices of the platform $\alpha1$ and 2 domains.

4.3. Minor histocompatibility antigens

HLA presents the major genetic barrier to stem cell transplantation. However, evidence that other genetic systems are involved includes GvHD and some degree of rejection even when transplanting with HLA identical siblings. A non HLA system which is thought to contribute to this is the minor histocompatibility antigen (mHA) system. Minor histocompatibility antigens comprise of peptides derived from proteins in which some degree of polymorphism exists such there may be differences between the patient and donor repertoires. These peptides can be presented to the immune system by both HLA class I and II antigens.

The best characterised minor antigens are the Y chromosome derived HY peptide and the autosomal HA1 to HA5 peptides. Minor histocompatibility antigens such as HA1 and HA2 have restricted tissue distribution and are present normally only on haematopoietic cells. Others such as HY are more ubiquitously distributed, expressed for instance on gut epithelium. HA1 and HA2 are expressed on leukaemic cells and some tumour cells, making them potential targets for cellular therapy. Minor HLA antigens are restricted by certain HLA types such as HLA-A2 for instance.

http://dx.doi.org/10.5772/54738

5. Cross-matching techniques

Crossmatching was developed in an attempt to identify recipients who are likely to develop acute vascular rejection of a graft from a given donor. This phenomenon, hyperacute rejection (HAR) [24], is a result of preformed antibodies against the donor; referred to as donor-specific antibodies (DSA). Such antibodies are usually formed as the result of previous exposure to HLA, generally through pregnancy, blood transfusion or previous transplantation [25]. There are other debated forms of developing anti-HLA Abs such as via microbial exposure but the above three are thought to be the most prevalent. Particularly relevant is the exposure of women during pregnancy, to their partner's HLA. This commonly results in direct sensitization against the partner, potentially making him an unsuitable living donor. HAR may also occur in blood group incompatible transplantation or rarely as a result of other non-HLA antibodies.

Preformed antibodies cause rejection by binding to HLA antigens expressed on the endothelium of vessels in the transplanted kidney, resulting in activation of the complement cascade with resultant thrombosis and infarction of the graft. HAR can occur immediately upon reperfusion of the donor kidney. This catastrophic outcome necessitates the immediate removal of the graft. Clearly avoiding HAR is desirable and crossmatching helps predict and hence prevent this [17].

There are different types of crossmatch tests available.

5.1. Complement-Dependent Cytotoxicity (CDC) crossmatch

A CDC crossmatch involves placing recipient serum (potentially containing donor-specific anti-HLA antibodies) onto donor lymphocytes (containing HLA antigens). A cytotoxic reaction (deemed 'positive') suggests the presence of preformed DSA.

CDC crossmatching was pioneered by Terasaki and colleagues in the 1960s [13, 17]. It identifies clinically significant donor specific HLA antibody mediated responses for a given recipient. Lymphocytes from the donor are isolated and separated into T and B cells. Serum from the recipient is mixed with the lymphocytes in a multi-well plate. Complement is then added (usually derived from rabbit serum). If donor-specific antibody is present and binds to donor cells, the complement cascade will be activated via the classical pathway resulting in lysis of the lymphocytes.

The read-out of the test is the percentage of dead cells relative to live cells as determined by microscopy. The result can thus be scored on the percentage of dead cells, with 0 correlating to no dead cells; scores of 2, 4 and 6 represent increasing levels of lysis. On this basis, a score of 2 is positive at a low level, consistent with approximately 20% lysis (generally taken as the cut-off for a positive result). A score of 8 represents all cells having lysed and indicates the strongest possible reaction. The use of a scoring system allows a semi-quantitative analysis of the strength of reaction. Another way to determine the strength of the reaction is to repeat the crossmatch using serial doubling dilutions of the recipient serum (often known as a 'titred crossmatch'). In this way, dilutions are usually performed to 1 in 2, 4, 8, 16, 32, 64 and so on.

In the situation of a high titre of high avidity DSA it may be that many dilutions are required for the test to become negative (e.g. 1 in 128). With antibody at a low level or one with a low affinity, a single dilution may be enough to render the crossmatch result negative. This may also give an indication as to the likelihood that a negative crossmatch could be achieved with a desensitization protocol.

The basic CDC crossmatch can be enhanced by the addition of antihuman globulin (AHG). This technique increases the sensitivity of the CDC crossmatch as a result of multiple AHG molecules binding to each DSA attached to thedonor cells thereby amplifying the total number of Fc receptors available for interaction with complement component 1, which increases the likelihood of complement activation and cell lysis.

It is also possible to have a negative crossmatch in the presence of a DSA and this can happen in the following conditions:

1. antibody titre is too low to cause complement activation
2. antibody is of a type that does not activate complement and
3. antigen for which the antibody is specific is expressed only at very low levels on the donor's lymphocytes.

A further consideration relates to variations in antibody levels in a given individual's serum samples, collected at different times. The most reactive serum is generally called the 'peak serum'. This may have been collected several years earlier, with the 'current serum' showing quite different reactivity. As an example, the peak serum may show a clear positive CDC crossmatch result, but as the antibody levels have fallen in subsequent sera, so too may the degree of cell lysis in the assay. This may render the CDC crossmatch negative. Nevertheless, the antibodies found in the peak sera may still be of relevance, indicating that re-exposure to the relevant antigen could initiate a memory response with the risk of early and aggressive rejection. For this reason, patients on transplant waiting lists have sera collected at frequent intervals; variations can be monitored and newly appearing HLA antibodies can be detected.

There are important differences in HLA expression between T and B cells, which influence the interpretation of the crossmatch. T cells do not constitutively express HLA class II so the result of a T-cell crossmatch generally reflects antibodies to HLA class I only. B cells on the other hand express both HLA class I and II, as well as a larger range of surface markers, icluding Fc receptors. Because of this, a positive B-cell crossmatch is more difficult to interpret than a positive T-cell cross match. It may be due to antibodies directed against HLA class I or II or both, or it may be due to antibody binding to other sites, that may or may not be clinically important. Hence, if the T- and B-cell crossmatches are positive the interpretation is that there may be either single or multiple HLA class I DSA/s or a mixture of HLA class I and II DSA. While a negative T-cell crossmatch in the setting of a positive B-cell crossmatch suggests either there may be one or more class II DSA/s but no class I antibodies or that there is a low-level DSA to a class I antigen with greater lysis of B cells relative to T cells. This is often due to the fact that B cells express higher levels of HLA class I than do T cells [26]. When class I complement fixing HLA DSA are present at a significant level one would expect both the T and B-cell crossmatches to be positive. A negative B-cell crossmatch in the presence of a positive T-cell crossmatch therefore suggests a technical error. This is not unusual as B cells tend to be less resilient than T cells and their viability can often be a concern in the assays.

5.2. Positive T-cell CDC crossmatch

Transplanting in the setting of a positive T-cell crossmatch, which is not due to an autoantibody, is likely to generate a very poor outcome. Patel and Terasaki described the outcomes of 30 such transplants [17]. Twenty four (24) patients lost their grafts immediately to HAR while another three lost their grafts within 3 months. It is not clear why the other three patients had less severe reactions but it may relate to false positive crossmatches generated by autoantibodies given that dithiothreitol (DTT) which cleaves the multimers of IgM antibodies was not used in their assays. Other possibilities include false positive tests or lower immunogenicity of the antibodies or antigens in those cases.

A recent study investigated whether IVIg or plasma exchange was more effective at desensitizing crossmatchpositive recipients so that they might be crossmatch-negative at the time of transplant [27]. While most patients were successfully desensitized there was a group of 10 patients who did not achieve a negative crossmatch but were still transplanted. Of this group 70% developed AMR with 50% losing their grafts. Given this data, even after reducing the antibody titre with a desensitization protocol before transplant, a persistent positive T-cell crossmatch remains an absolute contraindication to transplantation.

5.3. Positive B-cell CDC crossmatch

B-cell CDC crossmatching is not as predictive of HAR as the T-cell CDC crossmatch and there has been much controversy about its role [28]. Many centres do not perform B-cell crossmatching for cadaveric renal transplantation because of uncertainty about the significance of a positive result. The major limitation is a rate of false positive results of up to 50% [29]. In some cases this reactivity may be due to non-HLA molecules on the surface of the B lymphocytes, including the presence of Fc receptors. While a negative result is reassuring a positive result may mean a transplant is cancelled when it was safe to proceed. Another argument against the routine use of B-cell crossmatching is that antibodies to class II antigens are of less significance in generating antibody-mediated rejection. But recently it has been found that they are not so benign [30].

B-cell crossmatches are often performed as part of the immunologic assessment before live donor transplantation when there is more time to determine the significance of the result. Paired with information about the presence of DSA, determined by more specific means such as antigen-coated beads (Luminex, discussed below) the B-cell CDC crossmatch results may be more meaningful [31]. If a B-cell crossmatch is positive and there are no detectable antibodies to class I or II antigens, the result may be falsely positive while a positive result in the presence of detectable DSA signifies that the identified DSA may be functionally relevant in that it can activate complement and were associated with increased risk of rejection [32]. This has led to the suggestion that the B-cell

CDC crossmatch should not be used alone to determine transplant suitability and that it be interpreted only in the light of accompanying Luminex results [31].

5.4. The flow crossmatching technique

A flow crossmatch involves adding recipient's serum to donor lymphocytes and then incubating them with fluorescein-labelled antibodies against human IgG (antihuman IgG fluorescein isothicyanate [FITC]). This fluorescein-labelled antibody will bind to all the IgG antibodies in the recipient serum. If a DSA in this serum then binds to the donor lymphocytes, it will be detectable by flow cytometry.

Flow crossmatching is performed using the same initial base ingredients as CDC crossmatching (i.e. donor lymphocytes and recipient serum) and was first described in 1983 [33]. The two are mixed to allow antibody binding and after washing, fluoresceinated AHG is added to bind attached DSA and hence allow detection by flow cytometry. The read-out may be reported simply as positive or negative or can be further quantitated. Intensity of fluorescence above control, referred to as channel shifts, may be reported while another means of quantitation is to determine the number of dilutions of recipient serum required to generate a negative result.

The subtype of antibody can also be determined by the isotype specificity of the fluorescently labelled detection antibody. Hence if only IgG antibodies are of interest the detection antibody chosen will be of the type that binds only to IgG and not IgM or IgA [34]. Furthermore the subtype of IgG can be elucidated by choosing a detection antibody that binds only to IgG1, 2, 3 or 4. Refining the analysis in this way provides information about the likelihood of complement activation *in vivo* as IgG4 does not activate complement.

The role of flow crossmatching in the pre-transplant assessment is controversial. The significance of a positive result is mainly of interest when the CDC crossmatch is negative. In this setting the positive flow crossmatch is likely to be caused by a non-complement fixing antibody, a non-HLA antibody or a low-level antibody that is below the threshold of sensitivity of the CDC methodology. In patients who are not known to be sensitized several studies have suggested that a positive T- or B-cell flow crossmatch was not predictive of increased rejection rates or worse graft survival while in sensitized patients other studies have suggested inferior graft survival [30, 34-39]. A possible reason for this difference is that there would be a higher false positive rate in non-sensitized patients than in sensitized patients given that they are not expected to have a positive result. Another factor determining the significance of the result is the cut-off values used to determine a positive test [34]. These are not applied uniformly between centres and those that apply a very low cut-off value will increase sensitivity at the expense of specificity.

Some transplant clinicians do not use flow crossmatching as part of their pre-transplant assessment and rely on CDC crossmatching along with defining DSA by Luminex, otherwise known as 'virtual crossmatching'. Others contend that flow crossmatching adds important information on the strength of donor-specific antibody reactivity and should be considered in the context of donor-specific antibody results and CDC crossmatching to help develop an

http://dx.doi.org/10.5772/54738

overall opinion on the likelihood of immune complications. The area remains controversial and no clear recommendation can be made at this time.

5.5. Virtual crossmatching

Virtual crossmatching refers to the comparison of the anti- HLA antibodies of the recipient, derived from Luminex, with the HLA of the donor [40]. If there is a DSA present this would represent a positive virtual crossmatch. Antibodies are defined against HLA class I and II antigens. Synthetic microspheres (beads) coated with HLA antigens are commercially available for this testing. Beads may be coated with multiple HLA antigens for screening purposes or a single HLA antigen for defining specificity of antibodies more precisely. For the virtual crossmatch, multiple beads each coated with a single HLA antigen are mixed with recipient serum. Anti-HLA antibodies present bind to the beads and are detected by an isotype-specific (e.g. IgG) detection antibody via flow cytometry. Unique fluorochromes within the beads mark the HLA antigen specificity of each bead. This technique is as sensitive as flow crossmatching and provides the specificity of the antibody [41].

It has long been established that the presence of antibodies that react with human leucocytes portend worse long-term graft survival [42]. This information has been further refined by more sensitive antibody detection systems, particularly Luminex. It has been shown that recipients with DSA have worse graft survival than those with third party anti-HLA Abs (antibodies against HLA antigens that are not donor-specific) who in turn have reduced graft survival compared with recipients without any anti-HLA antibodies [43]. Therefore, the presence of a DSA suggests inferior graft survival compared with no DSA even in the presence of a negative CDC crossmatch [44].

Luminex testing offers significant advantages over CDC and flow crossmatch in terms of defining the HLA specificity of identified antibodies. The presence of a DSA detected by Luminex in the setting of a negative or positive CDC crossmatch appears to have prognostic importance in terms of graft survival and acute rejection risk; however, there are insufficient data to determine the significance of a DSA with a negative flow crossmatch [40, 44-46].

In each assay, negative control beads provide a minimum threshold for a positive result. Positive results can then be graded as weak, moderate or strong on the basis of the degree of fluorescence of the positive bead. This result can be scored as a median fluorescence index (MFI) or molecules of equivalent soluble fluorescence. The molecules of equivalent soluble fluorescence of a DSA have been shown to correlate with antibody titre and predict graft failure [47].

While Luminex testing has added significantly to the understanding of crossmatching, the methodology has some significant limitations that can make interpretation difficult. Limitations include possible interference by IgM antibodies, variable antigen density on beads, conformational changes to antibodies in the process of binding to the beads, and gaps in the HLA antibody repertoire in bead sets. [45, 48, 49].

5.6. Cellular crossmatching

All of the above-mentioned crossmatching techniques attempt to detect a donor-reactive antibody likely to result in acute or chronic antibody-mediated rejection. The presence of sensitization of the cellular arm of the immune system, particularly T cells, can be assessed by cytokine assays such as ELISPOTs. These assays detect the number of recipient T cells producing cytokines such as interferon gamma when encountering donor antigen presenting cells. The assays are conducted in plates coated with a capture antibody for the cytokine of interest. The mixed donor and recipient leucocytes are added to the plate and incubated. After washing to remove the cells the reaction is developed by adding a second antibody for the cytokine of interest and then stained for that antibody [50].

6. Conclusion

Understanding of the transplantation antigens and crossmatching is a vital tool in transplant. Crossmatching plays a key role in assessing immune compatibility between a donor and recipient. A positive T-cell CDC crossmatch would usually mean that a particular pairing should not proceed. But in some cases, a desensitization protocol may allow such a transplant to occur, avoiding hyperacute or early acute rejection. However they have inferior longterm graft outcomes compared with patients who are not sensitized to their donor. The advent of flow crossmatching and Luminex assays has allowed the detection of very lower titre, anti-HLA antibodies of uncertain clinical significance.

CDC crossmatching along with Luminex should be used in determining anti-HLA antibodies. The role of flow crossmatching is less clear and its help in decision making is unclear. The ideal future crossmatch will be highly sensitive in identifying DSA and provide accurate prediction of the functional significance of the antibody. This will hopefully allow differentiation between transplants that can safely proceed in the face of a clinically irrelevant DSA while providing clear prognostic information in the setting of more serious antibodies.

Further studies are required to better define the significance of very low-level DSA, non-complement fixing antibodies, IgM antibodies and non-HLA antibodies as well as the importance of assessing T cellular sensitization.

Author details

Bhadran Bose*, David W. Johnson and Scott B. Campbell

*Address all correspondence to: bhadranbose@yahoo.com

Department of Nephrology, Princess Alexandra Hospital, Brisbane, Australia

References

[1] Sanfilippo, F. and A. DB, *An interpretation of the major histocompatibility complex*. 3rd ed. Manual of clinical Immunology, ed. H.F. NR Rose, JL Fahey1986, Washington DC: Am Soc Microbiol.

[2] Roitt, I.M., B. J, and M. DK, *Immunology*. 5th ed1998, London: Churchill Livingston.

[3] Stern, L.J. and D.C. Wiley, *Antigenic peptide binding by class I and class II histocompatibility proteins*. Structure, 1994. 2(4): p. 245-51.

[4] Browning M and M.M. A, *HLA and MHC: Genes, Molecules and Function*1996, Oxford: Bios Scientific Publishers.

[5] Long, E.O. and S. Jacobson, *Pathways of viral antigen processing and presentation to CTL: defined by the mode of virus entry?* Immunology today, 1989. 10(2): p. 45-8.

[6] Yanagiya, A., et al., *Prolongation of second heart transplants in rats*. Transplantation, 1992. 54(4): p. 690-4.

[7] Norman, P.J. and P. Parham, *Complex interactions: the immunogenetics of human leukocyte antigen and killer cell immunoglobulin-like receptors*. Seminars in hematology, 2005. 42(2): p. 65-75.

[8] Marsh, S.G., et al., *An update to HLA nomenclature, 2010*. Bone marrow transplantation, 2010. 45(5): p. 846-8.

[9] Marsh, S.G., et al., *Nomenclature for factors of the HLA system, 2010*. Tissue antigens, 2010. 75(4): p. 291-455.

[10] Opelz, G., *Correlation of HLA matching with kidney graft survival in patients with or without cyclosporine treatment*. Transplantation, 1985. 40(3): p. 240-3.

[11] Terasaki, M., *Clinical Transplants*1992, Los Angles: UCLA Tissue Typing Laboratory.

[12] Sanfilippo, F., et al., *Benefits of HLA-A and HLA-B matching on graft and patient outcome after cadaveric-donor renal transplantation*. The New England journal of medicine, 1984. 311(6): p. 358-64.

[13] Terasaki, P.I. and J.D. McClelland, *Microdroplet Assay of Human Serum Cytotoxins*. Nature, 1964. 204: p. 998-1000.

[14] B, D., *Immunology of HLA vol. 1 Histocompatibility Testing 1987*1989, New York: Springer Verlag.

[15] Bidwell, J., *DNA-RFLP analysis and genotyping of HLA-DR and DQ antigens*. Immunology today, 1988. 9(1): p. 18-23.

[16] A, M., D. HGI, and J. JS, *PCR Strategies*1995, New York: Academic Press.

[17] Patel, R. and P.I. Terasaki, *Significance of the positive crossmatch test in kidney transplantation*. The New England journal of medicine, 1969. 280(14): p. 735-9.

[18] Cecka, J.M., *Calculated PRA (CPRA): the new measure of sensitization for transplant candidates.* American journal of transplantation : official journal of the American Society of Transplantation and the American Society of Transplant Surgeons, 2010. 10(1): p. 26-9.

[19] Deng, L. and R.A. Mariuzza, *Structural basis for recognition of MHC and MHC-like ligands by natural killer cell receptors.* Seminars in immunology, 2006. 18(3): p. 159-66.

[20] Middleton, D. and F. Gonzelez, *The extensive polymorphism of KIR genes.* Immunology, 2010. 129(1): p. 8-19.

[21] Tran, T.H., et al., *Analysis of KIR ligand incompatibility in human renal transplantation.* Transplantation, 2005. 80(8): p. 1121-3.

[22] Li, P., et al., *Crystal structure of the MHC class I homolog MIC-A, a gammadelta T cell ligand.* Immunity, 1999. 10(5): p. 577-84.

[23] Stephens, H.A., *MICA and MICB genes: can the enigma of their polymorphism be resolved?* Trends in immunology, 2001. 22(7): p. 378-85.

[24] Morimoto, T., et al., *Clinical application of arterialization of portal vein in living related donor partial liver transplantation.* Transplant international : official journal of the European Society for Organ Transplantation, 1992. 5(3): p. 151-4.

[25] Terasaki, P.I., *Humoral theory of transplantation.* American journal of transplantation : official journal of the American Society of Transplantation and the American Society of Transplant Surgeons, 2003. 3(6): p. 665-73.

[26] Pellegrino, M.A., et al., *B peripheral lymphocytes express more HLA antigens than T peripheral lymphocytes.* Transplantation, 1978. 25(2): p. 93-5.

[27] Stegall, M.D., et al., *A comparison of plasmapheresis versus high-dose IVIG desensitization in renal allograft recipients with high levels of donor specific alloantibody.* American journal of transplantation : official journal of the American Society of Transplantation and the American Society of Transplant Surgeons, 2006. 6(2): p. 346-51.

[28] Mahoney, R.J., S. Taranto, and E. Edwards, *B-Cell crossmatching and kidney allograft outcome in 9031 United States transplant recipients.* Human immunology, 2002. 63(4): p. 324-35.

[29] Le Bas-Bernardet, S., et al., *Identification of the antibodies involved in B-cell crossmatch positivity in renal transplantation.* Transplantation, 2003. 75(4): p. 477-82.

[30] Pollinger, H.S., et al., *Kidney transplantation in patients with antibodies against donor HLA class II.* American journal of transplantation : official journal of the American Society of Transplantation and the American Society of Transplant Surgeons, 2007. 7(4): p. 857-63.

[31] Eng, H.S., et al., *Anti-HLA donor-specific antibodies detected in positive B-cell crossmatches by Luminex predict late graft loss.* American journal of transplantation : official journal of

the American Society of Transplantation and the American Society of Transplant Surgeons, 2008. 8(11): p. 2335-42.

[32] Eng, H.S., et al., *Clinical significance of anti-HLA antibodies detected by Luminex: enhancing the interpretation of CDC-BXM and important post-transplantation monitoring tools.* Human immunology, 2009. 70(8): p. 595-9.

[33] Garovoy MRRM, et al., *Flow cytometry analysis: A high technology crossmatch technique facilitating transplantation.* Transplant Proceedings, 1983. XV(1939).

[34] Limaye, S., et al., *Improved graft survival in highly sensitized patients undergoing renal transplantation after the introduction of a clinically validated flow cytometry crossmatch.* Transplantation, 2009. 87(7): p. 1052-6.

[35] Bryan, C.F., et al., *Long-term graft survival is improved in cadaveric renal retransplantation by flow cytometric crossmatching.* Transplantation, 1998. 66(12): p. 1827-32.

[36] Christiaans, M.H., et al., *No advantage of flow cytometry crossmatch over complement-dependent cytotoxicity in immunologically well-documented renal allograft recipients.* Transplantation, 1996. 62(9): p. 1341-7.

[37] Ilham, M.A., et al., *Clinical significance of a positive flow crossmatch on the outcomes of cadaveric renal transplants.* Transplantation proceedings, 2008. 40(6): p. 1839-43.

[38] Karpinski, M., et al., *Flow cytometric crossmatching in primary renal transplant recipients with a negative anti-human globulin enhanced cytotoxicity crossmatch.* Journal of the American Society of Nephrology : JASN, 2001. 12(12): p. 2807-14.

[39] Kerman, R.H., et al., *Flow cytometry-detected IgG is not a contraindication to renal transplantation: IgM may be beneficial to outcome.* Transplantation, 1999. 68(12): p. 1855-8.

[40] Bielmann, D., et al., *Pretransplant risk assessment in renal allograft recipients using virtual crossmatching.* American journal of transplantation : official journal of the American Society of Transplantation and the American Society of Transplant Surgeons, 2007. 7(3): p. 626-32.

[41] Pei, R., et al., *Single human leukocyte antigen flow cytometry beads for accurate identification of human leukocyte antigen antibody specificities.* Transplantation, 2003. 75(1): p. 43-9.

[42] Terasaki, P.I., M. Kreisler, and R.M. Mickey, *Presensitization and kidney transplant failures.* Postgraduate medical journal, 1971. 47(544): p. 89-100.

[43] Terasaki, P.I., M. Ozawa, and R. Castro, *Four-year follow-up of a prospective trial of HLA and MICA antibodies on kidney graft survival.* American journal of transplantation : official journal of the American Society of Transplantation and the American Society of Transplant Surgeons, 2007. 7(2): p. 408-15.

[44] Amico, P., et al., *Clinical relevance of pretransplant donor-specific HLA antibodies detected by single-antigen flow-beads.* Transplantation, 2009. 87(11): p. 1681-8.

[45] Tambur, A.R., et al., *Perception versus reality?: Virtual crossmatch--how to overcome some of the technical and logistic limitations.* American journal of transplantation : official

journal of the American Society of Transplantation and the American Society of Transplant Surgeons, 2009. 9(8): p. 1886-93.

[46] Vaidya, S., et al., *Prediction of crossmatch outcome of highly sensitized patients by single and/ or multiple antigen bead luminex assay.* Transplantation, 2006. 82(11): p. 1524-8.

[47] Mizutani, K., et al., *The importance of anti-HLA-specific antibody strength in monitoring kidney transplant patients.* American journal of transplantation : official journal of the American Society of Transplantation and the American Society of Transplant Surgeons, 2007. 7(4): p. 1027-31.

[48] Morris, G.P., et al., *Virtual crossmatch by identification of donor-specific anti-human leukocyte antigen antibodies by solid-phase immunoassay: a 30-month analysis in living donor kidney transplantation.* Human immunology, 2010. 71(3): p. 268-73.

[49] Zachary, A.A., et al., *Naturally occurring interference in Luminex assays for HLA-specific antibodies: characteristics and resolution.* Human immunology, 2009. 70(7): p. 496-501.

[50] Augustine, J.J., et al., *Pre-transplant IFN-gamma ELISPOTs are associated with post-transplant renal function in African American renal transplant recipients.* American journal of transplantation : official journal of the American Society of Transplantation and the American Society of Transplant Surgeons, 2005. 5(8): p. 1971-5.

Chapter 18

CD4 T Lymphopenia, Thymic Function, Homeostatic Proliferation and Late Complications Associated with Kidney Transplantation

Philippe Saas, Jamal Bamoulid, Cecile Courivaud,
Jean-Michel Rebibou, Beatrice Gaugler and
Didier Ducloux

Additional information is available at the end of the chapter

http://dx.doi.org/10.5772/55330

1. Introduction

Chronic kidney disease represents a public health problem worldwide. The prevalence of chronic kidney disease lies between 3 to 16% according to different epidemiological studies [1-5]. This high prevalence is observed in both developed and developing countries [1-5]. Chronic kidney disease is responsible for increased risk of cardiovascular diseases and end-stage renal failure. In the United States, for instance, the number of patients exhibiting end-stage renal failure was around 150 000 in 1995, 360 000 in 2003, and is estimated to reach 650 000 in 2015 [6]. This exponential growth of the end-stage renal disease population has relevant implications for health care systems. The treatment option for these patients is dialysis or kidney transplantation. The number of end-stage renal failure patients treated by either dialysis or transplantation was around 209 000 in 1991 and 472 000 in 2004 (data from the US Renal Data System 2006, reported in [3]). The costs of Medicare for end-stage renal failure treatment represents 5% of total budget, while it serves only 0.7% of patients [6]. The same observation is true for Europe with the proportion of the total health care budget dedicated to the end-stage renal disease population varying from 0.7% in the United Kingdom to 1.8% in Belgium in 1994, while this population is only 0.022% to 0.04% of the general population, respectively [6]. In France, the REIN (for *Réseau Epidémiologie et Information en Néphrologie*) program, hosted by the Agence de BioMédecine, is dedicated to assess the number of French patients suffering from end-stage renal failure and how these patients are treated (*i.e.*, dialysis or transplantation). In 2009, 33 558 patients were dialyzed. This represents a frequency of 558 per million of inhabitants. At the same time, 29 181 patients received a kidney transplant (510 per million of inhabitants). During the last five years, the number of kidney transplantations per million of inhabitants in France was around 44. Currently, 8 397 patients with end-stage renal failure are awaiting transplantation among whom 4 043 are new patients. In 2010, only 2 893 kidney transplantations were performed in France (Agence de BioMédecine, REIN Annual Report 2010, [7]). Kidney transplantation has emerged as the best option for patients with end-stage renal failure, providing both a better quality of life and a better survival [8, 9]. Another advantage of renal transplantation over dialysis is its reduced cost. For instance, the 1-year cost per patient on maintenance hemodialysis exceeds US $52 000, whereas it is only a third (US $18 500) for kidney transplantation [6]. Overall, end-stage renal diseases are increasing worldwide. This corresponds to important expenses for health care systems that can be limited by preferentially selected kidney transplantation as therapeutic option. However, the severe lack of kidney transplant is a major obstacle preventing the full development of transplantation. This limits severely the number of end-stage renal disease patients who may benefit from this therapy. Moreover, this enforces the medical/scientific community involved in kidney transplantation to carefully select patients eligible for transplantation and to limit graft loss.

The use of nonspecific immunosuppressive drugs has significantly reduced the incidence of acute kidney graft rejection [10]. This led to a significant improvement in the first-year graft survival rates that are "almost close to perfect", as mentioned in [11]. However, the benefits of such immunosuppressive therapies on chronic rejection and overall long-term graft survival are uncertain [12, 13]. Long term graft survival remains unchanged over decades [13, 14]. Persistent excessive immunosuppression (also called over-immunosuppression) –related to these immunosuppressive drugs– exposes renal transplant recipients to long-term toxicities including: increased incidence of cancers, severe infectious complications and/or inflammatory "metabolic" diseases (for instance, diabetes, and accelerated atherosclerosis leading to cardiovascular diseases). The three major complications, cardiovascular diseases, infections and cancers, are reported to be the most common causes of patient death with functional graft. For instance, a recent study including 1 606 kidney transplant recipients reports that these three complications represent respectively 24%, 16%, and 12% of death with graft function [15]. Preventing these complications is a way to limit the loss of functional kidney graft and to ameliorate patient quality of life.

An enhanced risk of cancer after renal transplantation has been observed in the last decades [16-21], as advances in medicine have extended the life of renal transplant recipients. A meta-analysis including five studies of cancer risks in organ transplant recipients, involving 31 977 organ transplant recipients –among whom 97% have received a kidney graft– from Denmark, Finland, Sweden, Australia, and Canada illustrates perfectly the importance of malignancy occurrence after kidney transplantation. This study shows an increase in the incidence of cancers related to viral infections implicating Epstein-Barr virus (EBV), human herpesvirus 8 (HHV8), hepatitis viruses B and C (HBV and HCV), or related to *Helicobacter pylori* infections in renal transplant recipients when compared to the general population [16]. Nevertheless, increased incidence of cancers after transplantation is not restricted to virus-induced cancers, since other cancers such as kidney cancers, myeloma, leukemia, melanoma as well as bladder and thyroid cancers are more frequent in transplant recipients than in the general population [16]. Common epithelial cancers, such as breast and prostate cancers, occur at the same rate as for the general population [16]. But, despite similar incidence, a more aggressive course have been noticed in renal transplant recipients [22, 23]. Immunosuppression and its extent directly influence cancer occurrence after kidney transplantation [20, 24].

The incidence of cardiovascular diseases related to accelerated atherosclerosis associated with kidney transplantation [8, 25] is at least 3 to 5 times higher than in the general population [8]. Cardiovascular disease is reported to be the most common cause of death with functional graft ranging from 24% to 55% depending on the considered studies [8, 15, 26, 27]. Risk factors for cardiovascular diseases in renal transplant recipients are numerous including traditional and nontraditional factors. The main highly prevalent traditional risk factors of cardiovascular diseases are the following: tobacco use, physical inactivity, hypertension, diabetes, or dyslipidemia. Nontraditional cardiovascular risk factors related to a long history of end-stage renal failure, such as hyper-homocysteinemia, chronic inflammation or anemia, are also prevalent in renal transplant recipients [8, 15, 26, 28, 29]. Moreover, factors related to transplantation itself, including immunosuppression or rejection episodes as well as new-onset diabetes after transplant, impact on cardiovascular disease occurrence after kidney transplantation [8, 15, 26, 29, 30].

Altogether, it appears that over-immunosuppression is involved in both increased cancer occurrence and cardiovascular disease incidence observed after kidney transplantation. A greater understanding of risk factors leading to this excessive immunosuppression may help physicians in charge of end-stage renal failure patients to determine high-risk recipient profiles and optimize pre- and post-transplantation treatment strategies. In other words, identification of biomarkers predictive of immunosuppression-associated complications may improve late kidney transplantation outcome and patient selection. In this chapter, we will report the efforts of our laboratory to identify immunological factors that can predict the two main complications associated with kidney transplantation, namely cancer and accelerated atherosclerosis that leads to cardiovascular diseases. For many years, we had been focusing on $CD4^+$ T cell lymphopenia –a consequence of anti-thymocyte globulin (ATG) administration– and T cell reconstitution after this severe T cell depletion. The analysis was performed on non-invasive blood samples (*i.e.*, serum and PBMC) from a Caucasian population receiving transplantation from deceased donors. Persistent $CD4^+$ T cell lymphopenia is a potent biomarker for over-immunosuppression-associated complications (see below, §2). But, this biomarker is not a predictive one, and thus, recent works in our laboratory have tried to identify predictive biomarkers linked to prolonged $CD4^+$ T cell lymphopenia. Pre-transplant thymic function, assessed by TREC levels, can be such a biomarker (see §4).

2. Persistent CD4⁺ T cell lymphopenia, a biomarker for immunosuppression-associated complications

The first question to address is when $CD4^+$ T cell lymphopenia is encountered in renal transplant recipients. $CD4^+$ T cell lymphopenia in renal transplant recipients results mainly from ATG administration. $CD4^+$ T cell lymphopenia persists for several years in some transplanted patients [31, 32] despite a limited treatment duration (until 4 days). In addition to ATG, Campath-1H, a humanized anti-CD52 monoclonal antibody called Alemtuzumab, can be used as induction immunosuppression causing T cell depletion [33, 34].

Our group previously reported that persistent $CD4^+$ T cell lymphopenia after kidney transplantation is correlated with enhanced risks of cancers, including: skin cancers [35], monoclonal gammapathies [36], lymphomas as well as other non skin cancers, such as colon or lung cancers [37]. This persistent $CD4^+$ T cell depletion is also correlated with the increased incidence of opportunistic infections [38] and of atherosclerotic events [39]. On the opposite, $CD4^+$ T cell lymphopenia seems not to be associated with *de novo* genitourinary malignancies [40]. Recently, we associated prolonged $CD4^+$ T cell lymphopenia and renal transplant recipient mortality [41]. The two identified major causes of death in these patients were cancers and cardiovascular diseases [41]. Same data were observed by others in liver transplant recipients receiving ATG as induction therapy [42]. Overall, $CD4^+$ T cell lymphopenia represents an adequate biomarker for over-immunosuppression leading to immunosupression-associated complications, at least in patients receiving depletion therapy.

However, the limitations of using persistent $CD4^+$ T cell lymphopenia as a biomarker in clinical setting are the following: not all transplanted patients treated with ATG did develop a prolonged $CD4^+$ T cell lymphopenia [39, 41, 42] and this is not a predictive biomarker. Indeed, when a patient exhibits a prolonged $CD4^+$ T cell lymphopenia after ATG, how can physicians deal with it? Physicians can propose a more frequent clinical follow up in order, for instance, to detect earlier cancer occurrence. However, it will be difficult to prevent over-immunosuppression-associated complications. This is why the next step was to identify factors responsible for this prolonged severe $CD4^+$ T cell lymphopenia allowing us to distinguish patients that will develop prolonged $CD4^+$ T cell lymphopenia from patients that will not and to select the adequate immunosuppressive regimen. Indeed, ATG exerts a benefit over nondepleting induction therapy, especially for sensitized (high panel reactive antibodies, PRA) transplant patients. This is true not only for early acute graft rejection occurrence, but also for the preservation of allograft function [43, 44]. However, the ATG benefit is not similar for each patient [45, 46]. Thus, the choice of a complication risk level could vary according to the theoretical benefit of ATG. A high benefit of ATG may lead to accept a higher risk, whereas a slight benefit should lead to prefer a lower risk. Biomarkers, such as prolonged $CD4^+$ T cell lymphopenia, but rather those allowing us to predict this lymphopenia, may help to select ATG as an appropriate induction therapy. We imagine that these biomarkers identified in the setting of ATG can be transposed to other depleting therapies, such as Campath-1H/Alemtuzumab. Indeed, clinical studies are available regarding the prolonged $CD4^+$ T cell lymphopenia induced by Alemtuzumab administration [47], not always in the context of kidney transplantation [48, 49].

The identification of prolonged CD4⁺ T cell lymphopenia was a critical step in our search for biomarkers associated with over-immunosuppression. However, we need to go further and to identify factors present at the time of transplantation responsible for the persistent lymphopenia. This could limit the complications associated with kidney transplantation. We reasoned that factors that affect the duration, intensity or variability of CD4⁺ T cell reconstitution after ATG-induced T cell depletion can be useful biomarkers. Based on the literature, these factors can be the following: the thymic function/activity at time of transplantation and its capacity to regenerate, the capacity to respond to cytokines involved in homeostatic proliferation, and the variable sensitivity of CD4⁺ T cell subsets to ATG-induced lymphopenia. This will be discussed in the next paragraphs of this review, but before that we will quickly summarize the different steps involved in T cell reconstitution after profound depletion.

Based on studies performed in animal models (mainly mouse models), Mackall and colleagues proposed several years ago that T cell reconstitution after profound T cell depletion in Human arises from two main pathways: thymopoiesis (*i.e.*, the capacity of producing new T cells from hematopoietic stem cells) and homeostatic proliferation expansion of residual host lymphocytes that resist to depletion [50]. The latter pathway remains the major pathway early after hematopoietic cell transplantation, until donor-derived prothymocytes migrate to the recipient thymus, where they undergo maturation [51]. These two pathways are involved in T cell recovery after ATG-induced lymphopenia (see below, §3 and §4). Afterwards in this review, we will follow the chronological order of T cell reconstitution and list the factors involved in homeostatic proliferation and thymopoiesis that are critical for delayed or accelerated reconstitution. A third way of T cell reconstitution has been described in Human involving the extrathymic development, for instance in the tonsil [52]. This will not be discussed here. However, this is another interesting track to understand persistent CD4⁺ T cell lymphopenia after ATG in renal transplant recipients in the future.

3. The role of homeostatic proliferation expansion after CD4⁺ T cell depletion in the complications associated with over-immunosuppression

The first pathway of T cell reconstitution occurring after induction therapy-induced lymphopenia is the homeostatic proliferation of residual T cells, a compensatory process, also called lymphopenia-induced proliferation. We highly recommend a recent review on lymphodepletion and homeostatic proliferation [53]. How does this step influence T cell reconstitution after CD4⁺ T cell depletion? First, it depends on the residual T cells that persist after ATG. In consequence, we will start with a paragraph dealing with data reporting sensitivity and resistance to ATG-induced T cell death. Second, the capacity of residual T cells to respond to homeostatic factors present in the microenvironment and competition for such factors may impact on T cell recovery. Here, we will restrict the discussion on CD4⁺ T cells.

The CD4$^+$ T cell pool is constituted by different CD4$^+$ T cell subsets: naive CD4$^+$ T cells expressing CD45RA that have not encountered their antigens called also T helper (Th) 0 cells and memory/activated CD4$^+$ T cells expressing CD45RO$^+$. These cells can be divided into effector memory and central memory according to CD62L/CCR7 or CD62L/CD44 expression. Depending on the cytokine microenvironment in which naive CD4$^+$ T cells are primed, different Th subsets have been described: Th1, Th2, and Th17 (for a general scheme of Th cell differentiation, please refer to [54]). Moreover, this CD4$^+$ T cell pool contains regulatory T cells (Treg) that play a key role in the control and maintenance of tolerance [55, 56]. FoxP3$^+$ natural Treg (nTreg) are produced in the thymus while induced Treg (iTreg) are generated in the periphery from naive CD45RA$^+$ CD4$^+$ T cells in the presence of immunosuppressive cytokines: IL-10 for FoxP3^{neg} T regulatory 1 (Tr1) cells [57] or TGF-β for FoxP3$^+$ Th3 iTreg [58]. This CD4$^+$ T cell pool may vary after T cell depletion and reconstitution may affect this pool. Modifications of the CD4$^+$ T cell pool may have consequences on late complications associated with renal transplantation (see below, §3.3).

3.1. CD4$^+$ T cell subsets and sensitivity to anti-thymocyte globulin administration

Anti-thymocyte globulins are a complex mixture of antibodies with multiple specificities directed against different molecules expressed by T cells, but also non T cells [59, 60]. A thorough study in non human primates reported that ATG treatment induced a dose-dependent T cell depletion in the peripheral blood, as well as in the spleen and in the lymph nodes. Massive T cell apoptosis in secondary lymphoid organs was identified as the main mechanism implicated in T cell lymphopenia [61]. This supports that lymphocyte depletion is the major mechanism by which ATG preparation exerts its immunosuppressive effect. However, when considering T cell reconstitution, one has to evoke other mechanisms: *i*) the relative resistance of some T cell subsets to ATG that has the advantage to expand in the lymphopenic environment; *ii*) depletion-independent mechanisms [62]; *iii)* the elimination of non T cells that may participate to homeostatic proliferation.

It has been reported that CD4$^+$ T cells are more sensitive to ATG-induced depletion than CD8$^+$ T cells [62] and that the different CD4$^+$ T cell subsets are not equally sensitive to ATG-induced depletion [63, 64]. For instance, in a mouse model, Treg were spared by anti-lymphocyte serum (ALS) –an equivalent of ATG in mice– treatment [63]. This occurs by a mechanism dependent on OX40 signaling pathway present in Treg with a memory phenotype [65]. However, another study in mice reported that all CD4$^+$ T cell subsets are equally sensitive to mouse ATG, but that naive T cells expand very quickly after homeostatic proliferation with the acquisition of a memory phenotype [66]. This may explain why initial studies reported that memory phenotype T cells are more resistant than naive T cells to ATG-induced death. The same is maybe true for CD8$^+$ T cells that expand faster than CD4$^+$ T cells (as discussed in [67]). The hypothesis of a different susceptibility to ATG-induced death or an imbalance in CD4$^+$ T cell subset reconstitution is tantalizing to explain the relationship between CD4$^+$ T cell lymphopenia and accelerated atherosclerosis after kidney transplantation, since some Th subsets are pro-atherogenic while other are anti-atherogenic (see §3.3). Whether ATG or immune recovery following ATG-induced lymphopenia may differently affect CD4$^+$ Th subsets remains to be determined in renal transplant recipients. A study in renal transplant recipients suggested that Th2 subsets were less sensitive than Th1 subsets to ATG treatment [68]. However, other Th subsets –such as Th17, or the putative Th9 [69, 70] or Th22 [71, 72] subsets– have not been explored yet.

What are the arguments in favor of depletion-independent mechanisms that may influence $CD4^+$ T cell reconstitution after ATG-induced lymphopenia? The major mechanism is the induction of iTreg or the conversion of naive $CD4^+$ T cells into iTreg. In *in vitro* experiments, ATG has been reported to induce the conversion of iTreg from naive $CD25^-$ $CD4^+$ T cells [73]. The source of ATG (from rabbit or horse) may impact Treg conversion with only rabbit-derived ATG allowing Treg conversion [74]. An increase of Treg after rabbit ATG treatment has been reported *in vivo* in renal transplant recipients [75]. The same data were reported with mouse ATG in mice [64, 76]. ATG is constituted by a mixture of antibodies with multiple specificities (see below) and CD3-specific antibody has been shown to efficiently deplete T cells, and then in a second step, to favor conversion of residual naive $CD4^+$ T cells in iTreg *via* TGF-β [77, 78]. Whether CD3-specific antibodies present in ATG preparations are responsible for ATG-induced iTreg remains to be determined. In-depth analysis of Treg phenotype after ATG treatment using CD45RA, CD45RO, CD27 and CD31 markers suggests that Treg come from both thymus and peripheral expansion in adult renal transplant recipients, while they are mainly derived from thymus in pediatric patients [75]. Furthermore, ATG may also alter T cell migration [79] and naive T cells have to home to secondary lymphoid organs in order to maintain a stable population size [53]. A subset of stromal cells present in the secondary lymphoid organs, called fibroblastic reticular cells supports T cell survival *via* CCL19 [80]. Moreover, secondary lymphoid organs are an important source of IL-7 [80, 81], which participates to naive $CD4^+$ T cell expansion after lymphopenia (see below, §3.2). Thus, altered T cell homing in the secondary lymphoid organs after ATG may participate to delayed immune reconstitution. Transient CD3-specific antibody treatment resulting in T cell lymphopenia has been also shown to affect T cell homing by stimulating the accumulation of Th17 cells with regulatory functions in the small intestine [78]. This sustains the main role of "so-called" depletion-independent mechanisms after depleting antibody therapy in T cell homeostasis. We used the term "so-called", since these depletion independent-mechanisms may in fact correspond to bystander mechanisms related to depletion rather than really depletion-independent mechanisms.

3.2. $CD4^+$ T cell subsets and homeostatic proliferation after anti-thymocyte globulin administration

Lymphopenia-induced proliferation has been extensively studied in mice (for review [81]) and has been cleverly transposed to human setting [53]. T cell dynamics –including T cell replenishment by homeostatic proliferation or after thymopoiesis– are usually extrapolated from mice to humans and *vice versa*. These extrapolations are due to some common observations performed in both species. However, some major differences may exist, such as naive T cell lifespan: 7 to 11 weeks for mouse naive T cells *versus* 6 to 9 years for human naive T cells [82]. This will be also discussed later in this review when thymopoiesis will be evoked (see below, §4.1). In murine models, homeostatic proliferation after T cell depletion uses different kinetics (fast and slow), requires homeostatic cytokines (e.g., IL-7) and sometimes cognate antigen-driven interactions (*i.e.*, peptide/major histocompatibility complex [MHC] presentation by antigen-presenting cells) [81]. The requirements of homeostatic cytokines and contact with host MHC molecules vary depending on whether residual naive or memory T cells are considered.

Homeostatic proliferation is the first pathway to be triggered when peripheral T cells decline acutely. It can follow a fast (~ one cell division per 6-8 hours) or a slow (~one division per 24-36 hours) kinetics [53]. The fast kinetics is an antigen-specific process, and thus, only a smaller subset of T cells (*i.e.*, antigen-specific T cells) is concerned. These antigens may be rather foreign antigens including, for instance, latent viruses such as EBV or commensal bacteria, such as gut flora that favors homeostatic expansion of residual T cells in the gut [83]. Recent fascinating reports have described how commensal bacteria are involved in the regulation of the immune system in the gastro-intestinal tract [84, 85]. Interestingly, limited clinical manifestations involving the gastro-intestinal tract have been reported in renal transplant recipients. The slow homeostatic proliferation occurs in response to T cell depletion, can be self-antigen driven and implicates IL-7 [53]. Interleukin-7 is produced at a relatively constant level and a decrease in circulating T cell counts reduces IL-7 consumption, hence leading to enhanced levels of IL-7. This cytokine become then available for residual T cell expansion. High serum levels of IL-7 were found in transplanted patients with severe lymphopenia after treatment-induced depletion [86]. However, IL-7 levels decrease rapidly with lymphocyte recovery [86]. It was recently proposed that levels of IL-7 receptor (CD127) expression on reconstituting T cells rather than the absolute number of T cells may be responsible for the IL-7 availability [87]. Down-regulation of CD127 by increased levels of IL-7 causes termination of homeostatic proliferation [88]. Thus, IL-7 can be considered as a true regulator of the naive T cell pool size, driving homeostatic proliferation of $CD31^+$ $CD4^+$ recent thymic emigrants (RTE, see below, §4) with sustained CD31 expression [89]. Memory $CD4^+$ T cells –the dominant T cell subset following antibody-mediated T cell depletion [90]– express high levels of CD127 [81], and then compete with RTE for IL-7. Moreover, memory $CD4^+$ T cells expand more quickly during lymphopenia [53, 90]. While Treg are characterized by a low CD127 expression [91, 92], Treg may express high levels of CD127 upon activation [93] and may respond to IL-7 driven homeostatic proliferation [94]. To finish with the role of IL-7 in homeostatic proliferation, one has to mention that this cytokine is particularly available in secondary lymphoid organs attached to extracellular matrix after being synthesized by fibroblastic reticular cells [53, 80, 81]. This highlights the role of an adequate T cell homing to achieve an efficient T cell reconstitution. In addition, the strength of T cell receptor (TCR) affinity for peptide/MHC regulates homeostatic proliferation mediated by IL-7: the stronger is the TCR affinity, the less IL-7 concentration is necessary [95, 96]. Dependency on other cytokines (e.g., IL-15 or IL-21) for homeostatic proliferation expansion is less marked for $CD4^+$ T cells than for $CD8^+$ T cells. Thus, IL-7 levels after lymphopenia are a critical factor to be considered after depletion therapy, and competition of the different T cell subsets that resist to this therapy may occur. All these subsets do not expand with the same kinetics (see next paragraph). Cox *et al* [48] have studied the IL-7 pathway (circulating IL-7 levels and CD127 expression on T cells) in lymphopenic

http://dx.doi.org/10.5772/55330

multiple sclerosis patients receiving Campath-1H/Alemtuzumab treatment. No significant defect was observed [48]. Data are needed to confirm this observation in the context of kidney transplantation. This is particularly interesting since recombinant human IL-7 has been used in clinical trials [97] (see below, §4.3).

The kinetics of reconstitution after lymphopenia are dependent on the considered T cell subsets, with memory T cells expanding more rapidly than naive T cells and naive $CD8^+$ T cells undergoing faster proliferation rates than naive $CD4^+$ T cells [53, 62]. Furthermore, Th1 cell expansion is favored by homeostatic proliferation [98]. This sustains that the subsets of T cells that resist to depleting therapy play a major role in reconstitution. Antigen persistence such as latent viruses may favor T cell exhaustion [67], and the loss of T cell specificity participating to immunodeficiency. The picture is more complicated for Treg [53]. Initial works reported that in lymphopenic environment, Treg expand quickly and massively by homeostatic proliferation [98], as a mechanism to prevent unwanted autoimmune responses. "Spontaneous" conversion of naive $CD4^+$ T cells into iTreg in the lymphopenic environment [99] may also participate to this increase of Treg. Moreover, the sites (gut *versus* secondary lymphoid organs) may influence the speed (fast or slow) of recovery [53] and the T cell subset implicated in homeostatic proliferation [78]. A recent editorial suggests harnessing this homeostatic proliferation to favor transplantation tolerance [67].

3.3. Clinical implications of altered homeostatic proliferation in the setting of $CD4^+$ T cell lymphopenia

How can altered homeostatic proliferation after severe $CD4^+$ T cell depletion participate in increased cancer occurrence or accelerated atherosclerosis? Several features with clinical consequences for lymphopenic patients are associated with the preferential homeostatic proliferation of limited T cells: *i)* a limited TCR repertoire diversity leading to reduced immune responses against oncogenic virus or maybe tumor antigens explaining the increased incidence of cancers, *ii)* a shift from naive to memory/activated phenotype in the proliferating cells, *iii)* a competition for limiting levels of homeostatic cytokines (increasing TCR repertoire skewing, hence decreasing the capacity of the host to respond to antigen challenge), *iv)* a more delayed T cell recovery [100], a possibility to lose transplantation tolerance [101], to favor autoimmunity by expanding autoreactive memory T cells [102], or T cell exhaustion [67]. Presence of latent infectious antigens, such as cytomegalovirus CMV, may participate in T cell exhaustion and subsequent cancer occurrence [103]. Thus, homeostatic proliferation favors over-immunosuppression and the overall immunodeficiency leading to enhanced cancer incidence.

Homeostatic proliferation may also be implicated in accelerated atherosclerosis. Indeed, experiments performed in atherosclerosis prone apolipoprotein-E deficient or low density lipoprotein receptor deficient mice have distinguished pro-atherogenic from anti-atherogenic $CD4^+$ T cell subsets (for reviews, [104, 105]). One may hypothesize that ATG-induced $CD4^+$ T cell lymphopenia may favor a preferential expansion of pro-atherogenic Th1 cells in detriment of anti-atherogenic Treg (*i.e.*, nTreg and iTreg subsets). This remains to be determined in the future. Nevertheless, patients with end-stage renal disease awaiting kidney transplantation exhibit an inflammatory state including high circulating levels of C reactive protein (CRP)

[106, 107]. Thus, immune reconstitution after depletion therapy occurs in the context of inflammation and may favor Th1 subsets. In lymphopenic setting, Th1 have been reported to expand massively [98]. One can speculate that pro-inflammatory and pro-atherogenic Th subsets are favored over anti-atherogenic T cells in renal transplantation recipients receiving ATG treatment leading to increased incidence of cardiovascular diseases.

4. The role of thymic activity after $CD4^+$ T cell depletion in the complications associated with over-immunosuppression

The thymus participates more lately than homeostatic proliferation to immune reconstitution after profound T cell depletion. The role of the thymic function on immune reconstitution after profound T cell depletion has been studied in different clinical settings such as human immunodeficiency virus (HIV) infection or hematopoietic cell transplantation (for recent review [108]).

Different tools are available to discriminate recent thymic emigrants (RTE, reflecting thymic activity/output) from other lymphopenia-induced expanded T cells (*i.e.*, naive or memory/activated). Douek and colleagues reported that circulating T cell excision circle (TREC) levels are a direct reflect of thymic function [109]. These TREC correspond to the episomal DNA circles generated during the rearrangement of the VDJ genes of the TCR α- and β-chains. TREC are stably retained during cell division, but do not replicate, thus becoming diluted among the daughter cells. It is possible to distinguish sjTREC and βTREC generated during recombination of the TCR α-chain and β-chain, respectively. The proliferative ability of thymic progenitors within the thymus can be assessed by sjTREC/ βTREC ratio due to the sequential recombination of TCR β-chain, and then, of TCR α-chain after several divisions (for further explanations, please refer to a complete review on TREC [108]). Expression of surface markers –including CD45RA, CD31 or protein tyrosine kinase 7 (PTK7)– on circulating $CD4^+$ T cells has been shown to identify RTE and to attest to an efficient thymopoiesis [110, 111]. $CD31^+$ $CD4^+$ T cells contain higher sjTREC levels than their $CD31^{neg}$ counterpart [89]. However, maintenance of CD31 expression on $CD4^+$ T cells during IL-7-driven homeostatic proliferation can be observed [89]. This renders CD31 expression analysis as a less pertinent marker to interpret thymic activity.

A last concern is that the thymus involutes with age and injury, but keeps its capacity for renewal. This is well illustrated in clinical settings associated with T cell recovery [112] where the thymus expands and may become greater than the normal size with intense cellular density, as attested by computerized tomography [100]. Radiographic measurement of thymus by computer tomographs correlates with circulating TREC levels [113]. However, thymus renewal capacity declines with age (for a review [100]). In consequence, circulating TREC levels are inversely correlated with age [114]. Over the age of 45-50, thymic activity/output is reduced and naive T cell recovery may take until 5 years after severe iatrogenic lymphopenia [100]. Overall, tools are available to study the part of thymic output in T cell reconstitution after ATG-induced lymphopenia.

4.1. Altered thymic activity, a predictive biomarker of persistent CD4$^+$ T cell lymphopenia after anti-thymocyte globulins

Few data are available to date concerning the human thymic function and CD4$^+$ T cell recovery after kidney transplantation. Several years ago, Monaco *et al* reported that thymectomy prior to ATG prolongs T cell lymphopenia in mice [115], attesting for the role of thymus in T cell reconstitution after ATG. Stable frequencies of RTE –assessed by CD31, CD45RA CD4 phenotype– have been reported in renal transplant recipients 6 months after transplantation [116]. These authors concluded that uremia due to past history of end-stage renal failure has no impact on thymic activity [116]. Only 7 patients among the 48 analyzed have received depleting induction therapy [116]. This renders difficult to interpret the role of thymic activity in the context of lymphopenia. In contrast, Scarsi et al [47] reported a massive reduction of RTE one year post-transplantation after Campath-1H/Alemtuzumab administration. Prolonged selective CD4$^+$ T cell lymphopenia suggests that naive CD4$^+$ T cells –including RTE– are highly sensitive to ATG [31, 75] and that time is necessary for RTE "replenishment" after T cell depletion. Analysis of thymic function in a cohort of rheumatoid arthritis patients receiving Alemtuzumab 12 years before shows that circulating TREC levels are independent on patient age but correlate with CD4$^+$ T cell counts (*i.e.*, patients with lower TREC are still lymphopenic) and patients with normal CD4$^+$ T cell counts exhibit the same TREC levels than age-matched controls [49]. Thus, TREC and CD31 expression analysis can be used to monitor thymic function in the setting of kidney transplantation.

We recently identified the thymic activity (as assessed by circulating TREC levels) at the time of kidney transplantation as a major factor predicting CD4$^+$ T cell immune reconstitution after ATG administration [41, 117]. In a first patient cohort, we found a TREC value lower than 2 000 per 150 000 CD3$^+$ cells at the time of transplantation to be the best threshold for prediction of persistent post-ATG CD4$^+$ T cell lymphopenia [41]. Renal transplant recipients with lower TREC levels at the time of transplantation exhibited a higher morbidity and mortality risk due to cancers as well as cardiovascular diseases. Determination of circulating TREC levels at the time of transplantation may help to identify patients at high risk of persistent ATG-induced CD4$^+$ T cell lymphopenia and post-transplant cancer occurrence [41]. Moreover, in a second cohort of patients, the levels of TREC at the time of transplantation is predictive of cancer occurrence in renal transplantation recipients and correlate with naive CD45RA$^+$ CD4$^+$ T cell recovery 1-5 years after transplantation [117]. Thus, TREC analysis at the time of transplantation can be a useful predictive biomarker for over-immunosuppression-associated complications. This new biomarker could be a valuable tool to select induction treatment (ATG *versus* non depleting anti-CD25 antibodies). Renal transplant recipients with lower TREC levels at the time of transplantation should not be eligible for ATG treatment. This needs to be validated in prospective trials.

The maintenance of naive T cell pool appears critical to avoid complications associated with over-immunosuppression after kidney transplantation. A recent interesting study challenges some "dogma" on the role of thymic output in the maintenance of human naive T cell pool [118]. While thymic output is stable even with age in mice, in humans peripheral T cell proliferation may be the major mechanism contributing to the maintenance of naive T cell pool. Indeed, when the authors normalized the TREC content of peripheral $CD4^+$ T cells by the TREC content of single positive $CD4^+$ thymocytes (obtained from 45 children who underwent cardiac surgery), they observed that, in individuals older than 20, only around 10% of circulating naive T cells come from thymus while the majority are formed from peripheral naive T cell proliferation. The same data were obtained using *in vivo* kinetic labeling using deuterated water and mathematical modeling. This confirms that T cell dynamics differ in mice and humans (see above, §3.2) and challenges the data obtained with TREC analysis. However, a potential limitation of this work is that analyses have been performed in healthy volunteers (in steady state) [118] and not in lymphopenic patients. As mentioned before, the human thymus keeps the capacity for renewal [100], especially in case of profound T cell depletion. Nevertheless, this works reinforces the idea that thymic function in lymphopenic renal transplant recipients should be further explored using, for instance, more sophisticated approaches such as *in vivo* labeling using deuterated water.

4.2. Clinical implications of altered thymic function in the setting of $CD4^+$ T cell lymphopenia

How can altered thymic output after severe $CD4^+$ T cell depletion participate in increased cancer occurrence or accelerated atherosclerosis? A major role of thymus during T cell recovery is the reconstitution of a most diverse polyclonal T cell repertoire. Thus, renal transplant recipients with an impaired thymic function exhibiting a skewed T cell repertoire and are less equipped to respond to pathogens (including oncogenic viruses) or even to control tumors than patients presenting an efficient T cell reconstitution with a fully diverse TCR repertoire (for a review [100]). This may explained the increased occurrence of cancers in renal transplant recipients.

In patients with altered thymic function, homeostatic proliferation becomes the main contributor to T cell recovery, and thus, duration of lymphopenia is extended with uncontrolled pro-atherogenic $CD4^+$ T cell subset expansion leading to accelerated atherosclerosis (see above). Moreover, impaired thymic function and uncontrolled homeostatic proliferation may lead to immune exhaustion that aggravates immunodeficiency. In addition, impaired thymic output by limiting naive T cell production impacts highly on homeostatic proliferation. This explains why pre-transplant thymic function is a good and sensitive biomarker.

4.3. Perspectives: Toward a restoration of thymic function?

We recently identified impaired thymic function as a biomarker for increased occurrence of cancers and accelerated atherosclerosis related to persistent $CD4^+$ T cell lymphopenia [41, 117]. It remains interesting to localize the defect more accurately in order to propose a therapeutic restoration of this function. One hypothesis is that the defect is localized before the thymus for instance, in $CD34^+$ lymphoid precursors, as proposed for HIV [119]. This is a

http://dx.doi.org/10.5772/55330

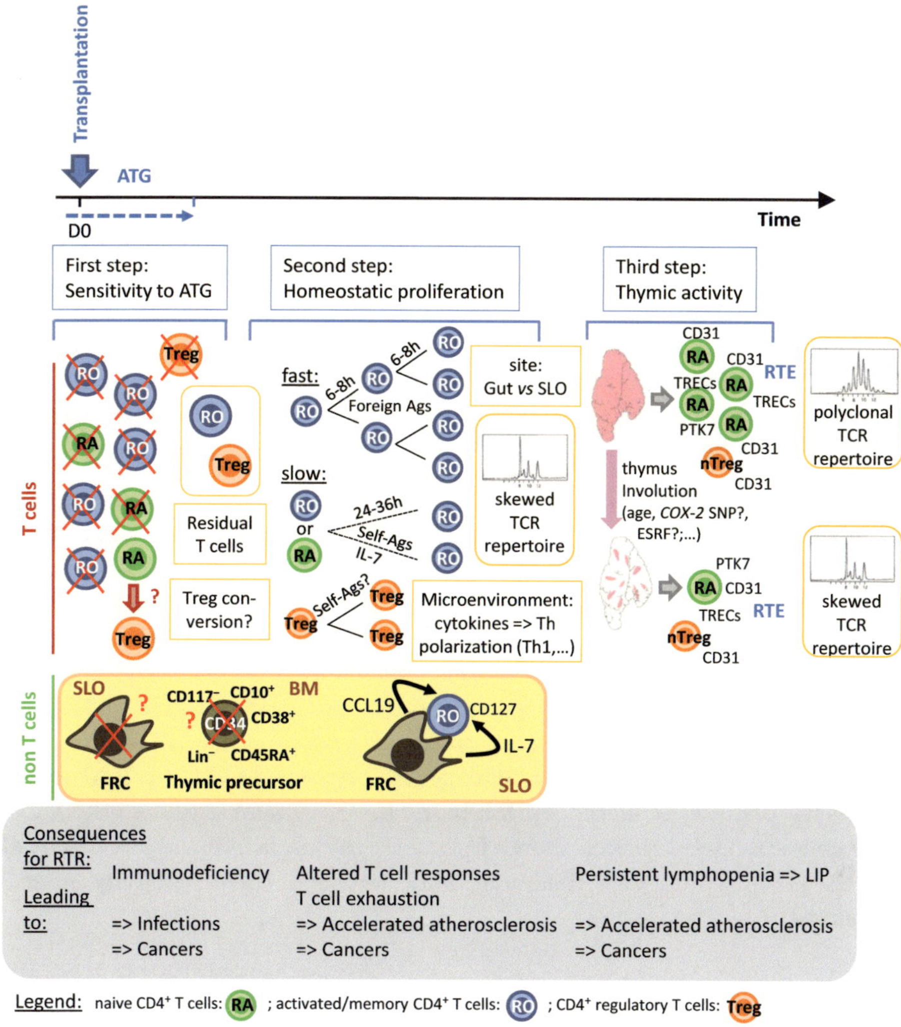

Figure 1. $CD4^+$ T cell recovery after anti-thymoglobulin (ATG)-induced depletion in renal transplant recipient (RTR) is dependent on three steps/stages: *i)* sensitivity to ATG; *ii)* cytokine and/or antigen-dependent homeostatic proliferation, a process called also lymphopenia-induced proliferation (LIP); *iii)* thymic activity. This figure identifies for each step critical parameters that may influence $CD4^+$ T cell recovery. Sensitivity to ATG depends on the considered $CD4^+$ T cell subsets. ATG may affect non T cells (lymphoid precursors or fibroblastic reticular cells [FRC] that in turn impact on T cell reconstitution). Non depletion mechanisms are illustrated by conversion of naive $CD4^+$ T cells into Treg. T cell recovery after depletion implicates first LIP. Kinetics of T cell proliferation depends on: the type of antigen (self antigens [Self-Ags] may induce a slow kinetic, whereas foreign antigens [Foreign Ags], including: EBV, CMV or commensal bacteria] may rather induce a fast kinetic – the average division time is given). The microenvironment and the site may also play a role. Cytokines such as IL-7 may participate in LIP, but also in helper T cell (Th) polarization. Finally, complete $CD4^+$ T cell recovery involves the thymus with production of new CD4+ T cells (called recent thymic emigrants [RTE]) allowing the reconstitution of a polyclonal TCR repertoire. Thymic function can be impacted by patient age, end stage renal failure (ESRF) duration, or maybe also by *COX-2* gene promoter single nucleotide polymorphisms (SNP). A dysfunction in each step may lead to complications in RTR (summarized in the gray box). *Other abbreviations used*: BM, bone marrow; D0, day 0 (*i.e.*, the day of transplantation); h, hour; SLO, secondary lymphoid organs; Th, T helper cells. The question mark represents a potential mechanism. For more details, please refer to the text.

possibility since ATG contains a mixture of antibodies with multiple specificities [59, 60], and thus, ATG may affect circulating thymic precursors. With this assumption in mind, we hypothesize that the capacity to regenerate hematopoiesis may impact thymic function. The *cyclo-oxygenase-2* (*COX-2*) gene promoter polymorphism at position -765 is responsible for the control of prostaglandin-E2 (PGE-2) synthesis and PGE-2 has been reported to be involved in lymphocyte reconstitution following depletion [120-122]. Indeed, COX-2 is expressed by thymic stroma [121], participates not only in thymocyte development [122], but also in accelerated hematopoiesis following myelotoxic injury [120]. We found that the *COX-2* gene promoter polymorphism at position -765 is associated with a higher risk of ATG-induced persistent CD4 T-cell lymphopenia. Pre-transplant TREC levels were higher in GG patients than in C carriers who have lower serum PGE-2 levels [123]. The possibility of selecting patients with low or high risk of immune reconstitution impairment through the *COX-2* gene promoter polymorphism could offer the opportunity to use ATG more safely. This suggests that ATG may affect T cell reconstitution before thymus.

Significant advances have been performed in the comprehension of endogenous thymus regeneration and several factors have been shown to increase thymic activity (for a recent review [108], see also Ref.[124] for IL-22). This is particularly interesting since recombinant human IL-7 has been used in clinical trials [97]. Administration of IL-7 results in an expansion of both naive and memory $CD4^+$ T cells and $CD8^+$ T cells with a tendency toward enhanced $CD8^+$ T cell expansion [97]. Lymphopenic or normal older hosts receiving IL-7 develop an expanded circulating T cell pool with increased T cell repertoire diversity [100]. Moreover, IL-7 administration exhibits a favorable toxicity profile [97], opening the perspective of potential future use in renal transplant recipients with severe prolonged $CD4^+$ T cell lymphopenia in case that this IL7 pathway is altered. Furthermore, IL-7 treatment of human thymus –*in vitro* or in a xenogeneic model– has been shown to increase thymic activity, as attested by elevated TREC levels [125]. Thus, IL-7 treatment may improve thymic activity after kidney transplantation.

5. Conclusion

We summarize in a Figure the different factors and critical steps involved in $CD4^+$ T cell reconstitution after depletion by ATG (Figure 1). Overall, the aim of this review was to report our experience on the identification of biomarkers ($CD4^+$ T cell lymphopenia after ATG and TREC levels at the time of transplantation) predicting transplantation-related complications (mainly atherosclerosis and cancer occurrence), and to propose to use these biomarkers in patient follow up and/or in immunosuppressive strategy design. Furthermore, we propose other "tracks" to improve the clinical relevance of these biomarkers, as well as to understand their implications in the occurrence of immunosuppression-associated complications. The efficacy of these identified biomarkers should be tested and validated in prospective clinical trials in order to select the appropriate immunosuppressive strategy. In the future, one could imagine that these biomarkers may help physicians to manage risks of cancers and cardiovascular diseases in renal transplant recipients.

http://dx.doi.org/10.5772/55330

Acknowledgements

We thank the Région de Franche-Comté for the LipSTIC grant (to P.S.)

Acknowledgements

We would like to thank Sarah Odrion for excellent editorial assistance and the Centre d'Investigation Clinique intégré en Biothérapies du CHU de Besançon (CBT-506) for its support. Our work in the fields was supported by grants from the Agence Nationale de la Recherche (Labex LipSTIC, ANR-11-LABX-0021 and ECellFrance consortium, ANR-11-INBS-0005), the Programme Hospitalier de Recherche Clinique 2011 (to D.D), the Fondation de France (Appel d'offre "Maladies cardiovasculaires" 2007, #2007 001859, to P.S.), the DHOS/INSERM/INCa (Appel d'offre Recherche Translationnelle 2008, to D.D. and P.S.), and the APICHU 2010 (SIGAL project to J.B.).

Author details

Philippe Saas[1,2,3,4], Jamal Bamoulid[1,2,5], Cecile Courivaud[1,2,5], Jean-Michel Rebibou[1,6,7], Beatrice Gaugler[1,2,3] and Didier Ducloux[1,2,4,5]

1 INSERM, UMR1098, France

2 Université de Franche-Comté, UMR1098, France

3 Etablissement Français du Sang Bourgogne Franche-Comté, Plateforme de BioMonitoring, France

4 CHU de Besançon, CIC-BT506, France

5 CHU de Besançon, Service de Néphrologie, Transplantation Rénale et Dialyse, France

6 Université de Bourgogne, UMR1098, Dijon, France

7 CHU de Dijon, Service de Néphrologie, Dijon, France

References

[1] Chadban SJ, Briganti EM, Kerr PG, Dunstan DW, Welborn TA, Zimmet PZ, Atkins RC. Prevalence of Kidney Damage in Australian Adults: The Ausdiab Kidney Study. J Am Soc Nephrol 2003;14(7 Suppl 2):S131-8.

[2] Cirillo M, Laurenzi M, Mancini M, Zanchetti A, Lombardi C, De Santo NG. Low Glomerular Filtration in the Population: Prevalence, Associated Disorders, and Awareness. Kidney Int 2006;70(4):800-6.

[3] Coresh J, Selvin E, Stevens LA, Manzi J, Kusek JW, Eggers P, Van Lente F, Levey AS. Prevalence of Chronic Kidney Disease in the United States. JAMA 2007;298(17): 2038-47.

[4] Sumaili EK, Krzesinski JM, Zinga CV, Cohen EP, Delanaye P, Munyanga SM, Nseka NM. Prevalence of Chronic Kidney Disease in Kinshasa: Results of a Pilot Study from the Democratic Republic of Congo. Nephrol Dial Transplant 2009;24(1):117-22.

[5] Zhang L, Zhang P, Wang F, Zuo L, Zhou Y, Shi Y, Li G, Jiao S, Liu Z, Liang W, Wang H. Prevalence and Factors Associated with Ckd: A Population Study from Beijing. Am J Kidney Dis 2008;51(3):373-84.

[6] Schieppati A, Remuzzi G. Chronic Renal Diseases as a Public Health Problem: Epidemiology, Social, and Economic Implications. Kidney Int Suppl 2005(98):S7-S10.

[7] Agence de BioMédecine. ABM: Rein Annual Report 2010. http://www.agence-biomedecine.fr/img/pdf/2012_Rapport_Rein_2010_v2.pdf (accessed 17 August 2012).

[8] Sarnak MJ, Levey AS, Schoolwerth AC, Coresh J, Culleton B, Hamm LL, McCullough PA, Kasiske BL, Kelepouris E, Klag MJ, Parfrey P, Pfeffer M, Raij L, Spinosa DJ, Wilson PW. Kidney Disease as a Risk Factor for Development of Cardiovascular Disease: A Statement from the American Heart Association Councils on Kidney in Cardiovascular Disease, High Blood Pressure Research, Clinical Cardiology, and Epidemiology and Prevention. Circulation 2003;108(17):2154-69.

[9] Schnuelle P, Lorenz D, Trede M, Van Der Woude FJ. Impact of Renal Cadaveric Transplantation on Survival in End-Stage Renal Failure: Evidence for Reduced Mortality Risk Compared with Hemodialysis During Long-Term Follow-Up. J Am Soc Nephrol 1998;9(11):2135-41.

[10] Sayegh MH, Carpenter CB. Transplantation 50 Years Later--Progress, Challenges, and Promises. N Engl J Med 2004;351(26):2761-6.

[11] Lamb KE, Lodhi S, Meier-Kriesche HU. Long-Term Renal Allograft Survival in the United States: A Critical Reappraisal. Am J Transplant 2011;11(3):450-62.

[12] McDonald S, Russ G, Campbell S, Chadban S. Kidney Transplant Rejection in Australia and New Zealand: Relationships between Rejection and Graft Outcome. Am J Transplant 2007;7(5):1201-8.

[13] Meier-Kriesche HU, Schold JD, Srinivas TR, Kaplan B. Lack of Improvement in Renal Allograft Survival Despite a Marked Decrease in Acute Rejection Rates over the Most Recent Era. Am J Transplant 2004;4(3):378-83.

http://dx.doi.org/10.5772/55330

[14] Meier-Kriesche HU, Schold JD, Kaplan B. Long-Term Renal Allograft Survival: Have We Made Significant Progress or Is It Time to Rethink Our Analytic and Therapeutic Strategies? Am J Transplant 2004;4(8):1289-95.

[15] Kahwaji J, Bunnapradist S, Hsu JW, Idroos ML, Dudek R. Cause of Death with Graft Function among Renal Transplant Recipients in an Integrated Healthcare System. Transplantation 2011;91(2):225-30.

[16] Grulich AE, van Leeuwen MT, Falster MO, Vajdic CM. Incidence of Cancers in People with HIV/AIDS Compared with Immunosuppressed Transplant Recipients: A Meta-Analysis. Lancet 2007;370(9581):59-67.

[17] Kasiske BL, Snyder JJ, Gilbertson DT, Wang C. Cancer after Kidney Transplantation in the United States. Am J Transplant 2004;4(6):905-13.

[18] Penn I. Tumors in Allograft Recipients. N Engl J Med 1979;301(7):385.

[19] Villeneuve PJ, Schaubel DE, Fenton SS, Shepherd FA, Jiang Y, Mao Y. Cancer Incidence among Canadian Kidney Transplant Recipients. Am J Transplant 2007;7(4): 941-8.

[20] van Leeuwen MT, Grulich AE, Webster AC, McCredie MR, Stewart JH, McDonald SP, Amin J, Kaldor JM, Chapman JR, Vajdic CM. Immunosuppression and Other Risk Factors for Early and Late Non-Hodgkin Lymphoma after Kidney Transplantation. Blood 2009;114(3):630-7.

[21] Webster AC, Craig JC, Simpson JM, Jones MP, Chapman JR. Identifying High Risk Groups and Quantifying Absolute Risk of Cancer after Kidney Transplantation: A Cohort Study of 15,183 Recipients. Am J Transplant 2007;7(9):2140-51.

[22] Fiebiger W, Kaserer K, Rodler S, Oberbauer R, Bauer C, Raderer M. Neuroendocrine Carcinomas Arising in Solid-Organ Transplant Recipients: Rare but Aggressive Malignancies. Oncology 2009;77(5):314-7.

[23] Barrett WL, First MR, Aron BS, Penn I. Clinical Course of Malignancies in Renal Transplant Recipients. Cancer 1993;72(7):2186-9.

[24] Dantal J, Hourmant M, Cantarovich D, Giral M, Blancho G, Dreno B, Soulillou JP. Effect of Long-Term Immunosuppression in Kidney-Graft Recipients on Cancer Incidence: Randomised Comparison of Two Cyclosporin Regimens. Lancet 1998;351(9103):623-8.

[25] Ojo AO. Cardiovascular Complications after Renal Transplantation and Their Prevention. Transplantation 2006;82(5):603-11.

[26] Kasiske BL, Guijarro C, Massy ZA, Wiederkehr MR, Ma JZ. Cardiovascular Disease after Renal Transplantation. J Am Soc Nephrol 1996;7(1):158-65.

[27] Ojo AO, Hanson JA, Wolfe RA, Leichtman AB, Agodoa LY, Port FK. Long-Term Survival in Renal Transplant Recipients with Graft Function. Kidney Int 2000;57(1): 307-13.

[28] Ducloux D, Motte G, Challier B, Gibey R, Chalopin JM. Serum Total Homocysteine and Cardiovascular Disease Occurrence in Chronic, Stable Renal Transplant Recipients: A Prospective Study. J Am Soc Nephrol 2000;11(1):134-7.

[29] Liefeldt L, Budde K. Risk Factors for Cardiovascular Disease in Renal Transplant Recipients and Strategies to Minimize Risk. Transpl Int 2010;23(12):1191-204.

[30] Ducloux D, Kazory A, Chalopin JM. Posttransplant Diabetes Mellitus and Atherosclerotic Events in Renal Transplant Recipients: A Prospective Study. Transplantation 2005;79(4):438-43.

[31] Louis S, Audrain M, Cantarovich D, Schaffrath B, Hofmann K, Janssen U, Ballet C, Brouard S, Soulillou JP. Long-Term Cell Monitoring of Kidney Recipients after an Antilymphocyte Globulin Induction with and without Steroids. Transplantation 2007;83(6):712-21.

[32] Muller TF, Grebe SO, Neumann MC, Heymanns J, Radsak K, Sprenger H, Lange H. Persistent Long-Term Changes in Lymphocyte Subsets Induced by Polyclonal Antibodies. Transplantation 1997;64(10):1432-7.

[33] Ciancio G, Burke GW, 3rd. Alemtuzumab (Campath-1h) in Kidney Transplantation. Am J Transplant 2008;8(1):15-20.

[34] Kaufman DB, Leventhal JR, Axelrod D, Gallon LG, Parker MA, Stuart FP. Alemtuzumab Induction and Prednisone-Free Maintenance Immunotherapy in Kidney Transplantation: Comparison with Basiliximab Induction--Long-Term Results. Am J Transplant 2005;5(10):2539-48.

[35] Ducloux D, Carron PL, Rebibou JM, Aubin F, Fournier V, Bresson-Vautrin C, Blanc D, Humbert P, Chalopin JM. CD4 Lymphocytopenia as a Risk Factor for Skin Cancers in Renal Transplant Recipients. Transplantation 1998;65(9):1270-2.

[36] Ducloux D, Carron P, Racadot E, Rebibou JM, Bresson-Vautrin C, Hillier YS, Chalopin JM. T-Cell Immune Defect and B-Cell Activation in Renal Transplant Recipients with Monoclonal Gammopathies. Transpl Int 1999;12(4):250-3.

[37] Ducloux D, Carron PL, Motte G, Ab A, Rebibou JM, Bresson-Vautrin C, Tiberghien P, Saint-Hillier Y, Chalopin JM. Lymphocyte Subsets and Assessment of Cancer Risk in Renal Transplant Recipients. Transpl Int 2002;15(8):393-6.

[38] Ducloux D, Carron PL, Racadot E, Rebibou JM, Bresson-Vautrin C, Saint-Hillier Y, Chalopin JM. CD4 Lymphocytopenia in Long-Term Renal Transplant Recipients. Transplant Proc 1998;30(6):2859-60.

[39] Ducloux D, Challier B, Saas P, Tiberghien P, Chalopin JM. CD4 Cell Lymphopenia and Atherosclerosis in Renal Transplant Recipients. J Am Soc Nephrol 2003;14(3): 767-72.

[40] Guichard G, Rebibou JM, Ducloux D, Simula-Faivre D, Tiberghien P, Chalopin JM, Bittard H, Saas P, Kleinclauss F. Lymphocyte Subsets in Renal Transplant Recipients with De Novo Genitourinary Malignancies. Urol Int 2008;80(3):257-63.

[41] Ducloux D, Courivaud C, Bamoulid J, Vivet B, Chabroux A, Deschamps M, Rebibou JM, Ferrand C, Chalopin JM, Tiberghien P, Saas P. Prolonged CD4 T Cell Lymphopenia Increases Morbidity and Mortality after Renal Transplantation. J Am Soc Nephrol 2010;21(5):868-75.

[42] Vrochides D, Hassanain M, Metrakos P, Tchervenkov J, Barkun J, Chaudhury P, Cantarovich M, Paraskevas S. Prolonged Lymphopenia Following Anti-Thymocyte Globulin Induction Is Associated with Decreased Long-Term Graft Survival in Liver Transplant Recipients. . Hippokratia 2012;16(1):66-70.

[43] Cai J, Terasaki PI. Induction Immunosuppression Improves Long-Term Graft and Patient Outcome in Organ Transplantation: An Analysis of United Network for Organ Sharing Registry Data. Transplantation 2010;90(12):1511-5.

[44] Willoughby LM, Schnitzler MA, Brennan DC, Pinsky BW, Dzebisashvili N, Buchanan PM, Neri L, Rocca-Rey LA, Abbott KC, Lentine KL. Early Outcomes of Thymoglobulin and Basiliximab Induction in Kidney Transplantation: Application of Statistical Approaches to Reduce Bias in Observational Comparisons. Transplantation 2009;87(10):1520-9.

[45] Brennan DC, Daller JA, Lake KD, Cibrik D, Del Castillo D. Rabbit Antithymocyte Globulin Versus Basiliximab in Renal Transplantation. N Engl J Med 2006;355(19): 1967-77.

[46] Noel C, Abramowicz D, Durand D, Mourad G, Lang P, Kessler M, Charpentier B, Touchard G, Berthoux F, Merville P, Ouali N, Squifflet JP, Bayle F, Wissing KM, Hazzan M. Daclizumab Versus Antithymocyte Globulin in High-Immunological-Risk Renal Transplant Recipients. J Am Soc Nephrol 2009;20(6):1385-92.

[47] Scarsi M, Bossini N, Malacarne F, Valerio F, Sandrini S, Airo P. The Number of Circulating Recent Thymic Emigrants Is Severely Reduced 1 Year after a Single Dose of Alemtuzumab in Renal Transplant Recipients. Transpl Int 2010;23(8):786-95.

[48] Cox AL, Thompson SA, Jones JL, Robertson VH, Hale G, Waldmann H, Compston DA, Coles AJ. Lymphocyte Homeostasis Following Therapeutic Lymphocyte Depletion in Multiple Sclerosis. Eur J Immunol 2005;35(11):3332-42.

[49] Anderson AE, Lorenzi AR, Pratt A, Wooldridge T, Diboll J, Hilkens CM, Isaacs JD. Immunity 12 Years after Alemtuzumab in RA: CD5+ B-Cell Depletion, Thymus-De-

pendent T-Cell Reconstitution and Normal Vaccine Responses. Rheumatology (Oxford) 2012;51(8):1397-406.

[50] Mackall CL, Hakim FT, Gress RE. T-Cell Regeneration: All Repertoires Are Not Created Equal. Immunol Today 1997;18(5):245-51.

[51] Moss P, Rickinson A. Cellular Immunotherapy for Viral Infection after HSC Transplantation. Nat Rev Immunol 2005;5(1):9-20.

[52] McClory S, Hughes T, Freud AG, Briercheck EL, Martin C, Trimboli AJ, Yu J, Zhang X, Leone G, Nuovo G, Caligiuri MA. Evidence for a Stepwise Program of Extrathymic T Cell Development within the Human Tonsil. J Clin Invest 2012;122(4):1403-15.

[53] Tchao NK, Turka LA. Lymphodepletion and Homeostatic Proliferation: Implications for Transplantation. Am J Transplant 2012;12(5):1079-90.

[54] Dong C. Th17 Cells in Development: An Updated View of Their Molecular Identity and Genetic Programming. Nat Rev Immunol 2008;8(5):337-48.

[55] Sakaguchi S, Miyara M, Costantino CM, Hafler DA. Foxp3+ Regulatory T Cells in the Human Immune System. Nat Rev Immunol 2010;10(7):490-500.

[56] Vignali DA, Collison LW, Workman CJ. How Regulatory T Cells Work. Nat Rev Immunol 2008;8(7):523-32.

[57] Groux H, O'Garra A, Bigler M, Rouleau M, Antonenko S, de Vries JE, Roncarolo MG. A CD4+ T-Cell Subset Inhibits Antigen-Specific T-Cell Responses and Prevents Colitis. Nature 1997;389(6652):737-42.

[58] Chen W, Jin W, Hardegen N, Lei KJ, Li L, Marinos N, McGrady G, Wahl SM. Conversion of Peripheral CD4+CD25- Naive T Cells to CD4+CD25+ Regulatory T Cells by TGF-Beta Induction of Transcription Factor Foxp3. J Exp Med 2003;198(12):1875-86.

[59] Bonnefoy-Berard N, Vincent C, Revillard JP. Antibodies against Functional Leukocyte Surface Molecules in Polyclonal Antilymphocyte and Antithymocyte Globulins. Transplantation 1991;51(3):669-73.

[60] Rebellato LM, Gross U, Verbanac KM, Thomas JM. A Comprehensive Definition of the Major Antibody Specificities in Polyclonal Rabbit Antithymocyte Globulin. Transplantation 1994;57(5):685-94.

[61] Preville X, Flacher M, LeMauff B, Beauchard S, Davelu P, Tiollier J, Revillard JP. Mechanisms Involved in Antithymocyte Globulin Immunosuppressive Activity in a Nonhuman Primate Model. Transplantation 2001;71(3):460-8.

[62] Cherkassky L, Lanning M, Lalli PN, Czerr J, Siegel H, Danziger-Isakov L, Srinivas T, Valujskikh A, Shoskes DA, Baldwin W, Fairchild RL, Poggio ED. Evaluation of Alloreactivity in Kidney Transplant Recipients Treated with Antithymocyte Globulin Versus Il-2 Receptor Blocker. Am J Transplant 2011;11(7):1388-96.

[63] Minamimura K, Gao W, Maki T. Cd4+ Regulatory T Cells Are Spared from Deletion by Antilymphocyte Serum, a Polyclonal Anti-T Cell Antibody. J Immunol 2006;176(7):4125-32.

[64] D'Addio F, Yuan X, Habicht A, Williams J, Ruzek M, Iacomini J, Turka LA, Sayegh MH, Najafian N, Ansari MJ. A Novel Clinically Relevant Approach to Tip the Balance toward Regulation in Stringent Transplant Model. Transplantation 2010;90(3): 260-9.

[65] Kroemer A, Xiao X, Vu MD, Gao W, Minamimura K, Chen M, Maki T, Li XC. Ox40 Controls Functionally Different T Cell Subsets and Their Resistance to Depletion Therapy. J Immunol 2007;179(8):5584-91.

[66] Sener A, Tang AL, Farber DL. Memory T-Cell Predominance Following T-Cell Depletional Therapy Derives from Homeostatic Expansion of Naive T Cells. Am J Transplant 2009;9(11):2615-23.

[67] Stock P, Kirk AD. The Risk and Opportunity of Homeostatic Repopulation. Am J Transplant 2011;11(7):1349-50.

[68] Weimer R, Staak A, Susal C, Streller S, Yildiz S, Pelzl S, Renner F, Dietrich H, Daniel V, Rainer L, Kamali-Ernst S, Ernst W, Padberg W, Opelz G. Atg Induction Therapy: Long-Term Effects on Th1 but Not on Th2 Responses. Transpl Int 2005;18(2):226-36.

[69] Dardalhon V, Awasthi A, Kwon H, Galileos G, Gao W, Sobel RA, Mitsdoerffer M, Strom TB, Elyaman W, Ho IC, Khoury S, Oukka M, Kuchroo VK. IL-4 Inhibits Tgf-Beta-Induced Foxp3+ T Cells and, Together with TGF-Beta, Generates IL-9+ IL-10+ Foxp3(-) Effector T Cells. Nat Immunol 2008;9(12):1347-55.

[70] Veldhoen M, Uyttenhove C, van Snick J, Helmby H, Westendorf A, Buer J, Martin B, Wilhelm C, Stockinger B. Transforming Growth Factor-Beta 'Reprograms' the Differentiation of T Helper 2 Cells and Promotes an Interleukin 9-Producing Subset. Nat Immunol 2008;9(12):1341-6.

[71] Duhen T, Geiger R, Jarrossay D, Lanzavecchia A, Sallusto F. Production of Interleukin 22 but Not Interleukin 17 by a Subset of Human Skin-Homing Memory T Cells. Nat Immunol 2009;10(8):857-63.

[72] Trifari S, Kaplan CD, Tran EH, Crellin NK, Spits H. Identification of a Human Helper T Cell Population That Has Abundant Production of Interleukin 22 and Is Distinct from T(H)-17, T(H)1 and T(H)2 Cells. Nat Immunol 2009;10(8):864-71.

[73] Lopez M, Clarkson MR, Albin M, Sayegh MH, Najafian N. A Novel Mechanism of Action for Anti-Thymocyte Globulin: Induction of CD4+CD25+Foxp3+ Regulatory T Cells. J Am Soc Nephrol 2006;17(10):2844-53.

[74] Feng X, Kajigaya S, Solomou EE, Keyvanfar K, Xu X, Raghavachari N, Munson PJ, Herndon TM, Chen J, Young NS. Rabbit ATG but Not Horse Atg Promotes Expan-

sion of Functional CD4+CD25highFoxp3+ Regulatory T Cells in Vitro. Blood 2008;111(7):3675-83.

[75] Gurkan S, Luan Y, Dhillon N, Allam SR, Montague T, Bromberg JS, Ames S, Lerner S, Ebcioglu Z, Nair V, Dinavahi R, Sehgal V, Heeger P, Schroppel B, Murphy B. Immune Reconstitution Following Rabbit Antithymocyte Globulin. Am J Transplant 2010;10(9):2132-41.

[76] Lu Y, Suzuki J, Guillioli M, Umland O, Chen Z. Induction of Self-Antigen-Specific Foxp3+ Regulatory T Cells in the Periphery by Lymphodepletion Treatment with Anti-Mouse Thymocyte Globulin in Mice. Immunology 2011;134(1):50-9.

[77] Perruche S, Zhang P, Liu Y, Saas P, Bluestone JA, Chen W. CD3-Specific Antibody-Induced Immune Tolerance Involves Transforming Growth Factor-Beta from Phagocytes Digesting Apoptotic T Cells. Nat Med 2008;14(5):528-35.

[78] Esplugues E, Huber S, Gagliani N, Hauser AE, Town T, Wan YY, O'Connor W, Jr., Rongvaux A, Van Rooijen N, Haberman AM, Iwakura Y, Kuchroo VK, Kolls JK, Bluestone JA, Herold KC, Flavell RA. Control of Th17 Cells Occurs in the Small Intestine. Nature 2011;475(7357):514-8.

[79] LaCorcia G, Swistak M, Lawendowski C, Duan S, Weeden T, Nahill S, Williams JM, Dzuris JL. Polyclonal Rabbit Antithymocyte Globulin Exhibits Consistent Immunosuppressive Capabilities Beyond Cell Depletion. Transplantation 2009;87(7):966-74.

[80] Link A, Vogt TK, Favre S, Britschgi MR, Acha-Orbea H, Hinz B, Cyster JG, Luther SA. Fibroblastic Reticular Cells in Lymph Nodes Regulate the Homeostasis of Naive T Cells. Nat Immunol 2007;8(11):1255-65.

[81] Boyman O, Letourneau S, Krieg C, Sprent J. Homeostatic Proliferation and Survival of Naive and Memory T Cells. Eur J Immunol 2009;39(8):2088-94.

[82] Zhang SL, Bhandoola A. Losing Trec with Age. Immunity 2012;36(2):163-5.

[83] Kieper WC, Troy A, Burghardt JT, Ramsey C, Lee JY, Jiang HQ, Dummer W, Shen H, Cebra JJ, Surh CD. Recent Immune Status Determines the Source of Antigens That Drive Homeostatic T Cell Expansion. J Immunol 2005;174(6):3158-63.

[84] Lathrop SK, Bloom SM, Rao SM, Nutsch K, Lio CW, Santacruz N, Peterson DA, Stappenbeck TS, Hsieh CS. Peripheral Education of the Immune System by Colonic Commensal Microbiota. Nature 2011;478(7368):250-4.

[85] Round JL, Lee SM, Li J, Tran G, Jabri B, Chatila TA, Mazmanian SK. The Toll-Like Receptor 2 Pathway Establishes Colonization by a Commensal of the Human Microbiota. Science 2011;332(6032):974-7.

[86] Bolotin E, Annett G, Parkman R, Weinberg K. Serum Levels of Il-7 in Bone Marrow Transplant Recipients: Relationship to Clinical Characteristics and Lymphocyte Count. Bone Marrow Transplant 1999;23(8):783-8.

[87] Hodge JN, Srinivasula S, Hu Z, Read SW, Porter BO, Kim I, Mican JM, Paik C, Degrange P, Di Mascio M, Sereti I. Decreases in Il-7 Levels During Antiretroviral Treatment of Hiv Infection Suggest a Primary Mechanism of Receptor-Mediated Clearance. Blood 2011;118(12):3244-53.

[88] Park JH, Yu Q, Erman B, Appelbaum JS, Montoya-Durango D, Grimes HL, Singer A. Suppression of IL7ralpha Transcription by IL-7 and Other Prosurvival Cytokines: A Novel Mechanism for Maximizing IL-7-Dependent T Cell Survival. Immunity 2004;21(2):289-302.

[89] Azevedo RI, Soares MV, Barata JT, Tendeiro R, Serra-Caetano A, Victorino RM, Sousa AE. IL-7 Sustains CD31 Expression in Human Naive CD4+ T Cells and Preferentially Expands the CD31+ Subset in a PI3K-Dependent Manner. Blood 2009;113(13): 2999-3007.

[90] Pearl JP, Parris J, Hale DA, Hoffmann SC, Bernstein WB, McCoy KL, Swanson SJ, Mannon RB, Roederer M, Kirk AD. Immunocompetent T-Cells with a Memory-Like Phenotype Are the Dominant Cell Type Following Antibody-Mediated T-Cell Depletion. Am J Transplant 2005;5(3):465-74.

[91] Liu W, Putnam AL, Xu-Yu Z, Szot GL, Lee MR, Zhu S, Gottlieb PA, Kapranov P, Gingeras TR, Fazekas de St Groth B, Clayberger C, Soper DM, Ziegler SF, Bluestone JA. CD127 Expression Inversely Correlates with Foxp3 and Suppressive Function of Human CD4+ T Reg Cells. J Exp Med 2006;203(7):1701-11.

[92] Seddiki N, Santner-Nanan B, Martinson J, Zaunders J, Sasson S, Landay A, Solomon M, Selby W, Alexander SI, Nanan R, Kelleher A, Fazekas de St Groth B. Expression of Interleukin (IL)-2 and IL-7 Receptors Discriminates between Human Regulatory and Activated T Cells. J Exp Med 2006;203(7):1693-700.

[93] Simonetta F, Chiali A, Cordier C, Urrutia A, Girault I, Bloquet S, Tanchot C, Bourgeois C. Increased CD127 Expression on Activated Foxp3+CD4+ Regulatory T Cells. Eur J Immunol 2010;40(9):2528-38.

[94] Simonetta F, Gestermann N, Martinet KZ, Boniotto M, Tissieres P, Seddon B, Bourgeois C. Interleukin-7 Influences Foxp3+CD4+ Regulatory T Cells Peripheral Homeostasis. PLoS One 2012;7(5):e36596.

[95] Kassiotis G, Zamoyska R, Stockinger B. Involvement of Avidity for Major Histocompatibility Complex in Homeostasis of Naive and Memory T Cells. J Exp Med 2003;197(8):1007-16.

[96] Kieper WC, Burghardt JT, Surh CD. A Role for TCR Affinity in Regulating Naive T Cell Homeostasis. J Immunol 2004;172(1):40-4.

[97] Sportes C, Babb RR, Krumlauf MC, Hakim FT, Steinberg SM, Chow CK, Brown MR, Fleisher TA, Noel P, Maric I, Stetler-Stevenson M, Engel J, Buffet R, Morre M, Amato RJ, Pecora A, Mackall CL, Gress RE. Phase I Study of Recombinant Human Interleu-

kin-7 Administration in Subjects with Refractory Malignancy. Clin Cancer Res 2010;16(2):727-35.

[98] Moxham VF, Karegli J, Phillips RE, Brown KL, Tapmeier TT, Hangartner R, Sacks SH, Wong W. Homeostatic Proliferation of Lymphocytes Results in Augmented Memory-Like Function and Accelerated Allograft Rejection. J Immunol 2008;180(6): 3910-8.

[99] Liang S, Alard P, Zhao Y, Parnell S, Clark SL, Kosiewicz MM. Conversion of CD4+ CD25- Cells into CD4+ CD25+ Regulatory T Cells in Vivo Requires B7 Costimulation, but Not the Thymus. J Exp Med 2005;201(1):127-37.

[100] Williams KM, Hakim FT, Gress RE. T Cell Immune Reconstitution Following Lymphodepletion. Semin Immunol 2007;19(5):318-30.

[101] Wu Z, Bensinger SJ, Zhang J, Chen C, Yuan X, Huang X, Markmann JF, Kassaee A, Rosengard BR, Hancock WW, Sayegh MH, Turka LA. Homeostatic Proliferation Is a Barrier to Transplantation Tolerance. Nat Med 2004;10(1):87-92.

[102] Monti P, Scirpoli M, Maffi P, Ghidoli N, De Taddeo F, Bertuzzi F, Piemonti L, Falcone M, Secchi A, Bonifacio E. Islet Transplantation in Patients with Autoimmune Diabetes Induces Homeostatic Cytokines That Expand Autoreactive Memory T Cells. J Clin Invest 2008;118(5):1806-14.

[103] Courivaud C, Bamoulid J, Gaugler B, Roubiou C, Arregui C, Chalopin JM, Borg C, Tiberghien P, Woronoff-Lemsi MC, Saas P, Ducloux D. Cytomegalovirus Exposure, Immune Exhaustion and Cancer Occurrence in Renal Transplant Recipients. Transpl Int 2012;25(9):948-55.

[104] Hansson GK, Hermansson A. The Immune System in Atherosclerosis. Nat Immunol 2011;12(3):204-12.

[105] Taleb S, Tedgui A, Mallat Z. Adaptive T Cell Immune Responses and Atherogenesis. Curr Opin Pharmacol 2010;10(2):197-202.

[106] Ducloux D, Bresson-Vautrin C, Kribs M, Abdelfatah A, Chalopin JM. C-Reactive Protein and Cardiovascular Disease in Peritoneal Dialysis Patients. Kidney Int 2002;62(4):1417-22.

[107] Ducloux D, Kazory A, Chalopin JM. Predicting Coronary Heart Disease in Renal Transplant Recipients: A Prospective Study. Kidney Int 2004;66(1):441-7.

[108] Toubert A, Glauzy S, Douay C, Clave E. Thymus and Immune Reconstitution after Allogeneic Hematopoietic Stem Cell Transplantation in Humans: Never Say Never Again. Tissue Antigens 2012;79(2):83-9.

[109] Douek DC, McFarland RD, Keiser PH, Gage EA, Massey JM, Haynes BF, Polis MA, Haase AT, Feinberg MB, Sullivan JL, Jamieson BD, Zack JA, Picker LJ, Koup RA.

Changes in Thymic Function with Age and During the Treatment of Hiv Infection. Nature 1998;396(6712):690-5.

[110] Haines CJ, Giffon TD, Lu LS, Lu X, Tessier-Lavigne M, Ross DT, Lewis DB. Human CD4+ T Cell Recent Thymic Emigrants Are Identified by Protein Tyrosine Kinase 7 and Have Reduced Immune Function. J Exp Med 2009;206(2):275-85.

[111] Kohler S, Thiel A. Life after the Thymus: CD31+ and CD31- Human Naive Cd4+ T-Cell Subsets. Blood 2009;113(4):769-74.

[112] Dion ML, Poulin JF, Bordi R, Sylvestre M, Corsini R, Kettaf N, Dalloul A, Boulassel MR, Debre P, Routy JP, Grossman Z, Sekaly RP, Cheynier R. Hiv Infection Rapidly Induces and Maintains a Substantial Suppression of Thymocyte Proliferation. Immunity 2004;21(6):757-68.

[113] Harris JM, Hazenberg MD, Poulin JF, Higuera-Alhino D, Schmidt D, Gotway M, McCune JM. Multiparameter Evaluation of Human Thymic Function: Interpretations and Caveats. Clin Immunol 2005;115(2):138-46.

[114] Gruver AL, Hudson LL, Sempowski GD. Immunosenescence of Ageing. J Pathol 2007;211(2):144-56.

[115] Monaco AP, Wood ML, Russell PS. Effect of Adult Thymectomy on the Recovery from Immunological Depression Induced by Anti-Lymphocyte Serum. Surg Forum 1965;16:209-11.

[116] Nickel P, Kreutzer S, Bold G, Friebe A, Schmolke K, Meisel C, Jurgensen JS, Thiel A, Wernecke KD, Reinke P, Volk HD. CD31+ Naive Th Cells Are Stable During Six Months Following Kidney Transplantation: Implications for Post-Transplant Thymic Function. Am J Transplant 2005;5(7):1764-71.

[117] Ducloux D, Bamoulid J, Courivaud C, Gaugler B, Rebibou JM, Ferrand C, Chalopin JM, Borg C, Tiberghien P, Saas P. Thymic Function, Anti-Thymocytes Globulins, and Cancer after Renal Transplantation. Transpl Immunol 2011;25(1):56-60.

[118] den Braber I, Mugwagwa T, Vrisekoop N, Westera L, Mogling R, de Boer AB, Willems N, Schrijver EH, Spierenburg G, Gaiser K, Mul E, Otto SA, Ruiter AF, Ackermans MT, Miedema F, Borghans JA, de Boer RJ, Tesselaar K. Maintenance of Peripheral Naive T Cells Is Sustained by Thymus Output in Mice but Not Humans. Immunity 2012;36(2):288-97.

[119] Sauce D, Larsen M, Fastenackels S, Pauchard M, Ait-Mohand H, Schneider L, Guihot A, Boufassa F, Zaunders J, Iguertsira M, Bailey M, Gorochov G, Duvivier C, Carcelain G, Kelleher AD, Simon A, Meyer L, Costagliola D, Deeks SG, Lambotte O, Autran B, Hunt PW, Katlama C, Appay V. HIV Disease Progression Despite Suppression of Viral Replication Is Associated with Exhaustion of Lymphopoiesis. Blood 2011;117(19):5142-51.

[120] Lorenz M, Slaughter HS, Wescott DM, Carter SI, Schnyder B, Dinchuk JE, Car BD. Cyclooxygenase-2 Is Essential for Normal Recovery from 5-Fluorouracil-Induced Myelotoxicity in Mice. Exp Hematol 1999;27(10):1494-502.

[121] Rocca B, Spain LM, Ciabattoni G, Patrono C, FitzGerald GA. Differential Expression and Regulation of Cyclooxygenase Isozymes in Thymic Stromal Cells. J Immunol 1999;162(8):4589-97.

[122] Rocca B, Spain LM, Pure E, Langenbach R, Patrono C, FitzGerald GA. Distinct Roles of Prostaglandin H Synthases 1 and 2 in T-Cell Development. J Clin Invest 1999;103(10):1469-77.

[123] Courivaud C, Bamoulid J, Ferrand C, Tiberghien P, Chalopin JM, Saas P, Ducloux D. The Cox-2 Gene Promoter Polymorphism -765 Delays CD4 T-Cell Reconstitution after Lymphocyte Depletion with Antithymocyte Globulins. Hum Immunol 2011;72(11):1060-3.

[124] Dudakov JA, Hanash AM, Jenq RR, Young LF, Ghosh A, Singer NV, West ML, Smith OM, Holland AM, Tsai JJ, Boyd RL, van den Brink MR. Interleukin-22 Drives Endogenous Thymic Regeneration in Mice. Science 2012;336(6077):91-5.

[125] Okamoto Y, Douek DC, McFarland RD, Koup RA. Effects of Exogenous Interleukin-7 on Human Thymus Function. Blood 2002;99(8):2851-8.

Chapter 19

Current and Future Directions in Antibody-Mediated Rejection Post Kidney Transplantation

Rashad Hassan and Ahmed Akl

Additional information is available at the end of the chapter

http://dx.doi.org/10.5772/55001

1. Introduction

Late graft loss remains a major obstacle to successful long-term kidney allograft transplantation. The factors contributing to late graft loss include immunological (cellular and/or antibody mediated injuries) and non-immunological (donor disease, recurrent disease, peri-transplant ischemia, viral infection or drug toxicity) factors (Smith et al., 2006).

For decades, T cells were considered as the primary contributors to acute as well as chronic rejection after organ transplantation.

The role of antibody in rejection of transplanted organs was the subject of debate in the early days of transplantation. Peter Gorer was the first to describe the role of antibody and Peter Medwar championing cell-mediated immunity. Following the death of Gorer's in 1961, the concept of antibody-mediated rejection faded into the background. However, by 1997 demonstration of the relative sensitivity and specificity of C4d staining in peritubular capillaries in identifying antibody mediated rejection raised the hope that a rigorous morphological classification could be devised.

Allo-antibodies to HLA class I or II and other antigens expressed by endothelium cause a variety of effects on renal transplants, ranging from acute to chronic rejection, and even apparent graft acceptance (accommodation). Recognition of these conditions and appropriate therapy requires demonstration of C4d in biopsies, commonly confirmed by tests for circulating allo-antibody (Lefaucheur et al., 2010).

Pre-existing (Amico et al., 2009) or post transplant (Cantarovich et al., 2011; Lefaucheur et al., 2010) development of donor specific antibodies (DSA) lead to Acute AMR occurred in 8% of kidney transplant patients. The 5-year graft survivals of patients who had an episode of AMR were significantly worse than that of the remaining transplant population. The relative risk

(RR) for graft loss for patients who had an episode of AMR was around 4 times as compared with patients without AMR. Importantly, even in patients without any episode of AMR, the presence of anti-HLA-DSA on the peak serum was still associated with a significantly lower graft survival as compared with patients without anti-HLA-DSA (Amico et al., 2009; Cantarovich et al., 2011; Lefaucheur et al., 2010).

The recently described entity of subclinical AMR (Gloor et al., 2006; Haas et al., 2007) in which progressive morphologic lesions are found on biopsy in the absence of overt clinical rejection may account for this different course. A recent study demonstrated that subclinical AMR is a frequent finding in patients with preformed HLA-DSA (31.1% at 3 months) and is associated with worse GFR at 1 year (Loupy et al., 2009). These progressive lesions lead to chronic humoral rejection, first described in 2001 (Regele et al., 2002) and now recognized to be a distinct cause of late graft dysfunction and loss (Gloor et al., 2007; Regele et al., 2002).

Antibody-mediated rejection has become clinically critical because this form of rejection is usually unresponsive to conventional anti-rejection therapy, and therefore, it has been recognized as a major cause of allograft loss. Although desensitization protocols have enabled transplantation across donor-specific antibody barriers in a growing number of cases (Haas et al., 2007; Jordan, 2006), these protocols are neither consistently efficacious nor standardized. It reflects an incomplete understanding of the pathogenesis of alloantibody-induced injury as a major cause of allograft loss. Furthermore, patients treated with these modalities persist in having a high risk of multiple AMR episodes and lower graft long term survival compared to antibody free patients.

2. Natural course

In 1968, when kidney transplant patients were first examined for the development of antibodies after graft failure, antibodies were detected in 11 (38%) of 29 patients who had rejected their grafts (Morris et al., 1969).

The fact that some patients in desensitization protocols developed AMR and others with similar levels of DSA at baseline did not, has remained unexplained due to the lack of detailed studies of these patients post transplant. Burns et al. (Burns et al., 2008) aimed to define the natural history of AMR in highly sensitized patients undergoing positive cross-match kidney transplantation. They found that the serum DSA level after transplantation was the major determinant of AMR. Patients who developed high levels of DSA within the first month after transplantation almost invariably developed acute humoral rejection (AHR), whereas those who maintained low levels were rejection-free. Importantly, more than half of the patients who had high levels of DSA at baseline did not develop high levels of DSA after transplantation. Almost all patients, including those who developed AMR, had a significant decrement or even disappearance of DSA early after transplantation (Gloor et al., 2004; Zachary et al., 2005). This finding that increases in DSA levels in AMR may be transient and self-limited in many patients presents difficulties in assessing the effectiveness of therapy aimed at treating AMR.

During the 12th International Histocompatibility workshop, a multicenter prospective study was initiated to test patients with functioning kidney transplants once for HLA antibodies post-transplantation. The 806 patients without HLA antibodies, had a subsequent 4 year graft survival of 81%, compared with 58% for 158 patients with HLA antibodies [the presence of anti-HLA antibodies led to 5% allograft loss every year; therefore, after 4 years, 20% of the grafts will be lost](Terasaki et al., 2007).

Among 512 patients followed for 1 year post-testing in Sao Paulo, 12% of antibody positive patients lost their grafts, whereas graft failure occurred in only 5.5% of those without HLA antibodies (P=0.03) (Campos et al., 2006). These results have been updated, demonstrating that at 3 years post-transplantation, patients without HLA antibodies had a 94% survival rate compared with 79% for those with HLA class II antibodies (Gerbase-DeLima et al., 2007).

In a large multicentre trial, HLA-specific antibodies were detected in 21% of patients with renal allografts and 14–23% of patients with heart, liver or lung allografts (Terasaki & Ozawa, 2004). Of 2,278 renal-allograft recipients who were followed prospectively, graft failure at 1 year occurred more frequently in patients who developed alloantibodies than in those who did not (8.6% versus 3.0%). Several studies have reported that de novo antibodies that are specific for graft HLA class I and class II molecules are a risk factor for premature graft loss as a consequence of renal and cardiac chronic arteriopathy (Michaels et al., 2003; Pelletier et al., 2002; Piazza et al., 2001).

For example, during a 5-year follow-up period, donor-reactive antibodies were present in 51% of patients with graft failure compared with 2% of stable control individuals. The presence of antibodies preceded graft failure in 60% of cases (Worthington et al., 2003). Worthington et al (Worthington et al., 2001) showed that among 12 patients who developed ELISA-detected HLA antibodies post-transplantation, 92% of the grafts failed, whereas among the 64 patients who remained negative, only 11% of the grafts failed (P<0.001).

So, circulating HLA-specific antibodies are typically present months to years before graft dysfunction, indicating that antibody-mediated graft injury might be slow to develop.

3. Pathogenesis and mechanism

The pathogenesis of late renal allograft loss is heterogeneous and difficult to diagnose.

How alloantibody and complement activation promote glomerulopathy, arteriopathy and fibrosis is incompletely clear. Only in the past 7 years, a potential role of alloantibodies for chronically deteriorating graft function has been postulated.

Alloantibodies are now appreciated as important mediators of acute and chronic rejection, differing in pathogenesis, or "nature," from T cell–mediated rejection.

Alloantibodies preferentially attack a different "location," namely the peritubular and glomerular capillaries, in contrast to T cells, which characteristically infiltrate tubules and arterial endothelium.

Antibody-mediated rejection generally has a worse prognosis and requires different approaches to treatment and prevention than the usual T cell–mediated rejection.

Antibody induces rejection acutely through the fixation of complement, resulting in tissue injury and coagulation. In addition, complement activation recruits macrophages and neutrophils, causing additional endothelial injury. Antibody and complement also induce gene expression by endothelial cells, which is thought to remodel arteries and basement membranes, leading to fixed and irreversible anatomical lesions that permanently compromise graft function.

3.1. Antigenic targets

The main antigenic targets of antibody-mediated rejection are MHC molecules (both class I and class II) (Erlich et al., 2001) and the ABO blood-group antigens (Race & Sanger, 1958). MHC class I molecules are found at the surface of all nucleated cells, including endothelial cells. By contrast, the distribution of MHC class II molecules is more limited. These molecules are constitutively expressed at the surface of B cells, dendritic cells (DCs) and microvascular endothelial cells (the last applies to humans but not mice) and are expressed by other cells depending on the stimuli that they have been exposed to and their transcriptional activation. The extreme polymorphism of MHC class I and class II polypeptides (more than 1,600 alleles in humans) aids their main function, which is antigen presentation to T cells.

Production of HLA specific alloantibodies depends on exposure to HLA molecules as a consequence of pregnancy, blood transfusion or transplantation. These antibodies are mainly of the IgG class. Blood-group antigens, most importantly the A and B antigens, are carbohydrate epitopes on glycolipids and glycoproteins that are present at the surface of most tissues, including erythrocytes and endothelial cells. Antibodies that are specific for A or B antigens arise 'naturally' in normal individuals who are not of the A and/or B blood group in response to antigens from the environment, and they are usually of the IgM class (Colvin & Smith, 2005).

Antibodies to class I MHC antigens can stimulate endothelial and smooth muscle proliferation and expression of FGF receptors (Bian & Reed, 2001). Soluble terminal complement components (C5b-9) trigger the production of FGF and PDGF by endothelial cells (Benzaquen et al., 1994). Thus antibodies and activated complement might induce gene products that promote endothelial activation and injury with consequent basement membrane duplication and arterial smooth muscle proliferation and thickening until finally, the characteristic atherosclerosis lesion of chronic rejection results in obstruction (Jin et al., 2002; Reed, 2003).

In addition to MHC molecules and blood-group antigens, minor histocompatibility antigens might also be targets of antibody-mediated rejection. Minor histocompatibility antigens, which were originally defined in mice by their ability to cause prompt skin-graft rejection, are also thought to be relevant as targets of graft-versus-host disease and as tumor antigens (Chao, 2004). In animal studies, non-MHC-specific antibodies can cause endothelial-cell apoptosis and graft rejection (Derhaag et al., 2000; Wu et al., 2002).

However, in humans, the molecular characterization of these antigens is limited.

MICA (MHC-class-I-polypeptide-related sequence A), one of the few potential endothelial-cell surface alloantigens, has been defined at the molecular level (Kooijmans-Coutinho et al., 1996).

MICA is a polymorphic non-classical MHC molecule. Antibody that is specific for MICA (MHC-class-I-polypeptide-related sequence A) can be detected in renal-allograft recipients and is associated with later rejection and graft loss (Mizutani et al., 2005; Sumitran-Holgersson et al., 2002) that was demonstrated by Zou and coworkers (Zou et al., 2007) who found that antibodies against minor histocompatibility antigens such as MICA may be associated with a poorer graft outcome.

Antibodies that recognize self-proteins might also contribute to graft injury. For example, autoantibody that is specific for the angiotensin II type 1 receptor, which is expressed by vascular smooth muscle, has been associated with severe hypertension, graft dysfunction and fibrinoid arterial necrosis of human renal allografts (Dragun et al., 2005).

Several studies have shown that circulating anti-HLA class I or II antibodies, either donor reactive (Worthington et al., 2003; Hourmant et al., 2005) or de novo non–donor reactive (Hourmant et al., 2005; Terasaki & Ozawa, 2005), are found in a substantial fraction of renal allograft recipients, and these are associated with later graft loss. Retrospective studies demonstrated that de novo appearance of DSA was associated with poor graft outcome (Colvin, 2007). One study in more than 2000 patients prospectively established the risk of circulating alloantibodies for graft survival after 1 and 2 years (Terasaki & Ozawa, 2005).

3.2. B- lymphocytes

B cells are not just plasma cell precursors, but represent an important population of antigen-presenting cells particularly efficient in the situation of a sensitized recipient, because they have specific immunoglobulin as an antigen-specific receptor on their surface, which leads to efficient uptake and presentation of donor antigens to T cells (Noorchashm et al., 2006). Indeed, an increased frequency of alloantigen-specific B cells in sensitized recipients has been reported (Zachary et al., 2007). Therefore, targeting these B cells will also interfere with activation of indirectly allo-reactive T cells, which play an important role in chronic allograft rejection.

In sensitized allograft recipients with DSA, sensitization has always occurred on the level of B and T cells; because B cells need T help to produce alloantibodies of IgG isotype as measured by the Luminex technology. Therefore, a combined pathogenesis of rejection must always be postulated, even if not all the pathologic criteria are fulfilled (Fehr et al., 2009).

However, failure to demonstrate DSA does not rule out a contribution of antibodies to the pathologic process, because absorption of antibodies by the allograft may result in a lack of circulating DSA (Martin et al., 2005). Alternatively, DSA against non-HLA antigens or HLA-DP could explain the missing ELISA reactivity in the presence of increased cytotoxic anti-B-cell reactivity and ongoing antibody-mediated rejection (Arnold et al., 2005; Opelz, 2005; Zou et al., 2007).

The combination of alloantibody, basement membrane multilamination, C4d, and duplication of the GBM has been termed the "ABCD tetrad" by Solez and colleagues (Solez et al., 2007).

3.3. Plasma cells

During AMR, it is likely that a portion of the DSA found in the serum is due to ongoing antibody production by pre-existing plasma cells. In addition, the observed increase in DSA during AMR suggests that conversion of allospecific memory B cells to plasma cells also may play a role. Unfortunately, no studies of the activity of memory B cells during AMR exist. Despite this, several groups have developed protocols to treat AMR based on their presumed impact on either B cells or plasma cells (Stegall & Gloor, 2010).

3.4. Presence of antibodies with good function

It is a common observation and "complaint" that some patients with HLA antibodies have excellent kidney graft function. The exact frequency of this occurrence has been documented to be about 20% in studies of 2658 patients with functioning grafts (Terasaki et al., 2007) Thus, at any transplant center roughly 20% of patients would likely have antibodies and good function.

According to prospective studies, when 158 patients with antibodies were followed for as long as 4 years, their graft survival was 58% as compared with 81% for 806 patients without antibodies (Terasaki et al., 2007).

Significantly, the presence of antibodies did not foretell immediate or certain graft failure. Studies by Worthington et al. (Worthington et al., 2007) have shown that the mean time from antibody development to failure for class I antibodies was 2.7 years and 3.9 years for class II antibodies. Additionally, antibodies causing humoral rejection may not appear until as many as may reach up to 13 years (Kamimaki et al., 2007), or even after 26 years (Weinstein et al., 2005) posttransplant. The reason for this long interval between antibody appearance and graft failure is the time needed for the endothelial walls of arteries to hypertrophy and close the lumen, or for the tubules to disappear because of peritubular capillary damage produced by antibodies (Shimizu et al., 2002). In both instances, defense mechanisms could be triggered as the endothelium is damaged and repair mechanisms are triggered (Jin et al., 2005).

4. Accommodation

Transplantation across an ABO barrier, which normally precipitates hyperacute rejection, has been done successfully in many centers, using special protocols to deplete naturally occurring anti–blood group antibodies.

The phenomenon of accommodation, in which the graft acquires resistance to humoral injury and continues to function well despite the continued presence of antibody against a target antigen expressed on graft endothelium, is well documented in ABO-incompatible kidney transplants (Park et al., 2003; Platt, 2002).

Alexandre and colleagues (Alexandre et al., 1987) initially observed accommodation in recipients of an ABO-incompatible renal allograft. Transient depletion of the circulating antibodies that are specific for these blood-group antigens at the time of transplantation allows immediate graft survival without hyperacute rejection.

A rebound of antibody concentrations (primarily IgM) within the first 10 days occurs together with rejection in 90% of cases. However, after 21 days, for the remaining grafts, there is no correlation between the occurrence of rejection and the antibody titre (Park et al., 2003; Shishido et al., 2001). Even if the antibody titre returns to pre-transplantation levels or higher, the grafts continue to function. It has been proposed that in these cases, complement regulatory proteins and/or other control mechanisms may interrupt the complement cascade distal to the generation of C4d, so the persistence of C4d on graft endothelium represents a marker for the arrest of the complement cascade rather than ongoing complement-mediated graft injury (Williams et al., 2004).

As suggested by Platt (Platt, 2002), careful histologic and immunohistologic study may help to answer this question and address any potential role of complement in the accommodation process. Accommodation in ABO-incompatible grafts is not due to a change in the nature of the antibody or loss of the target antigen in the graft, because C4d is deposited in the renal microcirculation.

At a cellular level, accommodation may occur via multiple mechanisms, including internalization, downregulation, inactivation, and inhibition of the target antigen (Colvin & Nickeleit, 2006; Colvin & Smith, 2005).

Studies in mice show that, in the absence of T-cell help, B cells that are exposed to incompatible carbohydrate antigens on allografts differentiate into cells that can produce non-complement-fixing antibody which potentially competes with complement-fixing antibody, and these B cells gradually become tolerant after prolonged exposure (Ogawa et al., 2004).

In HLA-mismatched grafts, alloantibodies can be found in the absence of clinical graft dysfunction, thereby fitting the definition of accommodation. However, patients with circulating HLA-specific antibody have a greater likelihood of later graft loss, indicating that, if accommodation occurs, then it is either transient or insufficient to prevent CAMR. Long-term, complete accommodation has not been documented for MHC molecules, and the phenomenon might therefore be partly determined by the nature of the antigen (Colvin & Smith, 2005). Accommodation may have different degrees of effectiveness and stability (gradations), ranging from none (hyperacute rejection), to minimal (acute rejection), substantial (chronic rejection), or complete (stable accommodation) (Colvin, 2007). The minimal features that indicate transformation from accommodation to rejection have yet to be defined and drugs that promote more effective accommodation would potentially be useful clinically.

5. Stages of antibody-mediated rejection

At a National Institutes of Health (United States) consensus conference, draft criteria were established for antibody-mediated rejection and for four theoretical stages in the development of CAMR (Takemoto et al., 2004) as shown in FIG. 1 (Colvin & Smith, 2005).

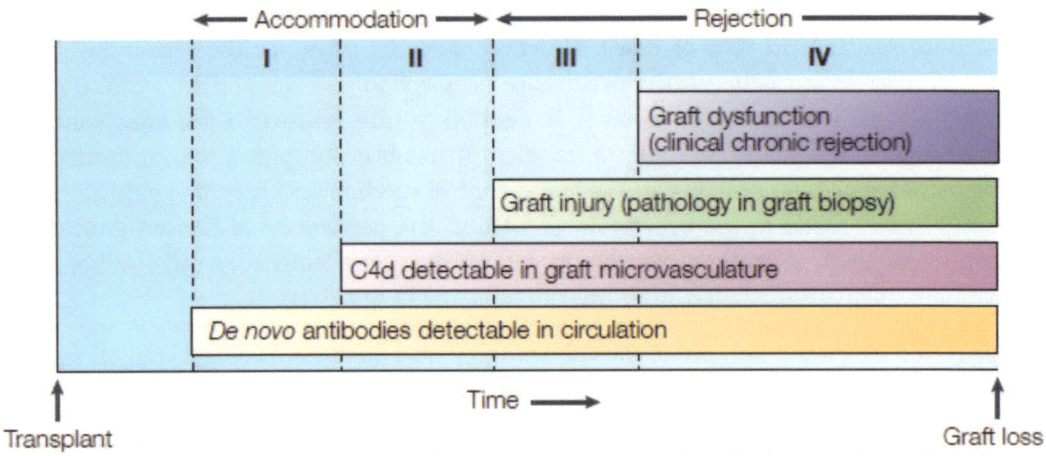

Figure 1. Proposed stages of antibody-mediated rejection (Reproduced with permission from Nature Publishing Group).

According to this model, the first evidence of an antibody-mediated response is the de novo generation of donor-reactive antibodies (stage I). In many circumstances and for unknown reasons, donor-reactive antibodies do not elicit AAMR.

The next stage (stage II) shows evidence of antibody reactivity and complement activation in the graft, with C4d deposition in peritubular or glomerular capillary endothelium. At this stage, there is no evidence of pathological or clinical injury in the graft. Both stage I and stage II fit the criteria for accommodation and are therefore not necessarily predestined to lead to graft injury. In stage III, in addition to positive staining for C4d, there are identifiable pathological changes, but graft function is still normal (that is, there is subclinical rejection). Finally, in stage IV, in addition to positive staining for C4d and pathological changes, graft dysfunction occurs. The interval between stages can be long and variable, and it is not known whether progression is inexorable (Colvin & Smith, 2005).

6. Pathology

The past 20 years have seen major advances in the understanding of the effects of anti-donor antibodies on renal allografts at various stages after transplantation. These advances have been due in large part to pathologic examination of both early and late renal allograft biopsies, including both routine histologic evaluation and immunohistology to detect complement split products.

6.1. Acute antibody mediated rejection

As pathologists have become increasingly adept at diagnosing antibody-mediated rejection (AMR) on allograft biopsies, substantial progress has been made in the treatment of AMR and in successful renal transplantation in recipients with pre-existing antibodies against donor blood group (ABO) and/or major histocompatibility (HLA) antigens. It has become critical to develop standardized criteria for the pathological diagnosis of AMR.

The diagnostic criteria for acute humoral rejection (AMR; acute antibody-mediated rejection). Patients with AHR present with an acute loss of graft function that often arises in the first few weeks after transplantation and cannot be distinguished from cell-mediated rejection on clinical grounds (Halloran et al., 1992; Takemoto et al., 2004). AMR can also develop years after transplantation, often triggered by a decrease in immunosuppression (iatrogenic, noncompliance, or malabsorption). Presensitization is the major risk factor, but most of the patients with AMR had a negative cross-match. AMR has occurred with all immunosuppression regimens, even profoundly depleting therapy (Lorenz et al., 2004). The first clue that circulating anti–class I HLA antibody caused a different pattern of acute rejection came from the studies of Halloran's group in Edmonton (Halloran et al., 1992). These investigators showed that neutrophils in peritubular capillaries (PTC) and glomerular capillaries are strongly associated with circulating anti-donor HLA antibodies. Other features, such as fibrinoid necrosis of arteries and microthrombi, are also more common. However, none of these features is specific.

The pathology of AMR has a wide spectrum and can easily be missed by histologic criteria alone. Renal biopsies may show acute cellular rejection, acute tubular injury, or thrombotic microangiopathy. Neutrophils in capillaries are characteristically but not always found. Macrophages are now recognized as a common intracapillary cell in AMR in kidney (Tinckam et al., 2005) and heart (Lepin et al., 2006) allografts. Typically, the PTC are dilated. Fibrinoid necrosis is found in a minority of cases (approximately 10 to 20%). A component of acute cellular rejection may also be present, as manifested by a prominent mononuclear infiltrate, tubulitis, or endarteritis. These lesions are generally not attributable to antibody alone. Treg cells (FOXP3+) are rarer in the infiltrate than in cell-mediated rejection, perhaps contributing to the poorer prognosis in AMR (Veronese et al., 2007). Microthrombi and interstitial hemorrhage also sometimes occur. The PTC and glomerular endothelium shows a variety of ultrastructural changes, including loss of fenestrations, detachment from the basement membrane, lysis, and apoptosis; complete destruction of capillaries can occur, leaving thickened laminated basement membranes (Liptak et al., 2005). Immunofluorescence (IF) curiously does not often show antibody or C3 deposition in the vessels. However, IF does show C4d in the majority of the PTC as a bright ring pattern, using a mAb in cryostat sections (Collins et al., 1999; Mauiyyedi et al., 2001, 2002). Immunohistochemistry (IHC) works in formalin-fixed, paraffin-embedded tissues with a polyclonal antibody (Lorenz et al., 2004). By immunoelectron microscopy, C4d is detected on the surface of the endothelial cells and in intracytoplasmic vesicles (Regele et al., 2002). Antibodies that react to non-C4d portions of the

C4 molecule do not show PTC deposition, arguing that what is detected in tissues is primarily C4d (Seemayer et al., 2006).

6.2. Chronic antibody mediated rejection

Chronic AMR is now included in the newest update of the Banff 07 classification of renal allograft pathology with the following criteria: [1]morphological changes as glomerular double contours compatible with transplant glomerulopathy (TPG) and severe PTC basement membrane multilayering, interstitial fibrosis and tubular atrophy with or without PTC loss, and fibrous intimal thickening in arteries without internal elastica duplication; [2] diffuse C4d deposition in PTCs; and [3] presence of DSA (Solez et al.,2008). Not all these criteria are always fulfilled in an individual patient at every given time point (Fehr et al., 2009).

PTC basement membrane multilayering correlates highly with TPG, and most of TPG have evidence of either C4d-positive staining or DSA. However, the proposed criteria do not apply to all situations of chronic active antibody-mediated rejection. Chronic AMR is distinct from acute AMR in that no acute inflammation (neutrophils, edema, necrosis, thrombosis) is present. However, cellular activity is often reflected by increased mononuclear cells in glomerular capillaries and PTC (Colvin, 2007). The Banff criteria require PTC C4d positivity for diagnosis of ABMR as well as microcirculation injury. However, C4d is not a sensitive marker of chronic ABMR, and in many patients with transplant glomerulopathy, C4d staining is negative in the presence of anti-HLA DSA. Therefore, the recent update of the Banff classification introduced the diagnostic category of "suspicious for ABMR." It is defined with the presence of morphologic evidence of antibody-mediated tissue injury and positive anti-HLA antibody with negative C4d, or PTC C4d positivity in the absence of alloantibody (Solez et al., 2008).

7. Markers of antibody mediated rejection

7.1. Histopathologic detection of C4d

Feucht et al. (Feucht et al., 1993) in Munich showed that peritubular capillary (PTC) C4d deposition in renal transplant biopsies is strongly associated with a poor prognosis and raised the possibility that antibodies were responsible. Currently, C4d has been adopted as a marker of antibody-mediated rejection (Racusen et al., 2003). The justification for the selection of C4d, a split product of C4, as a marker for AMR comes from its position in the cascade of complement activation. C4d, a split product of the classical pathway of complement activation, is present covalently bound on tissue near the sites of complement activation by alloantibody, e.g., vascular endothelial cell membrane.

C4d deposition in renal peritubular capillaries is strongly associated with circulating antibody to donor HLA class I or class II antigens (Bohmig et al., 2002; Haas et al., 2006) and is currently the best single marker of complement-fixing circulating antibodies to the endothelium.

7.2. C4d detection pitfalls

C4d is not a magic marker for antibody-mediated rejection and in many patients with transplant glomerulopathy. It is negative in the presence of anti-HLA DSA. Another issue with chronic active antibody-mediated rejection is non-HLA antibody induced rejection without complement fixation of C4d. Moreover, it was shown in many studies that focal C4d staining was not a reliable indicator of AMR (Kayler et al., 2008), and it is not a guarantee of AMR: diffuse C4d staining can occur with no morphologic injury or impaired outcome in ABO-incompatible allografts (Solez et al., 2008). Another important problem is the significance of positive C4d staining in the peritubular capillaries (PTC) and glomerular capillaries.

There are significant data to show that C4d positivity is usually long-lasting but is not permanent. C4d staining can change from negative to positive and vice versa within days to weeks. The detection of C4d signifies a humoral alloresponse in a subgroup of kidney transplants, which is often associated with signs of cellular rejection (Nickeleit et al., 2002). It is not clear how long C4d deposits persist in the absence of continued DSA production. One study reported that C4d deposits were no longer detectable on repeat biopsy performed 2–3 weeks after DSA (Mauiyyedi et al., 2002). If C4d staining misses some cases of antibody-mediated injury, and the presence of alloantibody does not identify which grafts are undergoing antibody-mediated damage, we need new methods for identifying which kidneys are being damaged by alloantibody.

7.3. Alternative markers (New diagnostic tools)

7.3.1. Endothelial-associated transcripts (ENDATs) as a new marker for CAMR

Recognizing the key role of endothelial changes in AMR, it was postulated by Sis and colleagues (Sis et al., 2009) that altered expression of endothelial genes in biopsies from patients with alloantibody would identify kidneys incurring antibody-mediated damage and at risk for graft loss, whether they were C4d+ or negative. They explored whether expression of endothelial genes was increased in biopsies manifesting antibody-mediated graft injury, and whether such changes could be seen in C4d negative as well as C4d positive biopsies. They identified 119 endothelial-associated transcripts (ENDATs) from literature, and studied their expression by microarrays in 173 renal allograft biopsies for cause.

Mean ENDAT expression was increased in all rejection but was higher in AMR than in T-cell-mediated rejection and correlated with histopathologic lesions of AMR, and alloantibody. Many individual ENDATs were increased in AMR and predicted graft loss. Kidneys with high ENDATs and antibody showed increased lesions of AMR and worse prognosis in comparison to controls. Only 40% of kidneys with high ENDAT expression and chronic AMR or graft loss were diagnosed by C4d positivity. High ENDAT expression with antibody predicts graft loss with higher sensitivity (77% versus. 31%) and slightly lower specificity (71% vs. 94%) than C4d. The results were validated in independent set of 82 kidneys. They concluded that in patients with alloantibodies, abnormalities in expression of endothelial genes identify not only C4d+ AMR but some kidney transplants developing antibody associated graft injury despite negative C4d staining and that ENDAT changes in renal transplants occur in rejection and in other forms of renal injury, and their impact on transplant glomerulopathy and graft loss is principally in patients with circulating HLA antibodies. The elevation of the ENDATs is of value in determining which biopsies for cause in patients with antibody may have antibody-mediated injury, even when they are C4d negative. Based on their study, the combined burden of C4d+ and C4d negative AMR accounts for the majority of graft losses in kidney transplants biopsied for clinical indications (17 of 26, 65%). ENDAT expression in biopsy provides a new tool for understanding the pathogenesis of late kidney graft loss and AMR, and for predicting graft outcomes and defining AMR even in C4d negative biopsies in patients with antibodies (Sis et al., 2009).

7.3.2. TRIB1as a new non-invasive marker for CAMR

The discovery of novel and less invasive surrogate biomarkers of acute cellular rejection, for which urine levels of Granzyme B and FOXP3 transcripts have been shown to have diagnostic and prognostic value (Muthukumar et al., 2005; Veale et al., 2006), has proved successful. Such an approach in the case of the different causes of late graft failure would facilitate the introduction of more targeted immunosuppression and thereby improve long-term outcome. Ashton-Chess and colleagues (Ashton-Chess et al., 2008) set out to discover novel minimally invasive biomarkers of more precise histologic diagnoses of late graft scarring. Using a literature gene-set comparison approach for late graft injury, they identified TRIB1, a human homolog of Drosophila tribbles, (Grosshans & Wieschaus, 2000) as a potentially informative biomarker. TRIB1 is a scarcely characterized member of the tribbles family that has been shown to be a potent regulator of cell signaling18 in various cells lines. It was determined that TRIB1 is expressed primarily by antigen-presenting cells (APC) and activated endothelial cells (EC). TRIB1 differs from the other minimally invasive biomarkers of transplant rejection described to date that are of T/NK cell origin, (Muthukumar et al., 2005; Seiler et al., 2007; Veale et al., 2006) in that it is expressed primarily by APC as well as EC.

They explored the potential of TRIB1 as a tissue, peripheral blood, and urine biomarker by measuring its mRNA profiles in graft biopsies, blood, and urine from healthy volunteers and kidney transplant recipients with different histologic and/or clinical diagnoses. For testing this, mRNA expression in 76 graft biopsies, 71 blood samples, and 11 urine samples were profiled from independent cohorts of renal transplant patients with different histologic diagnoses recruited at two European centers. TRIB1 but not TRIB2 or TRIB3 was found to be a potential blood and tissue (but not urine) biomarker of chronic antibody-mediated rejection. Moreover, TRIB1 mRNA in the blood was more specific and sensitive for diagnosing chronic AMR than TRIB1 mRNA in biopsies.

TRIB1 mRNA levels in peripheral blood mononuclear cells discriminated patients with chronic antibody-mediated rejection from those with other types of late allograft injury with high sensitivity and specificity, suggests TRIB1 to be a marker of an active immune response. Overall, these data support the potential use of TRIB1 as a biomarker of chronic antibody-mediated allograft failure.

http://dx.doi.org/10.5772/55001

8. Management of antibody mediated rejection

Unfortunately, no immunosuppressive standard for the prevention or therapy of alloantibody production has been established yet. Although based on very limited evidence, acute humoral rejections are frequently treated with a switch to tacrolimus, plasmapheresis or immunoadsorption, as well as T- and B-cell-depleting antibodies. However, the best therapeutic approach for C4d-positive, chronic humoral kidney rejection associated with an unfavourable prognosis remains completely unclear. Neither the dose nor the best drug combination for the therapy of an established humoral rejection is based on solid evidence. Although various immunosuppressive drugs can reduce the number of acute rejection ns via inhibition of the T-cell response, only very few data are available regarding immunosuppressive drugs affecting the humoral alloresponse after organ transplantation.

8.1. Intravenous immunoglobulins (IVIG)

The immunomodulatory effects of IVIG are multiple, and the exact mechanisms are not elucidated. However, effective alloantibody inhibition by IVIG was shown in the context of desensitization protocols only relying on high dose IVIG treatment (Jordan et al., 2003). IVIG inhibits mixed lymphocyte reactions and induces apoptosis mainly in B cells (Toyoda et al., 2004). There are numerous proposed mechanisms how IVIG exerts its immunomodulatory action. They include modification of circulating alloantibody concentration through induction of antiidiotypic circuits, antigen binding through the Fab part of the immunoglobulin molecule, Fc receptor-mediated interaction with antigen-presenting cells to block T- and B-cell activation, and inhibition of complement activity (Jordan et al., 2006).

In vivo, IVIG reduces the number of B cells and monocytes, and it reduces CD19, CD20 and CD40 expression by B cells, thereby modulating B-cell signaling (Jordan et al., 2003). IVIG inhibits binding of donor-reactive antibodies to target cells in ~80% of patients, indicating that the presence of blocking antibodies might explain the efficacy of IVIG, although the mechanism is not known (Jordan et al., 2003). Billing and colleagues (Billing et al., 2008) studied Six pediatric renal transplant recipients with CAMR and gave them four weekly doses of IVIG (1 g/kg body weight per dose), followed by a single dose of rituximab (375 mg/m2 body surface area) 1 week after the last IVIG infusion. Median glomerular filtration rate during 6 months before intervention dropped by 25 (range, 11–26) mL/ min/1.73m2 ($P<0.05$) and increased in response to antihumoral therapy by 21 (-14 to+30) 6 months ($P<0.05$) and by 19 (-14 to+_23) mL/min/1.73 m2 12 months ($P=0.063$) after start of treatment. Glomerular filtration rate improved or stabilized in 4 patients; the two non-responders had the highest degree of transplant glomerulopathy, the highest degree of C4d deposition in peritubular capillaries and pronounced interstitial inflammation. The treatment regimen was well tolerated. Another study conducted by Fehr and colleagues (Fehr et al., 2009) who reported four kidney allograft recipients suffering from chronic AMR 1 to 27 years post-transplant, who were treated with a combination of rituximab and intravenous immunoglobulin (IVIG) with improved kidney allograft function in all four patients, whereas donor-specific antibodies were reduced in 2 of 4 patients.

8.2. Rituximab

Rituximab, a chimeric monoclonal anti-CD20 antibody directed against B cells, prevents new antibody production by depletion of B cells as precursors of mature plasma cells in the circulation and the lymphoid tissue {although, some recent reports demonstrated that depletion in secondary and tertiary lymphoid structures is far less efficient and may not affect an ongoing localized humoral immune response (Genberg et al., 2006; Thaunat et al., 2008)}, prevention of B-cell proliferation, and induction of apoptosis and lysis of B cells through complement-dependent and -independent mechanisms (Salama & Pusey, 2006). Rituximab binds CD20 at the surface of precursor and mature B cells and leads to transient B-cell depletion, with typical B-cell recovery after 6–12 months in more than 80% of patients, although the degree of depletion is highly variable and is observed for up to 24 months in some individuals (Sureshkumar et al., 2007).An additional potential mechanism of action of rituximab is the direct targeting of CD20-positive cells that infiltrate the graft (Steinmetz et al., 2007). Preliminary studies indicate that rituximab decreases the concentration of pre-existing and post-transplantation antibodies (Gloor et al., 2003; Vieira et al., 2004). Conclusions and extrapolations from these studies are limited, because rituximab is usually combined with other therapies in these small and uncontrolled trials. The risk of bacterial infection as a result of immunoglobulin deficiency is also an important consideration. Based on the pathophysiologic condition of this rejection process and efficacy of rituximab in B cells and antibody-mediated autoimmune diseases (Eisenberg & Albert, 2006; Levesque & St Clair, 2008), a combination treatment with rituximab/IVIG represents a logical approach.

8.3. Mycophenolic acid and sirolimus

In a multicenter study, MMF in combination with cyclosporine resulted in significantly lower frequencies of HLA antibodies when compared with azathioprine and cyclosporine treatment (Terasaki & Ozawa, 2004). Moreover, MMF was described to be effective in inhibiting primary antigen-specific antibody responses in renal transplant patients (Rentenaar et al., 2002). Heidt et al (Heidt et al., 2008) stimulated purified human B cells devoid of T cells with CD40L expressing L cells, or by anti-CD40mAb with or without Toll-like receptor triggering, all in the presence of B-cell activating cytokines. These three protocols resulted in various degrees of B-cell stimulation. Then, they added four commonly used immunosuppressive drugs (tacrolimus, cyclosporin, mycophenolic acid [MPA], and rapamycin) to these cultures and tested a variety of parameters of B-cell activity including proliferation, apoptosis induction, and both IgM and IgG production. They found that MPA was extremely potent in inhibiting both proliferation and immunoglobulin production. Moreover, these effects persisted when MPA was added to already activated B cells, implying that an ongoing B-cell response may be dampened by MPA, whereas calcineurin inhibitors are ineffective. MPA levels used are lower than levels that are usually achieved physiologically.

In the same in vitro experiments, rapamycin, like MMF, was described to be extremely potent in inhibiting humoral responses. Rapamycin was the most effective drug tested, as it inhibited not only B-cell proliferation and immunoglobulin production, but also inhibited the number of immunoglobulin producing cells. None of the other drugs tested were capable of decreasing the number of immunoglobulin producing cells. By contrast, tacrolimus and cyclosporin marginally inhibited B-cell proliferation and immunoglobulin production, and the extent of inhibition depended on the degree of the B-cell stimulation.

8.4. Bortezomib

While the B cell-depleting anti-CD20 antibody rituximab is increasingly incorporated in treatment protocols of humoral rejection (Faguer et al., 2007), this reagent is neither effective in eliminating antibody-producing plasma cells (PC) – either newly created from memory or naïve B cells or from those that existed prior to transplant- nor does it decrease circulating antibody titers (Singh et al., 2009). For an effective blockade of alloantibody formation, a specific PC-depleting reagent would be desirable. Bortezomib (BZ), a selective inhibitor of the 26S proteasome, has been approved by FDA for the treatment of relapsed multiple myeloma. Mechanisms of BZ action include inhibition of NF-κ B and cytokine expression as well as induction of apoptosis as a result of activation of the terminal unfolded protein response (Meister et al., 2007). Susceptibility to BZ-induced apoptosis is related to the high immunoglobulin synthesis rate of PCs associated with accumulation of unfolded proteins/DRiPs inducing endoplasmatic reticulum stress (Meister et al., 2007). Moreover, BZ not only acted on the humoral response but also effectively inhibited the influx of MHC class II+ cells, monocytes/macrophages, CD8+ as well as CD4+ T cells. In animal models, Vogelbacher and colleagues (Vogelbacher et al., 2010) found that combination of Bortezomib and sirolimus inhibit the chronic active antibody-mediated rejection in experimental renal transplantation in the rat. In humans, data are lacking. In one case report, Bortezomib failed to treat CAMR even after treatment with rituximab and IVIG.

Perry and colleagues (Perry et al., 2009) described two sensitized patients with AMR treated in February 2007 using a combination of bortezomib and multiple plasmapheresis. Both patients had resolution of AMR and decreased serum DSA levels months after treatment. Neither developed transplant glomerulopathy. In a slightly different clinical setting, Everly and colleagues (Everly et al., 2008) used bortezomib to treat six patients who had combined AMR and cellular rejection occurring from 3 months to 7.5 years after transplant. All six patients showed resolution of AMR with a decrease in DSA levels after treatment. Unfortunately, three of the six patients developed transplant glomerulopathy. Flechner and coworkers (Flechner et al., 2010) treated 20 cases (16 kidney-only and 4 kidney-combined organ recipients) with AMR 19.8 months (range 1-71 months) posttransplant using a combined regimen of intravenous corticosteroids followed by a 2-week cycle on days 1-4-8-11 of plasmapheresis and 1.3 mg/m^2 bortezomib; then 0.5 mg/kg intravenous immunoglobulin four times. They found that the bortezomib-containing regimen demonstrated activity in AMR but seems to be most effective before the onset of significant renal dysfunction (serum creatinine <3 mg/dL) or proteinuria (<1 g/day).

Compared to rituximab, Waiser and colleagues (Waiser et al., 2012) found that patients with AMR treated with bortezomib had better graft survival At 18 months after treatment (P = 0.071) and renal function at 9 months was superior in patients treated with bortezomib as compared to rituximab-treated patients (P= 0.008). Whereas these early clinical experiences with proteasome inhibition are encouraging, the lack of controls is a major limitation in assessing true efficacy. In addition, since even successfully treated AMR can still result in the development of chronic transplant glomerulopathy, the prevention of AMR might be a more important goal of these types of therapies.

8.5. Eculizumab (Terminal complement inhibition with eculizumab)

Almost all episodes of AMR are accompanied by evidence of early complement activation as demonstrated by C4d staining of the peritubular capillaries (Burns et al., 2008). However, the exact role of complement in the pathogenesis of AMR is unclear. Eculizumab is a humanized monoclonal antibody with high affinity for C5 and thus blocks the activation of terminal complement. Eculizumab is approved by the FDA for the treatment of paroxysmal nocturnal hemoglobinuria. Locke et al. (Locke et al., 2009) reported the successful treatment of a patient with severe AMR using eculizumab. Stegall and colleagues reported their initial experience with eculizumab treatment at the time of transplant showing that blockade of terminal complement prevented the development of AMR in patients who developed high levels of DSA post transplant (Stegall et al., 2009). Stegall et al also examined the efficacy of eculizumab in the prevention AMR in sensitized renal transplant recipients with a positive crossmatch against their living donor (Stegall et al., 2011). The incidence of biopsy-proven AMR in the first 3 months posttransplant in 26 highly sensitized recipients of living donor renal transplants who received eculizumab posttransplant was compared to a historical control group of 51 sensitized patients treated with a similar plasma exchange-based protocol without eculizumab. The incidence of AMR was 7.7% in the eculizumab group compared to 41.2% in the control group ($P = 0.0031$). Eculizumab also decreased AMR in patients who developed high levels of DSA early after transplantation that caused proximal complement activation. With eculizumab, AMR episodes were easily treated with plasma exchange reducing the need for splenectomy. On 1-year protocol biopsy, transplant glomerulopathy was found to be present in 6.7% eculizumab-treated recipients and in 35.7% of control patients ($P = 0.044$).

Taken together, these studies suggest that terminal complement activation may play a critical role in the pathogenesis of early AMR. Thus, eculizumab may provide an attractive approach to the prevention of AMR.

8.6. Future therapies with new targets

8.6.1. B cells

Memory B cells are heterogeneous but have cell-surface markers (CD24, CD27, CD43 and CD79b) that are potential therapeutic targets (McHeyzer-Williams & McHeyzer-Williams, 2005). B cells also express TACI (transmembrane activator and calcium-modulating cyclophilin-ligand interactor), BCMA (B-cell maturation antigen) and BAFF receptor (B-cell-activating factor receptor), all of which are members of the TNF-receptor family that are triggered by the ligands BAFF and APRIL (a proliferation inducing ligand), which are expressed at the cell surface of DCs (Craxton et al., 2003). A soluble TACI–immunoglobulin fusion protein blocks B-cell development by inhibiting the interaction between B cells and DCs (Gross et al., 2001).

These cell-surface markers might be useful targets to prevent the development of B cells into plasma cells.

8.6.2. Plasma cells

Normal plasma cells express little or no CD20 and are therefore resistant to rituximab-mediated depletion. Several cell-surface molecules that are expressed by plasma cells might be considered as drug targets — syndecan-1 (CD138), CD38, $\alpha4\beta1$-integrin (CD49d–CD29) and CXC-chemokine receptor 4 (CXCR4) — although none of these is entirely plasma-cell specific. Plasma-cell longevity is thought to be an extrinsic phenomenon that is mediated by survival signals delivered by bone-marrow stromal cells (Colvin & Smith, 2005). Because the transcription factors BLIMP1 (B-lymphocyte-induced maturation protein 1) and XBP1 (X-box-binding protein 1) (as well as the repression of PAX5, paired box gene 5) are required to maintain plasma-cell function, their inhibition might result in the loss of plasma-cell function (Shapiro-Shelef & Calame, 2005).

8.6.3. Complement antagonists

Complement antagonists could prevent the acute pathological effects of complement activation. For example, soluble CR1 delays antibody-mediated rejection in xenograft models but is insufficient to prevent graft rejection completely (Azimzadeh et al., 2003). Other complement antagonists, such as C5-specific antibody, which blocks activation of C5 and formation of both C5a and the MAC, are in ongoing evaluation. Transgenic expression of human complement-regulatory proteins (DAF and CD59) in pigs has shown potency for preventing xenograft rejection (Menoret et al., 2004), but the relevance of these studies to allografts needs to be extended and tested.

9. Summary

Immunologic barriers once considered insurmountable are now consistently overcome to enable more patients to undergo organ transplantation. Alloantibodies are a substantial obstacle to short- and long-term graft survival. To prevent or reduce alloantibody titres, more insights are needed to improve our understanding of the regulation of B cells and the developmental and differentiation pathways of memory B cells and plasma cells.

Several important issues regarding AMR remain. First, the immunologic mechanisms responsible for the development of high levels of DSA are still unclear. The contribution of memory B cells versus the role of pre-existing PCs has important therapeutic implications since each may have a differential sensitivity to various agents.

Whereas several new therapeutic approaches have emerged, more extensive study and follow-up are needed to determine if these apparent advances will improve the outcomes of AMR.

Author details

Rashad Hassan* and Ahmed Akl

Mansoura Urology and Nephrology Center, Egypt

References

[1] Alexandre, GPJ.; Squifflet, JP.; De Bruyère, M.; Latinne, D.; Reding, R.; Gianello, P., et al. (1987). Present experience in a series of 26 ABO-incompatible living donor renal allografts. *Transplant Proc*, Vol., 19; pp. 4538–4544.

[2] Amico, P.; Honger, G.; Mayr, M.; Steiger, J.; Hopfer, H. & Schaub, S. (2009). Clinical relevance of pretransplant donor-specific HLA antibodies detected by single-antigen flow-beads. *Transplantation*, Vol., 87; pp. 1681–1688.

[3] Arnold, ML.; Pei, R.; Spriewald, B.& Wassmuth, R. (2005). Anti-HLA class II antibodies in kidney retransplant patients. *Tissue Antigens*, Vol., 65; pp. 370-378.

[4] Ashton-Chess, J.; Giral, M.; Mengel, M.; Renaudin, K.; Foucher, Y.; Gwinner, Wet., al. (2008). Tribbles-1 as a Novel Biomarker of Chronic Antibody-Mediated Rejection. *J Am Soc Nephrol*, Vol., 19; pp. 1116–1127.

[5] Azimzadeh, A.; Zorn, GL 3rd.; Blair, KS.; Zhang, JP.; Pfeiffer, S.; Harrison, RA., et al. (2003). Hyperacute lung rejection in the pig to-human model. 2. Synergy between soluble and membrane complement inhibition. *Xenotransplantation*, Vol., 10; pp. 120–131.

[6] Benzaquen, LR.; Nicholson-Weller, A. & Halperin, JA. (1994). Terminal complement proteins C5b-9 release basic fibroblast growth factor and platelet-derived growth factor from endothelial cells. *J Exp Med*, Vol., 179; pp. 985–992.

[7] Bian, H. & Reed, EF. (2001). Anti-HLA class I antibodies transduce signals in endothelial cells resulting in FGF receptor translocation, downregulation of ICAM-1 and cell proliferation. *Transplant Proc*, Vol., 33; pp. 311.

[8] Billing, H.; Rieger, S.; Ovens, J.; Süsal, C.; Melk, A.; Waldherr, R., et al. (2008). Successful treatment of chronic antibody-mediated rejection with IVIG and rituximab in pediatric renal transplant recipients. *Transplantation*, Vol., 86; pp. 1214–1221.

[9] Bohmig, GA.; Exner, M.; Habicht, A.; Schillinger, M.; Lang, U.; Kletzmayr, J., et al. (2002). Capillary C4d deposition in kidney allografts: A specific marker of alloantibody-dependent graft injury. *J Am Soc Nephrol*, Vol., 13; pp. 1091–1099.

[10] Burns, JM.; Cornell, LD.; Perry, DK.; Pollinger, HS.; Gloor, JM.; Kremers, WK., et al. (2008). Alloantibody levels and acute humoral rejection early after positive crossmatch kidney transplantation. *Am J Transplant*, Vol., 8; pp. 2684–2694.

[11] Campos, EF.; Tedesco-Silva, H.; Machado, PG.; Franco, M.; Medina-Pestana, JO. & Gerbase-DeLima, M. (2006). Post-transplant anti-HLA class II antibodies as risk factor for late kidney allograft failure. *Am J Transplant*, Vol., 6; pp. 2316-2320.

[12] Cantarovich, D.; De Amicis, S.; Akl, A.; Devys, A.; Vistoli, F.; Karam, G., et al. (2011). Posttransplant donor-specific anti-HLA antibodies negatively impact pancreas transplantation outcome. *Am J Transplant*, Vol., 11; pp. 2737-2746.

[13] Chao, NJ. (2004). Minors come of age: minor histocompatibility antigens and graft-versus-host disease. *Biol Blood Marrow Transplant*, Vol., 10; pp. 215–223.

[14] Collins, AB.; Schneeberger, EE.; Pascual, MA.; Saidman, SL.; Williams, WW.; Tolkoff-Rubin, N., et al. (1999). Complement activation in acute humoral renal allograft rejection: Diagnostic significance of C4d deposits in peritubular capillaries. *J Am Soc Nephrol*, Vol., 10; pp. 2208–2214.

[15] Colvin, RB. (2007). Antibody-mediated renal allograft rejection: Diagnosis and pathogenesis. *J Am Soc Nephrol*, Vol., 18; pp. 1046-1056.

[16] Colvin, RB. & Nickeleit, V. (2006). Renal transplant pathology. In: Heptinstall's Pathology of the Kidney, 6th Ed., edited by Jennette JC, Olson JL, Schwartz MM, Silva FG, Philadelphia, Lippincott-Raven, pp 1347–1490.

[17] Colvin, RB. & Smith, RN. (2005). Antibody-mediated organ-allograft rejection. *Nat Rev Immunol*, Vol., 5; pp. 807–817.

[18] Craxton, A.; Magaletti, D.; Ryan, EJ. & Clark, EA. (2003). Macrophage- and dendritic cell-dependent regulation of human B-cell proliferation requires the TNF family ligand BAFF. *Blood*, Vol., 101; pp. 4464–4471.

[19] Derhaag, JG.; Duijvestijn, AM.; Damoiseaux, JG. & van Breda Vriesman, PJ. (2000). Effects of antibody reactivity to major histocompatibility complex (MHC) and non-MHC alloantigens on graft endothelial cells in heart allograft rejection. *Transplantation*, Vol., 69; pp. 1899–1906.

[20] Dragun, D.; Müller, DN.; Bräsen, JH.; Fritsche, L.; Nieminen-Kelhä, M.; Dechend, R., et al. (2005). Angiotensin II type 1-receptor activating antibodies in renal-allograft rejection. *N Engl J Med*, Vol., 352; pp. 558–569.

[21] Eisenberg, R. & Albert, D. (2006). B-cell targeted therapies in rheumatoid arthritis and systemic lupus erythematosus. *Nat Clin Pract Rheumatol*,Vol., 2; pp. 20-27.

[22] Erlich, HA.; Opelz, G. & Hansen, J. (2001). HLA DNA typing and transplantation. *Immunity*, Vol., 14; pp. 347–356.

[23] Everly, MJ.; Everly, JJ.; Susskind, B.; Brailey, P.; Arend, LJ.; Alloway, RR., et al. (2008). Bortezomib provides effective therapy for antibody and cell-mediated rejection. *Transplantation*, Vol., 86; pp. 1754–1761.

[24] Faguer, S.; Kamar, N.; Guilbeaud-Frugier, C.; Fort, M.; Modesto, A.; Mari, A., et al. (2007). Rituximab therapy for acute humoral rejection after kidney transplantation. *Transplantation*, Vol., 83; pp. 1277–1280.

[25] Fehr, T.; Rüsi, B.; Fischer, A.; Hopfer, H.; Wüthrich, RP. & Gaspert, A. (2009). Rituximab and intravenous immunoglobulin treatment of chronic antibody-mediated kidney allograft rejection. *Transplantation*, Vol., 87(12); pp. 1837-1841.

[26] Feucht, HE.; Schneeberger, H.; Hillebrand, G.; Burkhardt, K.; Weiss, M.; Riethmuller, G., et al. (1993). Capillary deposition of C4d complement fragment and early renal graft loss. *Kidney Int*, Vol., 43; pp. 1333–1338.

[27] Flechner, SM.; Fatica, R.; Askar, M.; Stephany, BR.; Poggio, E.; Koo, A., et al. (2010). The role of proteasome inhibition with bortezomib in the treatment of antibody-mediated rejection after kidney-only or kidney-combined organ transplantation.*Transplantation*, Vol., 90; pp. 1486-1492.

[28] Genberg, H.; Hansson, A.; Wernerson, A.; Wennberg, L. & Tydén, G. (2006). Pharmacodynamics of rituximab in kidney allotransplantation. *Am J Transplant*, Vol., 6; pp. 2418-2428.

[29] Gerbase-DeLima, M.; Campos, EF.; Tedesco-Silva, H.; Machado, PG.; Franco, M.; Medina-Pestana, JO. (2006). Anti-HLA class II antibodies and chronic allograft nephropathy. Clin Transpl, p. 201-205.

[30] Gloor, JM.; Sethi, S.; Stegall, MD.; Park, WD.; Moore, SB.; DeGoey, S., et al. (2007). Transplant glomerulopathy: Subclinicalincidence and association with alloantibody. *Am J Transplant*, Vol., 7; pp. 2124–2132.

[31] Gloor, JM.; Cosio, FG.; Rea, DJ.; Wadei, HM.; Winters, JL.; Moore, SB.. et al. (2006). Histologic findings one year after positive crossmatch or ABO blood group incompatible living donor kidney transplantation. *Am J Transplant* , Vol., 6; pp. 1841–1847.

[32] Gloor, JM.; DeGoey, S.; Ploeger, N.; Gebel, H.; Bray, R.; Moore, SB., et al. (2004). Persistence of low levels of alloantibody after desensitization in crossmatch-positive living donor kidney transplantation. *Transplantation*, Vol., 78; pp. 221–227.

[33] Gloor, JM.; DeGoey, SR.; Pineda, AA.; Moore, SB.; Prieto, M.; Nyberg, SL., et al. (2003). Overcoming a positive crossmatch in living-donor kidney transplantation. *Am J Transplant*, Vol., 3; pp. 1017–1023.

[34] Gross, JA.; Dillon, SR.; Mudri, S.; Johnston, J.; Littau, A.; Roque, R., et al. (2001). TACI–Ig neutralizes molecules critical for B cell development and autoimmune disease: impaired B cell maturation in mice lacking BLyS. *Immunity*, Vol., 15; pp. 289–302.

[35] Grosshans, J. & Wieschaus, E. (2000). A genetic link between morphogenesis and cell division during formation of the ventral furrow in Drosophila. *Cell*, Vol., 101; pp. 523–531.

[36] Haas, M.; Montgomery, RA.; Segev, DL.; Rahman, MH.; Racusen, LC.; Bagnasco, SM., et al. (2007). Subclinical acute antibody-mediated rejection in positive cross-match renal allografts. *Am J Transpl*, Vol., 7; pp. 576–585.

[37] Haas, M.; Rahman, MH.; Racusen, LC.; Kraus, ES.; Bagnasco, SM.; Segev, DL., et al. (2006). C4d and C3d staining in biopsies of ABO- and HLA-incompatible renal allografts: Correlation with histologic findings. *Am J Transplant*, Vol., 6; pp. 1829–1840.

[38] Halloran, PF.; Schlaut, J.; Solez, K. & Srinivasa, NS. (1992). The significance of the anti-class I antibody response. II. Clinical and pathologic features of renal transplants with anti-class Ilike antibody. *Transplantation*, Vol., 53; pp. 550–555.

[39] Heidt, S.; Roelen, DL.; Eijsink, C.; van Kooten, C.; Claas, FH. & Mulder, A. (2008). Effects of immunosuppressive drugs on purified human B cells: evidence supporting the use of MMF and rapamycin. *Transplantation*, Vol., 86; pp. 1292–1300.

[40] Hourmant, M.; Cesbron-Gautier, A.; Terasaki, PI.; Mizutani, K.; Moreau, A.; Meurette, A., et al. (2005). Frequency and clinical implications of development of donor-specific and non-donor-specific HLA antibodies after kidney transplantation. *J Am Soc Nephrol*, Vol., 16; pp. 2804–2812.

[41] Jin, YP.; Jindra, PT.; Gong, KW.; Lepin, EJ. & Reed EF,. (2005). Anti-HLA class I antibodies activate endothelial cells and promote chronic rejection. *Transplantation*, Vol., 79(3 suppl); S19-21.

[42] Jin, YP.; Singh, RP.; Du, ZY.; Rajasekaran, AK.; Rozengurt, E. & Reed, EF. (2002). Ligation of HLA class I molecules on endothelial cells induces phosphorylation of Src, paxillin, and focal adhesion kinase in an actin-dependent manner. *J Immunol*, Vol., 168; pp. 5415–5423.

[43] Jordan, S. (2006). IVIG vs. plasmapheresis for desensitization: which is better? *Am J Transpl*, Vol., 6; pp. 1510–1511.

[44] Jordan, SC.; Vo, AA.; Peng, A.; Toyoda, M. & Tyan, D. (2006). Intravenous gammaglobulin (IVIG): A novel approach to improve transplant rates and outcomes in highly HLA-sensitized patients. *Am J Transplant*, Vol., 6; pp. 459-466.

[45] Jordan, SC.; Vo, AA.; Nast, CC. & Tyan, D. (2003). Use of high-dose human intravenous immunoglobulin therapy in sensitized patients awaiting transplantation: The Cedars-Sinai experience. *Clin Transpl*, pp. 193-198.

[46] Jordan, SC.; Vo, A.; Bunnapradist, S.; Toyoda, M.; Peng, A.; Puliyanda, D., et al. (2003). Intravenous immune globulin treatment inhibits crossmatch positivity and allows for successful transplantation of incompatible organs in living-donor and cadaver recipients. *Transplantation*, Vol., 76; pp. 631–636.

[47] Kamimaki, I.; Ishikura, K.; Hataya, H.; et al. (2007). A case of allograft dysfunction with antibody-mediated rejection developing 13 yr after kidney transplantation. *Clin Transplant*, Vol., 21(suppl 18); pp. 60.

[48] Kayler, LK.; Kiss, L.; Sharma, V.; Mohanka, R.; Zeevi, A.; Girnita, A., et al. (2008). Acute renal allograft rejection: Diagnostic significance of focal peritubular capillary C4d. *Transplantation*, Vol., 85; pp. 813–820.

[49] Kooijmans-Coutinho, MF.; Hermans, J.; Schrama, E.; Ringers, J.; Daha, MR.; Bruijn, JA., et al. (1996). Interstitial rejection, vascular rejection, and diffuse thrombosis of renal allografts. Predisposing factors, histology, immunohistochemistry, and relation to outcome. *Transplantation*, Vol., 61; pp. 1338–1344.

[50] Lefaucheur, C.; Loupy, A.; Hill, GS.; Andrade, J.; Nochy, D.; Antoine, C., et al. (2010). Preexisting donor-specific HLA antibodies predict outcome in kidney transplantation. *J Am Soc Nephrol*, Vol., 21; pp. 1398-1406.

[51] Lepin, EJ.; Zhang, Q.; Zhang, X.; Jindra, PT.; Hong, LS.; Ayele, P., et al. (2006). Phosphorylated S6 ribosomal protein: A novel biomarker of antibody-mediated rejection in heart allografts. *Am J Transplant*, Vol., 6; pp. 1560–1571.

[52] Levesque, MC. & St Clair, EW. (2008). B cell-directed therapies for autoimmune disease and correlates of disease response and relapse. *J Allergy Clin Immunol*, Vol., 121; pp. 13-21.

[53] Liptak, P.; Kemeny, E.; Morvay, Z.; Szederkenyi, E.; Szenohradszky, P.; Marofka, F., et al.(2005). Peritubular capillary damage in acute humoral rejection: An ultrastructural study on human renal allografts. *Am J Transplant*, Vol., 5; pp. 2870–2876.

[54] Locke, JE.; Magro, CM.; Singer, AL.; Segev, DL.; Haas, M.; Hillel, AT., et al. (2009). The use of antibody to complement protein C5 for salvage treatment of severe antibody-mediated rejection. *Am J Transplant*, Vol., 9; pp. 231–235.

[55] Lorenz, M.; Regele, H.; Schillinger, M.; Exner, M.; Rasoul-Rockenschaub, S.; Wahrmann, M., et al. (2004). Risk factors for capillary C4d deposition in kidney allografts: Evaluation of a large study cohort. *Transplantation*, Vol., 78; pp. 447–452.

[56] Loupy, A.; Suberbielle-Boissel, C.; Hill, GS.; Lefaucheur, C.; Anglicheau, D.;Zuber, J., et al. (2009). Outcome of subclinical antibodymediated rejection in kidney transplant recipients with preformed donor-specific antibodies. *Am J Transplant*, Vol., 9; pp. 2561–2570.

[57] Martin, L.; Guignier, F.; Bocrie, O.; D'Athis, P.; Rageot, D.; Rifle, G., et al. (2005). Detection of anti-HLA antibodies with flow cytometry in needle core biopsies of renal transplants recipients with chronic allograft nephropathy. *Transplantation*, Vol., 79; pp. 1459-1461.

[58] Mauiyyedi, S.; Crespo, M.; Collins, AB.; Schneeberger, EE.; Pascual, MA.; Saidman, SL., et al. (2002). Acute humoral rejection in kidney transplantation: II. Morphology,

immunopathology, and pathologic classification. *J Am Soc Nephrol*, Vol., 13; pp. 779-787.

[59] Mauiyyedi, S.; Pelle, PD.; Saidman, S.; Collins, AB.; Pascual, M.; Tolkoff-Rubin, NE., et al. (2001). Chronic humoral rejection: Identification of antibody-mediated chronic renal allograft rejection by C4d deposits in peritubular capillaries. *J Am Soc Nephrol*, Vol., 12; pp. 574–582.

[60] McHeyzer-Williams, LJ. & McHeyzer-Williams, MG. (2005). Antigen-specific memory B cell development. *Annu Rev Immunol*, Vol., 23; pp. 487–513.

[61] Meister, S.; Schubert, U.; Neubert, K.; Herrmann, K.; Burger, R.; Gramatzki, M., et al. (2007). Extensive immunoglobulin production sensitizes myeloma cells for proteasome inhibition. *Cancer Res*, Vol., 67; pp. 1783–1792.

[62] Ménoret, S.; Plat, M.; Blancho, G.; Martinat-Botté, F.; Bernard, P.; Karam, G., et al. (2004). Characterization of human CD55 and CD59 transgenic pigs and kidney xenotransplantation in the pig-to-baboon combination. *Transplantation*, Vol., 77; pp. 1468–1471.

[63] Michaels, PJ.; Espejo, ML.; Kobashigawa, J.; Alejos, JC.; Burch, C.; Takemoto, S., et al. (2003). Humoral rejection in cardiac transplantation: risk factors, hemodynamic consequences and relationship to transplant coronary artery disease. *J Heart Lung Transplant*, Vol., 22; pp. 58–69.

[64] Mizutani, K.; Terasaki, P.; Rosen, A.; Esquenazi, V.; Miller, J.; Shih, RN., et al. (2005). Serial ten-year follow-up of HLA and MICA antibody production prior to kidney graft failure. *Am J Transplant*, Vol., 5; pp. 2265–2272.

[65] Morris, PJ.; Mickey, MR.; Singal, DP. & Terasaki, PI. (1969). Serotyping for homotransplantation, XXII: specificity of cytotoxic antibodies developing after renal transplantation. *Br Med J*, Vol., 1; pp. 758-759.

[66] Muthukumar, T.; Dadhania, D.; Ding, R.; Snopkowski, C.; Naqvi, R.; Lee, JB., et al. (2005). Messenger RNA for FOXP3 in the urine of renal-allograft recipients. *N Engl J Med*, Vol., 353; pp. 2342–2351.

[67] Nickeleit, V.; Zeiler, M.; Gudat, F.; Thiel, G. & Mihatsch, MJ. (2002). Detection of the complement degradation product C4d in renal allografts: diagnostic and therapeutic implications. *J Am Soc Nephrol*, Vol., 13; pp. 242-251.

[68] Noorchashm, H.; Reed, AJ.; Rostami, SY.; Mozaffari, R.; Zekavat, G.; Koeberlein, B., et al. (2006). B cell-mediated antigen presentation is required for the pathogenesis of acute cardiac allograft rejection. *J Immunol*, Vol., 177; pp. 7715-7722.

[69] Ogawa, H.; Mohiuddin, MM.; Yin, DP.; Shen, J.; Chong, AS. & Galili, U. (2004). Mouse-heart grafts expressing an incompatible carbohydrate antigen. II. Transition from accommodation to tolerance. *Transplantation*, Vol., 77; pp. 366–373.

[70] Opelz, G. (2005). Collaborative Transplant Study. Non-HLA transplantation immunity revealed by lymphocytotoxic antibodies. *Lancet*, Vol., 365; pp. 1570-1576.

[71] Park, WD.; Grande, JP.; Ninova, D.; Nath, KA.; Platt, JL.; Gloor, JM., et al. (2003). Accommodation in ABO-incompatible kidney allografts, a novel mechanism of self-protection against antibody-mediated injury. *Am J Transplant*, Vol., 3; pp. 952–960.

[72] Pelletier, RP.; Hennessy, PK.; Adams, PW.; VanBuskirk, AM.; Ferguson, RM. & Orosz, CG. (2002). Clinical significance of MHC-reactive alloantibodies that develop after kidney or kidney–pancreas transplantation. *Am J Transplant*, Vol., 2; pp. 134–141.

[73] Perry, DK.; Burns, JM.; Pollinger, HS.; Amiot, BP.; Gloor, JM.; Gores, GJ., et al. (2009). Proteasome inhibition causes apoptosis of normal human plasma cells preventing alloantibody production. *Am J Transplant*, Vol., 9; pp. 201–209.

[74] Piazza, A.; Poggi, E.; Borrelli, L.; Servetti, S.; Monaco, PI.; Buonomo, O., et al. (2001). Impact of donor-specific antibodies on chronic rejection occurrence and graft loss in renal transplantation: posttransplant analysis using flow cytometric techniques. *Transplantation*, Vol., 71; pp. 1106–1112.

[75] Platt, JL. (2002). C4d and the fate of organ allografts. *J Am Soc Nephrol*, Vol., 13; pp. 2417–2419.

[76] Race, RR. & Sanger, R. (1958). Blood Groups in Man (*Blackwell Scientific*, Oxford,).

[77] Racusen, LC.; Colvin, RB.; Solez, K.; Mihatsch, MJ.; Halloran, PF.; Campbell, PM., et al. (2003). Antibody-mediated rejection criteria—an addition to the banff 97 classification of renal allograft rejection. *Am J Transpl*, Vol., 3; pp. 708–714.

[78] Reed, EF. (2003). Signal transduction via MHC class I molecules in endothelial and smooth muscle cells. *Crit Rev Immunol*, Vol., 23; pp. 109–128.

[79] Regele, H.; Bohmig, GA.; Habicht, A.; Gollowitzer, D.; Schillinger, M.; Rockenschaub, S., et al. (2002). Capillary deposition of complement split product C4d in renal allografts is associated with basement membrane injury in peritubular and glomerular capillaries: A contribution of humoral immunity to chronic allograft rejection. *J Am Soc Nephrol*, Vol., 13; pp. 2371–2380.

[80] Rentenaar, RJ.; van Diepen, FN.; Meijer, RT.; Surachno, S.; Wilmink, JM.; Schellekens, PT., et al. (2002). Immune responsiveness in renal transplant recipients: Mycophenolic acid severely depresses humoral immunity in vivo. *Kidney Int*, Vol., 62; pp. 319-328.

[81] Salama, AD. & Pusey, CD. (2006). Drug insight: Rituximab in renal disease and transplantation. *Nat Clin Pract Nephrol*, Vol., 2; pp. 221-230.

[82] Seemayer, CA.; Gaspert, A.; Nickeleit, V. & Mihatsch, MJ. (2006). C4d staining of renal allograft biopsies: Comparative analysis of different staining techniques. *Nephrol Dial Transplant*, Vol., 22; pp. 568–576.

[83] Seiler, M.; Brabcova, I.; Viklicky, O.; Hribova, P.; Rosenberger, C.; Pratschke, J., et al. (2007). Heightened expression of the cytotoxicity receptor NKG2D correlates with acute and chronic nephropathy after kidney transplantation. *Am J Transplant*, Vol., 7; pp. 423–433.

[84] Shapiro-Shelef, M. & Calame, K. (2005). Regulation of plasma-cell development. *Nature Rev Immunol*, Vol., 5; pp. 230–242.

[85] Shimizu, A.; Yamada, K.; Sachs, DH. & Colvin, RB. (2002). Persistent rejection of peritubular capillaries and tubules is associated with progressive interstitial fibrosis. *Kidney Int*, Vol., 61; pp. 1867-1879.

[86] Shishido, S.; Asanuma, H.; Tajima, E.; Hoshinaga, K.; Ogawa, O.; Hasegawa, A., et al. ABO-incompatible living-donor kidney transplantation in children. *Transplantation*. 2001; 72, 1037–42.

[87] Singh, N.; Pirsch, J. & Samaniego, M. (2009). Antibody-mediated rejection: treatment alternatives and outcomes. *Transplant Rev (Orlando)*, Vol., 23; pp. 34–46.

[88] Sis, B.; Jhangri, GS.; Bunnag, S.; Allanach, K.; Kaplan, B. & Halloran, PF. (2009). Endothelial Gene Expression in Kidney Transplants with Alloantibody Indicates Antibody-Mediated Damage Despite Lack of C4d Staining. *Am J Transplant*, Vol., 9(10); pp. 2312-2323.

[89] Smith, RN.; Kawai, T.; Boskovic, S.; Nadazdin, O.; Sachs, DH.; Cosimi, AB., et al. (2006). Chronic antibody mediated rejection of renal allografts: pathological, serological and immunologic features in nonhuman primates. *Am J Transplant*, Vol., 6(8), pp. 1790-1798.

[90] Solez, K.; Colvin, RB.; Racusen, LC.; Haas, M.; Sis, B.; Mengel, M., et al. (2008). Banff 07 classification of renal allograft pathology: updates and future directions. *Am J Transplant*, Vol., 8; pp. 753-760.

[91] Solez, K.; Colvin, RB.; Racusen, LC.; Sis, B.; Halloran, PF.; Birk, PE., et al. (2007). Banff '05 meeting report: Differential diagnosis of chronic injury and elimination of chronic allograft nephropathy ("CAN") in the Banff schema. *Am J Transplant*, Vol., 7; pp. 518–526.

[92] Stegall, MD.; Diwan, T.; Raghavaiah, S.; Cornell, LD.; Burns, J.; Dean, PG., et al. (2011). Terminal Complement Inhibition decreases Antibody-Mediated Rejection in Sensitized Renal Transplant Recipients. *Am J Transplant*, Vol., 11; pp. 2405–2413.

[93] Stegall, MD. & Gloor, JM. (2010). Deciphering antibody-mediated rejection: new insights into mechanisms and treatment. *Curr Opinion in Organ Transplant*, Vol., 15; pp. 8–10.

[94] Stegall, MD.; Diwan, T.; Burns, P., et al. (2009). Prevention of acute humoral rejection with C5 inhibition. *Am J Transplant*, Vol., 9 (s2):241.

[95] Steinmetz, OM.; Lange-Hüsken, F.; Turner, JE.; Vernauer, A.; Helmchen, U.; Stahl, RA., et al. (2007). Rituximab removes intrarenal B cell clusters in patients with renal vascular allograft rejection. *Transplantation*, Vol., 84; pp. 842-850.

[96] Sumitran-Holgersson, S.; Wilczek, HE.; Holgersson, J. & Soderstrom, K. (2002). Identification of the nonclassical HLA molecules, MICA, as targets for humoral immunity associated with irreversible rejection of kidney allografts. *Transplantation*, Vol., 74; pp. 268–277.

[97] Sureshkumar, KK.; Hussain, SM.; Carpenter, BJ.; Sandroni, SE. & Marcus, RJ. (2007). Antibody-mediated rejection following renal transplantation. *Expert Opin Pharmacother*, Vol., 8; pp. 913-921.

[98] Takemoto, SK.; Zeevi, A.; Feng, S.; Colvin, RB.; Jordan, S.; Kobashigawa, J., et al. (2004). National conference to assess antibody-mediated rejection in solid organ transplantation. *Am J Transplant*, Vol., 4; pp. 1033–1041.

[99] Terasaki, P.; Ozawa, M. & Castro, R. (2007). Four-year follow-up of a prospective trial of HLA and MICA antibodies on kidney graft survival. *Am J Transplant*, Vol., 7; pp. 408-415.

[100] Terasaki, PI. & Ozawa, M. (2005) Predictive value of HLA antibodies and serum creatinine in chronic rejection: Results of a 2-year prospective trial. *Transplantation*, Vol., 80; pp. 1194–1197.

[101] Terasaki, PI. & Ozawa, M. (2004). Predicting kidney graft failure by HLA antibodies: a prospective trial. *Am J Transplant*, Vol., 4; pp. 438–443.

[102] Thaunat, O.; Patey, N.; Gautreau, C.; Lechaton, S.; Fremeaux-Bacchi, V.; Dieu-Nosjean, MC., et al. (2008). B cell survival in intragraft tertiary lymphoid organs after rituximab therapy. *Transplantation*, Vol., 85; pp. 1648-1653.

[103] Tinckam, KJ.; Djurdjev, O.& Magil, AB. (2005). Glomerular monocytes predict worse outcomes after acute renal allograft rejection independent of C4d status. *Kidney Int*, Vol., 68; pp. 1866–1874.

[104] Toyoda, M.; Petrosyan, A.; Pao, A. & Jordan, SC. (2004). Immunomodulatory effects of combination of pooled human gammaglobulin and rapamycin on cell proliferation and apoptosis in the mixed lymphocyte reaction. *Transplantation*, Vol., 78; pp. 1134–1138.

[105] Veale, JL.; Liang, LW.; Zhang, Q.; Gjertson, DW.; Du, Z.; Bloomquist, EW., et al. (2006). Noninvasive diagnosis of cellular and antibody-mediated rejection by perforin and granzyme B in renal allografts. *Hum Immunol*, Vol., 67; pp. 777–786.

[106] Veronese, F.; Rotman, S.; Smith, RN.; Pelle, TD.; Farrell, ML.; Kawai, T., et al. (2007). Pathological and clinical correlates of FOXP3+ cells in renal allografts during acute rejection. *Am J Transplant*, Vol., 7; pp. 914-922.

[107] Vieira, CA.; Agarwal, A.; Book, BK.; Sidner, RA.; Bearden, CM.; Gebel, HM., et al. (2004). Rituximab for reduction of anti-HLA antibodies in patients awaiting renal transplantation: 1. Safety, pharmacodynamics, and pharmacokinetics. *Transplantation*, Vol., 77; pp. 542–548.

[108] Vogelbacher, R.; Meister, S.; Gückel, E.; Starke, C.; Wittmann, S.; Stief, A., et al. (2010). Bortezomib and sirolimus inhibit the chronic active antibody-mediated rejection in experimental renal transplantation in the rat. *Nephrol Dial Transplant*, Vol., 25; pp. 3764–3773.

[109] Waiser, J.; Budde, K.; Schütz, M.; Liefeldt, L.; Rudolph, B.; Schönemann, C., et al. (2012).Comparison between bortezomib and rituximab in the treatment of antibody-mediated renal allograft rejection. *Nephrol Dial Transplant*, Vol., 27; pp. 1246-1251.

[110] Weinstein, D.; Braun, WE.; Cook, D.; McMahon, JT.; Myles, J. & Protiva, D. (2005). Ultra-late antibody-mediated rejection 30 years after a living-related renal allograft. *Am J Transplant*, Vol., 5; pp. 2576-2581.

[111] Williams, JM.; Holzknecht, ZE.; Plummer, TB.; Lin, SS.; Brunn, GJ. & Platt, JL. (2004). Acute vascular rejection and accommodation: Divergent outcomes of the humoral response to organ transplantation. *Transplantation*, Vol., 78; pp. 1471–1478.

[112] Worthington, JE.; McEwen, A.; McWilliam, LJ.; Picton, ML. & Martin, S. (2007). Association between C4d staining in renal transplant biopsies, production of donor-specific HLA antibodies, and graft outcome. *Transplantation*, Vol., 83; pp. 398-403.

[113] Worthington, JE.; Martin, S.; Al-Husseini, DM.; Dyer, PA. & Johnson, RW. (2003). Posttransplantation production of donor HLA specific antibodies as a predictor of renal transplant outcome. *Transplantation*, Vol., 75; pp. 1034–1040.

[114] Worthington, JE.; Martin, S.; Dyer, PA. & Johnson, RW. (2001). An association between posttransplant antibody production and renal transplant rejection. *Transplant Proc*, Vol., 33; pp. 475-476.

[115] Wu, GD.; Jin, YS.; Salazar, R.; Dai, WD.; Barteneva, N.; Barr, ML., et al. (2002). Vascular endothelial cell apoptosis induced by anti-donor non-MHC antibodies: a possible injury pathway contributing to chronic allograft rejection. *J Heart Lung Transplant*, Vol., 21; pp. 1174–1187.

[116] Zachary, AA.; Kopchaliiska, D.; Montgomery, RA.; Melancon, JK. & Leffell, MS. (2007). HLA-specific B cells. II. Application to transplantation. *Transplantation*, Vol., 83; pp. 989-994.

[117] Zachary, AA.; Montgomery, RA. & Leffell, MS. (2005). Factors associated with and predictive of persistence of donor-specific antibody after treatment with plasmapheresis and intravenous immunoglobulin. *Hum Immunol*, Vol., 66; pp. 364–370.

[118] Zou, Y.; Stastny, P.; Süsal, C.; Döhler, B. & Opelz, G. (2007). Antibodies against MICA antigens and kidney-transplant rejection. *N Engl J Med*, Vol., 357; pp. 1293-1300.

Chapter 20

Advances in Antibody Mediated Rejection

Siddharth Sharma, Kimberley Oliver and
David W Mudge

Additional information is available at the end of the chapter

http://dx.doi.org/10.5772/54855

1. Introduction

Kidney transplantation is considered the treatment of choice for patients with end-stage renal disease, and is associated with improved survival, better quality of life and reduced costs when compared with dialysis.[1, 2] However, the renal transplantation waiting list is forever growing, out of proportion to the number of donors.[2, 3] Therefore it is all the more crucial to develop strategies to extend the life and functionality of every allograft.

Rejection is no longer considered as a primarily T-cell-mediated process. We are fast realising that inadequate control of the humoral arm of a recipient's immune system is the pathogenic factor primarily responsible for allograft dysfunction and loss. The destructive power of anti-Human Leucocyte Antigen (HLA) alloantibodies and their association with antibody-mediated rejection (ABMR) has been demonstrated and compelling evidence exists to show that donor-specific anti-HLA antibodies (DSAs) are largely responsible for the chronic deterioration of allografts, and may be a major contributor to the entity of chronic allograft nephropathy (CAN).

ABMR must now be considered to be a spectrum of diseases; which include indolent ABMR, C4d-negative ABMR, and transplant arteriopathy— in which DSAs have significant pathological effect. Also it has been shown that arteriosclerosis is accelerated in ABMR.[4-11]

A dynamic and progressive process of injury and repair that ultimately contributes to failure of the allograft is considered the hallmark of ABMR.[12]

It has been demonstrated that glomerular endothelial swelling, subendothelial widening, and early glomerular basement membrane duplication (precursor lesions) appear in the first weeks after transplantation in a substantial number of crossmatch-positive kidney transplant recipients.[13] Thus suggesting that the process of chronic antibody-mediated changes (transplant glomerulopathy) may occur earlier than previously reported.[12, 13] In addition, DSAs can emerge at any time after transplantation and need not be present prior to transplantation.[14] Another important issue is that DSAs may differ in terms of their pathogenicity and so have varying prognosis. [14]

Currently, treatment options for ABMR are aimed at antibody reduction and the inhibition of complement activation and injury. These include plasma exchange with low-dose IVIG, high-dose IVIG and rituximab for antibody reduction, and high-dose IVIG for complement and C3 convertase inhibition and the absorption of complement activation fragments (such as C3a, C5a and C4b). Eculizumab (monoclonal anti-C5 antibody) and inhibitors of C1 are likely to show benefit in the prevention and treatment of ABMR.

Advances in B-cell-directed immunotherapeutics will have a considerable impact on DSA production, and consequently ABMR and allograft loss.

This chapter reviews the current understanding of antibody mediated rejection, and details its diagnosis, and treatments, both those established in current routine clinical practice and those on the horizon.

2. Rejection

Over the past two decades, our thinking has changed from considering rejection as a primarily T-cell-mediated process (one that is now increasingly better managed in the era of more potent calcineurin inhibitors and broader use of T-cell depleting therapies), to the realization that insufficient control of the humoral arm of a recipient's immune system by current immunosuppressive regimens is now the pathogenic factor primarily responsible for allograft dysfunction and loss.[13, 15, 16] This has changed our perception about allograft losses which were deemed to be caused by calcineurin inhibitor (CNI) toxicity and chronic allograft nephropathy (CAN).

Furthermore, the growing incidence of transplantation across HLA and ABO barriers by using desensitisation programs, but in the face of known DSAs, has led to increased incidence and a wider variety of ABMR. We are now exposed to a greater spectrum of antibody-mediated graft injury.

3. Donor Specific Antibodies (DSAs)

Great advances have occurred in solid organ transplantation since the pioneering observation of Kissmeyer et al.[17] in the 1960s, of the deleterious impact of allo-antibodies in kidney grafts. About three decades later, the team of Edmonton described rejection episodes following kidney transplantation related to the presence of anti-HLA donor specific antibodies (DSA) [18]. The presence of DSAs and positive crossmatches with donors has long been considered a contraindication to proceeding with transplantation as ABMR and graft loss is highly likely

http://dx.doi.org/10.5772/54855

to occur in such situations[4]. However, recent data by Montgomery *et al.*[19] demonstrated a significant reduction in the risk of mortality among highly sensitized patients who underwent desensitization and transplantation compared with a well-controlled group of patients who remained on dialysis. These authors concluded that desensitization followed by living-donor transplantation offered significant survival benefit and that the survival advantage more than doubled by 8 years.

In addition to DSAs existing prior to transplant, it has been realised that they can emerge at any time after transplant, thus mediating allograft injury [14]. These *de novo* DSAs are different in their pathogenicity. They are active against class II HLA and are associated with a worse prognosis than DSAs against Class I HLA [14].

DSAs can cause all types of ABMR, including chronic ABMR, otherwise known as transplant glomerulopathy.[4, 5, 7-10, 20]

4. ABMR

The pathophysiology of ABMR is not fully understood, but is an area of rapidly expanding research. Several different patterns of allograft injury have been realised. These are initiated by DSAs which bind to HLA antigens or to other targets on the allograft endothelium.

As mentioned earlier, the pathogenicity of DSAs is influenced by the isotype of the heavy chain. Therefore, if DSAs are complement activating (IgG1 and IgG3), by binding IgG and activation of C1q the classic complement pathway is rapidly activated[21] resulting in rapid loss of graft. Alternatively, DSAs can bind to endothelial cell targets and stimulate cell proliferation (NK cells) or induce antibody-dependent cell- mediated cytotoxicity (ADCC) with interferon γ release.[4, 21]

Antibodies can also bind to HLA and other targets and incompletely activate the complement system (that is, no C5b-C9 membrane attack complex generation) without causing apparent injury. This process is referred to as accommodation.[22, 23] In addition, the long-term lack of ADCC may be related to IgG Fc polymorphisms that lead to the failure of activation of NK cells through FcγR (CD16)-dependent pathways[24] thus creating a greater degree of difficulty in assessing pathogenicity of DSAs.

Protocol biopsy studies have shown that substantial oscillations occur in a patient's humoral status during the first 12 months after kidney transplantation. These oscillations are characterized by fluctuations in DSAs, C4d deposition and scores for glomerulitis and/or capillaritis in a dynamic and multidirectional fashion.[12] Hence, the new concept that allograft injury is unlikely the result of a single episode of ABMR, but instead that it represents a dynamic process of injury and repair that begins early after transplantation and continues, unabated, at varying levels thereafter.[3, 12]

The most florid form of ABMR, hyperacute rejection, has been almost completely eliminated, owing to greatly improved crossmatching techniques between recipients and prospective donors, particularly technologies such as flow-cytometry. These tests are much more sensitive for detecting a problem due to potential DSAs than older methods such as cell-dependent cytotocity (CDC). With the waning of hyperacute rejection, the different manifestations of ABMR that have emerged are indolent ABMR and C4d –negative ABMR.

4.1. Indolent ABMR

Modern therapies can efficiently reverse acute renal dysfunction from ABMR, but they usually fail to deplete antibody-secreting plasma cells from the spleen and bone marrow of allograft recipients.[25] Hence, after a clinical episode of acute ABMR, DSAs remain in circulation and cause slowly progressive microvascular abnormalities without acute compromise of graft function, at least initially. This truncated form of antibody-mediated injury is called subclinical or indolent ABMR. [26, 27]

4.2. C4d-negative disease

In 1991, Feucht and co-workers discovered peritubular capillary deposition of C4d, an inactive product of the classic complement pathway [28] in the histology of cases of ABMR. This greatly improved the understanding and diagnosis of ABMR. It was called the "footprint" of antibody mediated tissue injury. It soon became a requisite to test for C4d in all transplant allograft biopsies. However, it has been recognised over time that C4d may only be the tip of the iceberg of the humoral process and that it was neither completely specific nor sufficiently sensitive for the diagnosis of ABMR[12, 29, 30].

C4d negative ABMR usually occurs more than 12 months after transplantation, but can occur acutely in highly sensitised patients with persistent DSAs (even after desensitisation).

There have been many theories put forth to explain the presence of microvascular inflammation on biopsy and presence of DSAs in circulation, without any evidence of complement deposition. One is the technical issues related to type of fixative used and different methods of C4d detection. Another is that some DSAs are poor at fixing complement. Also, some believe the existence of a complement-independent pathway.[4] Furthermore, it is thought that as a result of treatment of high risk patients, the clinical and histological presentation of ABMR has changed.[3]

4.3. Acceleration of arteriosclerosis

This phenomenon has been recognised for many decades. It is evidenced by monocytic and lymphocytic inflammation of the intima, myofibroblast proliferation and extracellular matrix deposition causing mild to severe intimal arteritis and compromise of the lumen. It is a major component of graft rejection but thought to be cell mediated. However, in 2003 Banff criteria, the v^3 lesions have been classified to reflect probable ABMR. More and more, studies have shown that even v^1 and v^2 lesions occur in ABMR.[31]

Studies suggest that in DSA-positive patients there is significant acceleration of arteriosclerosis.[11] Pathological examination demonstrated that while there is active ABMR, the intima is

http://dx.doi.org/10.5772/54855

hypercellular, laying down new collagen over older (usually originating from donor). Once ABMR is brought under control, the myofibroblasts stop proliferating, and the intima is no longer hypercellular. What is left behind is a lesion no different from simple arteriosclerosis of aging. This is termed "transplant arteriopathy".[11, 32]
Chronic Antibody Mediated Rejection First described in 2001[33], the natural history of chronic humoral rejection is now well known.[12, 29, 34] The presence of DSAs activates the classical complement pathway causing peritubular multilamination and transplant glomerulopathy. These gradually become irreversible and cause permanent graft dysfunction. The main challenges are when to initiate treatment and how to treat it, as it may be too late to slow or halt the progress of this injury.[34, 35]

5. Pathology of antibody-mediated rejection

Antibody-mediated rejection (ABMR) was described in the early 1990s but was not incorporated into the Banff classification until 2001. Now, due to an expanding spectrum of clinical disease, two phenotypes of acute antibody-mediated rejection have been postulated and the chronic form of ABMR is recognized as a leading cause of late allograft failure. The histology of acute and chronic ABMR remains non-specific however.

5.1. Acute antibody-mediated rejection

Three patterns of tissue injury reflect acute antibody-mediated damage. These are acute tubular injury (Figure 1), inflammation of glomerular and/or peritubular capillaries (so-called microcirculation inflammation) (Figure 2 and 3), and fibrinoid necrosis of arteries (v3 lesion) (Figure 4). Microcirculation inflammation may include a TMA-like pattern as well. It is immediately obvious that all three types are not specific for ABMR and may be encountered in a variety of clinical settings in the transplanted kidney. For example, the acute tubular injury pattern is similar to that produced by ischaemia and capillaritis can be seen in the setting of acute tubular necrosis or acute cellular rejection.

For these reasons, it was recommended that histology be correlated with C4d immunomicroscopy and donor-specific antibodies (DSA) status. The former is an inactive fragment, split from its parent molecule C4b during activation of the classical complement pathway, but due to covalent binding with the endothelium, able to persist at sites of complement activation. This covalent binding can be demonstrated with immunoperoxidase or immunofluorescent (Figure 5 and 6) techniques and serves as a marker of complement activation. Neither method is sensitive enough to detect all cases of ABMR.

A positive C4d result on renal biopsy shows linear, circumferential endothelial reaction in peritubular capillaries by either method, although the immunoperoxidase signal may be less intense by one grade. Interrupted, granular deposition is considered non-specific. Diffuse and focal linear reaction in peritubular capillaries appears to correlate with glomerulitis and presensitization [36], however an important caveat is the ABO-incompatible renal allograft. In this situation, diffuse linear C4d may be seen in the absence of tissue injury and graft dysfunction.

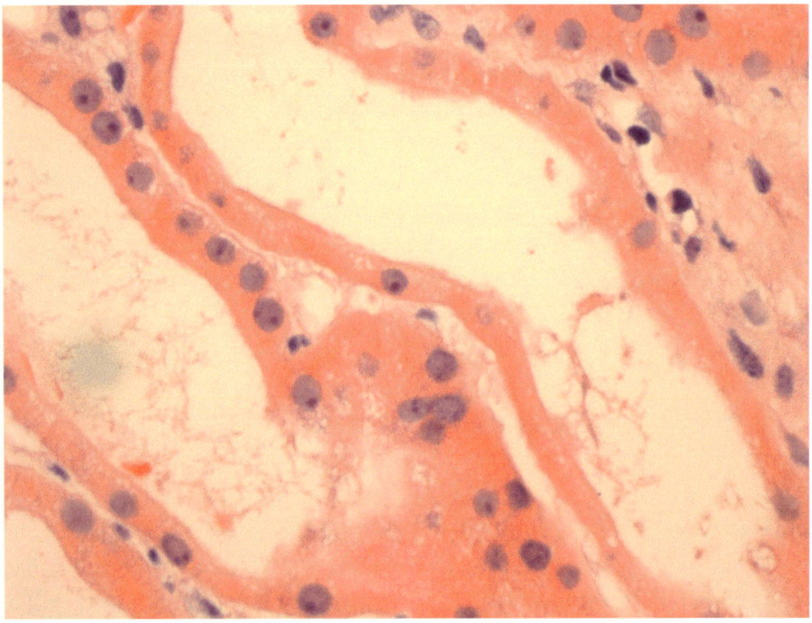

Figure 1. Acute tubular necrosis (ATN) in acute ABMR

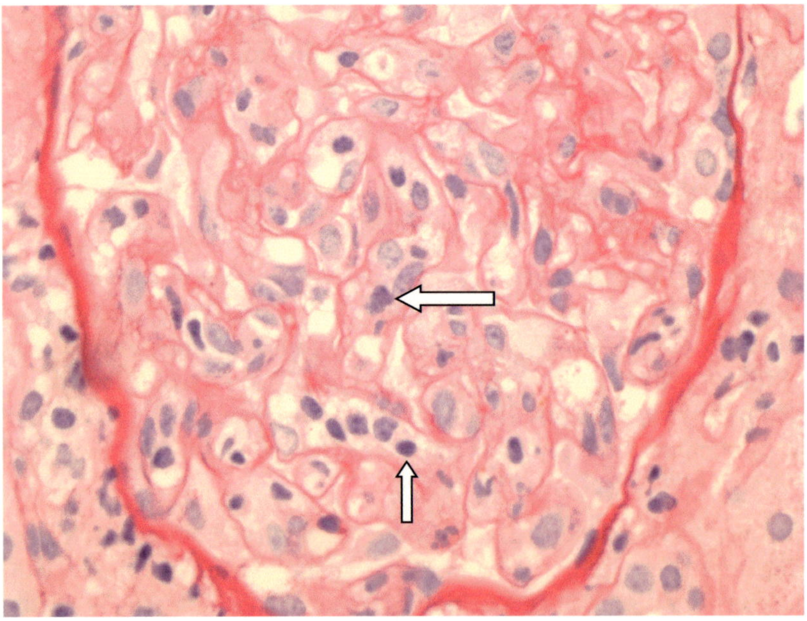

Figure 2. Glomerulitis (infiltration of capillary loops by monocytes [white arrows])

http://dx.doi.org/10.5772/54855

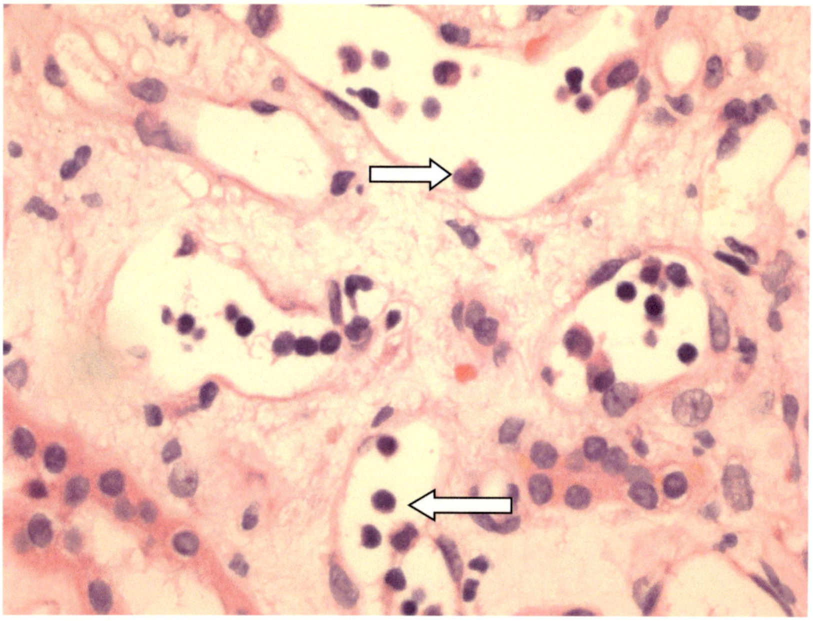

Figure 3. Peritubular Capillaritis (dilatation of capillaries and margination of monocytes [white arrows])

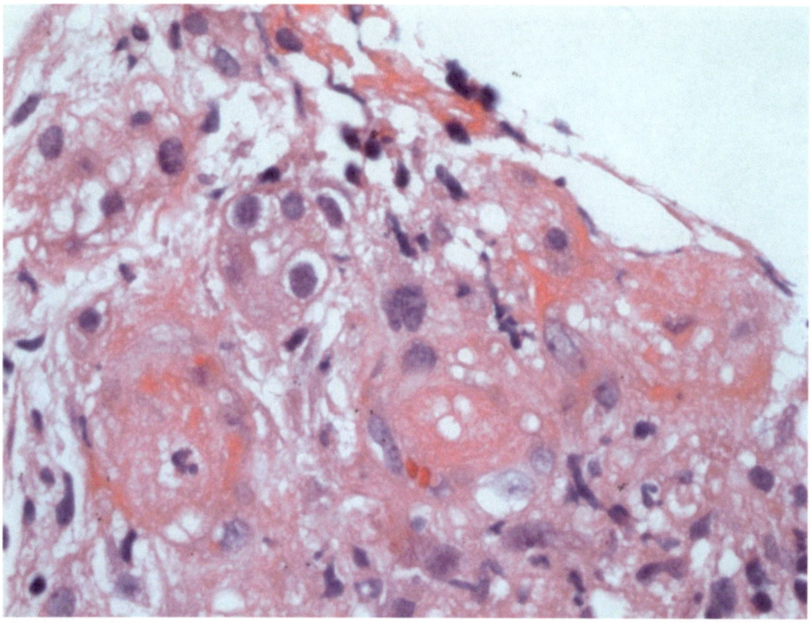

Figure 4. Fibrinoid necrosis of small arteries (v3 lesion)

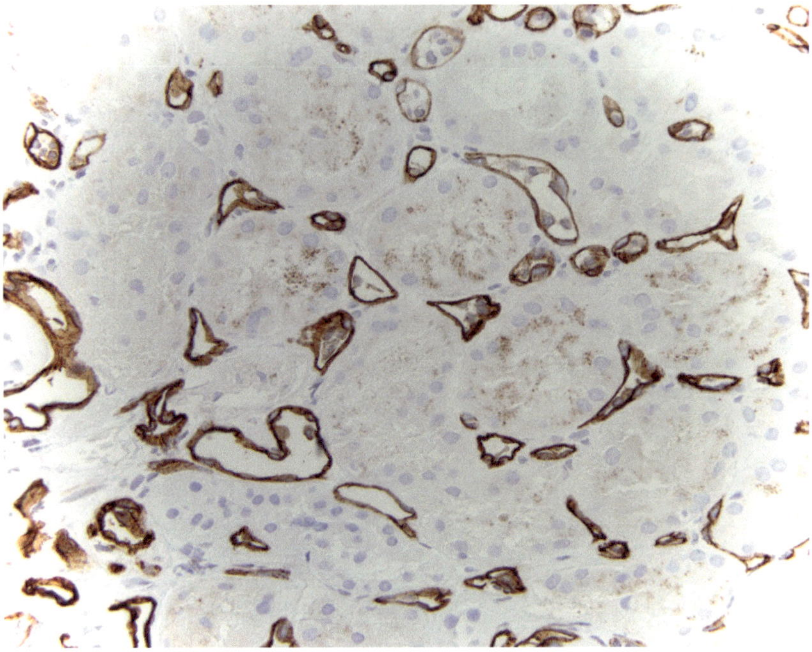

Figure 5. Diffuse C4d staining (immunoperoxidase method)

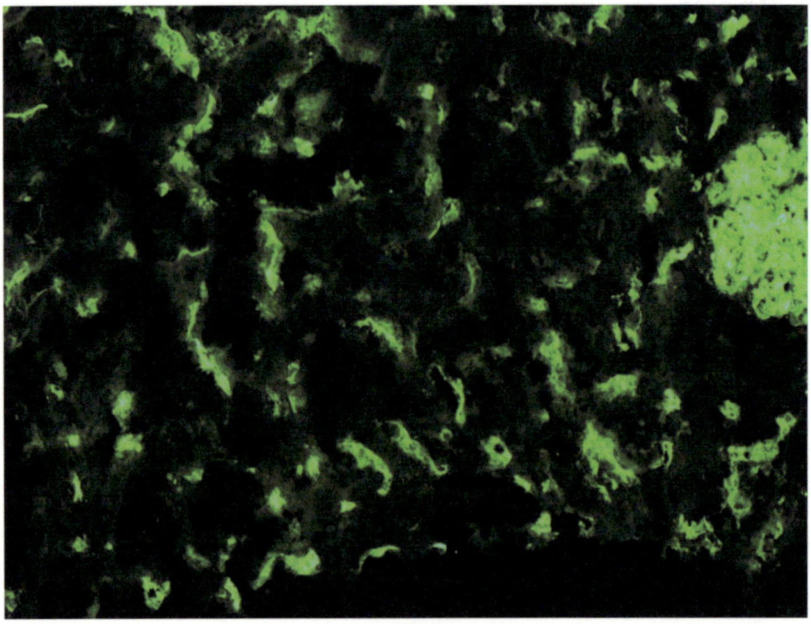

Figure 6. Diffuse C4d staining (immunofluorescence method)

The most recent Banff meeting update highlights two major phenotypes of ABMR. The first type appears early in the post-transplant period in a presensitized patient and is more likely to be C4d-positive. The second type develops late post-transplant, is due to de novo DSA development and is likely to be C4d-negative [36]. The second phenotype is an important factor in late graft loss[37]. It appears that Class II HLA molecules may be responsible and that much of the endothelial damage is mediated by NK cells and, to a lesser extent, monocytes and neutrophils (antibody-dependent cell-mediated cytotoxicity (ADCC) [38].

5.2. Chronic antibody-mediated rejection

Microcirculation Injury

The term "chronic ABMR" does not relate to a particular time post-transplantation, but rather to architectural remodelling which can affect all compartments of the biopsy. In addition, active ABMR may be superimposed on these changes. (Figure 7)

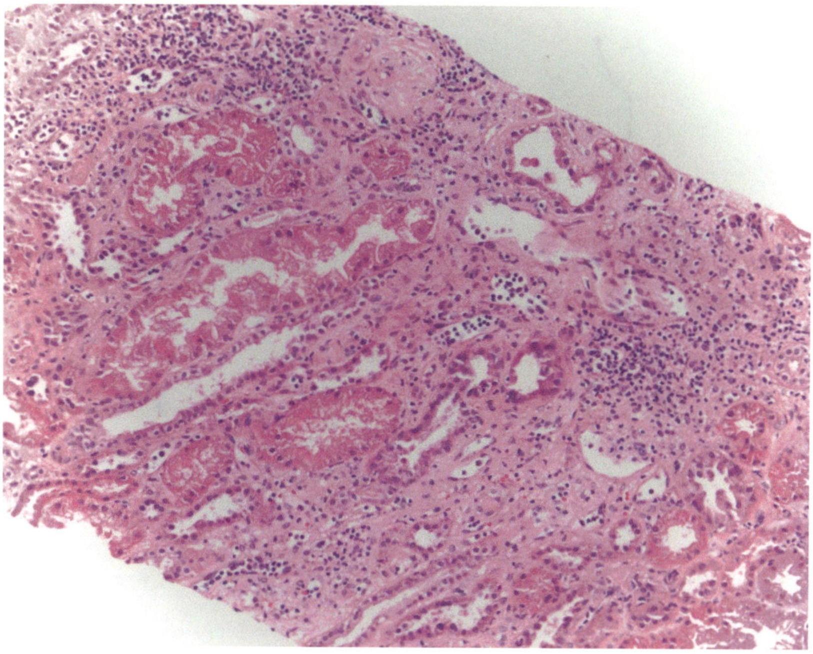

Figure 7. Active chronic ABMR. Severe peritubular capillaritis is seen in the setting of interstitial fibrosis (ci) and tubular atrophy (ct)

The hallmarks of chronic ABMR are transplant glomerulopathy (TG) and multilayering of peritubular capillary basement membranes, with or without transplant arteriopathy (TA) and interstitial fibrosis and tubular atrophy, indicating that the microcirculation is the main target of humoral attack. Transplant glomerulopathy manifests as double contours in silver-stained sections and is well demonstrated by electron microscopy (figure 8). There is widening of the subendothelial space by flocculent material and eventual duplication of the glomerular basement membrane. It has been shown in protocol biopsies that ultrastructural changes of endothelial cell injury such as cell activation and loss, can be detected within weeks of transplantation [39], pre-dating more permanent changes like mesangial matrix expansion and glomerular basement membrane duplication.

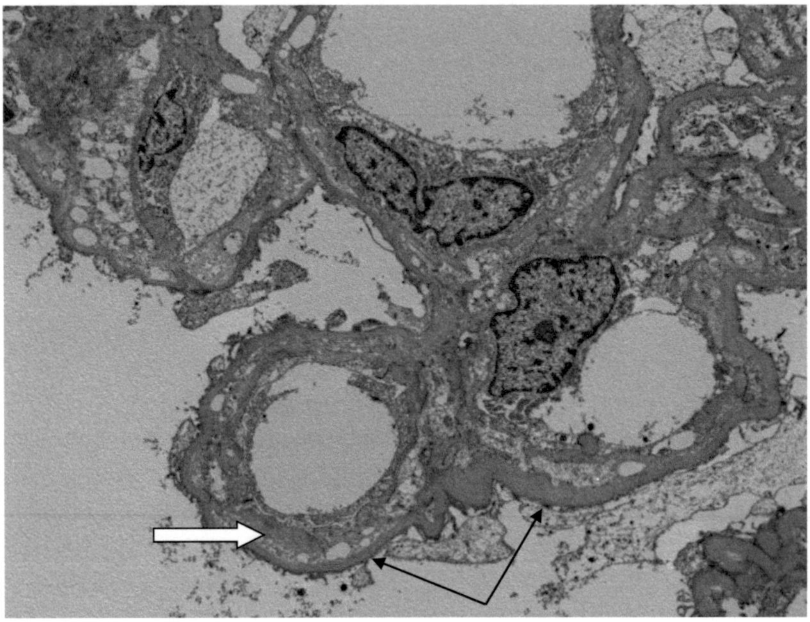

Figure 8. Electron microscopy showing a widened subendothelial space containing flocculent material (thick arrow). Duplication of the glomerular basement membrane is present (thin arrows).

Despite its close correlation with DSA, TG may not be specific for chronic ABMR, with significant numbers of TG cases reportedly due to hepatitis C and thrombotic microangiopathy [40]. Superimposed active antibody-mediated injury produces endocapillary proliferation and, together with double contour formation, a mesangiocapillary-like pattern in glomeruli (Figure 9). This is not accompanied by immunofluorescence findings typical of that type of glomerulonephritis and no diagnostic deposits are seen by electron microscopy.

The endothelium of peritubular capillaries can also display early ultrastructural evidence of damage before remodelling of the basement membrane occurs. Moderate to severe lamination (>5 layers of basement membrane) is seen in chronic ABMR whereas mild lamination (2-5 layers) may be due to causes other than antibody-mediated rejection in the transplant kidney and is also seen in native renal disease [39].

A study by Sis and co-workers [41] found that approximately 40% of cases with transplant glomerulopathy were C4d negative despite having circulating antibodies and showing high endothelial cell-associated transcript (ENDAT) expression. ENDATs represent altered gene expression due to the effects of alloantibody and are thought to be a sensitive indicator of ABMR. This same study reported a high percentage of graft loss when both antibodies and high ENDAT expression were present; graft loss was even higher when the biopsies showed diffuse C4d positivity as well. Although currently experimental, the detection of high ENDAT expression may prove useful in cases with circulation DSA and C4d-positivity on biopsy but lacking histologic evidence of tissue damage.

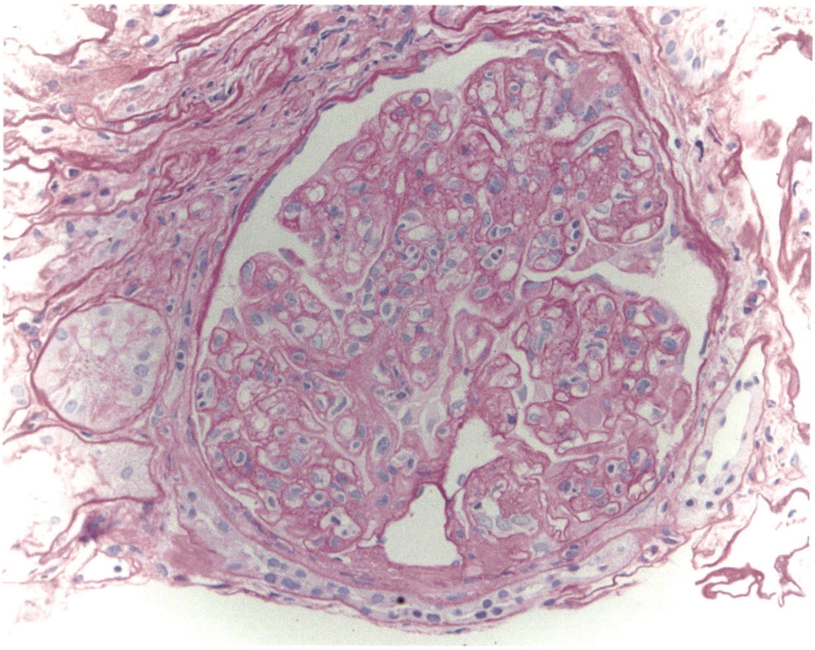

Figure 9. Active chronic ABMR. Glomerulitis is superimposed on changes of transplant glomerulopathy.

Vascular lesions

The lesion of Transplant Arteriopathy TA is characterized by expansion of the arterial intima by fibrous tissue and a variable amount of inflammation. Originally, TA was attributed to chronic T-cell mediated rejection (TCMR) but it more likely reflects generalized scarring seen in the aging kidney allograft, the causes of which include ABMR. A percentage of v1 and v2 lesions, also previously thought to be result of TCMR, may also be associated with DSA and microcirculation injury [31].

Scarring and hyalinosis

A cluster analysis of 234 indicated renal allograft biopsies by Sis and co-workers [31] revealed an association amongst arteriolar hyalinosis (ah), interstitial fibrosis (ci), tubular atrophy (ct) and transplant arteriopathy (cv). In the past, these features were thought to be the result of chronic calcineurin inhibitor use but it appears that they are non-specific and may be encountered in a variety of settings in the renal allograft, including ABMR. Arteriolar hyalinosis, in particular, is commonly encountered in the aging kidney, hypertensive nephrosclerosis and diabetic nephropathy.

6. Treatment

There has been significant development of newer and more specific therapies for ABMR. These are aimed at depleting B cells, antibodies and inhibiting complement, owing to the unique role of antibody and effector molecules in the process of ABMR. The therapeutic options include intensification of maintenance immunosuppression (e.g. tacrolimus and mycophenolate), plasmapheresis/plasma exchange, intravenous immunoglobulin (IVIg), corticosteroids and antilymphocyte antibodies. Rituximab, splenectomy, bortezomib, and eculizumab have also emerged as adjunctive or experimental therapies.

6.1. IVIg

The mechanism of action and the optimal dose of IVIg that should be administered in ABMR are poorly understood.[42], but it is thought to have an immunomodulatory effect. The proposed beneficial properties include compliment inhibition, suppression of immunoglobulin synthesis.[43, 44] High dose IVIg inhibits C3 convertase and the ability to absorb complement activation fragments (e.g. C3a,C5a and C4b).[45]

There have been retrospective studies reporting improved one year graft survival in cases of steroid and antithymocyte resistant ABMR treated with protocols incorporating IVIg and plasmapheresis/ plasma exchange.[46-49] The need to combine plasma exchange is however, unclear.[42]

6.2. Plasma exchange/plasmapheresis

Plasma exchange removes antibodies from the circulation. In the case of ABMR it is thought to be efficacious through the removal of DSAs. However, it does not suppress further production. In fact, it may stimulate rebound immunoglobulin production if used on its own. It is hence necessary to use it in conjunction with strategies which target antibody production (for example, the anti-CD20 monoclonal antibody rituximab). ABMR treatment protocols may utilise plasma exchange depending upon the antibody titre, the affinity of the antibody for the antigen, the dose of IVIg and use of other agents.[42]

6.3. Rituximab

This is a humanised mouse monoclonal antibody that targets CD20, which is expressed on the majority of B cells. However, most plasma cells lack CD20 and are unaffected by Rituximab. Hence, its role will be as an adjunctive treatment. A recent single centre study compared outcomes in 24 cases of ABMR treated with either high dose IVIg (2g/kg for four doses) versus plasmapheresis plus IVIg (100mg/kg) for four treatments followed by IVIg (2g/kg for four doses) and two doses of rituximab (375mg/m2). Improved 3-year survival (92% vs. 50%) and significantly reduced DSA at 3 months was observed in the plasmapheresis/IVIg/rituximab group.[6] It has also been seen to be effective when used as part of desensitization protocol in ABO- incompatible (ABOI) transplants, although there is concern over the cost of increased infections in recipients of such transplants. One study reported \patients who received B-cell depletion with rituximab as an induction agent had significant reductions in DSA generation and rates of chronic transplant glomerulopathy over 5 years compared with ABO-compatible low-risk transplant recipients who did not receive rituximab.[50]

6.4. Eculizumab

Drugs that inhibit compliment and C1 are likely to show benefit in the prevention and treatment of ABMR and currently they are many human trials being conducted to evaluate their effect.[3, 51]

Eculizumab is an antibody against complement protein C5, and hence, inhibits the formation of the membrane attack complex (MAC). It is approved for use in paroxysmal nocturnal hemoglobinuria (PNH) and has had promising results in treatment and ongoing management of atypical haemolytic uraemic syndrome, for which it has also recently been approved for use. It is, however, and extremely expensive therapy. A single case reported the use of eculizumab in combination with plasmapheresis/IVIg to rescue a renal allograft undergoing severe ABMR, and showed significant reduction in C5b-C9 (MAC) complex deposition in the kidney.[52]

6.5. Splenectomy

The role of splenectomy in treating ABMR is not yet known. Case reports have demonstrated that it may be useful as a rescue treatment in severe ABMR.[53] Majority of its use has been in preventing hyperacute rejection in ABOI transplants [54, 55]. There remains concern over the increased infection risk in splenectomised patients, particularly due to encapsulated organisms, and vaccination against Meningococcus and Pneumococcus is warranted where possible prior to splenectomy to mitigate this risk.

7. Conclusion

Significant progress has occurred in the understanding of ABMR. Diagnosis, classification and treatment of this process have evolved greatly. However, standardisation of diagnostic tests (DSA-testing), and development of evidence-based treatment guidelines is still lacking. Currently, protocols are individualised among different centres and based largely on anecdotal and/or local experience. ABOI and HLA desensitisation protocols (not detailed in this chapter) also need to gain excellent long term results to justify the tremendous cost involved in order to reduce the growing number of sensitised potential recipients on the waiting list. Paired donor exchange programs, although fraught with major logistic as well as some ethical and occasionally legal concerns, may be part of the solution to provide allografts to some of these difficult-to-transplant individuals in order to improve their quality and quantity of life. Such recipients, after successful transplantation, will be at increased risk of ABMR and will need good monitoring and treatment strategies to enable successful long-term outcomes.

Author details

Siddharth Sharma[1], Kimberley Oliver[2] and David W Mudge[1]

*Address all correspondence to: siddharth_sharma@health.qld.gov.au

1 University of Queensland at Princess Alexandra Hospital, Queensland, Australia

2 Department of Anatomical Pathology, Princess Alexandra Hospital, Queensland, Australia

References

[1] Evans, R.W., et al., The quality of life of patients with end-stage renal disease. N Engl J Med, 1985. 312(9): p. 553-9.

[2] Port, F.K., et al., Comparison of survival probabilities for dialysis patients vs cadaveric renal transplant recipients. JAMA, 1993. 270(11): p. 1339-43.

[3] Loupy, A., G.S. Hill, and S.C. Jordan, The impact of donor-specific anti-HLA antibodies on late kidney allograft failure. Nat Rev Nephrol, 2012. 8(6): p. 348-57.

[4] Colvin, R.B., Antibody-mediated renal allograft rejection: diagnosis and pathogenesis. J Am Soc Nephrol, 2007. 18(4): p. 1046-56.

[5] Lefaucheur, C., et al., Preexisting donor-specific HLA antibodies predict outcome in kidney transplantation. J Am Soc Nephrol, 2010. 21(8): p. 1398-406.

[6] Lefaucheur, C., et al., Comparison of combination Plasmapheresis/IVIg/anti-CD20 versus high-dose IVIg in the treatment of antibody-mediated rejection. Am J Transplant, 2009. 9(5): p. 1099-107.

[7] Solez, K., et al., Banff '05 Meeting Report: differential diagnosis of chronic allograft injury and elimination of chronic allograft nephropathy ('CAN'). Am J Transplant, 2007. 7(3): p. 518-26.

[8] Sis, B., et al., Transplant glomerulopathy, late antibody-mediated rejection and the ABCD tetrad in kidney allograft biopsies for cause. Am J Transplant, 2007. 7(7): p. 1743-52.

[9] Gloor, J.M., et al., Transplant glomerulopathy: subclinical incidence and association with alloantibody. Am J Transplant, 2007. 7(9): p. 2124-32.

[10] Solez, K., et al., Banff 07 classification of renal allograft pathology: updates and future directions. Am J Transplant, 2008. 8(4): p. 753-60.

[11] Hill, G.S., et al., Donor-specific antibodies accelerate arteriosclerosis after kidney transplantation. J Am Soc Nephrol, 2011. 22(5): p. 975-83.

[12] Loupy, A., et al., Significance of C4d Banff scores in early protocol biopsies of kidney transplant recipients with preformed donor-specific antibodies (DSA). Am J Transplant, 2011. 11(1): p. 56-65.

[13] Einecke, G., et al., Antibody-mediated microcirculation injury is the major cause of late kidney transplant failure. Am J Transplant, 2009. 9(11): p. 2520-31.

[14] Hidalgo, L.G., et al., De novo donor-specific antibody at the time of kidney transplant biopsy associates with microvascular pathology and late graft failure. Am J Transplant, 2009. 9(11): p. 2532-41.

[15] Gaston, R.S., et al., Evidence for antibody-mediated injury as a major determinant of late kidney allograft failure. Transplantation, 2010. 90(1): p. 68-74.

[16] Sellares, J., et al., Understanding the causes of kidney transplant failure: the dominant role of antibody-mediated rejection and nonadherence. Am J Transplant, 2012. 12(2): p. 388-99.

[17] Kissmeyer-Nielsen, F., et al., Hyperacute rejection of kidney allografts, associated with pre-existing humoral antibodies against donor cells. Lancet, 1966. 2(7465): p. 662-5.

[18] Halloran, P.F., et al., The significance of the anti-class I response. II. Clinical and pathologic features of renal transplants with anti-class I-like antibody. Transplantation, 1992. 53(3): p. 550-5.

[19] Montgomery, R.A., et al., Desensitization in HLA-incompatible kidney recipients and survival. N Engl J Med, 2011. 365(4): p. 318-26.

[20] Lefaucheur, C., et al., Clinical relevance of preformed HLA donor-specific antibodies in kidney transplantation. Contrib Nephrol, 2009. 162: p. 1-12.

[21] Smith, R.N. and R.B. Colvin, Chronic alloantibody mediated rejection. Semin Immunol, 2012. 24(2): p. 115-21.

[22] Jordan, S.C., M. Toyoda, and A.A. Vo, Regulation of immunity and inflammation by intravenous immunoglobulin: relevance to solid organ transplantation. Expert Rev Clin Immunol, 2011. 7(3): p. 341-8.

[23] Platt, J.L., Antibodies in transplantation. Discov Med, 2010. 10(51): p. 125-33.

[24] Jordan, S.C., et al., B-cell immunotherapeutics: emerging roles in solid organ transplantation. Curr Opin Organ Transplant, 2011. 16(4): p. 416-24.

[25] Loupy, A., et al., Combined posttransplant prophylactic IVIg/anti-CD 20/plasmapheresis in kidney recipients with preformed donor-specific antibodies: a pilot study. Transplantation, 2010. 89(11): p. 1403-10.

[26] Haas, M., et al., Subclinical acute antibody-mediated rejection in positive crossmatch renal allografts. Am J Transplant, 2007. 7(3): p. 576-85.

[27] Lerut, E., et al., Subclinical peritubular capillaritis at 3 months is associated with chronic rejection at 1 year. Transplantation, 2007. 83(11): p. 1416-22.

[28] Feucht, H.E., et al., Vascular deposition of complement-split products in kidney allografts with cell-mediated rejection. Clin Exp Immunol, 1991. 86(3): p. 464-70.

[29] Loupy, A., et al., Outcome of subclinical antibody-mediated rejection in kidney transplant recipients with preformed donor-specific antibodies. Am J Transplant, 2009. 9(11): p. 2561-70.

[30] Sis, B. and P.F. Halloran, Endothelial transcripts uncover a previously unknown phenotype: C4d-negative antibody-mediated rejection. Curr Opin Organ Transplant, 2010. 15(1): p. 42-8.

[31] Sis, B., et al., Cluster analysis of lesions in nonselected kidney transplant biopsies: microcirculation changes, tubulointerstitial inflammation and scarring. Am J Transplant, 2010. 10(2): p. 421-30.

[32] Hill, G.S., D. Nochy, and A. Loupy, Accelerated arteriosclerosis: a form of transplant arteriopathy. Curr Opin Organ Transplant, 2010. 15(1): p. 11-5.

[33] Mauiyyedi, S., et al., Chronic humoral rejection: identification of antibody-mediated chronic renal allograft rejection by C4d deposits in peritubular capillaries. J Am Soc Nephrol, 2001. 12(3): p. 574-82.

[34] Colvin, R.B., Pathology of chronic humoral rejection. Contrib Nephrol, 2009. 162: p. 75-86.

[35] Fehr, T., et al., Rituximab and intravenous immunoglobulin treatment of chronic antibody-mediated kidney allograft rejection. Transplantation, 2009. 87(12): p. 1837-41.

[36] Mengel, M., et al., Banff 2011 Meeting report: new concepts in antibody-mediated rejection. Am J Transplant, 2012. 12(3): p. 563-70.

[37] Mengel, M., et al., Phenotypes of antibody-mediated rejection in organ transplants. Transpl Int, 2012. 25(6): p. 611-22.

[38] Hidalgo, L.G., et al., NK cell transcripts and NK cells in kidney biopsies from patients with donor-specific antibodies: evidence for NK cell involvement in antibody-mediated rejection. Am J Transplant, 2010. 10(8): p. 1812-22.

[39] Wavamunno, M.D., et al., Transplant glomerulopathy: ultrastructural abnormalities occur early in longitudinal analysis of protocol biopsies. Am J Transplant, 2007. 7(12): p. 2757-68.

[40] Baid-Agrawal, S., et al., Overlapping pathways to transplant glomerulopathy: chronic humoral rejection, hepatitis C infection, and thrombotic microangiopathy. Kidney Int, 2011. 80(8): p. 879-85.

[41] Sis, B., et al., Endothelial gene expression in kidney transplants with alloantibody indicates antibody-mediated damage despite lack of C4d staining. Am J Transplant, 2009. 9(10): p. 2312-23.

[42] Takemoto, S.K., et al., National conference to assess antibody-mediated rejection in solid organ transplantation. Am J Transplant, 2004. 4(7): p. 1033-41.

[43] Reinsmoen, N.L., et al., Pretransplant donor-specific and non-specific immune parameters associated with early acute rejection. Transplantation, 2008. 85(3): p. 462-70.

[44] Vo, A.A., et al., Analysis of subcutaneous (SQ) alemtuzumab induction therapy in highly sensitized patients desensitized with IVIG and rituximab. Am J Transplant, 2008. 8(1): p. 144-9.

[45] Lai, C.H., et al., Antibody testing strategies for deceased donor kidney transplantation after immunomodulatory therapy. Transplantation, 2011. 92(1): p. 48-53.

[46] Glotz, D., et al., Suppression of HLA-specific alloantibodies by high-dose intravenous immunoglobulins (IVIg). A potential tool for transplantation of immunized patients. Transplantation, 1993. 56(2): p. 335-7.

[47] Rocha, P.N., et al., Beneficial effect of plasmapheresis and intravenous immunoglobulin on renal allograft survival of patients with acute humoral rejection. Transplantation, 2003. 75(9): p. 1490-5.

[48] Tyan, D.B., et al., Intravenous immunoglobulin suppression of HLA alloantibody in highly sensitized transplant candidates and transplantation with a histoincompatible organ. Transplantation, 1994. 57(4): p. 553-62.

[49] Montgomery, R.A., et al., Plasmapheresis and intravenous immune globulin provides effective rescue therapy for refractory humoral rejection and allows kidneys to be successfully transplanted into cross-match-positive recipients. Transplantation, 2000. 70(6): p. 887-95.

[50] Kohei, N., et al., Chronic antibody-mediated rejection is reduced by targeting B-cell immunity during an introductory period. Am J Transplant, 2012. 12(2): p. 469-76.

[51] Stegall, M.D., et al., Terminal complement inhibition decreases antibody-mediated rejection in sensitized renal transplant recipients. Am J Transplant, 2011. 11(11): p. 2405-13.

[52] Locke, J.E., et al., The use of antibody to complement protein C5 for salvage treatment of severe antibody-mediated rejection. Am J Transplant, 2009. 9(1): p. 231-5.

[53] Locke, J.E., et al., The utility of splenectomy as rescue treatment for severe acute antibody mediated rejection. Am J Transplant, 2007. 7(4): p. 842-6.

[54] Alexandre, G.P., et al., Human ABO-incompatible living donor renal homografts. Neth J Med, 1985. 28(6): p. 231-4.

[55] Alexandre, G.P., et al., Present experiences in a series of 26 ABO-incompatible living donor renal allografts. Transplant Proc, 1987. 19(6): p. 4538-42.

Chapter 21

Tolerance in Renal Transplantation

Marco Antonio Ayala-García, Beatriz González Yebra,
Éctor Jaime Ramirez Barba and Eduardo Guaní Guerra

Additional information is available at the end of the chapter

http://dx.doi.org/10.5772/54734

1. Introduction

Tolerance in human transplantation can be defined in two ways [1]. Clinical tolerance (also referred to as clinical operational tolerance [2]) is the survival of a foreign organ or tissue (allogeneic or xenogeneic) in a normal recipient in the absence of immunosuppression [1]. Immune tolerance is the absence of a detectable immune response against a functional organ or tissue in the absence of immunosuppression [1].

Early evidence demonstrating that adult mice could be tolerant of skin grafts after the induction of neonatal tolerance by the introduction of splenocytes intraperitoneally was shown by Brent and Medawar, in 1953 [3]. The central role of the thymus in mediating cellular immunity and graft rejection was established by JFAP Miller, who showed that nude mice tolerated skin allografts because of a marked deficiency of lymphocytes [4]. Conversely, there have been recent studies that show that spleen transplantation in pigs or dogs has a tolerogenic effect on renal transplantation [5, 6]. On the basis of the promising results obtained in these animal models, several tolerogenic protocols have been attempted in humans, but most have failed to achieve robust and stable tolerance after renal transplantation. This is due to that the transplantation immunobiology is very complex, because of the involvement of several components such as antibodies, antigen presenting cells, helper and cytotoxic T cell subsets, immune cell, surface molecules, signaling mechanisms and cytokines; which play a role in the alloimmune response.

2. The alloimmune response

The allogeneic immune response has largely been attributed to the recognition of donor antigens, presented in the context of human leukocyte antigen (HLA) molecules to T cells, which in turn direct a huge array of cellular and humoral responses, causing tissular damage and graft rejection. This type of response is mediated by the adaptative branch of the immune system [7].

The immune system can be divided in two components, the innate and adaptative immunity. The innate immunity, refers to a nonspecific response that involves the recruitment of diverse components of the immune system such as, macrophages, neutrophils, natural killer cells (NK cells), cytokines, several cellular receptors, complement components, cytokines, Toll-like receptors (TLRs), and antimicrobial peptides (AMP's). The adaptative immunity, which involves recognition of specific antigen, conferring both specificity and a memory effect [8]. Data suggest that initial allograft injury (such as ischemia) may initiate an innate immune response (Figure 1A), thus contributing to acute and chronic allograft rejection. Furthermore, this inflammatory response may initiate and expand the adaptive immune response to the point where the different HLA antigens come into play for the first time [9]. Some immunologist choose not to divide the alloimmune response in adaptative and innate branches; nevertheless, they are closely related and dependent on each other.

The main and strongest responses to alloantigens are mediated by host T cells, which recognize peptide antigens presented by antigen presenting cells (APCs) in the context of HLA. The phenomenon by which the recipient immune system reacts with donor antigens that are considered to be "non-self" is called allorecognition. Foreign or donor antigen presentation to T cells may occur by either direct or indirect pathways [10] (Figure 2A).

2.1. Direct allorecogniton pathway

The direct allorecognition pathway involves recognition of intact donor HLA molecules on the donor cells, usually APCs. This seems to contradict the classic self-HLA restriction property of T cells, since the peptide being recognized is presented in a non-self HLA, and to date, two models have been proposed to explain this discrepancy [11].

The "high determinant density" model proposes that the transplanted organ carries a variable number of passenger APCs in the form of interstitial dendritic cells (DCs). Such APCs have a high density of allo-HLA molecules and are capable of directly stimulating the recipient's T cells. Given the very high ligand density, the affinity of alloreactive T cell receptors required to generate an optimal alloimmune response can be significantly lower compared to that required for self-HLA peptide complex [12].

In the "multiple binary complex" model, peptides derived from endogenous proteins that are bound into the groove of donor HLA molecules play a role. These peptides are derived from the same normal cellular proteins that are present even in the recipient. However, the differences in the allo-HLA groove causes a different set of peptides to be presented from homologous proteins. These peptides can be recognized by the recipient T cells. Therefore, even a single HLA mismatch between the donor and the recipient would be able to stimulate a large number of alloreactive T cells [13].

This pathway is thought to be the dominant pathway involved in the early alloimmune response (acute graft rejection), as the relative number of T cells that proliferate on contact with allogeneic or donor cells is extraordinarily high compared with the number of clones that target antigen presented by self-APCs [14].

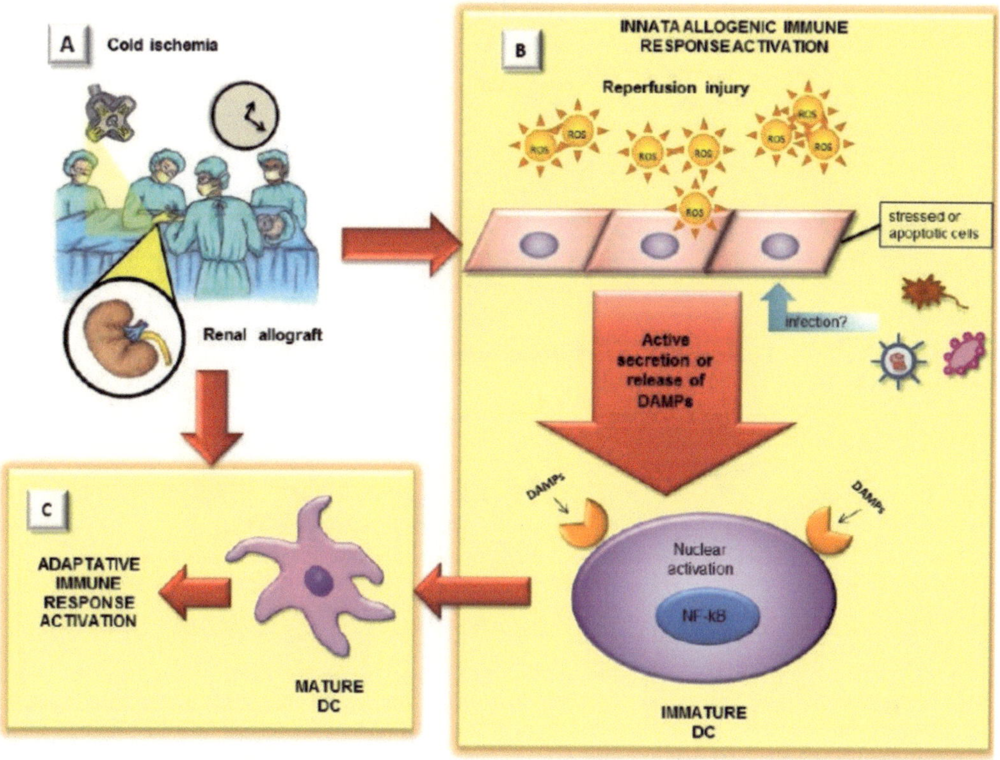

Figure 1. The alloimmune response: (A) ischemia may initiate an innate immune response, (B) which contributes to acute and chronic allograft rejection. The initial allograft injury, during reperfusion, is associated with generation of DAMPs for maturation of donor-derived and recipient-derived dendritic cells, (C) which represents the bridge to the development of an adaptive alloimmune response that results in rejection. Abbreviations: DAMPs, Damage-Associated Molecular Patterns; NF- κβ, Nuclear Factor- кappa beta; DC, Dendritic Cell.

2.2. Indirect allorecognition pathway

In the indirect pathway, T cells recognize processed alloantigen presented as peptides by self-APCs (host-APCs) [11]. The basic premise for indirect allorecognition as a mechanism involved in allograft rejection is shedding of donor HLA molecules from the graft. These HLA molecules are then taken up by recipient APCs and presented to CD4+ T cells. Interestingly, there is also evidence that demonstrates that recipient DCs can acquire and process intact donor HLA molecules from donor cell debris and stimulate CD8+ T cells by cross priming. Therefore, both CD4+ and CD8+ T cells mediate indirect allorecognition [11]. The indirect pathway is postulated to play a dominant role in chronic allograft rejection [15].

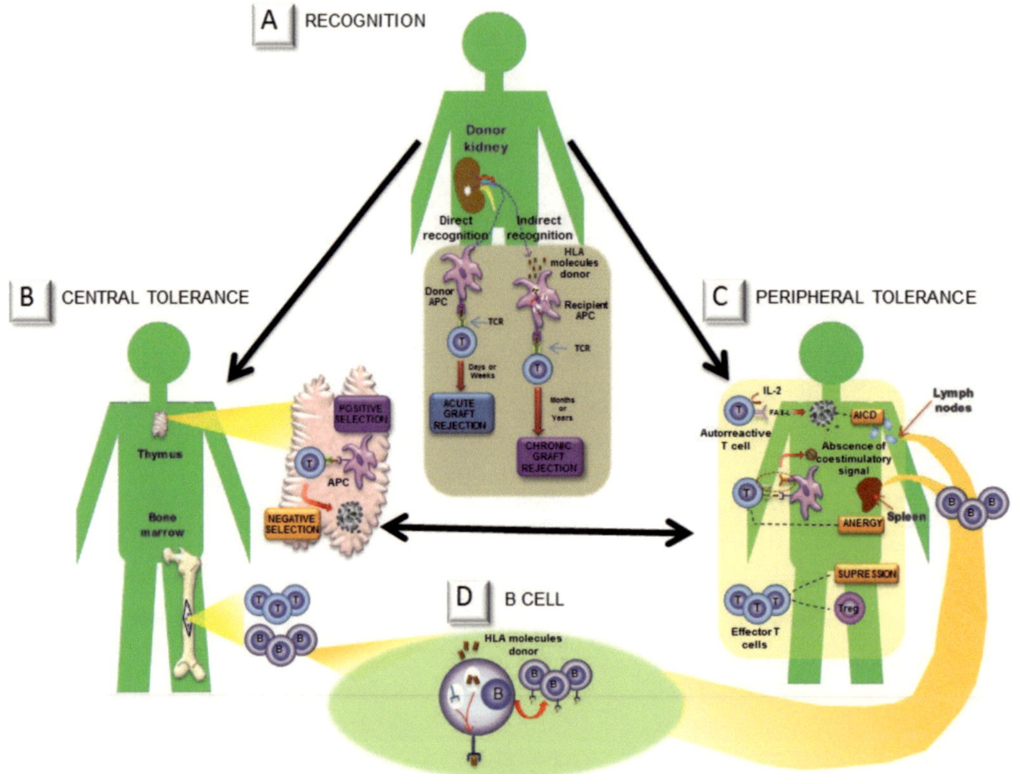

Figure 2. A). Allorecognition process. Two pathways lead to T-cell activation, the direct pathway and the indirect pathway. The mechanisms of tolerance are: (B) Central tolerance in which T cells migrate from the bone marrow to the thymus where they are educated, such that those recognizing self-antigens are deleted, and (C) Peripheral mechanisms of tolerance for self-reactive T cells including AICD, anergy, and suppression by T_{reg}. (D) B-cell awaiting the proper stimulus of a T-cell to initiate the production of alloantibodies. Two possible scenarios ensure tolerance: deletion of these self-reactive B cells and receptor editing, which is a process by which a new receptor with altered specificity is generated through another sequence of B cell receptor gene rearrangements. Abbreviations: HLA, Human Leukocyte Antigen; APC, Antigen Presenting Cells; TCR, T-cell Receptor; T, T-cell; T reg, regulatory T cells; B, B-cell; IL-2; Interleukin-2; AICD, Activation-Induced Cell Death.

2.3. Other allorecognition pathways

A third mode of allorecognition, which Lechler's group has termed the "semi-direct" pathway, has been recently proposed [16]. This model is based on the transfer of intact HLA molecules between cells. DCs have been shown to acquire intact HLA class I and II molecules from exosomes secreted by other DCs and to prime both naïve CD8+ and CD4+ T cells, thereby inducing an alloimmune response [17,18].

Another mechanism of allorecognition involves NK cells. NK cells may recognize HLA classical and non-classical type I molecules through interactions with cell surface receptors called killer cell immunoglobulin-like receptors (KIR, formerly named killer inhibitory receptors) that recognize classical HLA class I molecules [19] and CD94/NKG2 receptors that recognize non-classical HLA class I molecules. Currently, the role of NK cell-mediated cytotoxicity in allograft rejection remains controversial, but recent data shows that NK cells are potent alloreactive cells when fully activated with IL-15 and can mediate potent acute skin rejection, at least in a murine model [20]. While reports continue to provide evidence supporting a role for NK cells in promoting rejection, there are a growing number of studies that illustrate an alternative role for NK cells in promoting allograft survival and tolerance [21].

2.4. Activation of T cells

Through their specific antigen receptors, T cells are capable of recognizing external antigens and initiating immune responses. These reactions may be characterized predominantly by cell-mediated reactions in which effector immune cells play a major role; or by humoral reactions in which the stimulation of B cells (Figure 2D) may induce antibody responses. The T cells orchestrate both the initiation and the propagation of immune responses, largely through the secretion of protein mediators termed cytokines and chemokines. Moreover, recent findings suggest that a novel subtype of T cells, named regulatory T cells, have an important role in achieving allograft tolerance [22]. These facts make T cells important targets for immunosuppresive therapy and tolerance induction protocols.

T cells require two separate signals before activation occurs. The first signal is antigen specific and is provided by the interaction of a T cell receptor (TCR) with a peptide antigen presented within the antigen binding groove of HLA molecules on the surface of APCs (Figure 2A). These are HLA class I molecules in the case of CD8+ T cells and class II molecules in the case of CD4+ T cells. The second, costimulatory, signal is provided by the interaction of T cell surface molecules with their ligands on APCs, being the most important the B7[1]-CD28 and CD40-CD154 interactions. The first signal in the absence of the second signal may lead to T cell inactivation, anergy, or failure of a Th1 (T helper cell-1) response with a switch to a Th2 (T helper cell-2) response [23].

The Th1/Th2 response refers to the pattern of cytokines produced by T helper cells. Th1 cells produce interleukin-12 (IL-12) and interferon gamma (IFN-gamma) inducing macrophage activation leading to delayed-type hypersensitivity responses. The Th1 response has been implicated in acute allograft rejection. Th2 cells produce IL-4, IL-5, IL-10, and IL-13, and provide help for B cell function [24]. IL-4 is a growth factor for B cells and antibody production, and also can directly inhibit T cell maturation along the Th1 pathway [25]. Such responses have been associated with allograft tolerance, but are mainly implicated in clearing parasitic infections and the presentation of allergic diseases.

Once the binding of CD4/CD8 co-receptors stabilizes the immunologic synapse between the T cell and the APC, tyrosine-based activation motifs on the CD3 complex leads to the phosphorylation of a series of intracellular proteins, resulting in the activation of a variety of enzymes including calcineurin, and the activation of transcription factors, such as nuclear factor of activated T cells (NFAT) and NF-κβ, permitting the transcription of different genes,

1 B7-1 (or CD80) and B7-2 (or CD86).

including HLA class I and IL-2 [26]. There are other important events implicated in the activation of T cells, including leukocyte migration and the interaction of chemokines with their receptors.

3. Transplantation tolerance

The alloimmune response can be divided into central and peripheral tolerance, according to the mechanisms that induce a tolerance state. These are related and not exclusive [27] (Figure 2).

3.1. Central tolerance

Central tolerance is the most important means by which T and B autoreactive lymphocytes are eliminated in a process termed clonal deletion. T and B cells mature and are educated in the thymus and the bone marrow, respectively (Figure 2B).

Immature T lineage cells emerge from hematopoietic progenitors in the bone marrow and enter the thymus without expressing either the TCR or coreceptors. Since they lack CD4 and CD8 antigens, these cells are called double-negative (DN) cells or thymocytes. T cell selection begins after DN cells have undergone a TCR-mediated rearrangement process and up-regulated both CD4 and CD8 antigens, thus becoming double-positive (DP) cells [28]. From here, the thymocyte's fate is determined by the nature of its interaction with self-peptides that are presented on the self-HLA molecules of thymic stromal cells. This process is called "the affinity-avidity model". If a T cell reacts too strongly with self-antigens presented on bone marrow–derived APCs, it is eliminated by apoptosis or negative selection in the thymus [29]. Thymocytes with TCRs that interact with self HLA/peptides with lesser avidity, are positively selected and evolve into mature T cells that express either the CD4 or CD8 receptor (single positive T cells). The cells with very low avidity interactions fail to induce survival signals and die within the thymus. At the end of the process, only 3% of the total number of $CD4^{+}CD8^{+}$ DP cells are exported from the thymus, having developed into single positive $CD4^{+}$ or $CD8^{+}$ cells [30].

Currently, it is not completely understood how many peripheral tissue-specific antigens are expressed and presented in the thymus to ensure central T-cell tolerance to antigens that will be encountered in the periphery eventually. The expression of peripheral proteins in the thymus (such as insulin, thyroglobulin, and renal autoantigens) is driven in part by a gene called AIRE (autoimmune regulator). Mutations in the AIRE gene result in a disease known as autoimmune polyglandular syndrome type I. Interestingly, only certain organs and systems are involved, and within these, only particular parts of the organ tend to be affected, confirming that additional mechanisms must be involved to maintain systemic tolerance [31].

B cells undergo a similar process, as they are tested for reactivity to self-antigens before they enter the periphery. Immature B cells, developing in the bone marrow, test antigen through their antigen receptor, a surface IgM called the B cell receptor (BCR). If signaling through the BCR is sufficiently weak, immature B cells can be rendered permanently unresponsive or anergic. However, if immature B cells are strongly self-reactive, there are two possible scenarios to ensure tolerance. The first is deletion of these self-reactive B cells. The second is receptor editing, a process by which a new receptor with altered specificity is generated through another sequence of B cell receptor gene rearrangements [32].

3.2. Peripheral tolerance

Besides the deletion process of autoreactive cells occurring during central tolerance, some T or B cells with self-reactivity may escape from the thymus or bone marrow, making the loss of self-tolerance easier. However, several mechanisms, collectively named peripheral tolerance, can control or eliminate such cells. Peripheral tolerance involves deletion and apoptosis, anergy, and regulation or suppression (Figure 2C).

3.2.1. Deletion and apoptosis

This mechanism is used to eliminate activated T cells specific for self-antigen. The programmed cell death, or apoptosis, is also termed activation-induced cell death (AICD). This process is mediated by the interaction of Fas (CD95) with its ligand (Fas-L or CD95L) on T cells, and can occur in developing thymocytes as well as mature T cells [33]. IL-2 can activate the STAT 5 signaling pathway through the IL-2 receptor (IL-2R), which in turn potentiates the up-regulation of Fas-L and the down-regulation of Bcl2 expression on T cells, thus promoting AICD. Conversely, IL-15 acts as a growth and survival factor for T cells [34, 35]. Since augmented AICD can induce tolerance through elimination of populations of reactive lymphocytes [36], certain tolerogenic models which use IL-15 antagonists and IL-2 agonists during transplantation havere-sulted in donor-specific tolerance [37]. Further research on this topic is needed before considering this peripheral mechanism as a therapeutic approach.

3.2.2. Anergy

The hyporesponsiveness of T or B cells to further antigenic stimulation, also called anergy, is a process that can result from antigenic stimulation in the absence of costimulation. In the case of T cells, complete activation requires the presentation of peptide on the HLA molecule to the TCR (first signal), and costimulatory signals, such as the B7-CD28 and CD40-CD154 interactions (second signal). The second signal is required to induce the multiple pathways that will lead to the activation of IL-2 gene transcription, ultimately inducing T cell activation and proliferation. However, it has been shown that IL-2 production and subsequent signaling through its receptor, IL-2R, is necessary for T cells to escape anergy, since blocking IL-2/IL-2R engagement even after stimulation through the TCR and CD28 still results in induction of T cell anergy [38].

As with T cell activation, B cell activation requires two signals. In this context, naïve B cells can be anergized if their surface immunoglobulins bind to self-antigens (first signal) in the absence of the additional necessary T cell signals (second or costimulatory signal) [39].

3.2.3. Regulation or suppression

A third mechanism of peripheral tolerance is regulation or suppression of immune responses to self or foreign antigens. Perhaps, the regulatory T cells (Treg cells) are the most important and well documented effectors of this mechanism to date. These cells control the type and magnitude of the immune response to foreign antigen to ensure that the host remains undamaged. Treg cells are also integral to maintaining a lack of response to self-antigens or tolerance [40].

There are two subsets of Treg cells."Natural" Treg cells, are a thymus-derived population that constitute about 10% of the CD4 population. Natural Treg cells express CD4, CD25, CTLA4, and GITR on their surface [41], and express transcription factor Foxp3 intracellularly [42]. The importance of Foxp3 as the orchestrator of the molecular programs involved in mediating Treg function has been highlighted by diseases such as IPEX syndrome (immune dysfunction, polyendocrinopathy, enteropathy and X-linked inheritance), in which a mutation in the Foxp3 gene has been described [43].

The other subset of T_{reg} cells, commonly termed "adaptative" T_{reg} cells, develops in the periphery, in a thymic-independent manner, following antigen encounter under particular circumstances, namely exposure to transforming growth factor-β (TGF-β). This leads to the expression of Foxp3; the hallmark of T_{reg} cells [44]. Data suggesting the role of these cells in immunologic tolerance has been obtained from different studies in which patients with normal graft function reportedly possess a smaller T_{reg} population compared with patients having chronic allograft rejection, suggesting that T_{reg} cells may prevent damage and graft loss [45]. Other groups have shown that certain immunosuppressive protocols are more permissive than others in generating these populations [46].

The mechanisms by which Treg cells exert their effects are not completely understood. There have been two main mechanisms proposed. One mechanism requires cell contact between CD4+CD25+ Treg and responder cells and interaction between CTLA-4 and GITR molecules [47], while the other mechanism involves the induction of suppression or regulation by newly generated suppressor T cells in a cytokine-dependent manner through IL-10 and/or TGF β [48, 49]. Although promising, there is still too much to learn, before using this subset of cells for tolerance induction in renal transplantation.

In addition to T_{reg} cells, there are other cell phenotypes with regulatory properties, such as $CD8^+$ T cells and certain NK populations [50]. $CD8^+$ T cells with regulatory/suppressive properties have been named "veto cells". Such cells maintain peripheral tolerance by attacking alloreactive T cells which are present in bone marrow with increased frequency, and may be responsible in part for the reduction in graft versus host disease and the induction of chimerism seen in some bone marrow transplant models [51].

4. Tolerogenic strategies in renal transplantation

Tolerance in renal transplantation is an exceptional finding. Approximately 100 cases of tolerance in renal transplantation have been reported to date, mainly in patients who were not compliant with their immunosuppressive regimens or in individuals who had previously received a bone marrow transplant for hematological disorders [52]. At the present time, in looking for tolerance in renal transplantation, physicians in clinical practice have implemented protocols and surgical procedures in which tolerance was the planned objective before the transplant.

4.1. Strategies and protocols

Protocols in which tolerance in renal transplantation was the planned objective before the transplant may be divided into three subgroups, namely molecule-based, cell-based, and total lymphoid irradiation.

4.1.1. Molecule-based protocols

The molecule-based group includes all cases in which the induction of tolerance was attempted through administration of presumed tolerogenic drugs. These tolerogenic drugs include polyclonal antithymocyte globulin antibodies and anti-CD25 monoclonal antibodies. Anti-CD25 monoclonal antibodies competitively inhibit IL-2R-dependent T cell activation, while the polyclonal antithymocyte globulin antibodies are directed against lymphocyte antigens. The goal of the induction treatment was the nonspecific removal of clones of immune cells responsible for rejection before contact with foreign donor antigens occured. Once the donor antigens were in place after implantation of the new kidney, repletion of immune cells occured, favored by the homeostatic expansion triggered by leukocyte depletion. In addition, minimization of maintenance immunosuppression was implemented to further reduce the anti donor response with just enough treatment to prevent irreversible immune damage to the graft, but not with such heavy treatment that the donor specific clonal exhaustion-deletion process was precluded [53].

4.1.2. Cell-based protocols

In the cell-based group, patients received a donor-cell infusion of highly enriched CD34+ hematopoietic progenitor cells mixed with CD3+ T cells, [54] ie, patients received heavy conditioning regimens in association with the perioperative infusion of immunomodulatory cells, such as transplant-acceptance inducing cells. Afterward, maintenance immunosuppression was given for a few months until complete withdrawal, when possible. Overall, although these trials demonstrated that the infusion of transplant-acceptance inducing cells is feasible, major concerns remain regarding the efficacy and safety of such an approach. Whether this approach confers any benefit in the establishment of minimal immunosuppression in renal transplantation patients when compared with the protocols currently in use is unclear. Lastly, the optimal dose and timing of cell infusions, along with the most appropriate concomitant immunosuppression regimen, remains to be determined [55,56].

Patients who received renal transplantation after bone marrow transplantation from the same donor are also included in this group. Bone marrow transplantation, when successful, generally results in the total replacement of the recipient's bone marrow with the donor's bone marrow hematopoietic cells, a condition referred to as full chimerism [57]. Experimental data have confirmed that the infusion of donor-derived bone marrow cells can prolong allograft survival by still incompletely understood mechanisms [58]. However, the translation of this model from animals to humans has remained a very challenging task. In particular, an immunosuppression-free state has been achieved only sporadically after living-related donor renal transplantation, whereas similar findings have never been documented after deceased donor renal transplantation [57,59–63]. In some studies, the perioperative infusion of donor bone marrow seems to reduce the incidence of acute and chronic rejection, [57,60,61] and to improve graft function when infused not only systemically but also intrathymically [62,63].

4.1.3. Total lymphoid irradiation protocols

Total lymphoid irradiation was originally developed as a nonmyeloablative treatment for Hodgkin disease [64]. This treatment modality was first used about 40 years ago to induce prolonged renal allograft survival. However, total lymphoid irradiation has significant short- and long-term effects on lymphocyte subpopulations through suppression of activated T cells and the IL-2 pathway. Importantly, as the doses of radiation required for total lymphoid irradiation to be effective are high, with 10 doses of total lymphoid irradiation (80 to 120 cGy) targeted to the lymph nodes, spleen, and thymus, [54] its clinical application is limited by the toxicity that occurs with such high doses. With the advent of more effective immunosuppressive drugs and cytolytic therapy with antithymocyte globulin and monoclonal antibodies, the use of total lymphoid irradiation has declined considerably and is mainly applied, as stated earlier, as a nonmyeloablative preparative regimen of total lymphoid irradiation in combination with the infusion of donor-derived cells to induce a state of lymphohematopoietic chimerism [65-71].

4.2. Surgical procedures

Currently, Japan has a serious shortage of cadaveric organs. As a result ABO incompatible living kidney transplantation is being performed [72–76].

Between 2001 and 2004, the ABO-incompatible living kidney transplantation procedure used a 1-week pretransplant immunosuppression with tacrolimus/mycophenolate mofetil/methylprednisolon. During this period, splenectomy was performed in all cases and the short–term outcome was excellent [77]. Graft survival was 93.5% at three years and 91.3% at five years in these patients [78].

The spleen is involved in the production of B lymphocytes and IgM, so splenectomy can result in decreased antibody content and increased tolerance [79]. This effect could be considered analogous to the effect of rituximab (anti-CD20+ monoclonal antibody), [80,81] which prevents acute rejection mediated by antibodies, resulting in a tolerogenic effect. Conversely, recent studies show the important role of the spleen for the induction and maintenance of regulatory CD4+CD25+ T cells, which are important for self-tolerance [82,83]. This immune regulatory mechanism is known as non-specific suppression of acti-

http://dx.doi.org/10.5772/54734

vation and differentiation, and is the result of the release of anti-inflammatory cytokines [84,85]. Therefore, upon splenectomy, the activity of regulatory T cells is presumably affected, and this may simulate the mechanisms of action of some currently used immunosuppressant drugs, such as basiliximab and daclizumab (chimeric monoclonal antibodies that selectively affect T lymphocytes) [86].

5. Conclusion

Despite advances in understanding the cellular and molecular mechanisms of the alloimmune response, tolerance induction in renal transplantation remains an important clinical challenge. In clinical practice, prevention of graft rejections has combined tolerance mechanisms, such as suppression of activated T cells, inhibition the IL-2 pathway, decreased antibody production, and t chimerism. However, no completely satisfactory results have been achieved. The reason for these seemingly insurmountable challenges stems from the properties of the alloimmune response, which are not yet completely understood.

Acknowledgements

We thank Andrea Liliana López Flores, University of Guanajuato; for the preparation of drawings and we to thank Daniel Tafoya Arellano, University Quetzalcoatl of Irapuato; to help carry out this chapter.

Author details

Marco Antonio Ayala-García[1], Beatriz González Yebra[2], Éctor Jaime Ramirez Barba[3] and Eduardo Guaní Guerra[4]

*Address all correspondence to: eduardoguani@yahoo.com.mx

1 Hospital Regional de Alta Especialidad del Bajío and HGSZ No. 10 del Instituto Mexicano del Seguro Social Delegación Guanajuato, México

2 Hospital Regional de Alta Especialidad del Bajío and Department of Molecular Biology, University of Guanajuato, México

3 University of Guanajuato, México

4 Hospital Regional de Alta Especialidad del Bajío, México

References

[1] Rossini AA, Greiner DL, Mordes JP. Induction of immunologic tolerance for transplantation. Physiological Reviews 1999;79(1) 99-141.

[2] Ashton-Chess J, Giral M, Brouard S, et al. Spontaneous operational tolerance after immunosuppressive drug withdrawal in clinical renal allotransplantation. Transplantation 2007; 84(10) 1215–1219.

[3] Billingham RE, Brent L, Medawar PB. Activity acquired tolerance of foreign cells. Nature 1953; 172(4379) 603-606.

[4] Miller JFAP. Effect of neonatal thymectomy on the immunological responsiveness of the mouse. Proc R Soc Series B 1962; 156(964) 415-428.

[5] Dor FJ, Tseng YL, Kuwaki K, et al. Immunological unresponsiveness in chimeric miniature swine following MHC-mismatched spleen transplantation. Transplantation 2005; 80(12) 1791-804.

[6] Ayala-García MA, Soel JM, Díaz E, et al. Induction of tolerance in renal transplantation using splenic transplantation: experimental study in canine model. Transpl P 2010; 42(1) 376-380.

[7] Chinen J, Buckley RH. Transplantation immunology: solid organ and bone marrow. J Allergy Clin Immunol 2010; 125(2) S324-S335.

[8] Chaplin DD. Overview of the human immune response. J Allergy Clin Immunol 2006; 117(2) S430-S435.

[9] Land W, Messmer K. The impact of ischemia/reperfusion injury on specific and non-specific, early and late chronic events after organ transplantation. Transplantation Rev 1996; 10 (2) 108-253.

[10] Bharat A, Mohanakumar T. Allopeptides and the alloimmune response. Cell Immunol 2007; 248(1) 31–43.

[11] Game DS, Lechler RI. Pathways of allorecognition: implications for transplantation tolerance. Transpl Immunol 2002; 10(2-3) 101-108.

[12] Portoles P, Rojo JM, Janeway CA Jr. Asymmetry in the recognition of antigen: self class II MHC and non-self class II MHC molecules by the same T-cell receptor. J Mol Cell Immunol 1989; 4(3) 129-137.

[13] Sherman LA, Chattopadhyay S. The molecular basis of allorecognition. Annu Rev Immunol 1993;11 385-402.

[14] Matzinger P, Bevan MJ. Hypothesis: Why do so many lymphocytes respond to major histocompatibility antigens? Cell Immunol 1977; 29(1) 1-5.

[15] Heeger PS. T-cell allorecognition and transplant rejection: a summary and update. Am J Transplant 2003; 3(5) 525-533.

[16] Jiang S, Herrera O, Lechler RI. New spectrum of allorecognition pathways: implications for graft rejection and transplantation tolerance. Curr Opin Immunol 2004; 16(5) 550-557.

[17] Andre F, Chaput N, Schartz NE, et al. Exosomes as potent cell-free peptide-based vaccine. I. Dendritic cell-derived exosomes transfer functional MHC class I/peptide complexes to dendritic cells. J Immunol 2004; 172(4) 2126-2136.

[18] Thery C, Duban L, Segura E, et al. Indirect activation of naive CD4+ T cells by dendritic cell-derived exosomes. Nat Immunol 2002; 3(12) 1156-1162.

[19] Boyington JC, Brooks AG, Sun PD. Structure of killer cell immunoglobulin-like receptors and their recognition of the class I MHC molecules. Immunol Rev 2001; 181 66–78.

[20] Kroemer A, Xiao X, Degauque N, et al. The innate NK cells, allograft rejection, and a key role for IL-15. J Immunol 2008; 180(12) 7818-7826.

[21] Gill RG. NK cells: elusive participants in transplantation immunity and tolerance. Curr Opin Immunol 2010; 22(5) 649-654.

[22] Hwang I, Ki D. Receptor-mediated T cell absorption of antigen presenting cell-derived molecules. Front Biosci 2011; 16 411-421.

[23] Van der Merwe PA, Dushek O. Mechanisms for T cell receptor triggering. Nat Rev Immunol 2011; 11(1) 47-55.

[24] Fietta P, Delsante G. The effector T helper cell triade. Riv Biol 2009; 102(1) 61-74.

[25] Sayegh MH, Akalin E, Hancock WW, et al. CD28-B7 blockade after alloantigenic challenge in vivo inhibits Th1 cytokines but spares Th2. J Exp Med 1995; 181(5) 1869-1874.

[26] Auphan N, DiDonato JA, Rosette C, et al. Immunosuppression by glucocorticoids: inhibition of NF-kappa B activity through induction of I kappa B synthesis. Science 1995; 270(5234) 286-290.

[27] Dong VM, Womer KL, Sayegh MH. Transplantation tolerance. Pediatr transplant 1999; 3(3) 181-192.

[28] Coutinho A, Caramalho I, Seixas E, et al. Thymic commitment of regulatory T cells is a pathway of TCR-dependent selection that isolates repertoires undergoing positive or negative selection. Curr Top Microbiol Immunol 2005; 293 43-71.

[29] Sprent J, Lo D, Er-Kai G, et al. T cell selection in the thymus. Immunol Rev 1988; 101 172-190.

[30] Egerton M, Scollay R, Shortman K. Kinetics of mature T cell development in the thymus. Proc Natl Acad Sci U S A 1990; 87(7) 2579-2582.

[31] Peterson P, Org T, Rebane A. Transcriptional regulation by AIRE: molecular mechanisms of central tolerance. Nat Rev Immunol 2008; 8(12) 948–957.

[32] Russell DM, Dembić Z, Morahan G, et al. Peripheral deletion of self-reactive B cells. Nature 1991; 354(6351) 308–311.

[33] Ju S-T, Panka DJ, Cui H, et al. Fas(CD95)/FAsL interactions required for programmed cell death after T-cell activation. Nature 1995; 373(6513) 444-448.

[34] Van Parijs L, Refali Y, Lord JC, et al. Uncoupling IL-2 signals that regulate T cell proliferation, survival, and Fas-mediated activation-induced cell death. Immunity 1999; 11 281-288.

[35] Li XC, Demirci G, Ferrari-Lacraz S, et al. IL-15 and IL-2: a matter of life and death for T cells in vivo. Nat Med 2001; 7(1) 114-118.

[36] Zheng XX, Sanchez-Fuevo A, Sho M, et al. Favorably tipping the balance between cytopathic and regulatory T cells to create transplantation tolerance. Immunity 2003; 19(4) 503-514.

[37] Ferrari-Lacraz S, Zheng XX, Kim YS, et al. An antagonist IL-15/Fc protein prevents costimulation blockade-resistant rejection. J Immunol 2001; 167(6) 3478-3485.

[38] Wells AD. New insights into the molecular basis of T cell anergy: anergy factors, avoidance sensors, and epigenetic imprinting. J Immunol 2009; 182(12) 7331–7341.

[39] Yarkoni Y, Getahun A, Cambier JC. Molecular underpinning of B-cell anergy. Immunol Rev 2010; 237(1) 249-263.

[40] Seyfert-Margolis V, Feng S. Tolerance: is it achievable in pediatric solid organ transplantation? Pediatr Clin North Am 2010; 57(2) 523-538.

[41] Shimizu J, Yamazaki S, Takahashi T, et al. Stimulation of CD25(+)CD4(+) regulatory T cells through GITR breaks immunological self-tolerance. Nat Immunol 2002; 3(2) 135-142.

[42] Hori S, Nomura T, Sakaguchi S. Control of regulatory T cell development by the transcription factor Foxp3. Science 2003; 299(5609) 1057-1061.

[43] Taguchi O, Nishizuka Y. Self tolerance and localized autoimmunity. Mouse models of autoimmune disease that suggest tissue-specific suppressor T cells are involved in self tolerance. J Exp Med 1987; 165(1) 146-156.

[44] Maynard CL, Hatton RD, Helms WS, et al. Contrasting roles for all-trans retinoic acid in TGF-beta-mediated induction of Foxp3 and Il10 genes in developing regulatory T cells. J Exp Med 2009; 206(2) 343-357.

[45] Louis S, Brandeau C, Giral M, et al. Contrasting CD25hiCD4+T cells/FOXP3 patterns in chronic rejection and operational drug-free tolerance. Transplantation 2006; 81(3) 398-407.

[46] Lopez M, Clarkson MR, Albin M, et al. A novel mechanism of action for anti-thymocyte globulin: induction of CD4+CD25+foxp3+ regulatory T cells. J Am Soc Nephrol 2006; 17(10) 2644-2646.

[47] Thornton AM, Shevach EM. CD4+CD25+ immunoregulatory T cells suppress polyclonal T cell activation in vitro by inhibiting interleukin 2 production. J Exp Med 1998; 188(2) 287-296.

[48] Levings MK, Bacchetta R, Schulz U, et al. The role of IL-10 and TGF-beta in the differentiation and effector function of T regulatory cells. Int Arch Allergy Immunol 2002; 129(4) 263–276.

[49] Kingsley CI, Karim M, Bushell AR, et al. CD25+CD4+ regulatory T cells prevent graft rejection: CTLA-4- and IL-10-dependent immunoregulation of alloresponses. J Immunol 2002; 168(3) 1080-1086.

[50] Cosmi L, Liotta F, Lazzeri E, et al. Human CD8+CD25+ thymocytes share phenotypic and functional features with CD4+CD25+ regulatory thymocytes. Blood 2003; 102(12) 4107-4114.

[51] Womer KL. Transplantation tolerance. Saudi J Kidney Dis Transpl 2005; 16(4) 498-505.

[52] Orlando G, Hematti P, Stratta R, et al. Clinical Operational Tolerance After Renal Transplantation. Current Status and Future Challenges. Ann Surg 2010; 252(6) 915–928.

[53] Starzl TE, Murase N, Abu-Elmagd K, et al. Tolerogenic immunosuppression for organ transplantation. Lancet 2003; 361(9368) 1502–1510.

[54] Scandling, JD, Busque S, Shizuru JA, et al. Induced Immune Tolerance for Kidney Transplantation. N Engl J Med 2011;365(14) 1359-1360.

[55] Hutchinson JA, Brem-Exner BG, Riquelme P, et al. A cell-based approach to the minimization of immunosuppression in renal transplantation. Transplant Int 2008; 21(8) 742–754.

[56] Hutchinson JA, Riquelme P, Brem-Exner BG, et al. Transplant acceptanceinducing cells as an immune-conditioning therapy in renal transplantation. Transplant Int 2008; 21(8) 728–741.

[57] Delis S, Ciancio G, Burke GW, et al. Donor bone marrow transplantation, chimerism and tolerance. Transplant Immunol 2004; 13(2) 105–115.

[58] Sykes M. Hematopoietic cell transplantation for tolerance induction: animal models to clinical trials. Transplantation 2009; 87(3) 309–316.

[59] Barber WH, Mankin JA, Laskow DA, et al. Long-term results of a controlled prospective study with transfusion of donor-specific bone marrow in 57 cadaveric renal allograft recipients. Transplantation 1991; 51(1) 70–75.

[60] Mathew JM, Garcia-Morales RO, Carreno M, et al. Immune responses and their regulation by donor bone marrow cells in clinical organ transplantation. Transplant Immunol 2003; 11(3-4) 307–321.

[61] Ciancio G, Burke GW, Moon J, et al. Donor bone marrow infusion in deceased and living donor renal transplantation. Yonsei Med J 2004; 45(6) 998–1003.

[62] Trivedi HL, Vanikar AV, Vakil JM, et al. A strategy to achieve donor-specific hyporesponsiveness in cadaver renal allograft recipients by donor haematopoietic stem cell transplantation into the thymus and periphery. Nephrol Dial Transplant 2004; 19(9) 2374–2377.

[63] Trivedi HL, Shah VR, Vanikar AV, et al. High-dose peripheral blood stem cell infusion: a strategy to induce donor-specific hyporesponsiveness to allografts in pediatric renal transplant recipients. Pediatr Transplant 2002; 6(1) 63–68.

[64] Comerci GD, Williams TM, Kellie S. Immune tolerance after total lymphoid irradiation for heart transplantation: immunosuppressant-free survival for 8 years. J Heart Lung Transplant 2009; 28(7) 743–745.

[65] Fudaba Y, Spitzer TR, Shaffer J, et al. Myeloma responses and tolerance following combined kidney and nonmyeloablative marrow transplantation: in vivo and in vitro analyses. Am J Transplant 2006; 6(9) 2121–2133.

[66] Buhler LH, Spitzer TR, Sykes M, et al. Induction of kidney allograft tolerance after transient lymphohematopoietic chimerism in patients with multiple myeloma and end-stage renal disease. Transplantation 2002; 74(10) 1405–1409.

[67] Spitzer TR, Delmonico F, Tolkoff-Rubin N, et al. Combined histocompatibility leukocyte antigen-matched donor bone marrow and renal transplantation for multiple myeloma with end stage renal disease: the induction of allograft tolerance through mixed lymphohematopoietic chimerism. Transplantation 1999; 68(4) 480–484.

[68] Kawai T, Cosimi AB, Spitzer TR, et al. HLA-mismatched renal transplantation without maintenance immunosuppression. N Engl J Med 2008; 358(4) 353–361.

[69] BurlinghamWJ, Jankowska-Gan E, VanBuskirk A, et al. Loss of tolerance to a maternal kidney transplant is selective for HLA class II: evidence from transvivo DTH and alloantibody analysis. Hum Immunol 2000; 61(12) 1395–1402.

[70] Millan MT, Shizuru JA, Hoffmann P, et al. Mixed chimerism and immunosuppressive drug withdrawal after HLA-mismatched kidney and hematopoietic progenitor transplantation. Transplantation 2002; 73(9) 1386–1391.

[71] Scandling JD, Busque S, Dejbakhsh-Jones S, et al. Tolerance and chimerism after renal and hematopoietic-cell transplantation. N Engl J Med 2008; 358(4) 362–368.

[72] Takahashi K, Yagisawa T, Sonda K, et al. ABO-incompatible kidney transplantation in a singlecenter trial. Transplant Proc 1993; 25(1) 271–273.

[73] Tanabe K, Takahashi K, Sonda K, et al. ABO-incompatible living kidney donor transplantation: results and immunological aspects. Transplant Proc 1995; 27(1) 1020–1023.

[74] Tanabe K, Takahashi K, Sonda K, et al. Long-term results of ABO-incompatible living kidney transplantation: a single-center experience. Transplantation 1998; 65(2) 224–228.

[75] Toma H, Tanabe K, Tokumoto T. Long-term outcome of ABO-incompatible renal transplantation. Urol Clin North Am 2001; 28(4) 769–780.

[76] Gloor JM, Lager DJ, Moor SB, et al. ABO-incompatible kidney transplantation using both A2 and non-A2 living donors. Transplantation 2003; 75(7) 971–977.

[77] Tanabe K, Tokumoto T, Ishida H, et al. Excellent outcome of ABO-incompatible living kidney transplantation under pretransplant immunosuppression with tacrolimus, mycophenolate mofetil, and steroids. Transplant Proc 2004; 36(7) 2175–2177.

[78] Kazunari Tanabe, Hideki Ishida, Tomokazu Shimizu, et al. Evaluation of Two Different Preconditioning Regimens for ABO-Incompatible Living Kidney Donor Transplantation. Contrib Nephro 2009; 162 61–74.

[79] Olivera SO, Mederos CON, Faedo BF. Cirugía conservadora de la función esplénica en el adulto joven. Rev Cubana Cir 1995; 34(2). http://scielo.sld.cu/scielo.php?script=sci_arttext&pid=S0034-74931995000200012&lng=es (accessed 31 July 2012)

[80] Venetz JP, Pascual M. New treatments for acute humoral rejection of kidney allografts. Expert Opin Investig Drugs 2007; 16(5) 625-633.

[81] Golshayan D, Pascual M. Tolerance-inducing immunosuppressive strategies in clinical transplantation. Drugs 2008; 68(15) 2113-2130.

[82] Chosa E, Hara M, Watanabe A, et al. Spleen plays an important role in maintaining tolerance after removal of the vascularized heart graft. Transplantation 2007; 83(9) 1226-1233.

[83] Sakakura M, Wada H, Tawara I, et al. Reduced Cd4+Cd25+ T cells in patients with idiopathic thrombocytopenic purpura. Thromb Res 2007; 120(2) 187-193.

[84] Bradley BA. Prognostic assays for rejection and tolerance in organ transplantation. Transplant Immunology 2005; 14(3-4) 193-201.

[85] Waldmann H, Adams E, Fairchild P, et al. Regulation and privilege in transplantation tolerance. J Clin Immunol 2008; 28(6) 716-725.

[86] Halloran PF. Immunosuppressive drugs for kidney transplantation. N Engl J Med 2004; 351(26) 2715-2729.